Use Dr. Netter's famous illustrations
as your intuitive and interactive study guide!

New!

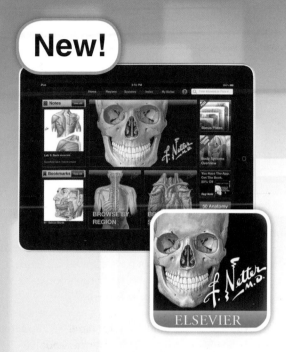

Netter's Anatomy Atlas for iPad™

Frank H. Netter, MD

The new standard for human anatomy!

Netter's Anatomy Atlas for iPad™ places the complete set of the **531 Netter Plates from the 5th edition Atlas of Human Anatomy** right at your fingertips. Enhanced with a suite of **quizzing and customization features**, you'll have the ideal review tool you can truly make your own!

- **Locate anatomic structures and views quickly.**

- **Make the Atlas your own** by customizing individual labels (on/off/highlight).

- **Tap Muscle Info buttons** to review **attachments, innervations, actions, and blood supply.**

- **Take label quizzes** to test your memory of terminology.

- **Prep for boards and test your understanding of clinical anatomy** with **50 anatomy questions** from **USMLEConsult.com.**

- **Use "My Netter" bookmarks and notes** to organize and personalize your studies.

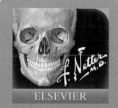

DOWNLOAD TODAY
FROM THE iTUNES™ APP STORE!

RC/AE
11-GCRch-2757

iPad™ and iTunes® are registered trademarks of Apple.

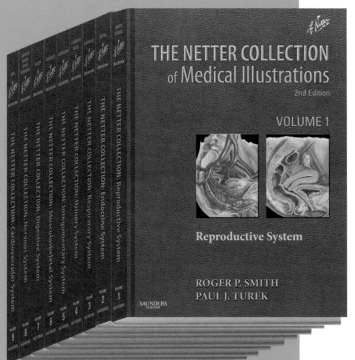

Netter's Illustrated Human Pathology

UPDATED EDITION

L. Maximilian Buja, MD
The University of Texas Health Science Center at Houston

Gerhard R. F. Krueger, MD, PhD
The University of Texas Health Science Center at Houston

Illustrations by Frank H. Netter, MD

SAUNDERS
ELSEVIER

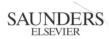

Elsevier Inc.
1600 John F. Kennedy Boulevard
Suite 1800
Philadelphia, PA 19103-2899

Netter's Illustrated Human Pathology
Updated Edition

ISBN: 978-0-323-22089-7

Notice

Knowledge and best practice in this field are constantly changing. As new research and experience broaden our understanding, changes in research methods, professional practices, or medical treatment may become necessary.

Practitioners and researchers must always rely on their own experience and knowledge in evaluating and using any information, methods, compounds, or experiments described herein. In using such information or methods they should be mindful of their own safety and the safety of others, including parties for whom they have a professional responsibility.

With respect to any drug or pharmaceutical products identified, readers are advised to check the most current information provided (i) on procedures featured or (ii) by the manufacturer of each product to be administered, to verify the recommended dose or formula, the method and duration of administration, and contraindications. It is the responsibility of practitioners, relying on their own experience and knowledge of their patients, to make diagnoses, to determine dosages and the best treatment for each individual patient, and to take all appropriate safety precautions.

To the fullest extent of the law, neither the Publisher nor the authors, contributors, or editors, assume any liability for any injury and/or damage to persons or property as a matter of products liability, negligence or otherwise, or from any use or operation of any methods, products, instructions, or ideas contained in the material herein.

ISBN: 978-0-323-22089-7

Content Strategist: Elyse O'Grady
Content Development Manager: Marybeth Thiel
Publishing Services Manager: Patricia Tannian
Project Manager: Carrie Stetz

Printed in China

Last digit is the print number: 9 8 7 6 5 4 3 2

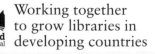

Working together
to grow libraries in
developing countries

www.elsevier.com • www.bookaid.org

DEDICATION

We dedicate this book to our families—especially our wives,
Donna Buja and Barbara Krueger.

Their encouragement and support have been inspirational
and fundamental in our work and our lives.

PREFACE

Netter's Atlas of Human Pathology is intended to provide students with a clear, concise, and compelling presentation of the pathologic basis of the most common human diseases. Pathology is a science and medical discipline that deals with the causes (etiology), mechanisms (pathophysiology), and interrelated anatomical, functional, and clinical manifestations of disease. Pathology is a vast field encompassing all of human disease and expanding geometrically to include information from rapidly evolving advances in the basic biomedical sciences, particularly the elucidation of the human genome. However, understanding human disease will always require a clear understanding of the ultimate expression of disease as anatomical changes in tissues and organs (pathologic anatomy). Therefore, this Atlas provides readily understandable representations of common human diseases, concentrating on pathologic anatomy and relating the anatomical changes to the functional and clinical manifestations of disease and their underlying causes and mechanisms.

The initial chapter covers basic pathologic changes encountered in organs and tissues in many disease processes, including degeneration and atrophy; apoptosis and necrosis; acute and chronic inflammation; immunologic reactions; regeneration, hypertrophy, and hyperplasia; and dysplasia and neoplasia. The following 12 chapters deal with diseases of specific organ systems: the cardiovascular system; respiratory system; gastrointestinal system; liver, gallbladder, and pancreas; kidneys and urinary system; male and female reproductive systems; integumentary (skin) system; hematopoietic and lymphatic systems; bones, joints, and soft tissues; endocrine system; and nervous system. Each chapter begins with a concise summary of the various pathologic processes and diseases to be presented in the chapter. The main body of each chapter consists of illustrations of pathologic processes and diseases accompanied by concise text aimed at clarifying and expanding the information presented in the illustrations. Comparative data about similar disease processes are summarized in tables.

The Atlas is designed to complement a comprehensive textbook of pathology or a course syllabus by providing a vivid visual framework and companion for the study of the causes, pathophysiology, and natural history of disease. The Atlas also can be used as an adjunct when studying gross and microscopic pathology specimens in the laboratory. Additionally, the Atlas can serve as an introduction to new subject matter and as a review after appropriate detail has been learned. Thus, the Atlas is meant to be a useful learning aid for students involved in their first human pathology course and a review for students, medical residents, physicians, and other health care professionals at subsequent stages of their careers.

The distinguishing element of this Atlas is the brilliantly conceived and executed medical illustrations of the famous physician-artist, Frank H. Netter, MD. As a result of a long and productive career, Dr. Netter has left a legacy of a vast collection of medical art familiar to physicians and other health care professionals throughout the world. Dr. Netter's insight into and understanding of structure-function relations has produced compelling and memorable depictions of the fundamental features of disease processes.

The Netter illustrations are the core of the Atlas. However, in some cases, the Netter drawings have been supplemented with gross photographs and photomicrographs to enhance and complete the picture. The chapters on general pathology, skin, and hematologic disorders use gross and microscopic photographs to illustrate these pathologic processes. Through the combination and integration of the Netter illustrations, gross and microscopic photographs, tables, and text, our goal is to present students with an Atlas that enhances their knowledge, understanding, and appreciation of the pathologic basis of human disease. Pathology is the fundamental bridging discipline linking the basic biomedical sciences to clinical medicine. Therefore, our ultimate goal is for our students to use their knowledge of pathology to become scientifically grounded, effective physicians and health care professionals.

L. Maximilian Buja, MD
Gerhard R.F. Krueger, MD, PhD

ABOUT THE ARTISTS

Frank H. Netter, MD, was born in 1906, in New York City. He studied art at the Art Student's League and the National Academy of Design before entering medical school at New York University, where he received his MD degree in 1931. During his student years, Dr. Netter's notebook sketches attracted the attention of the medical faculty and other physicians, allowing him to augment his income by illustrating articles and textbooks. He continued illustrating as a sideline after establishing a surgical practice in 1933, but he ultimately opted to give up his practice in favor of a full-time commitment to art. After service in the United States Army during World War II, Dr. Netter began his long collaboration with the CIBA Pharmaceutical Company (now Novartis Pharmaceuticals). This 45-year partnership resulted in the production of the extraordinary collection of medical art so familiar to physicians and other medical professionals worldwide.

In 2005, Elsevier Inc. purchased the Netter Collection and all publications from Icon Learning Systems. There are now over 50 publications featuring the art of Dr. Netter available through Elsevier Inc. (in the US: www.us.elsevierhealth.com/Netter and outside the US: www.elsevier-health.com)

Dr. Netter's works are among the finest examples of the use of illustration in the teaching of medical concepts. The 13-book Netter Collection of Medical Illustrations, which includes the greater part of the more than 20,000 paintings created by Dr. Netter, became and remains one of the most famous medical works ever published. The Netter Atlas of Human Anatomy, first published in 1989, presents the anatomical paintings from the Netter Collection. Now translated into 16 languages, it is the anatomy atlas of choice among medical and health professions students the world over.

The Netter illustrations are appreciated not only for their aesthetic qualities, but, more importantly, for their intellectual content. As Dr. Netter wrote in 1949, "… clarification of a subject is the aim and goal of illustration. No matter how beautifully painted, how delicately and subtly rendered a subject may be, it is of little value as a medical illustration if it does not serve to make clear some medical point." Dr. Netter's planning, conception, point of view, and approach are what inform his paintings and what makes them so intellectually valuable.

Frank H. Netter, MD, physician and artist, died in 1991.

Learn more about the physician-artist whose work has inspired the Netter Reference collection: http://www.netterimages.com/artist/netter.htm

Carlos Machado, MD, was chosen by Novartis to be Dr. Netter's successor. He continues to be the main artist who contributes to the Netter collection of medical illustrations.

Self-taught in medical illustration, cardiologist Carlos Machado has contributed meticulous updates to some of Dr. Netter's original plates and has created many paintings of his own in the style of Netter as an extension of the Netter collection. Dr. Machado's photorealistic expertise and his keen insight into the physician/patient relationship informs his vivid and unforgettable visual style. His dedication to researching each topic and subject he paints places him among the premier medical illustrators at work today.

Learn more about his background and see more of his art at: http://www.netterimages.com/artist/machado.htm

ABOUT THE AUTHORS

L. Maximilian Buja, MD, is Professor of Pathology and Laboratory Medicine and holds the H. Wayne Hightower Distinguished Professorship in the Medical Sciences and the Distinguished Chair in Pathology and Laboratory Medicine at The University of Texas Health Science Center at Houston. He also is Executive Vice President for Academic Affairs, having previously served as Dean of the Medical School and Chairman of the Department of Pathology and Laboratory Medicine at The University of Texas Health Science Center at Houston. He is certified by the American Board of Pathology. Dr. Buja's scholarly interests are centered on cardiovascular pathology and general principles of disease. Teaching has always been an important part of Dr. Buja's professional career, and he remains active in the teaching of pathology to medical students, residents, fellows, and graduate students. Dr. Buja's investigative career encompasses research on the pathogenesis and manifestations of cardiac and vascular diseases, including atherosclerosis, ischemic heart disease, and cardiomyopathies. He has published extensively in his areas of interest. He continues to pursue studies of cardiomyocyte and vascular cell injury and repair.

Gerhard R.F. Krueger, MD, PhD, is Adjunct Professor of Internal Medicine and Pathology and Laboratory Medicine at The University of Texas Health Science Center at Houston. Dr. Krueger formerly served as the Head of the Immunopathology Laboratory, Institute of Pathology, University of Cologne, and as Dean of the University of Cologne Medical School. He holds certificates from the German Board of Pathology and the American Board of Pathology. Throughout his career, Dr. Krueger has been actively engaged in the practice of pathology and the teaching of pathology to medical students, residents, fellows, and graduate students. Dr. Krueger's investigative career encompasses research in immunopathology, including the pathogenesis of diseases related to herpes viruses and the pathogenesis of lymphomas and other lymphoproliferative diseases. His work has led to an extensive number of publications. His most recent studies have involved computer modeling of T-cell proliferation and differentiation under normal and pathologic conditions.

ACKNOWLEDGMENTS

Our motivation for preparing this Atlas is our mutual passion for the science and practice of pathology and our desire to impart our understanding and appreciation of pathology to students of medicine and other health care fields. Our commitment to pathology was forged early in our careers, including the time we spent at the National Institutes of Health in the early 1970s doing research and training in pathology. Therefore, we want to acknowledge the teachers and mentors who were instrumental in the early stages of our careers, including Dr. Harold Stewart for Dr. Krueger and Dr. Buja, Dr. Victor Ferrans and Dr. William Roberts for Dr. Buja, Dr. Thelma B. Dunn and Dr. Costan W. Berard for Dr. Krueger, and others too numerous to mention. We also want to acknowledge our professional colleagues over the years who have inspired and taught us much. Also, we recognize our students, including medical students and pathology residents, who have challenged us and inspired us to constantly improve as teachers of pathology and medicine.

We thank and appreciate the colleagues and students who have reviewed the draft chapters. Their constructive comments have served to significantly improve the work. We also thank Jean Long, Executive Assistant, for her assistance with assembly of the text. We also acknowledge the review and constructive suggestions we received from Donna Hansel, MD, PhD, of Johns Hopkins University; Richard Sobonya, MD, of the University of Arizona; and Steven Spitalnik, MD, of Columbia University.

Many of Dr. Frank Netter's illustrations were originally included in the comprehensive multivolume work *The Netter Collection of Medical Illustrations*, which resulted from Dr. Netter's long-standing collaboration with the Ciba-Geigy Corporation, now Novartis Pharmaceuticals, Inc. We acknowledge the influence of The Netter Collection series and the contributions of its collaborating authors, who provided extensive descriptive information relevant to the illustrated material. The Collection series served as an important resource for our Atlas.

Finally, we acknowledge our indebtedness to Frank H. Netter, MD, whose incredible ability to capture the structure-function relations at the core of diseases has provided the creative stimulus and drive for our work in developing this Atlas. We have strived to provide explanatory text, photographs, and tables to enhance Dr. Netter's pictorial insights into disease. We feel fortunate and privileged to have had the opportunity to help extend Dr. Netter's legacy to future generations of physicians and health care professionals.

L. Maximilian Buja, MD
Gerhard R.F. Krueger, MD, PhD

CONTENTS

CONTENTS

CONTENTS

CONTENTS

CONTENTS

CHAPTER 9: INTEGUMENTARY SYSTEM (SKIN)

CONTENTS

CHAPTER 11: BONES, JOINTS, AND SOFT TISSUES

CHAPTER 12: ENDOCRINE SYSTEM

CONTENTS

CONTENTS

CONTENTS

CHAPTER 1

GENERAL REACTION PATTERNS

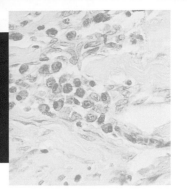

Pathologic anatomy, gross and microscopic, is the science of identifying and interpreting morphologic patterns and relating them to the physiologic and pathologic functions of a living organism. Pathology thus helps to elucidate the pathogenesis of diseases and to determine their classification. To correctly register morphologic changes, students of pathology must possess a solid knowledge of the normal composition and appearance of cells and tissues (i.e., normal anatomy and histology). Deviations from such normal appearances require pathologic interpretation. The student also should bear in mind 2 basic principles of pathologic anatomy:

1. All morphologic changes represent a dose-dependent effect in a "time-space window." That is, first, below a lower-dose threshold of functional alterations, no morphologic lesions occur despite the patient's apparent illness, and, second, there is a time delay between the occurrence of a functional disturbance and the development of morphologic changes (called morphogenesis). Space refers to the fact that morphologic lesions are most extensive at the site of "toxic impact" and become less severe (and possibly less typical) with increasing distance. This should be kept in mind when taking biopsies for pathologic evaluation.

2. Whatever the quality of injury, the living organism reacts with a limited number of patterns. There are variations to these patterns, which may provide us with clues to the etiology of the injury, but no entirely new reactions can be expected, even when a new pathologic agent (such as human immunodeficiency virus) arises.

Therefore, however clear pathologic anatomical lesions seem to be, the final evaluation with regard to the disease must result from a clinicopathologic correlation, i.e., from the careful evaluation of all the physical, biochemical, and anatomical findings.

GENERAL REACTION PATTERNS

This chapter covers 5 complex reaction patterns that apply equally to all cells, tissues, and organ systems:

1. Degeneration and atrophy
2. Apoptosis and necrosis
3. Inflammation and immunity
4. Regeneration, hypertrophy, and hyperplasia
5. Dysplasia, atypia, and neoplasia

Degeneration is the morphologic cell response to acute injury (i.e., reversible injury), which does not cause immediate cell death. **Atrophy** of individual cells or of their organized groups (tissues and organs) indicates a persistently catabolic metabolism that is not immediately lethal. **Apoptosis** and **necrosis** are distinct forms of cell death after irreversible cell injury. **Inflammation** is a microvascular response characterized by alterations in blood circulation (hyperemia, prestasis, and stasis), increased vascular permeability, exudation of blood fluids (edema, fibrinous exudates), margination and emigration of blood cell components, and passive expulsion of red blood corpuscles (hemorrhage). Activation of the immune system may result in different morphologic forms of inflammation depending on the nature of the initiating antigen (exogenous or autoimmune, soluble or particulate) and the reacting component of the immune system (T-cell or B-cell system). **Regeneration**, **hypertrophy**, and **hyperplasia** are forms of functional or structural repair or both of damaged cells and tissues. **Neoplasia** ("new growth") is a disturbance of physiologic growth regulation with persistent activity of growth-promoting factors or loss of proliferation inhibition functions (or of physiologic apoptosis). It leads to benign or malignant tumorous growth patterns independent of or at the expense of surrounding cells and tissues.

All reaction patterns vary according to differences in composition of the reacting tissue or organ (e.g., extent of vascularization, amount of connective tissue, amount and distribution of parenchymatous cells and their respective regenerative potential) and to the quality and quantity of the (exogenous or endogenous) stimulus. Because the normal tissue composition is known and additional reactive changes can be observed with the unaided eye or with the help of a microscope, the character of the pathologic change reveals the nature of the stimulus and thus of the etiologic agent. Meticulous morphologic interpretation therefore contributes to the elucidation of the etiology and pathogenesis of diseases. This is the essential task and responsibility of the practitioner of general pathology.

The following figures provide examples of the 5 reaction patterns in different tissues and organs.

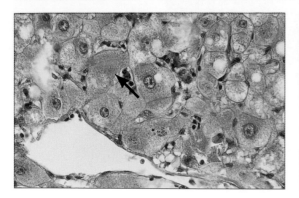

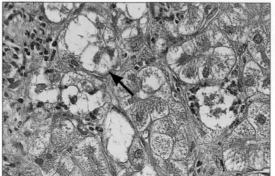

Hepatocellular damage with ballooning degeneration (**right**) and proteinaceous degeneration (**left**) of hepatocytes. Note swollen hepatocytes with clear cytoplasm or with eosinophilic cytoplasmic condensation (arrows).

Fatty degeneration of hepatocytes (**left**) and of renal tubular cells (**right**), Sudan red stain. Note the cytoplasmic fat droplets staining red in Sudan red (arrows).

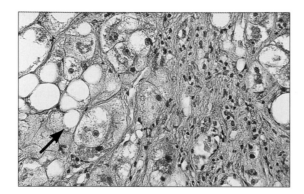

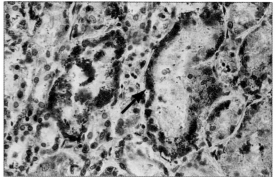

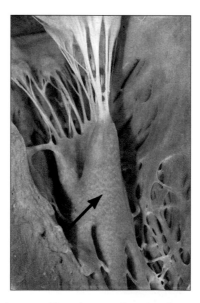

Gross features of fatty degeneration of cardiac muscle.
Note fatty streaks in papillary muscle (arrow).

FIGURE 1-1   DEGENERATION

Degeneration, the reversible cell response to injury, has 2 major forms: cellular swelling (proteinaceous, **hydropic** or **ballooning degeneration**) and fatty degeneration (fatty change or **steatosis**). Ultrastructurally, cells show bleb formation, loss of microvilli, loss of intracellular attachments, and swelling of mitochondria and endoplasmic reticulum with granular and fibrillar disaggregation of nuclear chromatin. Fat vacuoles result from disintegration of lipid membranes (**fat phanerosis**) or accumulation of metabolic lipids (**fat thesaurosis**). Causes include trauma, chemical injury,

metabolic and nutritional factors (hypoxidosis, toxic metabolites, malnutrition), and infectious or immunologic injuries. Enhanced influx of calcium ions into the cell and inactivation of the **sodium pump** (increase of intracellular sodium and loss of potassium) result in increased intracellular water (swelling). Under certain conditions (e.g., sustained **acidosis**, **hypercalcemia**), degenerating cells may accumulate precipitated calcium salts, leading to **dystrophic calcification**.

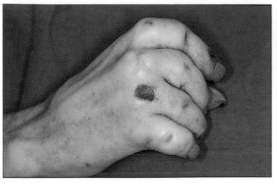

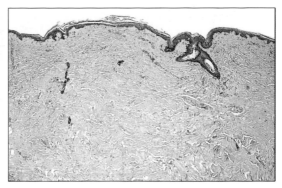

Atrophy of skin in patient with scleroderma, thinning, contraction, and ulceration of epidermis (**left**). Thinning of epidermis and loss of skin appendages with fibrosis (**right**).

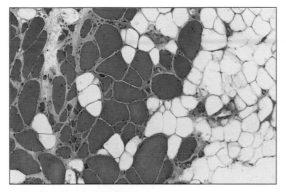

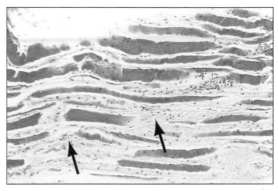

Atrophy of skeletal muscle secondary to inherited muscular dystrophy, with replacement of skeletal muscle by fat tissue, cross section (**left**), interstitial deposition of proteinaceous material in amyloidosis (arrow), longitudinal section (**right**).

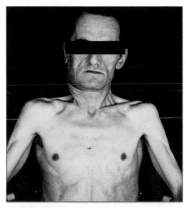

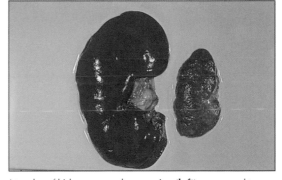

Atrophy of kidney, normal organ size (**left**) compared to end-stage inflammatory disease (**right**).

Systemic atrophy of the entire body (cachexia) in a patient with metastatic tumor.

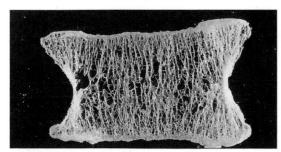

Atrophy of trabecular bone (osteoporosis of vertebra).

FIGURE 1-2   ATROPHY

Atrophy of cells or tissues indicates a catabolic metabolism that is not immediately lethal. Cells and organs shrink with or without accumulation of metabolic products (e.g., **lipofuscin, brown atrophy**). Tissue atrophy may be symmetric, with reduction of all tissue components, or asymmetric, with reduction of only some components. Symmetric atrophy is commonly caused by reduced blood supply or old age, whereas asymmetric atrophy suggests a variety of causes, such as decreased workload, nutritional deficiencies, decreased neural or endocrine stimulation, and chronic low-level injury (radiation, chemical toxins). Cellular atrophy (associated with reduction of functional activity) can be reversible on restoration of normal environmental conditions. **Cachexia** or **wasting syndrome** refers to systemic catabolic changes and symmetric atrophy of the entire body such as that accompanying advanced tumors or chronic consumptive infections (e.g., tuberculosis, acquired immunodeficiency syndrome [AIDS]).

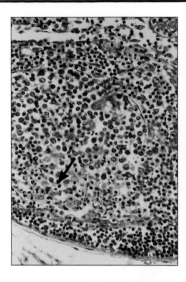

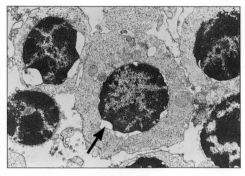

(**Left**) Apoptotic lymphocytes in thymic involution. Note the multiple pyknotic and fragmented nuclei (arrow).

(**Right**) Apoptotic lymphocytes following steroid treatment.

(**Left**) Necrosis of septic infarct in kidney; note yellow area (arrow).

(**Right**) Coagulation (fibrinoid) necrosis of small renal arteries; note the homogeneous pink stain of vessel walls (arrow).

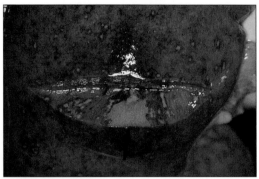

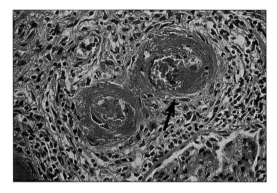

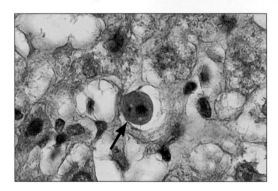

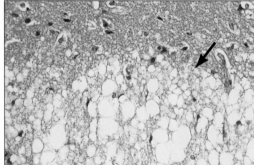

(**Left**) Apoptotic hepatocyte in viral hepatitis representing a **councilman body** (arrow).

(**Right**) Liquification necrosis of cerebral cortex, in case of insulin shock; note the laminar loss of structure in the lower part of the figure (arrow).

FIGURE 1-3 APOPTOSIS AND NECROSIS

Apoptosis (programmed cell death) serves the process of physiologic cell turnover in development and aging and the disposal of damaged or functionally incapable cells. It follows the specific stimulation of cell membrane receptors (**Fas receptor**) or genomic damage and is initiated by activation of endonucleases and caspases, DNA fragmentation, and mitochondrial disruption. In light microscopy, the key morphologic change is nuclear condensation and fragmentation followed by cell shrinkage, engulfment, and further disposal by macrophages. Electron microscopy reveals compartmentalization and dissolution of cytoplasmic organelles. Apoptosis is observed in the lymphocyte turnover in antigenically stimulated germinal centers (apoptotic cells in **germinal center macrophages**, i.e., **tingible body macrophages**), developing tissues during ontogenesis, other fast-growing tissues including cancer, virus infection, ionizing radiation, and hormonal or toxic conditions.

Necrosis, which follows irreversible cell and tissue injury, starts with cell membrane damage, swelling, denaturation, and coagulation of intracellular proteins with breakdown of organelles. Later stages are accompanied by nuclear **pyknosis** (shrinkage with condensation), loss of the nuclear membrane, and dissolution of nuclei. **Coagulative necrosis** occurs in tissues with normal protein content, and **liquefaction necrosis** occurs in tissues poor in protein (brain, fat tissue). Necrosis arises from enzymatic autodigestion (**autolysis** = self digestion; **heterolysis** = digestion of adjacent cells and tissues by enzymes released from dying cells). Breakdown products induce chemotaxis and cause a neutrophilic inflammation serving the disposal of necrotic debris. Common causes of necrosis are **ischemia**, physical trauma, chemical toxins, complex biologic injuries (toxins from infections, arthropods, snakes, plants), and immunologic factors.

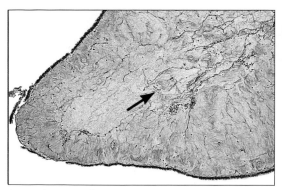

Serous rhinitis in allergic nasal polyp; note the severe edematous swelling of the stroma (arrow).

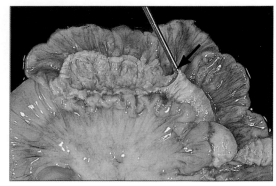

Pseudomembranous enteritis (serofibrinous exudate) in small intestine of baby with staphylococcal food poisoning; note the loose yellowish membranes covering the mucosa (arrow).

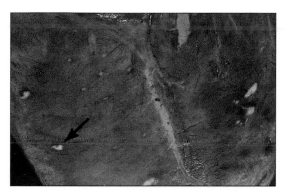

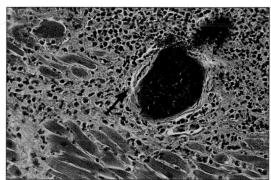

Suppurative myocarditis with abscess formation and bacterial colonies, gross (**left**) and microscopic (**right**); note the well-circumscribed yellow necroses (arrow) and fine granular bacterial colonies (arrow).

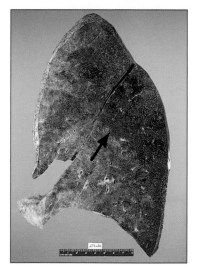

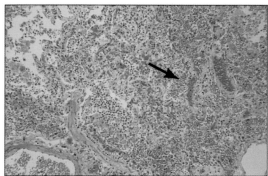

Bronchopneumonia (hemorrhagic), gross (**left**) and microscopic (**right**); note the prominent extravasation of erythrocytes (arrow).

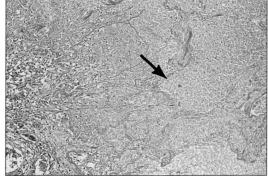

Necrotizing pneumonia, microscopic view; note the pale granular destruction of lung tissue (arrow).

FIGURE 1-4   ACUTE INFLAMMATION

Acute inflammation describes alterations in microvascular circulation (**hyperemia**, **peristasis**, and **stasis**) with increased vascular permeability and exudation of fluids (**edema**, **fibrinous exudates**). After additional toxic effects, local thrombosis or necrosis may complicate the reaction. The type of inflammatory response is determined by the nature of the etiologic agent and its distribution in the body and by the composition of the reacting tissue. Acute neutrophilic inflammation (**suppurative inflammation**) is commonly caused by bacterial infection. Acute viral infection causes lymphocytic infiltrations (stimulation of the immune system by viruses, virus-infected cells, or both). Bacterial (or fungal) toxins may induce necrosis or **abscesses** by **exotoxins** or hemorrhage by **endotoxins**. **Endotoxemia** and a systemic inflammatory response can lead to **circulatory shock**.

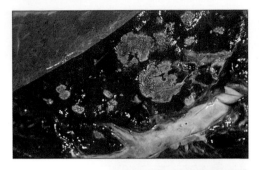

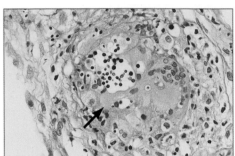

Granulomatous (fungal) pneumonitis, gross (**left**) and microscopic (**right**) with fungal organisms (*Histoplasma* sp. red in PAS stain) in giant cells (arrows).

Chronic (lymphocytic) gastritis in autoimmune disease; note the interstitial lymphoplasmacytic infiltration of the mucosa (arrow).

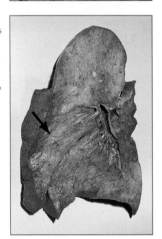

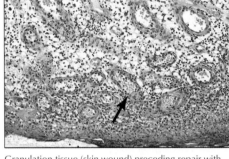

Granulation tissue (skin wound) preceding repair with fibrosis; note the edematous stroma with mixed inflammatory infiltration and proliferation of capillaries (arrow).

Severe chronic fibrosing pneumonitis ("carnification"), gross appearance; note the firm, pale condensation of lung tissue and sharp cutting edges (arrows).

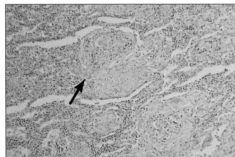

Fibrosing granulomatous pneumonitis in autoimmune disease (Wegener granulomatosis); note the fibrosing granulomas and the surrounding interstitial lymphocytic infiltration with progressive fibrosis (arrow).

Chronic atrophic enteritis (Crohn's) with mucosal atrophy in a patient with Crohn's disease; note the fibrous thickening of the terminal ileum with loss of mucosal structure (arrow).

FIGURE 1-5   CHRONIC INFLAMMATION

Chronic inflammation follows the initiation of repair ("organization") of acute inflammation and is characterized by activation of the immune system and of **phagocytosis** with subsequent proliferation of new capillaries and fibroblasts, production of collagen, and scarring. Lymphohistiocytic infiltration accompanied by capillaries in an edematous stroma and increasing numbers of fibroblasts is called **granulation tissue**. When inflammation involves a significant T-cell immune response, as in tuberculosis, salmonellosis, or yersiniosis, granuloma formation may result. The form and course of noninfectious inflammation depends on the toxic dose and duration of the pathologic stimulus. For example, acute low-dose radiation (sun exposure) causes hyperemia, a higher dose (sunburn) causes hyperemia and **edema**, and a very high dose (sunburn grade III) causes necrosis and secondary inflammation. Chronic low-dose exposure (sun or other radiation) causes mild persistent edema followed by atrophy and fibrosis.

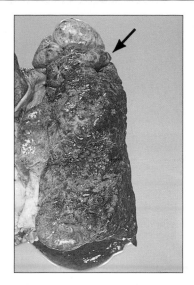

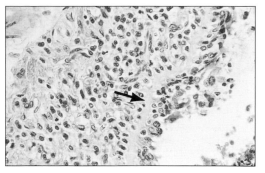

Type I (allergic) reaction, bronchial asthma with prominent bullous emphysema of the lung (**left**), and typical eosinophilic bronchitis with sclerosis of epithelial basement membrane (**right**) (arrow).

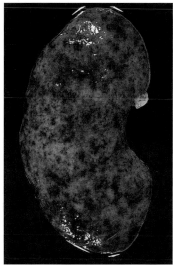

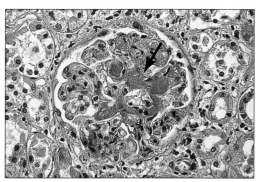

Type II (toxic) reaction, necrotizing glomerulitis and vasculitis with fibrinoid necrosis in patient with panarteritis nodosa, gross (**left**) and microscopic features (**right**); note the homogeneous red necroses of glomerular vessels and arteries (arrow).

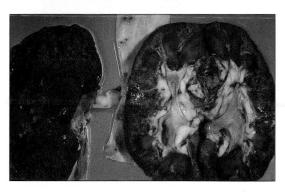

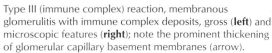

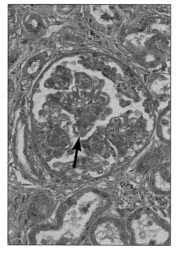

Type III (immune complex) reaction, membranous glomerulitis with immune complex deposits, gross (**left**) and microscopic features (**right**); note the prominent thickening of glomerular capillary basement membranes (arrow).

FIGURE 1-6   IMMUNOLOGIC INFLAMMATION: B CELL

The morphology of immunologically induced inflammation depends on the initiating antigen and the reacting component of the immune system (Table 1-1). Type I B-cell immune reaction (allergy type) is characterized by increased vascular permeability with edema, platelet aggregation, and infiltration by eosinophils (e.g., **allergic rhinitis**, **asthma bronchiale**). Type II B-cell reaction causes lysis of the antigenic target cell or necrosis of tissue components (e.g., **autoimmune hemolytic anemia**, **nephrotoxic glomerulonephritis**). Type III B-cell immune reactions or immune complex reactions are characterized by accumulations of

TABLE 1-1   BASIC TYPES OF B-CELL AND T-CELL IMMUNOREACTIONS*

Gell and Coombs Type	Alias	Mechanism
B-cell reactions		
Type I IR	Allergic IR Atopic IR Anaphylactic IR	Cytophilic antibodies (e.g., IgE) bind to mast cells; antigen binding to these cell-bound antibodies causes mast cell degranulation with release of vasoactive mediators (e.g., histamine), which initiate the microvascular inflammatory response (thrombocytes and eosinophils cooperate).
Type II IR	Toxic or cytotoxic IR	Complement-binding antibodies (on antigen binding) activate complement cascade, members of which initiate inflammatory response by activating cell chemotaxis and phagocytosis, ultimately causing toxic cell and tissue damage.
Type III IR	Immunocomplex IR	Persistence of antigen-antibody complexes are recognized by the immune system as foreign and induce the production of secondary anticomplex antibodies (i.e., anti-antibodies, such as rheumatoid factor); these bind and activate complement and cause tissue lesion through complement components (see above).
T-cell reactions		
Type IV IR	Cell-mediated IR T-cell cytotoxic IR CTL response	a. Direct destruction of target antigenic cells by binding of CTL, Fas-related induction of apoptosis, and/or release of perforin and granzymes b. T-cell cytokine response activation of macrophages: granulomatous (e.g., IFN-γ, TNF) reaction c. T-cell cytokine response activation of mast cells: basophil reaction (e.g., IL-3, IL-5) d. T-cell cytokine response: activation of vasoproliferative factors (e.g., IL-3, IL-8)

*CTL indicates cytotoxic T lymphocytes; Fas, cellular apoptosis receptor; Ig, immunoglobulin; IL, interleukin; IFN, interferon; IR, immunoreaction; TNF, tumor necrosis factor.

FIGURE 1-6   IMMUNOLOGIC INFLAMMATION: B CELL (CONTINUED)

antigen-antibody complexes and in situ complement activation with subsequent serofibrinous exudates; thickening of basement membranes; and slow, secondary development of granulation tissue at the site of immune complex deposition (e.g., **membrano-** **proliferative glomerulonephritis**, certain lesions in **lupus erythematosus**, and **rheumatoid arthritis**). More acute reactions cause acute vasculitis with or without microhemorrhage (**Arthus-type reaction**).

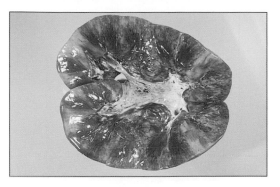

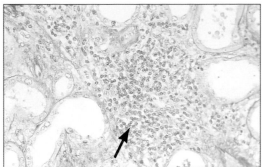

Kidney transplant rejection (lymphocytic), gross appearance of kidney (**left**), interstitial lymphocytic infiltration with tubular damage (**right**, arrow).

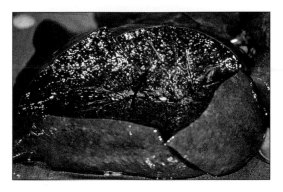

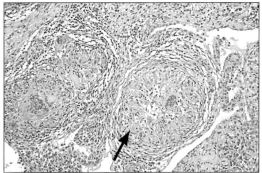

Granulomatous pneumonitis showing gross (**left**) and microscopic (**right**) features of pulmonary tuberculosis; note the well-circumscribed granulomas with giant cells and central (caseous) necrosis (arrow).

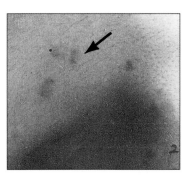

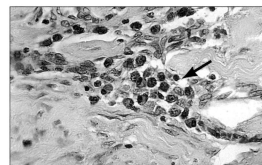

Basophil reaction of skin following recluse spider bites (**left**, arrow), microscopy of dermal vessels (**right**).

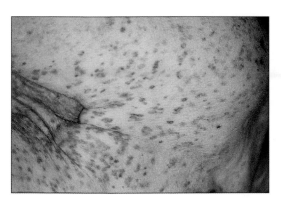

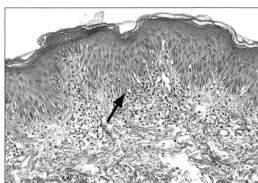

Eczematous skin reaction, gross features (**left**) and dermal microscopy (**right**); note the diffuse thickening of the skin with hyperkeratosis and focal epidermotropic inflammatory infiltrate (arrow).

FIGURE 1-7   IMMUNOLOGIC INFLAMMATION: T CELL

T-cell immune reactions are divided into the **lymphocytotoxic reaction** (classic type IV reaction or **tuberculin-type cellular immune reaction**), the **granulomatous reaction,** the **basophil reaction (Jones-Mote–type reaction)**, and the **contact allergy–**type reaction (Table 1-1). The lymphocytotoxic reaction is brought about by direct action of cytotoxic T lymphocytes on the cellular antigen, as in acute transplant rejection. Granulomatous reactions are initiated by T-cell–induced accumulation and

activation of phagocytes with typical tissue reactions in certain infectious diseases such as tuberculosis. Basophil reactions are caused by secretion of specific T-cell cytokines with attraction of basophils to the site of the antigen deposit. This can be seen in certain arthropod reactions, such as spider bites. The contact allergy–type reaction with production of vasoproliferative factors and other cytokines is caused by antigens such as heavy metals. Eczema is characteristic of contact allergy–type reaction.

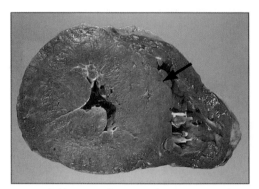

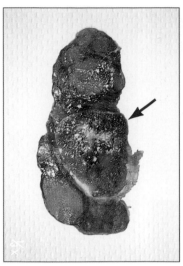

Myocardial hypertrophy (coronal section); note the concentric thickening of the left ventricular myocardium (arrow).

Nodular hypertrophy of thyroid gland (nonfunctioning goiter), gross (**left**) and hypertrophy of the thyroid follicles (**right**); note the striking enlargement of thyroid follicles in microscopy (arrow).

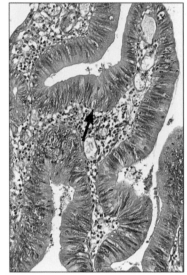

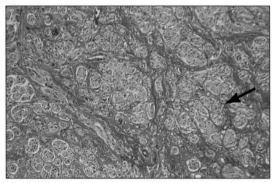

Neural hyperplasia (traumatic neuroma), regenerative proliferation of nerve fibers without functional reconstitution (arrow).

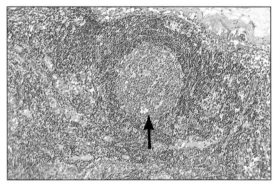

Follicular hyperplasia in lymph node with prominent germinal centers (arrow).

Intestinal glandular hyperplasia (in columnar cells of polyp); note the stratification of glandular epithelial and increase of nuclei (arrow).

FIGURE 1-8   HYPERTROPHY AND HYPERPLASIA

Regeneration, **hypertrophy**, and **hyperplasia** are forms of functional or structural repair or both of damaged cells and tissues. Regeneration may be complete with restitution of normal structure and function or incomplete. Hypertrophy is an increase in cell mass without cell division (i.e., increase in functional units such as organelles, nuclear ploidy). There are at least 2 identified stimuli for hypertrophy: mechanical triggers (i.e., stretching of cardiac or skeletal muscles) and trophical triggers (i.e., neuroendocrine activation). Compensation for structural or functional deficiency or both by hypertrophy remains limited, and degenerative changes occur when hypertrophic cells can no longer compensate for the increased burden.

Hyperplasia results from an increase in cell division and may follow or coincide with hypertrophy in nonpostmitotic tissues. It is initiated by growth factors produced by cells adjacent to the functionally or structurally damaged area. Hyperplasia compensates for a decrease or loss of cellular function or is a response to increased functional requirement. Examples are hyperplastic intestinal crypts in chronic inflammation, follicular hyperplasia of a lymph node in antigenic stimulation, and axonal proliferation after trauma (**traumatic neuroma**). Positive effects of hyperplasia are limited by the extent of the blood supply to the newly formed tissue. When hyperplasia becomes out of balance with vascularization, focal degeneration, hypoxidotic necroses, or both occur.

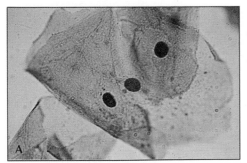

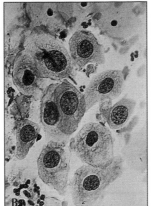

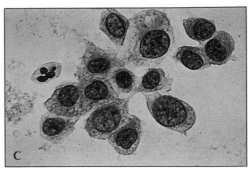

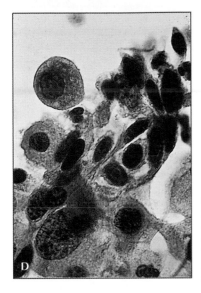

Cytology of touch preps of cervix uteri showing (**A**) normal surface epithelia, (**B**) epithelia from area of dysplasia, (**C**) epithelia with atypia indicative of carcinoma in situ (not yet invasive), and (**D**) overt carcinoma.

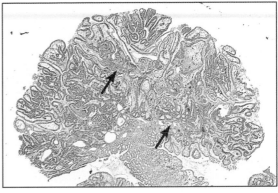

Intestinal adenoma with focal atypia (arrow) in large intestine.

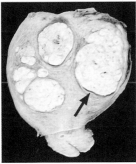

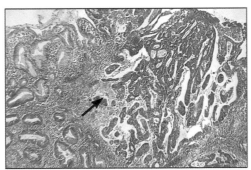

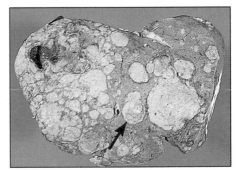

(**Left**) Corpus uteri showing multiple benign fibroleiomyomas. (**Middle**) Atypical glands (arrow) invading mucosa of gastric antrum, indicating carcinomatous transformation. (**Right**) Extensive metastases in liver of testicular tumor (seminoma).

FIGURE 1-9   DYSPLASIA AND NEOPLASIA

Dysplasia refers to restitution or tissue growth with altered features. **Atypia** refers to cellular changes. Dysplasia describes an abnormal structural regeneration that may become malignant, such as the adenomatous polyp of the colon. Typical dysplastic changes can be observed in proliferating mucosa of intestinal polyps (**adenomas**) or in the cervix uteri with chronic inflammation and mucosal regeneration. They are characterized by irregular glandular patterns, occasionally with some loss of cellular polarity. Cellular atypia indicating malignant potential is characterized by nuclear enlargement with hyperchromasia (**polyploidy** and **aneuploidy**) with increase in the nuclear/cytoplasmic ratio and irregular nucleoli, loss of cell polarity and contact inhibition, and increased and atypical mitotic figures.

Neoplasia ("new growth") results from a disturbance of physiologic growth regulation with persistent activity of growth-promoting factors or loss of proliferation inhibition functions (or of physiologic apoptosis). It leads to tumorous growth patterns independent of or at the expense of surrounding cells and tissues. Benign neoplasias (tumors), such as the uterine myoma in the figure, exhibit expansive growth with compression and atrophy of surrounding tissues but no true invasion or metastasis. Benign tumors are often designated by their tissue of origin with the affix *-oma,* such as myoma, hemangioma, and neurinoma. Although "benign," such tumors can cause severe disturbances and death when they interfere with the function of other organs, such as by compression (as a meningioma compresses the brain) or obstruction of canalicular structures.

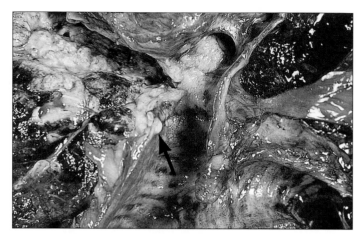
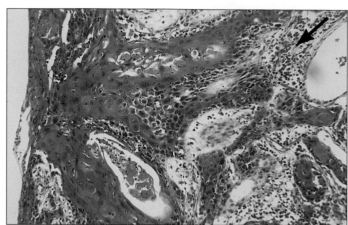

Squamous cell carcinoma of bronchus, gross (**left**) and microscopic (**right**); note the disorganized growth of squamous epithelium with loss of differentiation and cellular atypia (arrows).

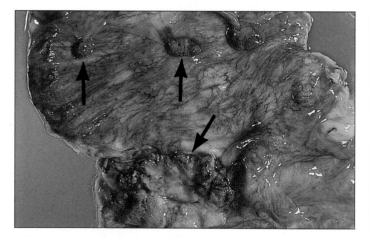
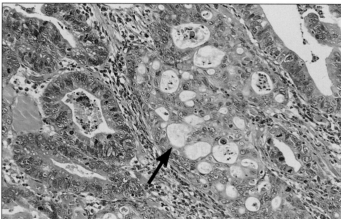

Adenocarcinoma of colon, gross (**left**); also note three polyps at the upper margin (arrows); adenocarcinoma, microscopic (**right**); note disorganized cribriform glands (arrow).

FIGURE 1-10   MALIGNANT TUMORS

Malignant tumors grow progressively at the expense of other tissues and cause death by damaging vital organs or by causing cachexia and infections. Malignancy is morphologically defined by cellular atypia, invasive and destructive growth, and meta-static spread via lymphatic vessels, hematogenously, or within other canalicular systems and body cavities. Malignant tumors of epithelial origin are **carcinomas**. Tumors of mesenchymal origin are **sarcomas** (e.g., squamous cell carcinoma, adenocarcinoma,

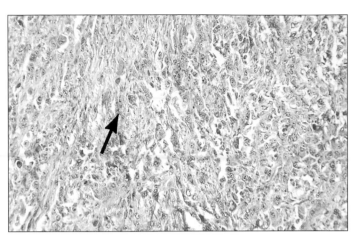 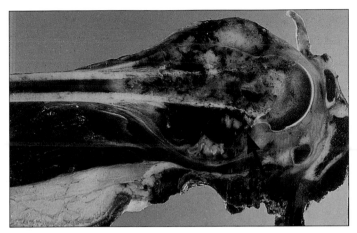

Osteogenic sarcoma of femur, gross (**left**) and microscopic (**right**) showing poorly differentiated atypical osteoblasts and focal bone formation (arrows).

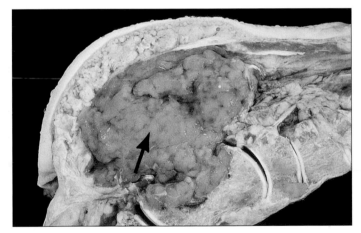 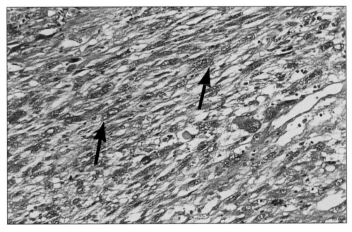

Rhabdomyosarcoma of foot, gross (**left**) and microscopic (**right**) showing poorly differentiated and atypical rhabdomyoblasts (arrow).

FIGURE 1-10   MALIGNANT TUMORS (CONTINUED)

fibrosarcoma, osteosarcoma). There are exceptions to this nomenclature, such as **malignant lymphomas** and **leukemias** for hemolymphatic malignancies and **astrocytoma**, **ependymoma**, **glioblastoma**, and others for malignant brain tumors. The degree of malignancy of a given tumor is assessed by tumor **classifica-**tion and **staging**, the histologic tumor type, its degree of differen-tiation, and its local invasion and metastatic spread. Classification and staging determine the choice of treatment and the patient's prognosis.

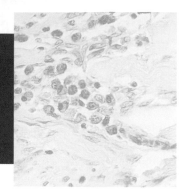

CHAPTER 2
CARDIOVASCULAR SYSTEM

Cardiovascular diseases are common and important causes of morbidity and mortality worldwide, particularly in industrialized countries. In spite of significant advances in primary prevention and therapy, cardiovascular disease, primarily the complications of atherosclerosis and hypertension (HTN), is still the leading cause of mortality in the United States.

CONGENITAL HEART DISEASE

Congenital malformations of the heart and major blood vessels are produced during embryologic development of the cardiovascular system in the early fetus. They usually arise from randomly occurring defects in embryogenesis, but they sometimes develop as a result of intrauterine infections, such as rubella, or as components of genetic abnormalities such as trisomy 21 (Down syndrome) or cytogenetic disorders of sex chromosomes (Turner syndrome). The 3 major pathophysiologic categories of congenital heart disease are those causing a **left-to-right shunt** of blood across the circulation (e.g., ventricular septal defect [VSD], atrial septal defect [ASD], patent ductus arteriosus [PDA]), a **right-to-left shunt** (e.g., tetralogy of Fallot), and **obstruction** without a shunt (e.g., coarctation of the aorta).

ATHEROSCLEROTIC DISEASES

Atherosclerosis develops as an inflammatory response of the vessel wall to chronic, multifactorial injury produced by hyperlipidemia, HTN, products of cigarette smoke, diabetes mellitus, and other predisposing factors. The pathogenesis of intimal lesions involves endothelial dysfunction, influx of macrophages and T lymphocytes, vascular smooth muscle proliferation, accumulation of oxidized low-density lipoprotein, and deposition of collagen and elastic tissue. The resultant **fibrous (atheromatous) plaques** are raised intimal lesions with a fibrous cap and a core containing variable amounts of necrotic, lipid-rich debris, fibrous tissue, calcification, and vascularization from ingrowth of vessels from the vasa vasorum. The plaques involve the aorta and its major distributing branches, including the coronary, cerebral, and iliofemoral arteries, with a propensity for localization adjacent to branch points.

Progression of disease leads to luminal narrowing and the development of complicated lesions as a result of surface ulceration, intraplaque hemorrhage, and superimposed thrombosis. The frequently abrupt transition to a clinically overt state can present as **coronary (ischemic) heart disease** manifest as angina pectoris, myocardial infarction, or sudden cardiac death; **cerebrovascular disease** with transient ischemic attacks or cerebral infarcts (stroke); rupture-prone **abdominal aortic aneurysm;** or iliofemoral atherosclerosis, predisposing to **gangrene** of the lower extremities.

CORONARY (ISCHEMIC) HEART DISEASE

The underlying pathologic substrate for clinically apparent myocardial ischemia is **coronary atherosclerosis** in at least 90% of cases. Narrowing of one or more of the coronary arteries to less than 25% of the luminal area can be slowly progressive, giving rise to recurrent episodes of **angina pectoris.** Acute changes in plaques associated with platelet aggregation and vasospasm can precipitate myocardial ischemia, ventricular fibrillation, and **sudden cardiac death.** Sudden luminal occlusion due to **thrombosis of an ulcerated plaque** can give rise to an acute **myocardial infarct,** usually of the left ventricle (LV), in the distribution of the occluded coronary artery. Myocardial necrosis begins in the ischemic subendocardial myocardium and progresses in a wave-front fashion over a period of 3 or 4 hours to involve the subepicardial myocardium. Myocardial infarcts undergo organization into granulation tissue over approximately 2 to 3 weeks and complete healing as fibrous scars in 2 to 3 months. Larger healed infarcts can develop into **ventricular aneurysms.** During the first week to 10 days when healing is minimal, myocardial infarcts are susceptible to developing **external rupture,** giving rise to cardiac tamponade; rupture across the interventricular septum, producing a **VSD;** or **rupture of a papillary muscle,** giving rise to mitral regurgitation. However, such life-threatening complications occur in only approximately 5% of cases. A massive acute myocardial infarct involving 40% or more of the LV can give rise to fatal **cardiogenic shock.** As myocardium is lost from one or more acute myocardial infarcts, congestive heart failure (CHF) may ensue.

HYPERTENSIVE DISEASE

Hypertension results from excessive arteriolar constriction and peripheral vascular resistance in relation to the blood volume and, when sustained, leads to hypertensive cardiovascular disease as well as predisposing to atherosclerotic disease. Most patients have **primary** or **essential HTN** due to a complex of genetic and environmental influences. Approximately 10% of patients have **secondary HTN** due to renal, endocrine, or other disease processes. **Slowly progressive ("benign") hypertensive disease** presents as mild to moderate blood pressure increase and leads to concentric hypertrophy of the LV and progressive damage to the microvasculature in the form of **hyaline arteriolosclerosis.** A leading complication is the development of hemorrhagic stroke. **Rapidly progressive ("malignant") HTN** is characterized by marked increase of blood pressure; prominent microvascular damage in the form of **hyperplastic arteriolosclerosis** and **fibrinoid necrosis;** and rapid progression to renal failure, cardiac failure, cerebral edema, and hemorrhagic stroke.

CONGESTIVE HEART FAILURE

Congestive heart failure has many causes that lead to a common final pathway of failure of the heart's pumping function to provide sufficient blood to meet the metabolic demands of the perfused organs of the body. Initially, compensation to an increased stress is accomplished by **ventricular hypertrophy,** but when the reserve capacity is exceeded, cardiac failure ensues. Most cases begin as **failure of the LV** as manifest by fatigue and progressive pulmonary congestion. **Failure of the right ventricle** (RV) leads to increased central venous pressure, hepatic congestion, pleural and pericardial effusions, and pitting edema of the lower extremities. **Cor pulmonale** refers to isolated right heart hypertrophy and failure due to pulmonary vascular or parenchymal disease.

ANEURYSMS

An aneurysm is an external bulging of a vascular structure. **Severe atherosclerosis** is the cause of the relatively common abdominal aortic aneurysm as well as aneurysms of the descending thoracic aorta and iliofemoral arteries. **Medial degenerative disease,** also known as *cystic medial necrosis*, gives rise to dissecting hematoma (aneurysm) with origin in the ascending thoracic aorta (type A) or the transverse or descending thoracic aorta (type B), as well as nondissecting aneurysms of the ascending thoracic aorta. Medial degeneration develops as a result of a genetic defect, as in Marfan syndrome and Ehlers-Danlos syndrome, or as a result of hemodynamic stress accelerated by HTN. Both dissecting and nondissecting aneurysms are prone to external rupture leading to exsanguination. Infections of a major artery can give rise to **mycotic (mushroomlike) aneurysms. Cardiovascular syphilis** is a form of tertiary syphilis with ascending aortic aneurysm.

VALVULAR HEART DISEASE

Acute rheumatic fever (RF) is an acute multisystem disorder involving the skin, joints, brain, and heart that is triggered by an autoimmune reaction after streptococcal pharyngitis. Most of the inflammation resolves without consequence except for the distortion and subsequent wear and tear on the cardiac valves, particularly the mitral and aortic valves, giving rise months to years later to **chronic rheumatic heart disease** (RHD).

Infective endocarditis (IE) of the valvular or mural endocardium results from infection with microorganisms (bacteria, fungi, or rickettsia) that gain access to the bloodstream through the gastrointestinal tract, skin, surgical instrumenta-

tion, or other means. Key clinical features of IE are fever and cardiac murmur, and positive blood cultures are confirmatory of the diagnosis. **Acute IE** is produced by highly virulent organisms, such as *Staphylococcus aureus*, involving a previously normal valve, whereas **subacute IE** is characterized by a more indolent clinical course with infection produced by a less virulent organism, such as *Streptococcus viridans*, often involving a previously diseased valve. In both acute and subacute IE, the infected vegetations produce destruction and incompetence of valves, CHF, and emboli to other organs.

A large variety of entities can produce valvular dysfunction, but the following figure prominently into the differential diagnosis. **Mitral valve stenosis** is virtually always due to RHD. **Mitral valve incompetence (regurgitation)** results from RHD, IE, or **mitral valve prolapse** due to myxomatous degeneration. **Aortic valvular stenosis** results from chronic RHD involving a tricuspid valve, age-related (senile) sclerosis and calcification of a tricuspid valve, or fibrosis and calcification of a congenitally bicuspid valve. **Aortic valvular incompetence** can develop from valvular lesions, such as IE, or aortic aneurysms producing distortion of the aortic annulus. Pulmonary and tricuspid valvular disease is produced by congenital defects and, less commonly, acquired causes.

MYOCARDIAL AND PERICARDIAL DISEASES

Myocarditis and **pericarditis** may be induced by infection with microorganisms (viruses, rickettsiae, bacteria, fungi, and protozoa) or noninfectious, immune-mediated processes. Bacterial infections produce neutrophil-rich suppurative inflammation. Viral infections are associated with lymphohistiocytic infiltrates. Granulomatous inflammation may represent sarcoidosis or tuberculous infection. Myocarditis can produce heart failure or sudden death from arrhythmia. Pericardial involvement is often manifest as fibrinous pericarditis with a pericardial effusion.

Cardiomyopathies are diseases of the heart muscle. Etiologically, primary cardiomyopathies are intrinsic diseases of the heart muscle, and secondary cardiomyopathies develop as a component of a defined disease process usually originating extrinsic to the myocardium. Pathophysiologically, cardiomyopathies are classified as dilated (congestive), hypertrophic, or restrictive. **Dilated (congestive) cardiomyopathy** is characterized by progressive eccentric hypertrophy, cardiomegaly, and CHF. The condition may have a genetic basis or occur because of an acquired condition, such as viral myocarditis or long-term alcoholism. **Hypertrophic cardiomyopathy** is due to mutations in contractile protein genes and includes the classic idiopathic hypertrophic subaortic stenosis (IHSS) as well as other variants. **Restrictive cardiomyopathy** typically has a relatively normal-sized heart coupled with evidence of cardiac failure due to infiltration of the myocardium by amyloid material or severe fibrosis.

Primary tumors of the heart occur at least 10 times less frequently than **metastatic tumors** of the heart, and most are benign. The most common primary tumor of the heart in adults is the **myxoma**, which usually occurs in the left atrium and presents with symptoms mimicking mitral stenosis. The most common primary tumor of the heart in infants and children is the **rhabdomyoma**, which can produce a mass effect in the myocardium as well as ventricular cavity obstruction.

TABLE 2-1   CONGENITAL MALFORMATIONS OF THE HEART AND MAJOR VESSELS

A. **Left-to-Right Shunts of the Circulation**   Ventricular septal defect (VSD), membranous type; ventricular septal defect (VSD), muscular type; patent ductus arteriosus (PDA); atrial septal defect (ASD), ostium secundum (patent foramen ovale) type; atrial septal defect (ASD), sinus venosus type (with partial anomalous pulmonary drainage of right pulmonary veins into right atrium); atrial septal defect (ASD), ostium primum type (partial endocardial cushion defect); atrioventricular septal defects (endocardial cushion defects), including complete atrioventricular canal defect; anomalous left coronary artery arising from pulmonary trunk; ruptured sinus of Valsalva aneurysm; other.
B. **Right-to-Left Shunts of the Circulation**   Tetralogy of Fallot; tricuspid atresia with ASD, VSD and/or PDA; total anomalous pulmonary venous connection (TAPVC) with ASD or PDA; transposition of the great vessels (congenital complete transposition of the great vessels) with VSD, ASD and/or PDA; persistent ductus arteriosus; aorticopulmonary septal defect; other.
C. **Obstruction of the Circulation Without Shunt**   Coarctation of the aorta, "infantile" form with tubular hypoplasia and "adult" postductal form; aortic arch and great vessel anomalies producing vascular rings around the trachea and esophagus; pulmonary stenosis; aortic valvular dysplasia and/or stenosis; supravalvular aortic stenosis; discrete subvalvular aortic stenosis; hypoplastic left heart syndrome; other.
D. **Other Lesions**   Ebstein's anomaly of the tricuspid valve; coronary artery anomalies, including origin of the left and right coronary arteries from a single right coronary ostium; other.

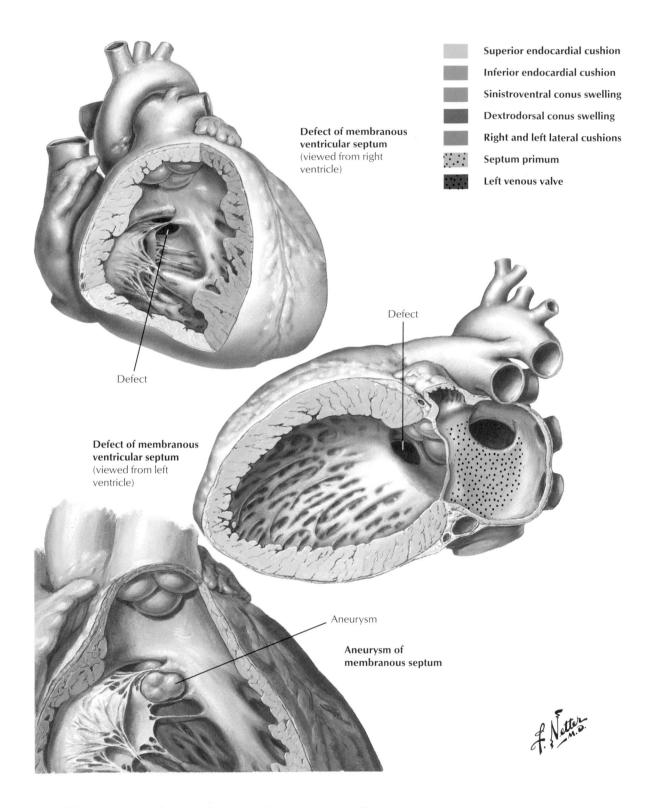

Defect of membranous ventricular septum (viewed from right ventricle)

Superior endocardial cushion
Inferior endocardial cushion
Sinistroventral conus swelling
Dextrodorsal conus swelling
Right and left lateral cushions
Septum primum
Left venous valve

Defect

Defect

Defect

Defect of membranous ventricular septum (viewed from left ventricle)

Aneurysm

Aneurysm of membranous septum

f. Netter M.D.

FIGURE 2-1 VENTRICULAR SEPTAL DEFECT: MEMBRANOUS TYPE

Congenital heart disease results from malformations of the heart and major vessels that develop during embryogenesis and are present at birth. A general classification of congenital malformations of the heart and major vessels is presented in Table 2-1. The **ventricular septal defect** (VSD) is the most common malformation presenting in infancy and childhood. Most VSDs result from defective closure of the membranous interventricular septum,

although some are located in the muscular interventricular septum. As a result of the left-to-right shunt, patients present with systolic murmur, CHF, and progressive pulmonary HTN. If not surgically corrected, pulmonary arterial pressure reaches the systemic level, and the shunt becomes predominantly right to left, leading to late onset of cyanosis (**Eisenmenger syndrome**).

Patent ductus arteriosus

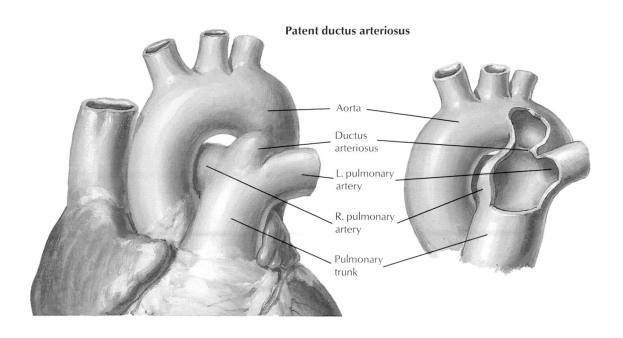

Aorta

Ductus arteriosus

L. pulmonary artery

R. pulmonary artery

Pulmonary trunk

Aberrant right subclavian artery

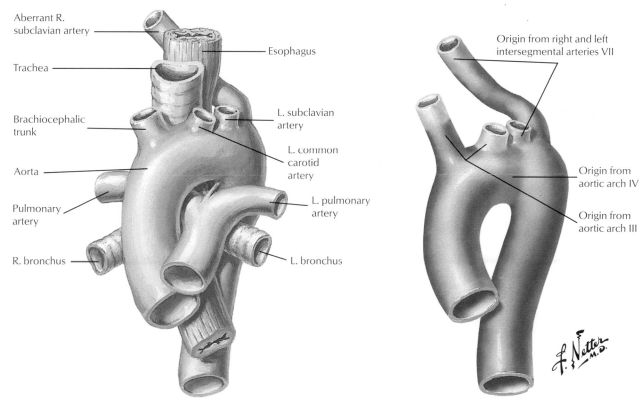

Aberrant R. subclavian artery

Trachea

Brachiocephalic trunk

Aorta

Pulmonary artery

R. bronchus

Esophagus

L. subclavian artery

L. common carotid artery

L. pulmonary artery

L. bronchus

Origin from right and left intersegmental arteries VII

Origin from aortic arch IV

Origin from aortic arch III

FIGURE 2-2   PATENT DUCTUS ARTERIOSUS

The **ductus arteriosus** is an arterial connection between the origin of the left pulmonary artery and the aorta that normally closes within hours after birth. Failure of this connection to close results in PDA. PDA is another type of high-pressure left-to-right shunt producing symptomatic disease in infants and children. Other anomalies of the aortic arch system, such as an **aberrant right subclavian artery,** give rise to anatomic variations of the normal pattern of origin of the great arteries. Some of these anomalies produce vascular rings that can compress the trachea and esophagus.

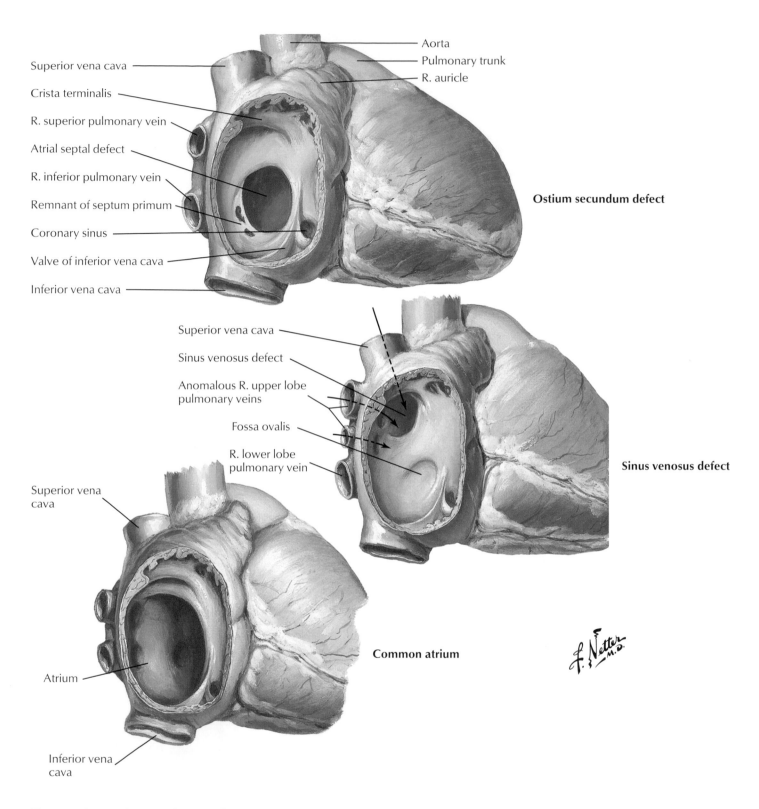

Superior vena cava

Crista terminalis

R. superior pulmonary vein

Atrial septal defect

R. inferior pulmonary vein

Remnant of septum primum

Coronary sinus

Valve of inferior vena cava

Inferior vena cava

Aorta

Pulmonary trunk

R. auricle

Ostium secundum defect

Superior vena cava

Sinus venosus defect

Anomalous R. upper lobe pulmonary veins

Fossa ovalis

R. lower lobe pulmonary vein

Sinus venosus defect

Superior vena cava

Atrium

Inferior vena cava

Common atrium

F. Netter
M.D.

FIGURE 2-3 ATRIAL SEPTAL DEFECTS

Ostium secundum defect, the most common atrial septal defect (ASD), is located in the middle portion of the interatrial septum in the region of the foramen ovale. This ASD occurs as a result of defective formation of septum primum and septum secundum tissue, which leads to failure of the ostium secundum to close. **Sinus venosus defect**, located high in the interatrial septum, is the result of defective incorporation of the sinus venosus into the RV.

This ASD is associated with anomalous drainage of the right upper lobe pulmonary veins into the right atrium. Failure of formation of the septum primum and septum secundum results in a **common atrium**. Because left-to-right shunting occurs at low pressure, patients with ASDs tend to have pulmonary HTN and become symptomatic later in childhood or as adults in contrast to the usual course of patients with VSDs and PDAs.

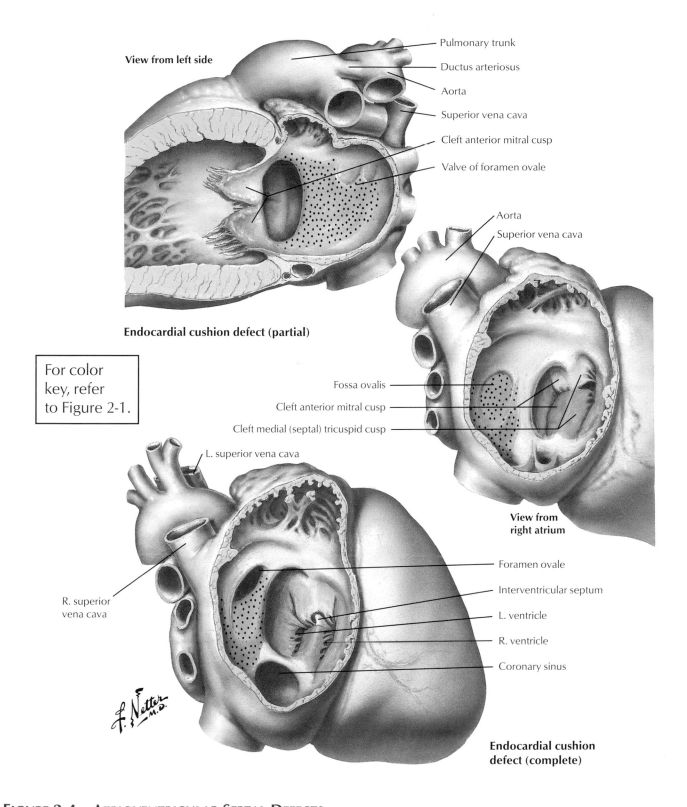

View from left side

Pulmonary trunk

Ductus arteriosus

Aorta

Superior vena cava

Cleft anterior mitral cusp

Valve of foramen ovale

Endocardial cushion defect (partial)

For color key, refer to Figure 2-1.

Aorta

Superior vena cava

Fossa ovalis

Cleft anterior mitral cusp

Cleft medial (septal) tricuspid cusp

View from right atrium

L. superior vena cava

R. superior vena cava

Foramen ovale

Interventricular septum

L. ventricle

R. ventricle

Coronary sinus

Endocardial cushion defect (complete)

FIGURE 2-4　ATRIOVENTRICULAR SEPTAL DEFECTS

Atrioventricular septal defects (AVSDs) result from significantly defective formation of endocardial cushion tissue. The ASD component is low in the interatrial septum because of failure of closure of the ostium primum. The VSD component is in the region of the membranous interventricular septum. The **partial endocardial-cushion defect** is composed of an ostium primum type of ASD, a defective mitral valve with a cleft in the anterior leaflet, and subtle anomalies in the LV, but it is associated with a closed membranous interventricular septum. The **complete endocardial-cushion defect**, also called a **persistent common atrioventricular canal**, consists of a large ostium primum ASD, a membranous VSD, and an abnormal common atrioventricular valve straddling the AVSD.

21

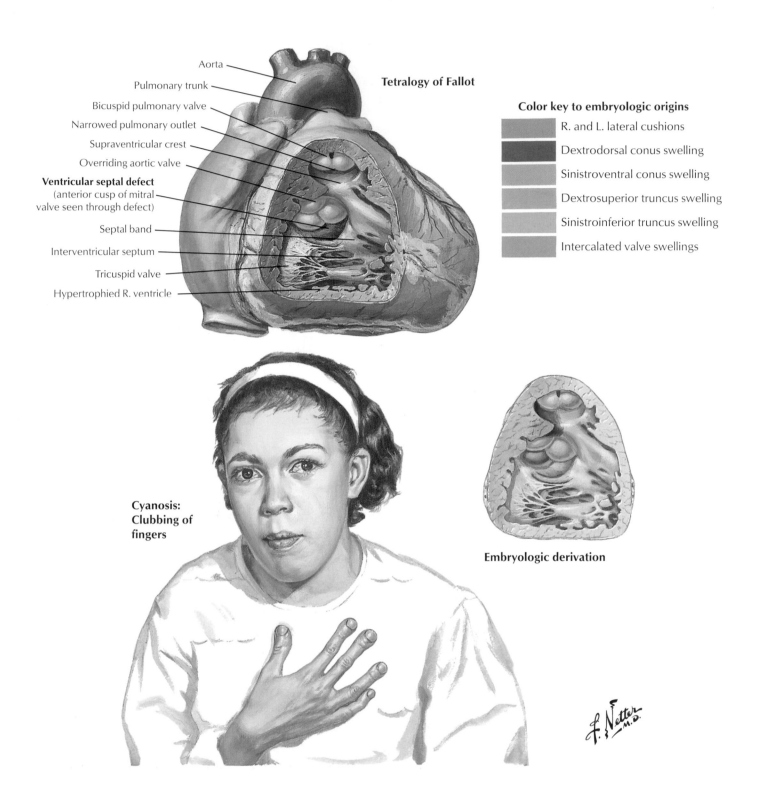

Aorta

Pulmonary trunk

Bicuspid pulmonary valve

Narrowed pulmonary outlet

Supraventricular crest

Overriding aortic valve

Ventricular septal defect
(anterior cusp of mitral
valve seen through defect)

Septal band

Interventricular septum

Tricuspid valve

Hypertrophied R. ventricle

Tetralogy of Fallot

Color key to embryologic origins

R. and L. lateral cushions

Dextrodorsal conus swelling

Sinistroventral conus swelling

Dextrosuperior truncus swelling

Sinistroinferior truncus swelling

Intercalated valve swellings

**Cyanosis:
Clubbing of
fingers**

Embryologic derivation

FIGURE 2-5　TETRALOGY OF FALLOT

The **tetralogy of Fallot** is the most common form of cyanotic congenital heart disease, a state characterized by a right-to-left shunt with **cyanosis** at the time of presentation (i.e., cyanotic congenital heart disease). Depending on the severity of the defects, the presentation may occur in infancy (**blue baby syndrome**) but is not usually apparent until at least early childhood.

The 4 components of the tetralogy of Fallot are (1) VSD; (2) obstruction of the right ventricular outflow tract, usually as a result of subpulmonic, infundibular stenosis; (3) an aorta that overrides the VSD; and (4) right ventricular hypertrophy. Complete surgical correction of the tetralogy of Fallot includes closure of the VSD and expansion of the right ventricular outflow tract.

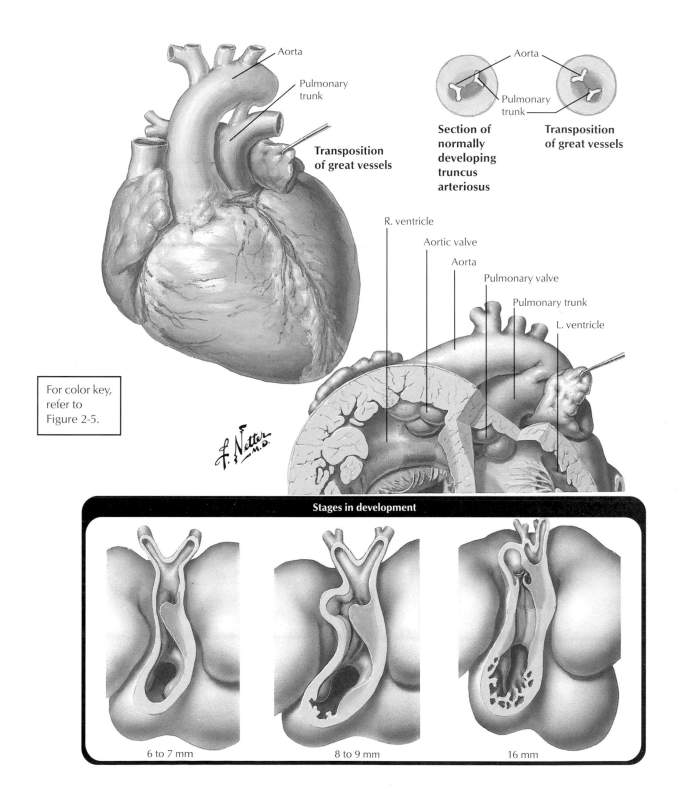

Aorta

Pulmonary trunk

Transposition of great vessels

Aorta

Pulmonary trunk

Section of normally developing truncus arteriosus

Transposition of great vessels

R. ventricle

Aortic valve

Aorta

Pulmonary valve

Pulmonary trunk

L. ventricle

For color key, refer to Figure 2-5.

Stages in development

6 to 7 mm   8 to 9 mm   16 mm

FIGURE 2-6   TRANSPOSITION OF THE GREAT VESSELS

Transposition of the great vessels, or more specifically, congenitally complete transposition of the great vessels, is a condition in which the aorta takes origin anteriorly from the RV and the pulmonic trunk arises posteriorly from the LV. Transposition of the great vessels is compatible with postnatal life only when the anomaly occurs in association with one or more other defects, usually VSD, ASD, or PDA. The lower diagram shows the embryological development of transposition. Normally, two pairs of truncal swellings develop. In transposition, the wrong pair of truncal swellings becomes involved in partitioning the truncus, resulting in the abnormal position of the great vessels.

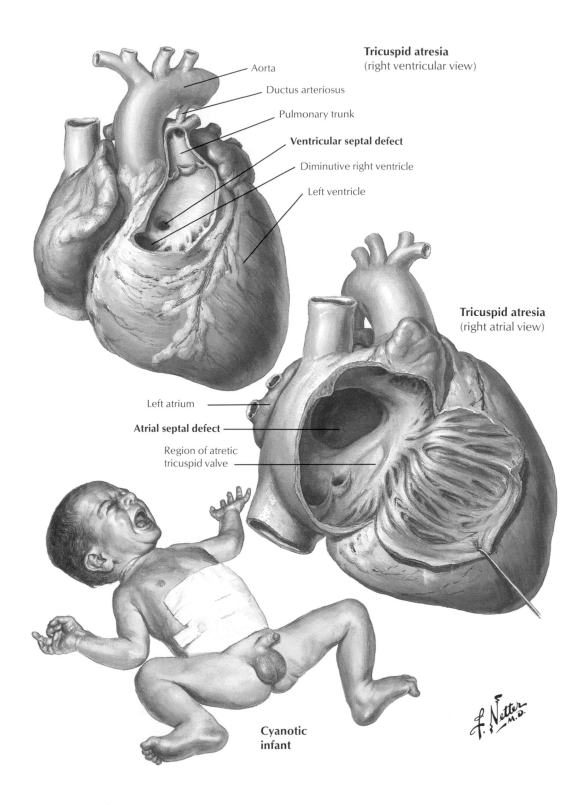

Tricuspid atresia
(right ventricular view)

Aorta

Ductus arteriosus

Pulmonary trunk

Ventricular septal defect

Diminutive right ventricle

Left ventricle

Tricuspid atresia
(right atrial view)

Left atrium

Atrial septal defect

Region of atretic
tricuspid valve

**Cyanotic
infant**

FIGURE 2-7   TRICUSPID ATRESIA

Tricuspid atresia, a severe complex anomaly of the right side of the heart with underdevelopment (hypoplasia) of the RV and a right-to-left shunt through an ASD, a VSD, or a PDA, results in severe **cyanotic heart disease** in infants. Next to transposition of the great vessels, it is the most common cause of severe cyanosis in the neonatal period, and the degree of cyanosis is usually more marked than in cases of transposition.

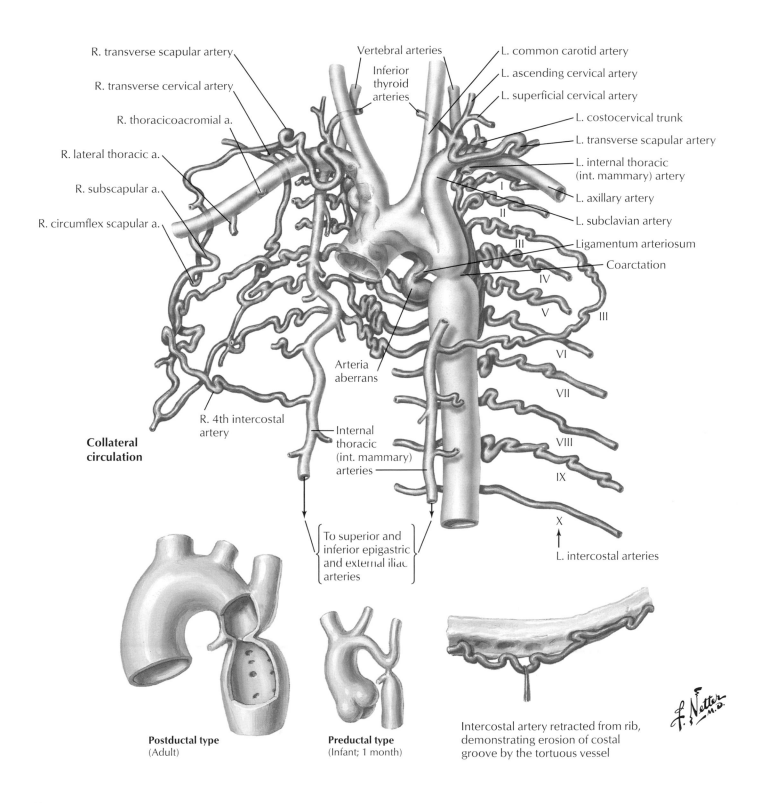

R. transverse scapular artery

R. transverse cervical artery

R. thoracicoacromial a.

R. lateral thoracic a.

R. subscapular a.

R. circumflex scapular a.

Collateral circulation

R. 4th intercostal artery

Vertebral arteries

Inferior thyroid arteries

Arteria aberrans

Internal thoracic (int. mammary) arteries

To superior and inferior epigastric and external iliac arteries

L. common carotid artery

L. ascending cervical artery

L. superficial cervical artery

L. costocervical trunk

L. transverse scapular artery

L. internal thoracic (int. mammary) artery

L. axillary artery

L. subclavian artery

Ligamentum arteriosum

Coarctation

L. intercostal arteries

Postductal type
(Adult)

Preductal type
(Infant; 1 month)

Intercostal artery retracted from rib, demonstrating erosion of costal groove by the tortuous vessel

FIGURE 2-8   COARCTATION OF THE AORTA

Coarctation of the aorta is a common obstructive congenital anomaly. There are 2 major types: (1) an **infantile form**, with tubular hypoplasia of the aortic arch proximal to a PDA, typically resulting in clinical problems in early childhood; and (2) an **adult postductal form**, in which there is a discrete ridgelike infolding of the aorta, just opposite the closed ductus arteriosus (the ligamen-tum arteriosum). The postductal type of coarctation leads to the development of an extensive collateral circulation (top image) to bypass the obstruction. The patient presents with HTN in the upper extremities and normal pressures in the lower extremities. Rib notching (produced by the enlarged collateral arteries) is seen on chest radiograph.

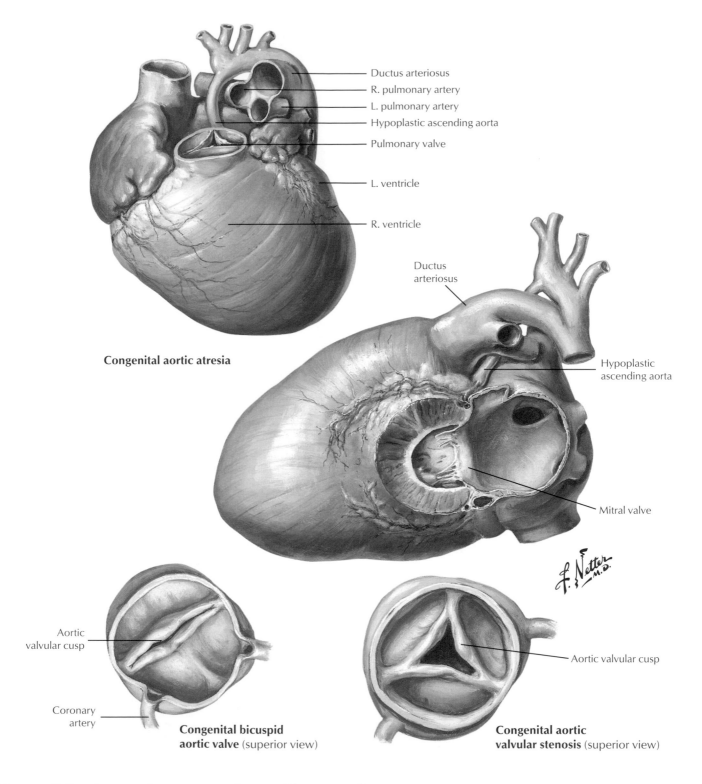

Ductus arteriosus
R. pulmonary artery
L. pulmonary artery
Hypoplastic ascending aorta
Pulmonary valve

L. ventricle

R. ventricle

Congenital aortic atresia

Ductus arteriosus

Hypoplastic ascending aorta

Mitral valve

Aortic valvular cusp

Coronary artery

Congenital bicuspid aortic valve (superior view)

Aortic valvular cusp

Congenital aortic valvular stenosis (superior view)

FIGURE 2-9 AORTIC ATRESIA AND AORTIC VALVULAR STENOSIS

Left ventricular outflow tract (LVOT) obstruction can result from **aortic stenosis** or **atresia**. In severe congential aortic malformation, LVOT obstruction leads to underdevelopment (hypoplasia) of the LV and ascending aorta. There is a dense, porcelainlike endocardial fibroelastosis of the diminutive LV. The ductus arteriosus is open. This constellation of anomalies constitutes the **hypoplastic left heart syndrome**, a condition that is fatal in the first several days of postnatal life when the ductus closes, unless high-risk surgery is performed. Less severe congenital aortic stenoses are compatible with longer survival. The congenital bicuspid aortic valve occurs in approximately 1% to 2% of the population and can give rise to aortic stenosis in adulthood because of hemodynamic turbulence that leads to fibrosis and calcification.

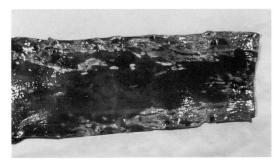

Aorta with fatty streaks

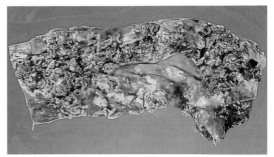

Aorta with fibrous (atheromatous) plaques

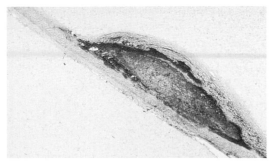

Oil red O stain of fibrous plaque showing lipid-rich core (red) and fibrous cap (low magnification)

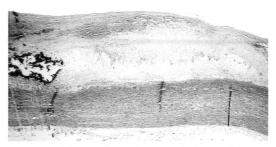

Histology of fibrous plaque showing calcification (blue), lipid core (pale), and fibrous cap (low magnification)

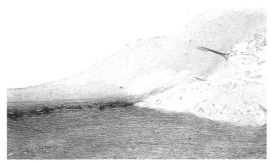

Fibrous cap and lipid core of fibrous plaque (medium magnification)

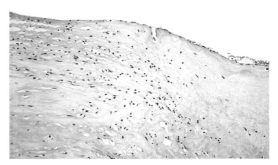

Fibrous cap containing inflammatory cells (medium magnification)

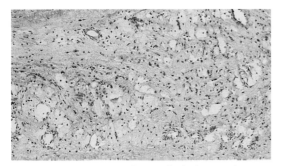

Core of plaque containing foam cells (high magnification)

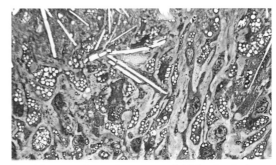

Special preparation to demonstrate lipid droplets in foam cells and cholesterol crystals (high magnification)

FIGURE 2-10   ATHEROSCLEROSIS

Atherosclerosis, the most prevalent and important form of arteriosclerosis, is a disease that typically affects the aorta and its major muscular distributing branches. The lesion of established atherosclerosis is the atherosclerotic (fibrous or atheromatous) plaque (gross photo, upper right). The fatty streak is the most obvious precursor lesion (gross photo, upper left). The photomicrographs show the features of atherosclerotic plaques, including fibrous capsule and lipid-rich core containing foam cells and cholesterol crystals.

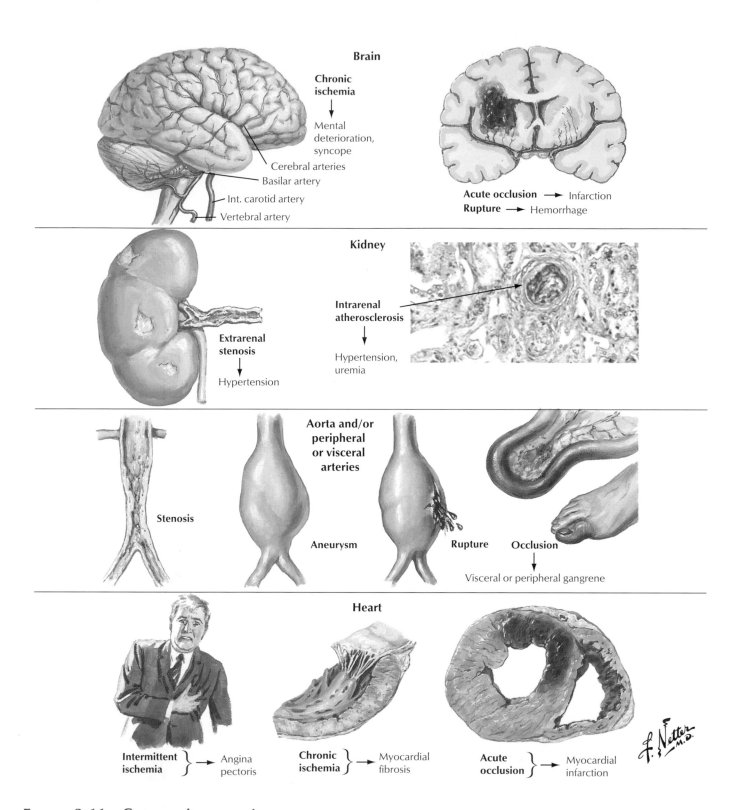

FIGURE 2-11 CRITICAL AREAS OF ATHEROSCLEROSIS

The major pathologic and clinical effects of **atherosclerosis** involve the brain, the kidneys, the aorta, the peripheral and visceral arteries, and the heart. According to the response to injury hypothesis, atherosclerosis develops as a response of the vessel wall to multifactorial and repetitive injury. Genetic susceptibility, environmental factors, and endogenous metabolic alterations are risk factors that participate in the pathogenesis of atherosclerosis and the formation of **atherosclerotic plaques** in vessels. Atherosclerosis progresses asymptomatically for years until a clinical threshold is reached. The onset of symptoms may be gradual or abrupt. The major treatable risk factors for development of atherosclerosis are a diet high in saturated fats and cholesterol, HTN, cigarette smoking, and diabetes mellitus.

Atherogenesis: Unstable Plaque Formation

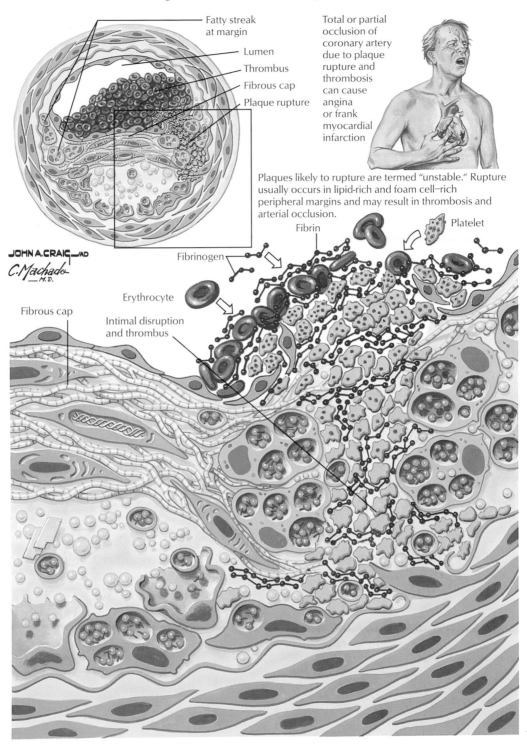

Fatty streak at margin

Lumen

Thrombus

Fibrous cap

Plaque rupture

Total or partial occlusion of coronary artery due to plaque rupture and thrombosis can cause angina or frank myocardial infarction

Plaques likely to rupture are termed "unstable." Rupture usually occurs in lipid-rich and foam cell–rich peripheral margins and may result in thrombosis and arterial occlusion.

Fibrin

Platelet

Fibrinogen

Erythrocyte

Fibrous cap

Intimal disruption and thrombus

JOHN A. CRAIG _AD
C. Machado _M.D.

FIGURE 2-12   PATHOLOGIC CHANGES IN CORONARY ARTERY DISEASE

Coronary heart disease (**atherosclerotic** or **ischemic heart disease**), dysfunction and damage to the heart muscle resulting from coronary artery disease (CAD), is usually due to **coronary atherosclerosis**. Coronary atherosclerosis leads to progressive luminal narrowing of one or more of the coronary arteries by atherosclerotic plaques; these frequently have calcification. Coronary reserve is such that angina pectoris usually does not develop until there is at least 75% narrowing of the cross-sectional area. Most symptomatic disease is associated with the development of secondary changes in the plaques, especially surface ulceration, intraplaque hemorrhage, and thrombosis. Coronary thrombi can organize, leading to recanalization of the lumen. Nonatheromatous causes of myocardial ischemia include congenital coronary anomaly, coronary dissection, **coronary vasculitis** (Kawasaki disease, polyarteritis nodosa, and others), or a systemic hemodynamic problem, such as severe shock or profound anemia.

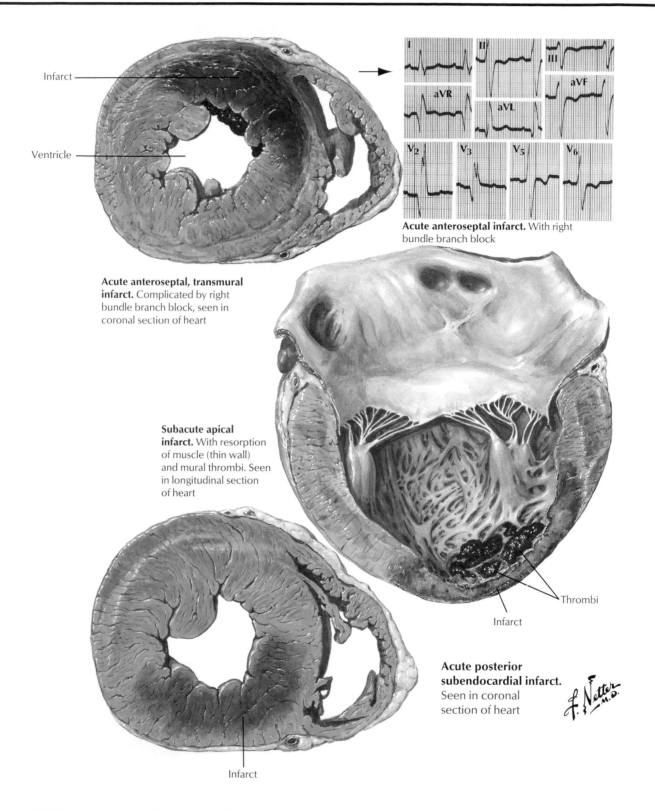

Infarct

Ventricle

Acute anteroseptal, transmural infarct. Complicated by right bundle branch block, seen in coronal section of heart

Acute anteroseptal infarct. With right bundle branch block

Subacute apical infarct. With resorption of muscle (thin wall) and mural thrombi. Seen in longitudinal section of heart

Thrombi

Infarct

Acute posterior subendocardial infarct. Seen in coronal section of heart

Infarct

FIGURE 2-13 ACUTE AND SUBACUTE MYOCARDIAL INFARCTS

Angina pectoris, which is due to myocardial ischemia of short duration (approximately 15 minutes), results in reversible myocardial injury. Myocardial infarction, the death of heart muscle due to prolonged, severe ischemia, usually involves the LV. **Myocardial necrosis** generally begins after 45 minutes of severe ischemia and extends from the subendocardium into the subepicardium in a wave-front fashion over a period of approximately 3 to 4 hours. **Subendocardial (intramural) myocardial**

infarcts are limited to the inner half of the wall. **Transmural myocardial infarcts** extend into the outer half of the wall. Lesions of the left anterior descending coronary system give rise to **anterior** and **anteroseptal myocardial infarcts**; lesions of the right coronary artery give rise to **inferior** (**posteroapical**) and **posterior myocardial infarcts**. Lesions of the left circumflex coronary artery give rise to **lateral myocardial infarcts**.

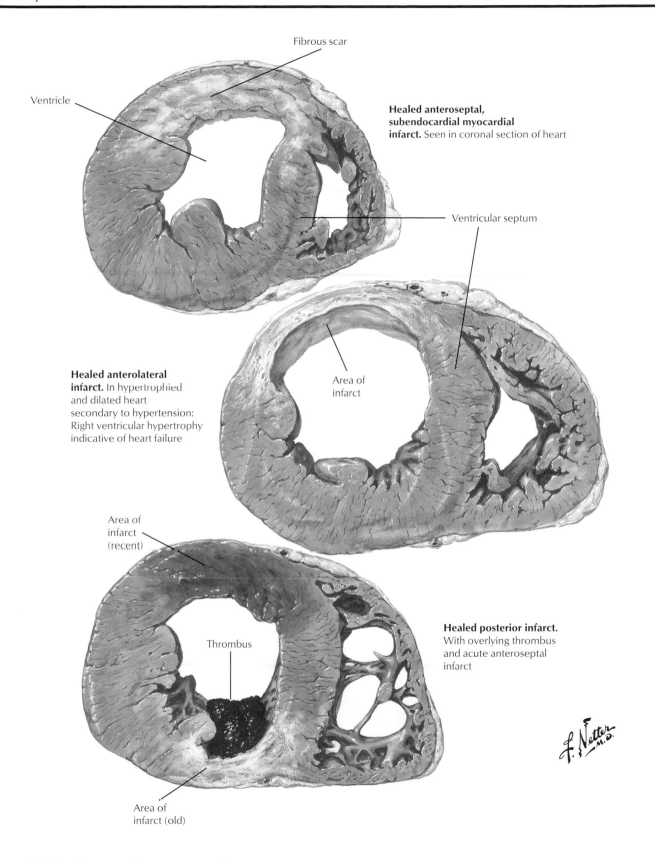

Fibrous scar

Ventricle

Healed anteroseptal, subendocardial myocardial infarct. Seen in coronal section of heart

Ventricular septum

Healed anterolateral infarct. In hypertrophied and dilated heart secondary to hypertension: Right ventricular hypertrophy indicative of heart failure

Area of infarct

Area of infarct (recent)

Thrombus

Healed posterior infarct. With overlying thrombus and acute anteroseptal infarct

Area of infarct (old)

FIGURE 2-14   HEALED MYOCARDIAL INFARCTS

Acute myocardial infarction may result in death due to pump failure or **ventricular fibrillation**. If the patient survives, the infarct undergoes organization and healing. During the first 2 to 3 weeks, the necrotic myocardium is gradually replaced by granulation tissue; during the next 2 to 3 months, the granulation tissue is converted to fibrous scar. This illustration shows various patterns of healed myocardial infarcts. During healing, the thinned infarcted wall may expand to form a ventricular aneurysm. Mural thrombi can form over the infarct and give rise to systemic emboli.

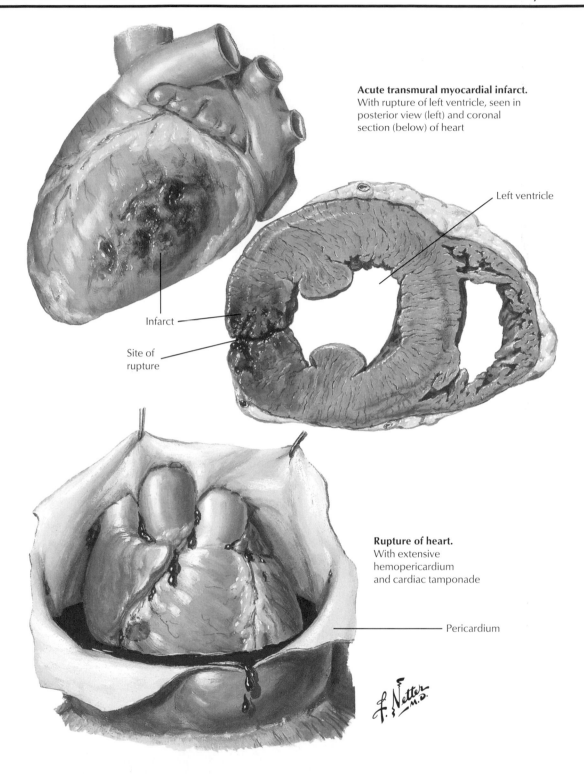

Acute transmural myocardial infarct.
With rupture of left ventricle, seen in
posterior view (left) and coronal
section (below) of heart

Left ventricle

Infarct

Site of
rupture

Rupture of heart.
With extensive
hemopericardium
and cardiac tamponade

Pericardium

FIGURE 2-15 RUPTURE OF MYOCARDIAL INFARCTS

Less than 5% of acute myocardial infarcts rupture. These ruptures involve **transmural myocardial infarcts** that may rupture during the first 7 to 10 days after onset. Patients at highest risk are those with persistent HTN during their infarcts and those with infarcts in regions without fibrosis; typically, these are first infarcts. Over time, a dissection track develops from the left ventricular chamber through the necrotic myocardium, and the completed process results in abrupt development of **hemopericardium**, **cardiac tamponade**, and electromechanical dissociation (electrical rhythm on electrocardiogram [ECG] but no effective cardiac output). This is generally fatal. In some cases, the intramural dissection occurs slowly enough for a pericardial inflammatory reaction to occur and seal off a region of pericardium, containing the rupture. This gives rise to a wide-mouthed pseudoaneurysm that, unlike true aneurysms, is prone to late rupture. Other severe complications of acute myocardial infarction involve rupture of infarcted interventricular septum to produce a VSD and rupture of the head or entire trunk of an infarcted papillary muscle. These complications lead to systolic murmurs and cardiac failure.

Causes of Secondary Hypertension That May Be Amenable to Surgery

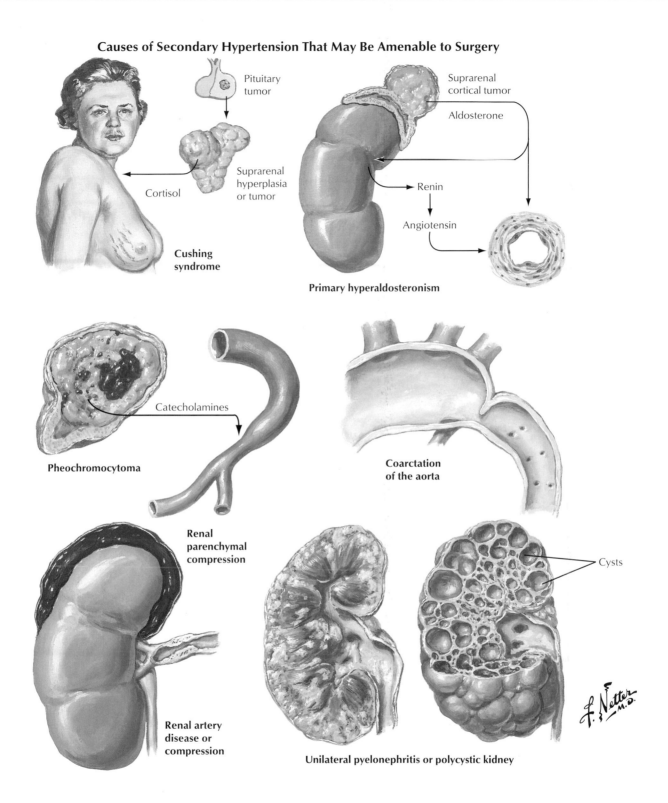

Pituitary tumor

Cortisol

Suprarenal hyperplasia or tumor

Cushing syndrome

Suprarenal cortical tumor

Aldosterone

Renin

Angiotensin

Primary hyperaldosteronism

Catecholamines

Pheochromocytoma

Renal parenchymal compression

Coarctation of the aorta

Cysts

Renal artery disease or compression

Unilateral pyelonephritis or polycystic kidney

FIGURE 2-16   CAUSES OF HYPERTENSION

Increase of systemic arterial pressure greater than the normal values of 120 mm Hg systolic and 80 mm Hg diastolic leads to a constellation of changes known as **hypertensive cardiovascular disease**. The pathophysiologic basis of HTN is excessive arteriolar constriction leading to increased peripheral vascular resistance. This may be exacerbated by factors promoting increased cardiac output. The fundamental etiology of HTN is unknown in most patients, although genetic predisposition and certain environmental influences, particularly high sodium intake, are known to be important factors. This condition is known as essential, idiopathic, or primary HTN. In approximately 10% of patients, HTN is secondary to a recognizable lesion or disease. Parenchymal renal disease and renovascular disease are the most common of these entities that are amenable to surgical treatment. Endocrine disorders and coarctation of the aorta are less common.

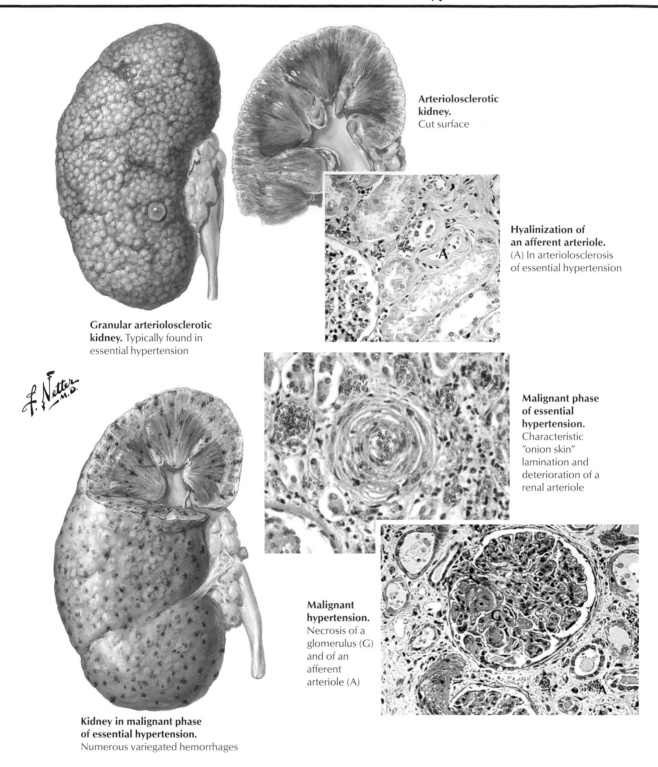

Arteriolosclerotic kidney. Cut surface

Granular arteriolosclerotic kidney. Typically found in essential hypertension

Hyalinization of an afferent arteriole. (A) In arteriolosclerosis of essential hypertension

Malignant phase of essential hypertension. Characteristic "onion skin" lamination and deterioration of a renal arteriole

Malignant hypertension. Necrosis of a glomerulus (G) and of an afferent arteriole (A)

Kidney in malignant phase of essential hypertension. Numerous variegated hemorrhages

FIGURE 2-17   THE KIDNEYS IN HYPERTENSION: BENIGN AND MALIGNANT

The natural history of HTN follows 2 general patterns. **Benign HTN** is characterized by mild to moderate increase of blood pressure and an asymptomatic period of several years before the inevitable onset of symptoms and end-organ damage (hence, the condition is not truly benign). **Malignant HTN** is characterized by marked increase of blood pressure and rapid progression over a few weeks to end-organ failure. Most patients with essential HTN follow the benign pattern, although it may accelerate to malignant HTN. The characteristic vascular lesion of benign essential HTN is widespread hyaline arteriolosclerosis manifest by thickening of the walls of the small arteries and arterioles by amorphous eosinophilic material composed of degenerated smooth cells and deposited plasma proteins. **Hyaline arteriolosclerosis** with associated small cortical scars (hyaline arteriolonephrosclerosis) is commonly seen in the kidneys. Hyperplastic arteriolosclerosis, marked luminal narrowing by cellular intimal proliferation in a lamellar, "onionskin" pattern, is the characteristic lesion of malignant HTN. In severe malignant HTN, fibrinoid necrosis of the glomerular arterioles occurs. An associated ischemic injury develops rapidly, leading to petechial hemorrhages in multiple organs, including the kidneys (hyperplastic arteriolonephrosclerosis).

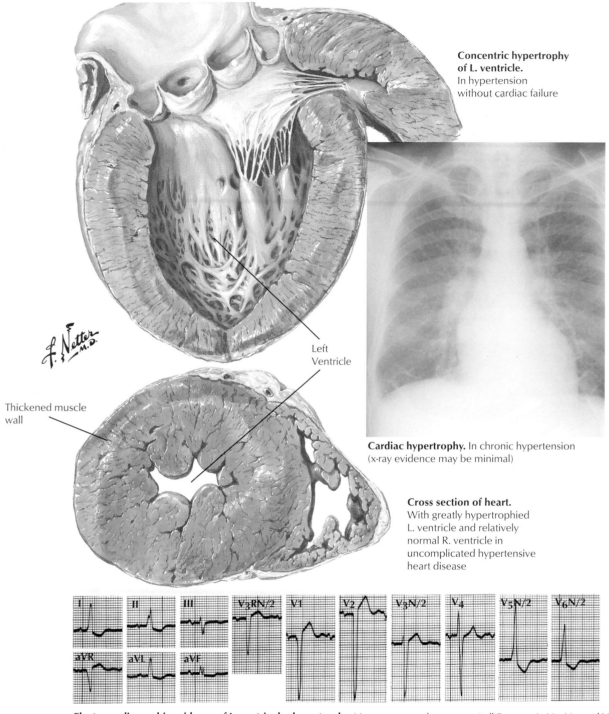

Concentric hypertrophy of L. ventricle. In hypertension without cardiac failure

Left Ventricle

Thickened muscle wall

Cardiac hypertrophy. In chronic hypertension (x-ray evidence may be minimal)

Cross section of heart. With greatly hypertrophied L. ventricle and relatively normal R. ventricle in uncomplicated hypertensive heart disease

Electrocardiographic evidence of L. ventricular hypertrophy. May or may not be present (tall R waves in V$_4$, V$_5$, and V$_6$; deep S waves in V$_3$R, V$_1$, V$_2$, III, and VR; depressed ST and inverted T in V$_5$, V$_6$, I, II, aVL, and aVF)

FIGURE 2-18   THE HEART IN HYPERTENSION: CONCENTRIC HYPERTROPHY

Hypertension, even of moderate degree, leads rapidly to **cardiac hypertrophy**, a compensatory increase of mass of the LV. The typical pattern of concentric hypertrophy of the LV, characterized by a thick wall and a relatively small chamber volume, is produced by a pressure load (afterload) on the ventricle. The heart size on cardiac silhouette is relatively normal, but the ECG shows increased voltage. When the limits of compensation are reached, the patient may have progressive cardiac decompensation accompanied by cardiac dilation. Cardiac hypertrophy is an independent risk factor for ventricular arrhythmias and sudden cardiac death.

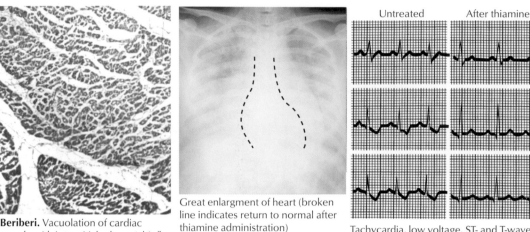

Beriberi. Vacuolation of cardiac muscle with interstitial edema (chiefly on right side)

Great enlargment of heart (broken line indicates return to normal after thiamine administration)

Untreated   After thiamine

Tachycardia, low voltage, ST- and T-wave abnormalities; return to normal after thiamine

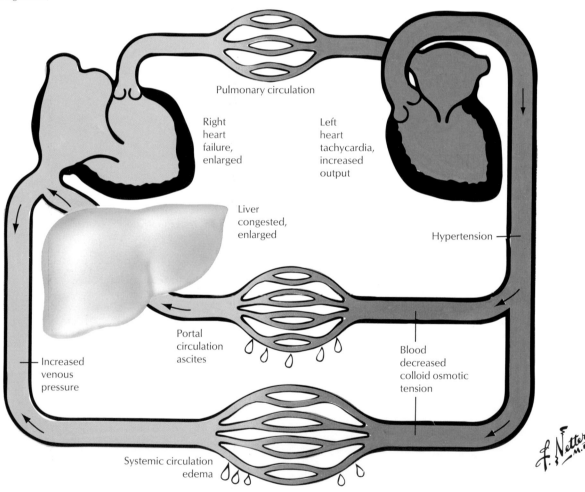

Pulmonary circulation

Right heart failure, enlarged

Left heart tachycardia, increased output

Liver congested, enlarged

Hypertension

Portal circulation ascites

Blood decreased colloid osmotic tension

Increased venous pressure

Systemic circulation edema

FIGURE 2-19   PATHOPHYSIOLOGY OF HEART FAILURE

Heart failure is a state in which the heart fails as a pump to provide sufficient volume of circulating blood to meet the metabolic demands of the body. Because the dominant symptoms usually result from pulmonary or systemic venous congestion, the condition is termed **congestive heart failure** (**CHF**). Most commonly, heart failure is of the low cardiac output variety, but some conditions, including thiamine deficiency (beriberi), thyrotoxicosis, and severe anemia, produce cardiac failure with an increased circulating blood volume (high output cardiac failure), as shown here. The failure may be left-sided, right-sided, or combined left- and right-sided heart failure. This illustration shows the major manifestations of failure of the left and right ventricles. Cardiac transplantation or an artificial heart is the last therapeutic option. The most common conditions necessitating cardiac transplantation are end-stage ischemic heart disease (ischemic cardiomyopathy) and dilated (congestive) cardiomyopathy.

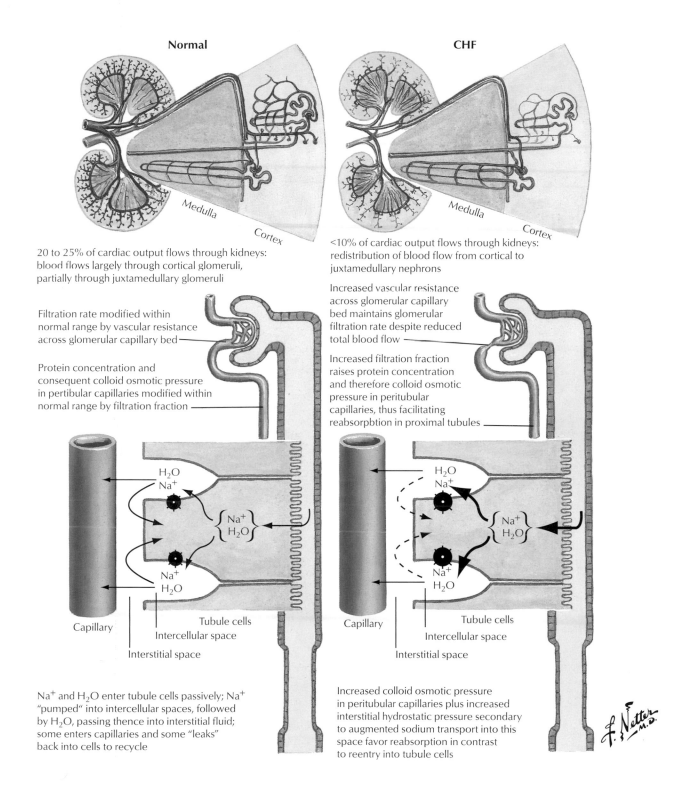

Normal

20 to 25% of cardiac output flows through kidneys: blood flows largely through cortical glomeruli, partially through juxtamedullary glomeruli

Filtration rate modified within normal range by vascular resistance across glomerular capillary bed

Protein concentration and consequent colloid osmotic pressure in pertibular capillaries modified within normal range by filtration fraction

H_2O
Na^+

Na^+
H_2O

Na^+
H_2O

Capillary

Tubule cells
Intercellular space
Interstitial space

Na^+ and H_2O enter tubule cells passively; Na^+ "pumped" into intercellular spaces, followed by H_2O, passing thence into interstitial fluid; some enters capillaries and some "leaks" back into cells to recycle

CHF

<10% of cardiac output flows through kidneys: redistribution of blood flow from cortical to juxtamedullary nephrons

Increased vascular resistance across glomerular capillary bed maintains glomerular filtration rate despite reduced total blood flow

Increased filtration fraction raises protein concentration and therefore colloid osmotic pressure in peritubular capillaries, thus facilitating reabsorpbtion in proximal tubules

H_2O
Na^+

Na^+
H_2O

Na^+
H_2O

Capillary

Tubule cells
Intercellular space
Interstitial space

Increased colloid osmotic pressure in peritubular capillaries plus increased interstitial hydrostatic pressure secondary to augmented sodium transport into this space favor reabsorption in contrast to reentry into tubule cells

Medulla
Cortex

Medulla
Cortex

f. Netter M.D.

FIGURE 2-20   THE KIDNEYS IN CONGESTIVE HEART FAILURE

Abnormal renal function is important in the pathophysiology of **CHF**. In response to impaired left ventricular output, renal blood flow is decreased and redistributed from cortical to juxtamedullary nephrons. The subsequent increased glomerular vascular resistance produces increases in filtration fraction and colloid osmotic pressure in peritubular capillaries and also an increase in interstitial hydrostatic pressure secondary to augmented sodium transport, leading to increased sodium and water retention in the peritubular capillaries. The sodium and water retention contribute to the development of edema associated with CHF.

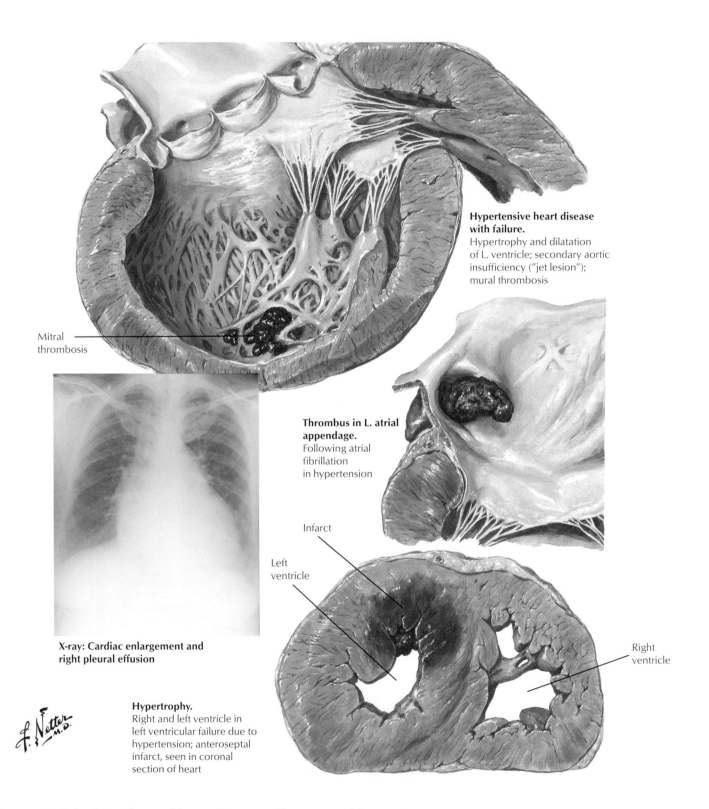

Hypertensive heart disease with failure.
Hypertrophy and dilatation of L. ventricle; secondary aortic insufficiency ("jet lesion"); mural thrombosis

Mitral thrombosis

Thrombus in L. atrial appendage.
Following atrial fibrillation in hypertension

Infarct

Left ventricle

Right ventricle

X-ray: Cardiac enlargement and right pleural effusion

Hypertrophy.
Right and left ventricle in left ventricular failure due to hypertension; anteroseptal infarct, seen in coronal section of heart

FIGURE 2-21   LEFT-SIDED HEART FAILURE: ECCENTRIC HYPERTROPHY

Most cases of CHF result from diseases that affect the LV initially or primarily, most commonly HTN and CAD. In response to chronic stress, the affected part of the heart undergoes compensatory hypertrophy. When the heart reaches a critical weight of 550 g, reserve is lost and progressive cardiac decompensation ensues. Heart failure results in progressive ventricular dilatation superimposed on the hypertrophy, which produces a pattern of so-called **eccentric hypertrophy**, as shown here. A severe acute load on the heart can produce failure and cardiac dilatation without previous hypertrophy. Stress of the atria can result in atrial fibrillation and formation of mural thrombi. The frequent coexistence of HTN and CAD can result in myocardial infarction of the hypertrophied LV.

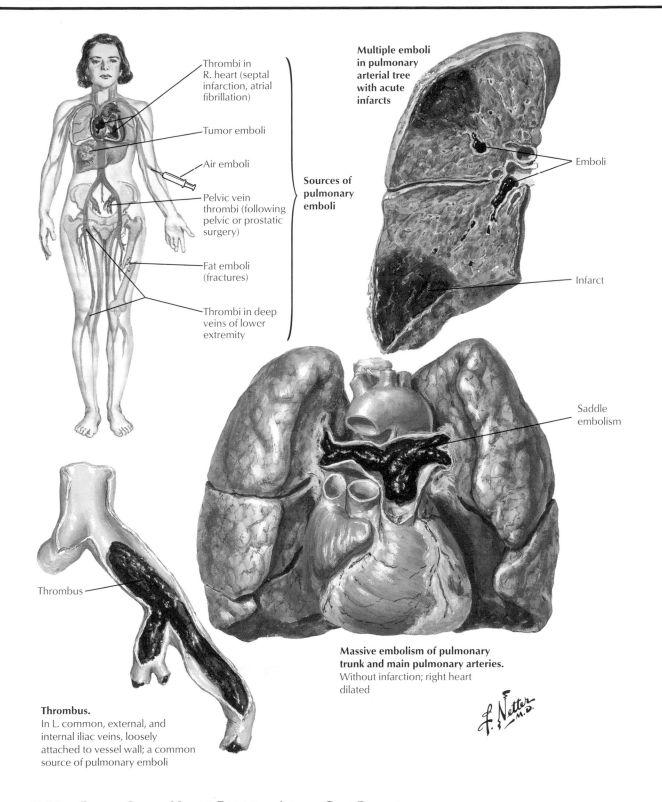

Thrombi in R. heart (septal infarction, atrial fibrillation)

Tumor emboli

Air emboli

Pelvic vein thrombi (following pelvic or prostatic surgery)

Fat emboli (fractures)

Thrombi in deep veins of lower extremity

Sources of pulmonary emboli

Multiple emboli in pulmonary arterial tree with acute infarcts

Emboli

Infarct

Saddle embolism

Massive embolism of pulmonary trunk and main pulmonary arteries. Without infarction; right heart dilated

Thrombus

Thrombus. In L. common, external, and internal iliac veins, loosely attached to vessel wall; a common source of pulmonary emboli

FIGURE 2-22   RIGHT-SIDED HEART FAILURE: ACUTE COR PULMONALE

Cor pulmonale, the selective or primary impairment of the right heart (RV and right atrium) due to HTN in the pulmonary circulation, is caused by pulmonary vascular or parenchymal disease. Acute strain on the right heart is produced by a massive thromboembolus or by multiple segmental thromboemboli in the pulmonary trunk. A **thromboembolus** of sufficient magnitude may cause sudden death because the obstruction of the pulmonary vasculature produces pulmonary HTN and acute right-sided heart failure coupled with an impaired return of blood to the left heart

with consequent decreased systemic and coronary perfusion and secondary left-sided heart failure. A thromboembolus usually does not result in pulmonary infarction. Because of the dual circulation from the pulmonary arteries and bronchial arteries, most **segmental thromboemboli** do not produce pulmonary infarcts. Pulmonary infarcts do occur in the presence of thromboemboli and impaired systemic circulation associated with preexistent CHF.

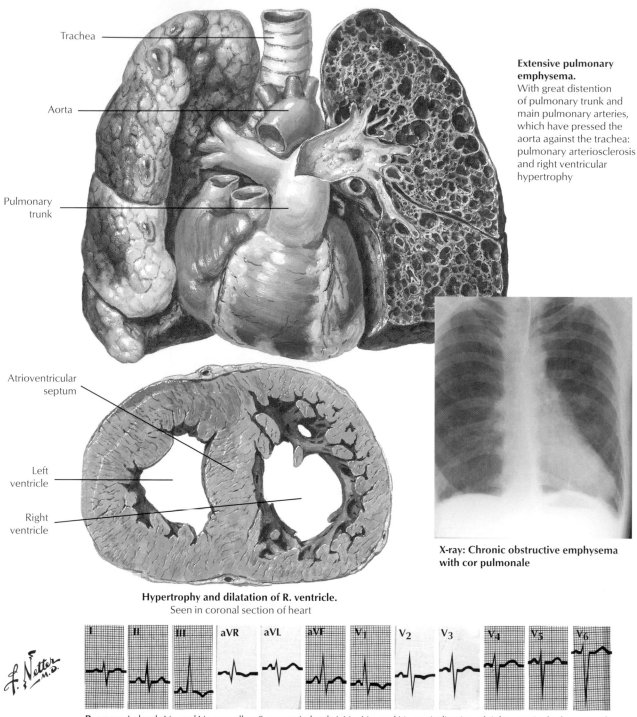

Trachea

Aorta

Pulmonary
trunk

**Extensive pulmonary
emphysema.**
With great distention
of pulmonary trunk and
main pulmonary arteries,
which have pressed the
aorta against the trachea:
pulmonary arteriosclerosis
and right ventricular
hypertrophy

Atrioventricular
septum

Left
ventricle

Right
ventricle

Hypertrophy and dilatation of R. ventricle.
Seen in coronal section of heart

**X-ray: Chronic obstructive emphysema
with cor pulmonale**

R waves. In leads V_1 and V_2 as well as S, waves in leads I, V_4, V_5, and V_6 are indicative of right ventricular hypertrophy.
Prominent P waves in leads II, III, aVF, V_1, and V_2 suggest right atrial enlargment.

FIGURE 2-23   RIGHT-SIDED HEART FAILURE: CHRONIC COR PULMONALE

Chronic cor pulmonale typically develops in response to recurring pulmonary thromboembolic disease or chronic pulmonary parenchymal diseases, particularly chronic **bronchitis** and **emphysema**. The heart exhibits significant hypertrophy and dilatation of the RV with a normal-sized LV (unless the patient has other diseases, such as systemic HTN or CAD).

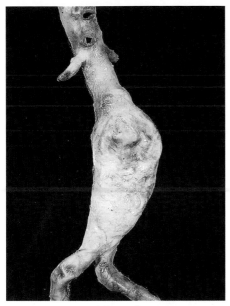

Aneurysm. Lower abdominal aorta

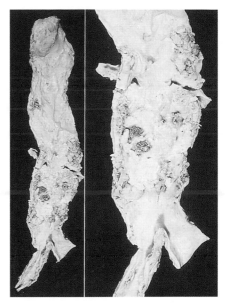

Severe atherosclerosis. In the aorta between the renal arteries and the bifurcation

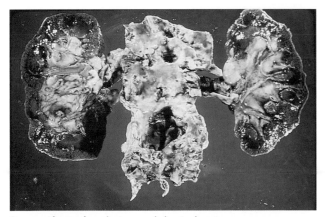

Severe atherosclerosis. Lower abdominal aorta

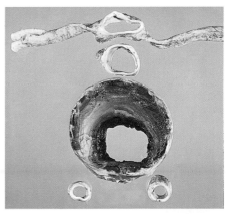

Lower abdominal aorta. Cross section showing mural thrombus in aneurysmal segment

FIGURE 2-24   AORTIC ATHEROSCLEROSIS

Atherosclerosis of the aorta is typically most severe in the lower abdominal aorta between the origin of the renal arteries and the aortic bifurcation. The frequent occurrence of abdominal **atherosclerotic aortic aneurysms** is due to the medial weakening that accompanies the severe atherosclerosis. Less frequently, the entire abdominal aorta and the descending thoracic aorta form a **thoracoabdominal atherosclerotic aortic aneurysm**. **Aortic root** and **ascending aorta atherosclerotic aneurysms** are secondary to

end arteriolitis of the vasa vasorum produced years previously by systemic infection by *Treponema pallidum* (syphilitic or luetic aortitis), unless proven otherwise. **Atherosclerotic aneurysms of the iliofemoral arteries** also occur. The cavity of the atherosclerotic aneurysm frequently fills with unorganized mural thrombus, and the expanding aneurysms become increasingly susceptible to external rupture and life-threatening exsanguinations.

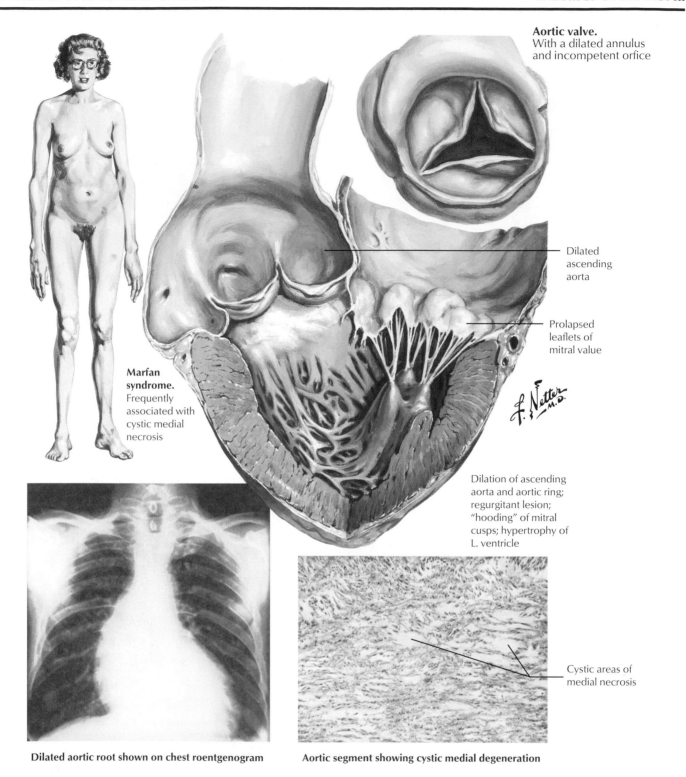

Aortic valve.
With a dilated annulus and incompetent orfice

Dilated ascending aorta

Prolapsed leaflets of mitral value

Marfan syndrome. Frequently associated with cystic medial necrosis

Dilation of ascending aorta and aortic ring; regurgitant lesion; "hooding" of mitral cusps; hypertrophy of L. ventricle

Cystic areas of medial necrosis

Dilated aortic root shown on chest roentgenogram

Aortic segment showing cystic medial degeneration

FIGURE 2-25　CYSTIC MEDIAL DEGENERATION OF THE AORTA

Primary degenerative disease of the aortic media manifests as cystic medial degeneration, also called cystic medial necrosis. The lesions, which consist of foci of an acid mucopolysaccharide (glycosaminoglycan)–rich ground substance, are devoid of smooth muscle cells and elastic fibers. Severe cystic medial degeneration develops as a component of genetic diseases of connective tissue, specifically, the Marfan syndrome and certain subtypes of the Ehlers-Danlos syndrome. Severe disease gives rise to **annuloaortic ectasia**, a progressive aneurysmal dilatation of the aortic root, with accompanying aortic valvular incompetence. Myxomatous degeneration of the mitral valve typically develops, which leads to mitral valvular prolapse and mitral incompetence. The aortic and mitral regurgitation place a volume load (preload) on the LV, which causes dilatation and hypertrophy (eccentric hypertrophy). The weakened and dilated aorta is prone to medial dissection or to focal perforation with external rupture and fatal exsanguination.

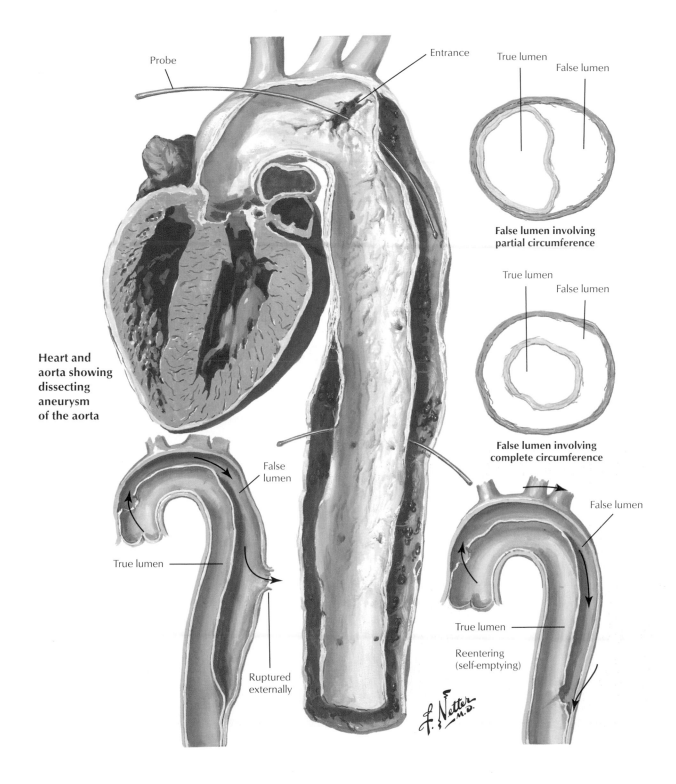

Probe

Entrance

True lumen

False lumen

**False lumen involving
partial circumference**

True lumen

False lumen

**False lumen involving
complete circumference**

Heart and
aorta showing
dissecting
aneurysm
of the aorta

False
lumen

True lumen

Ruptured
externally

False lumen

True lumen

Reentering
(self-emptying)

*f. Netter
M.D.*

FIGURE 2-26   DISSECTING ANEURYSM OF THE AORTA

The effects of HTN with excessive hemodynamic trauma on a weakened aortic wall can lead to the formation of a **hematoma** in the media. The hematoma dissects longitudinally to split the media, which creates a dissecting hematoma or a **dissecting aneurysm**, a double-barreled aorta with true and false lumens. In most cases, a proximal intimal tear allows blood to enter the false lumen under systemic pressure. In **type A dissections**, the proximal intimal tear is in the ascending thoracic aorta, whereas in **type B dissections**, the proximal intimal tear is in the aortic arch or the descending thoracic aorta. Type A dissections, which are prone to external rupture into the mediastinum or pericardial cavity, necessitate surgical intervention. Some dissections develop distal tears and become chronic with the potential for late rupture. Blood pressure control is key in the treatment of any aortic dissection.

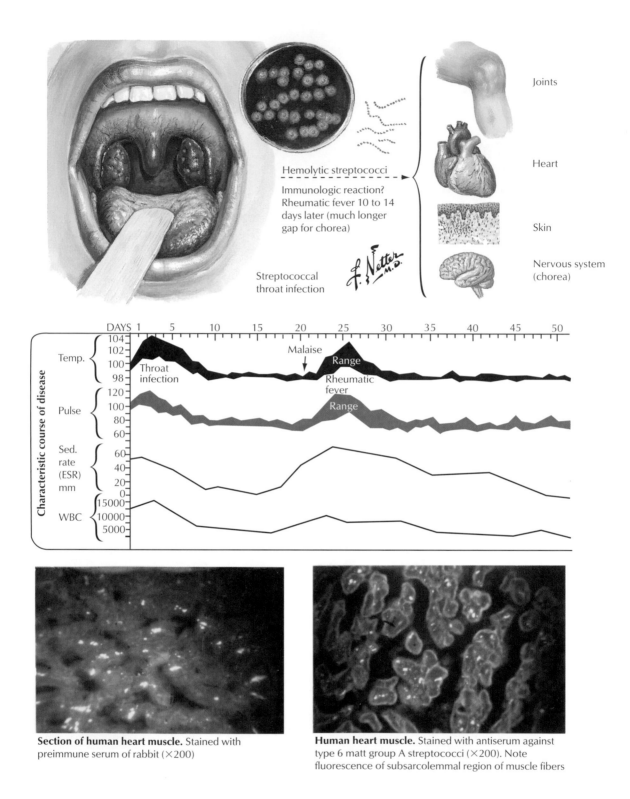

Section of human heart muscle. Stained with preimmune serum of rabbit (×200)

Human heart muscle. Stained with antiserum against type 6 matt group A streptococci (×200). Note fluorescence of subsarcolemmal region of muscle fibers

FIGURE 2-27 RHEUMATIC FEVER

Acute RF is a multisystem immunologic illness often resulting in chronic rheumatic heart disease (RHD). RF generally affects children between the ages of 5 and 15 years. Ten to 14 days after infection with **group A β-hemolytic streptococci**, patients have multisystem manifestations, including skin rash (erythema annulare), subcutaneous nodules, migratory polyarthritis involving the larger joints of the extremities, and acute cardiac failure

with mitral regurgitation. In some cases, central nervous system involvement manifests as spontaneous uncoordinated movements of the extremities (Sydenham chorea). The **autoimmune attack** of the target tissues of the host, which involves both humoral (antibody-mediated) and cellular (activated T lymphocytes) mechanisms, is a result of an immunologic reaction against the streptococci.

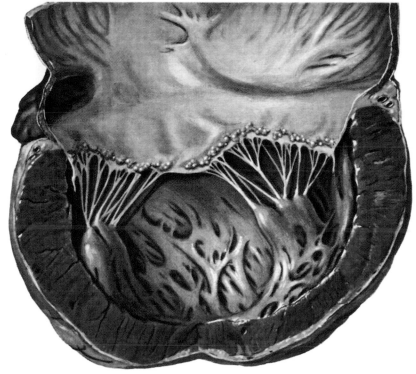

Acute rheumatic heart disease. Rheumatic vegetations on mitral valve

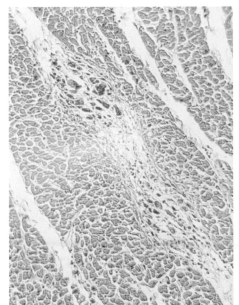

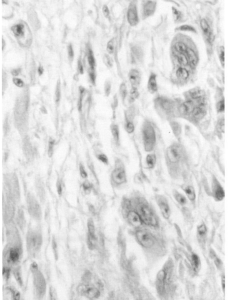

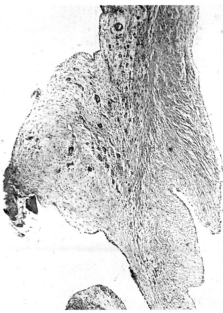

Characteristic distribution of myocardial Aschoff bodies. In interstitial tissue between fascicles of muscle

Well-developed Aschoff body. Composed of the variety of cells, including multinucleated Aschoff cells

Photomicrograph of mitral valve in acute rheumatic endocarditis. Swelling along line of closure of the valve cusp represents healing of vegetative material, some of which still caps the summit of the swelling

FIGURE 2-28   RHEUMATIC HEART DISEASE

The basic tissue lesion of acute RF consists of fibrinoid necrosis of connective tissue accompanied by inflammatory cellular infiltrates composed of lymphocytes and macrophages. Acute RHD is produced by inflammation of all components of the heart (pancarditis) composed of fibrinous pericarditis, perivascular nodular foci of fibrinoid degeneration of collagen with surrounding granulomatous inflammation (**Aschoff bodies**), and similar inflammation of the mural endocardium and cardiac valves. The cardiac **valvular lesions** consist of small, nodular, wartlike fibrin thrombi (verrucae) along the line of closure of the valves, particularly the mitral and aortic valves. The cardiac inflammation leads to depressed myocardial contractile function and dilatation of the cardiac chambers, particularly the LV, and associated mitral valvular regurgitation.

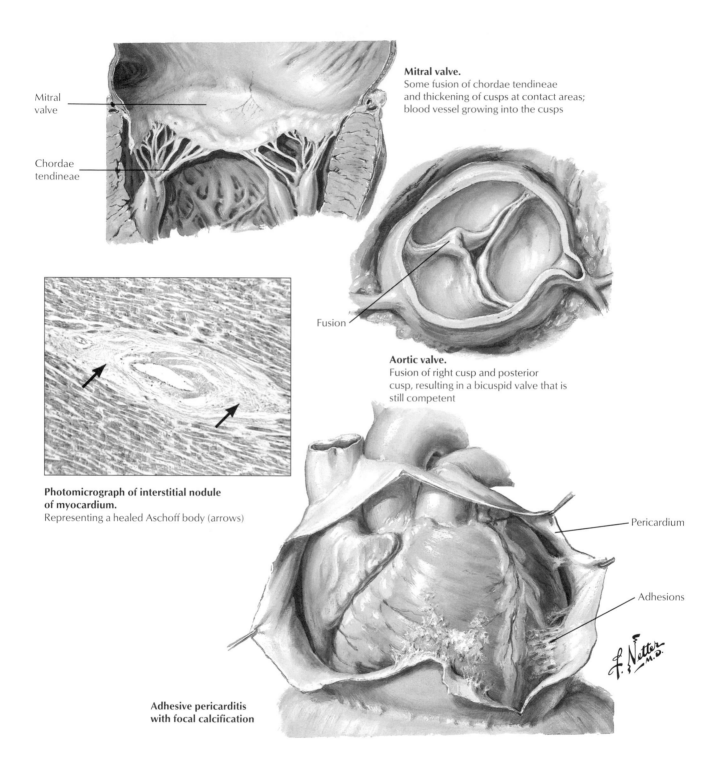

Mitral valve

Chordae tendineae

Mitral valve.
Some fusion of chordae tendineae and thickening of cusps at contact areas; blood vessel growing into the cusps

Fusion

Aortic valve.
Fusion of right cusp and posterior cusp, resulting in a bicuspid valve that is still competent

Photomicrograph of interstitial nodule of myocardium.
Representing a healed Aschoff body (arrows)

Pericardium

Adhesions

Adhesive pericarditis with focal calcification

FIGURE 2-29　CHRONIC RHEUMATIC HEART DISEASE

The heart manifests chronic residua at the sites of previous inflammation, including **fibrous adhesions**, which partially obliterate the pericardial space; perivascular scars in the myocardium; and alterations of the **cardiac valves** produced by the process of organization and healing. The inflammation of the cardiac valves elicits a granulation tissue response with ingrowth of small blood vessels (neovascularization) and fibroblasts, collagen production, diffuse fibrous thickening, and, later,

dystrophic calcification. The organization and healing of the fibrinous verrucae lead to the partial or complete **fusion** of one or more of the **commissures** between adjacent leaflets. These changes distort the anatomy and function of the valves. A vicious cycle of increased hemodynamic turbulence and wear and tear ensues, leading to progressive distortion of valvular anatomy and function, until months to years after the acute RF, the patient becomes symptomatic with chronic RHD.

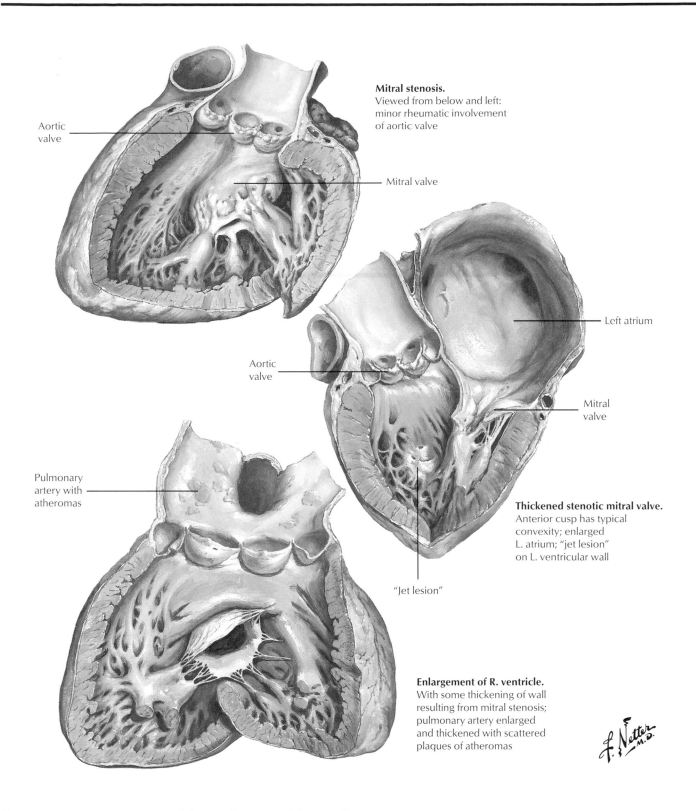

Mitral stenosis.
Viewed from below and left: minor rheumatic involvement of aortic valve

Aortic valve

Mitral valve

Left atrium

Aortic valve

Mitral valve

Thickened stenotic mitral valve.
Anterior cusp has typical convexity; enlarged L. atrium; "jet lesion" on L. ventricular wall

Pulmonary artery with atheromas

"Jet lesion"

Enlargement of R. ventricle.
With some thickening of wall resulting from mitral stenosis; pulmonary artery enlarged and thickened with scattered plaques of atheromas

f. Netter
M.D.

FIGURE 2-30   RHEUMATIC HEART DISEASE: MITRAL STENOSIS

Chronic RHD accounts for nearly all cases of **mitral stenosis**. **Stenosis** and **incompetence** of the mitral and aortic valve are produced by obstruction of the orifice and regurgitation of blood across the orifice, respectively. In rheumatic mitral stenosis, the shortening and thickening of the mitral leaflets, the fusion and thickening and the shortening of the chordae tendineae, and the fusion of the commissures results in a greatly reduced orifice. This "dam-in-the-stream" effect leads to increased left atrial pressure

with subsequent atrial dilatation, formation of atrial mural thrombi, and atrial fibrillation. Increased pulmonary venous pressure, pulmonary congestion, increased pulmonary arterial pressure, and right heart strain leads to **right ventricular hypertrophy and dilatation** and functional **tricuspid regurgitation**. There is a characteristic opening snap and diastolic rumbling murmur at the cardiac apex.

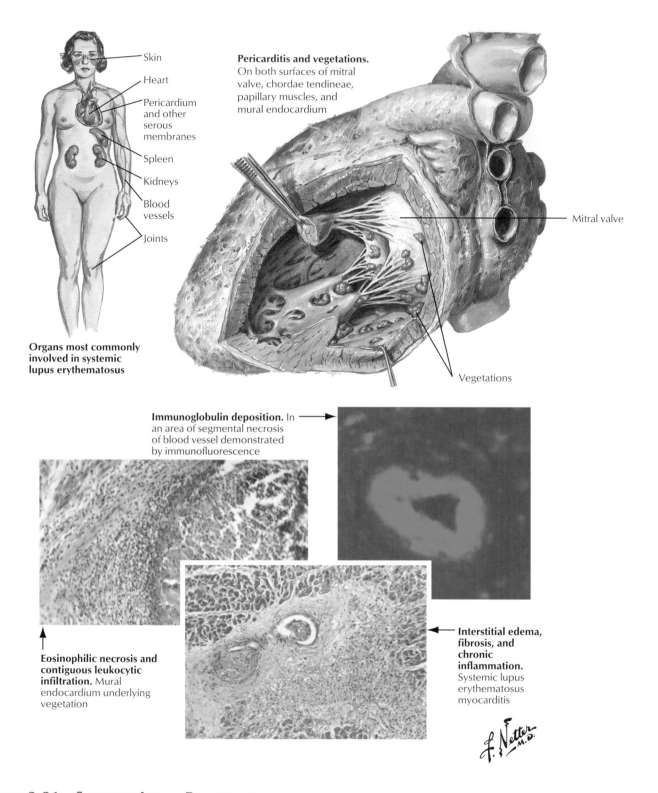

Skin

Heart

Pericardium and other serous membranes

Spleen

Kidneys

Blood vessels

Joints

Organs most commonly involved in systemic lupus erythematosus

Pericarditis and vegetations. On both surfaces of mitral valve, chordae tendineae, papillary muscles, and mural endocardium

Mitral valve

Vegetations

Immunoglobulin deposition. In an area of segmental necrosis of blood vessel demonstrated by immunofluorescence

Eosinophilic necrosis and contiguous leukocytic infiltration. Mural endocardium underlying vegetation

Interstitial edema, fibrosis, and chronic inflammation. Systemic lupus erythematosus myocarditis

FIGURE 2-31   SYSTEMIC LUPUS ERYTHEMATOSUS

Systemic lupus erythematosus can produce pancarditis with fibrinous pericarditis and pericardial effusion, multifocal lympho-histiocytic myocarditis, and mural and valvular endocarditis. Valvular inflammation can be extensive, leading to fibrinous verrucae on the upper and lower surfaces of the valvular leaflets, particularly those of the mitral valve. This valvular pathology is known as the **atypical verrucous endocarditis of Libman and Sacks**. Healing of the inflammation leads to progressive valvular deformity, including fibrous adhesions of the posterior mitral leaflet to the adjacent left ventricular wall with resultant mitral stenosis or regurgitation or both.

Sarcoidosis

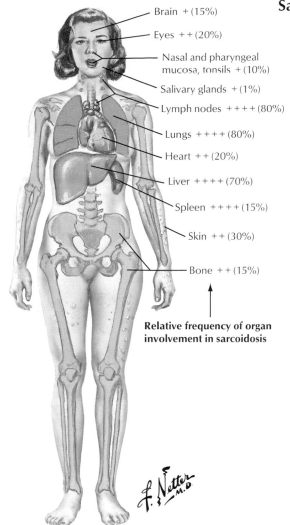

Brain + (15%)

Eyes + + (20%)

Nasal and pharyngeal mucosa, tonsils + (10%)

Salivary glands + (1%)

Lymph nodes + + + + (80%)

Lungs + + + + (80%)

Heart + + (20%)

Liver + + + + (70%)

Spleen + + + + (15%)

Skin + + (30%)

Bone + + (15%)

Relative frequency of organ involvement in sarcoidosis

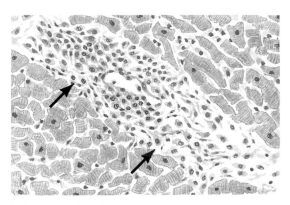

Perivascular infiltration.
Chiefly of histiocytes in cardiac interstitium (arrows)

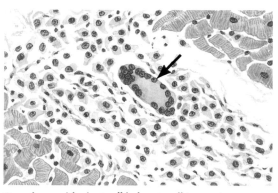

Granuloma with giant cell in heart wall (arrows)

Scleroderma

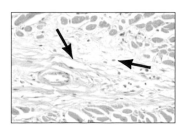

Extensive fibrosis (arrows) between and around cardiac muscle fibers and in arterial wall with only moderate lymphocytic and histiocytic infiltration

---

FIGURE 2-32   MYOCARDITIS IN SARCOIDOSIS AND SCLERODERMA

Progressive systemic **sclerosis** (**scleroderma**) can produce interstitial myocarditis and progressive myocardial fibrosis. **Sarcoidosis** can produce extensive replacement of the myocardium by multiple granulomas with multinucleated giant cells derived from macrophages and associated fibrosis. The process may involve the cardiac conduction system as well as the working myocardium.

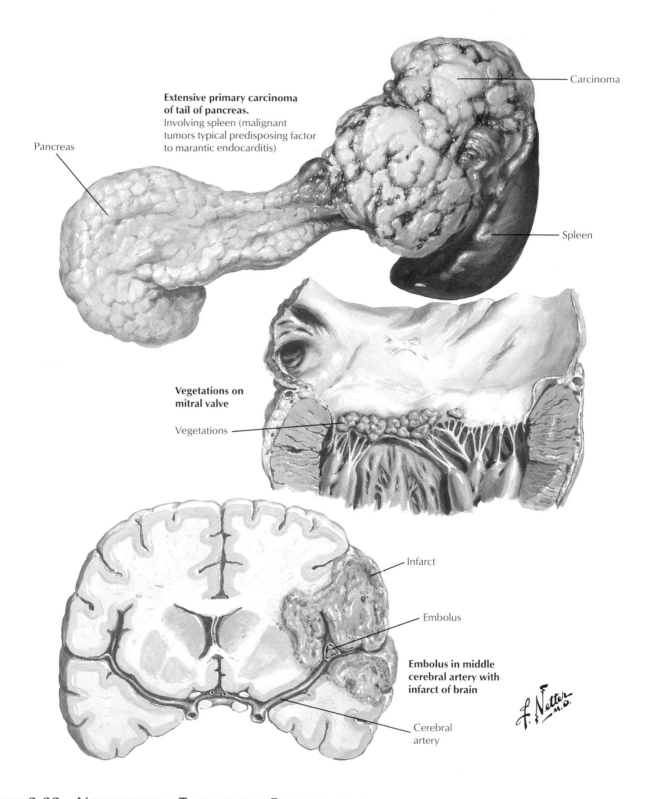

Extensive primary carcinoma of tail of pancreas. Involving spleen (malignant tumors typical predisposing factor to marantic endocarditis)

Pancreas

Carcinoma

Spleen

Vegetations on mitral valve

Vegetations

Infarct

Embolus

Embolus in middle cerebral artery with infarct of brain

Cerebral artery

FIGURE 2-33   NONBACTERIAL THROMBOTIC ENDOCARDITIS

Nonbacterial thrombotic endocarditis (NBTE) consists of sterile thrombi that form as vegetations on the superior surfaces of the leaflets of the aortic, mitral, tricuspid, and pulmonic valves as a result of mild inflammation and associated surface endothelial damage. The lesions are frequently associated with disseminated intravascular coagulation. Predisposing illnesses are those that initiate a systemic reaction, including serious infections, shock of various causes, and extensive burns. The valvular lesions also develop with chronic wasting states, particularly in association with malignant tumors, leading to the pseudonym *marantic endocarditis*. The valvular lesions can be clinically silent or can give rise to serious symptoms due to embolization of the vegetations. After acute illness, the valvular lesions form fibrous tags along the line of closure of the valvular leaflets (Lambl excrescences).

Common Portals of Bacterial Entry in Bacterial Endocarditis

Dental infections

Genitourinary infections

Cutaneous infections

Pulmonary infections

Bloodstream

Mild residual changes of rheumatic mitral valve disease

Bicuspid aortic valve (congenital or acquired)

Tetralogy of Fallot

Small ventricular septal defect (probe): "jet lesion" opposite

Coarctation of aorta and/or patent ductus (arrow)

Common Predisposing Lesions

FIGURE 2-34 INFECTIVE ENDOCARDITIS: PORTALS OF ENTRY AND PREDISPOSING FACTORS

Infective (bacterial) endocarditis results from direct infection of the valvular or mural endocardium by bacteria or other microorganisms, including fungi and rickettsia. The bacteria or other microorganisms enter the bloodstream from the site of a local infection of the skin, the lungs, the genitourinary system, or the oral cavity. Sometimes there is no obvious site of infection. Some medical or dental procedures may lead to the seeding of the bloodstream with microorganisms. Whether IE follows an acute hectic course or a subtle subacute course depends on whether the virulence of the microorganism is high (*Staphylococcus aureus*, gram-negative bacteria, fungi, and others) or low (*Streptococcus viridans* and others), the presence or absence of a preexisting valvular or congenital defect, and the presence or absence of systemic conditions in the host (chronic alcoholism, intravenous drug abuse, immunosuppression).

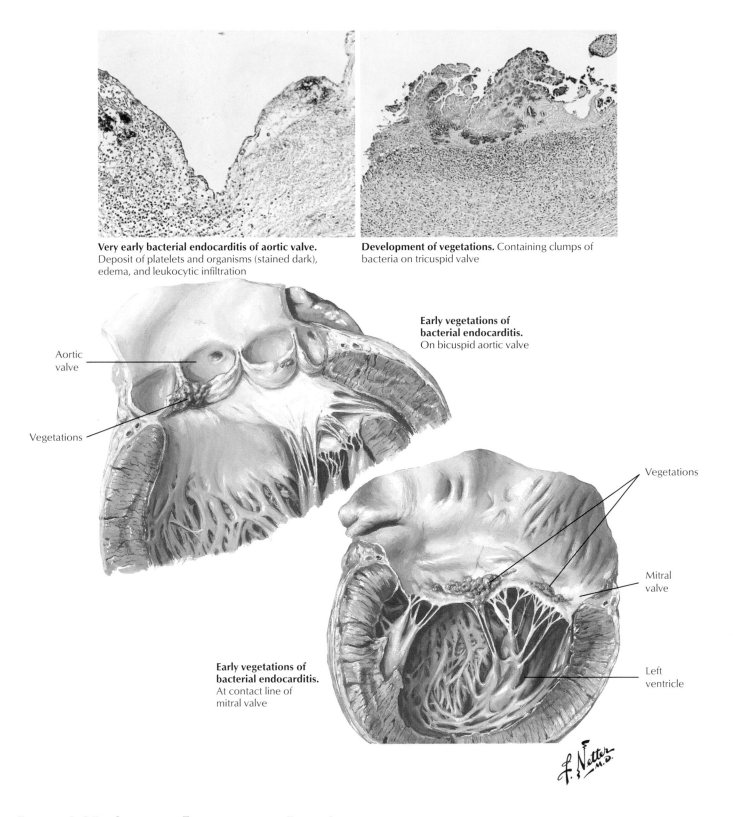

Very early bacterial endocarditis of aortic valve. Deposit of platelets and organisms (stained dark), edema, and leukocytic infiltration

Development of vegetations. Containing clumps of bacteria on tricuspid valve

Early vegetations of bacterial endocarditis. On bicuspid aortic valve

Aortic valve

Vegetations

Early vegetations of bacterial endocarditis. At contact line of mitral valve

Vegetations

Mitral valve

Left ventricle

f. Netter M.D.

FIGURE 2-35   INFECTIVE ENDOCARDITIS: EARLY LESIONS

Infective endocarditis generally involves the cardiac valves, unless a congenital cardiac defect, which predisposes to **mural endocarditis**, is present at the site of a jet lesion. As part of a generalized inflammatory reaction to a bacteremia (or fungemia etc), small thrombi form over foci of endothelial damage on the endocardium, producing lesions similar to those of **marantic**

endocarditis. These thrombi, which are sterile initially, become seeded with microorganisms rapidly, and the influx of neutrophils incites an accelerated inflammatory reaction. The surface thrombi grow to become vegetations. The toxic products of the bacteria and neutrophils produce necrosis of the valvular leaflets, which stimulates further suppurative inflammation.

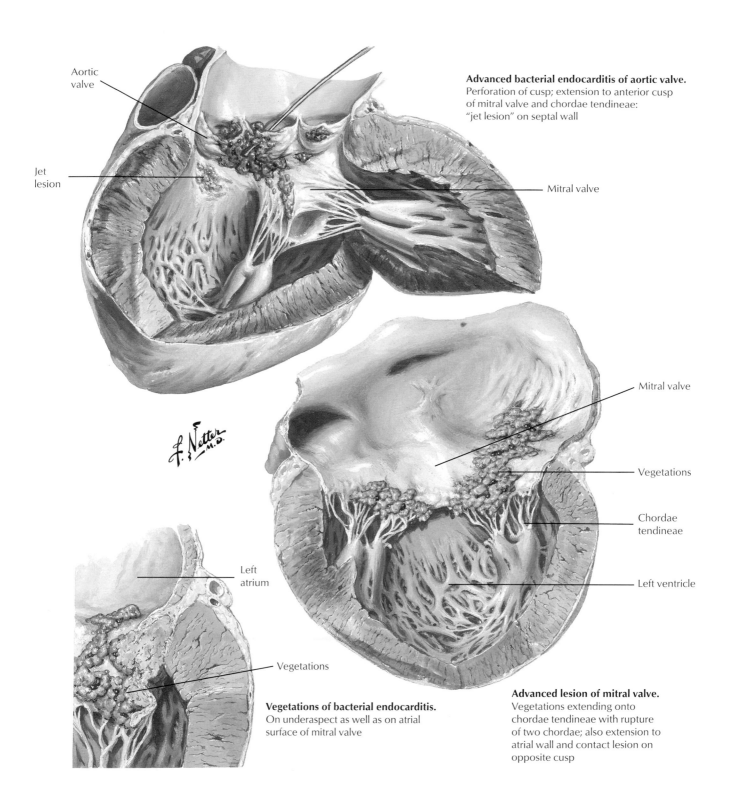

Advanced bacterial endocarditis of aortic valve. Perforation of cusp; extension to anterior cusp of mitral valve and chordae tendineae: "jet lesion" on septal wall

Aortic valve

Jet lesion

Mitral valve

Mitral valve

Vegetations

Chordae tendineae

Left ventricle

Left atrium

Vegetations

Vegetations of bacterial endocarditis. On underaspect as well as on atrial surface of mitral valve

Advanced lesion of mitral valve. Vegetations extending onto chordae tendineae with rupture of two chordae; also extension to atrial wall and contact lesion on opposite cusp

FIGURE 2-36   INFECTIVE ENDOCARDITIS: ADVANCED LESIONS

Progression of the inflammation can lead to the perforation of a valve leaflet or it can spread onto the chordae tendineae, leading to chordal rupture. The inflammation may also invade the valvular annulus, producing a valvular ring abscess. Generally, there is permanent damage to one or more of the cardiac valves, which leads to progressive valvular incompetence and cardiac failure. A major goal of clinical management is to make the diagnosis and institute high-dose intravenous antibiotic therapy to sterilize the vegetations and prevent the spread of the infection beyond the valve leaflets.

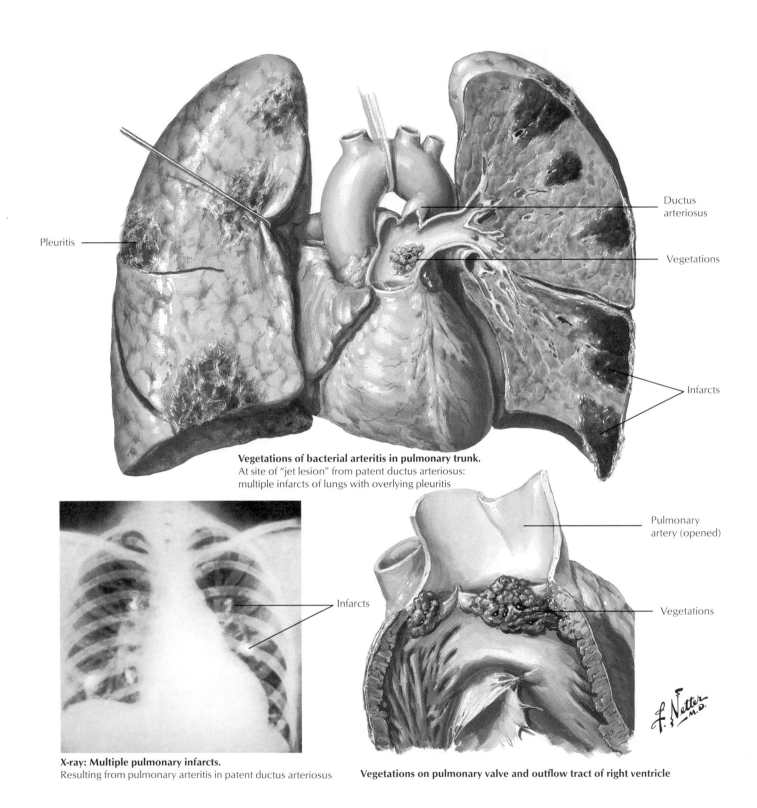

Pleuritis

Ductus arteriosus

Vegetations

Infarcts

Vegetations of bacterial arteritis in pulmonary trunk.
At site of "jet lesion" from patent ductus arteriosus:
multiple infarcts of lungs with overlying pleuritis

Infarcts

Pulmonary artery (opened)

Vegetations

X-ray: Multiple pulmonary infarcts.
Resulting from pulmonary arteritis in patent ductus arteriosus

Vegetations on pulmonary valve and outflow tract of right ventricle

FIGURE 2-37   INFECTIVE ENDOCARDITIS: RIGHT-SIDED INVOLVEMENT

Infection of the right-sided mural endocardium can occur at the site of a "**jet lesion**" produced by a **ventricular septal defect** with left-to-right shunting. Infection of the right-sided cardiac valves is also a complication of intravenous drug abuse with contaminated needles and foreign material. The patient may present with severe pneumonia due to seeding of the lungs with infected vegetations.

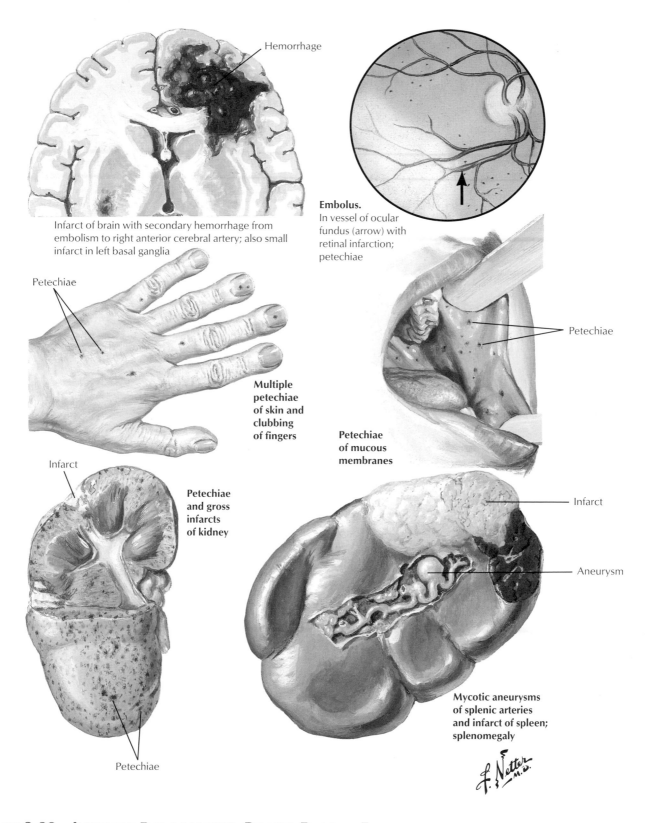

Infarct of brain with secondary hemorrhage from embolism to right anterior cerebral artery; also small infarct in left basal ganglia

Hemorrhage

Embolus. In vessel of ocular fundus (arrow) with retinal infarction; petechiae

Petechiae

Petechiae

Multiple petechiae of skin and clubbing of fingers

Petechiae of mucous membranes

Infarct

Petechiae and gross infarcts of kidney

Infarct

Aneurysm

Mycotic aneurysms of splenic arteries and infarct of spleen; splenomegaly

Petechiae

FIGURE 2-38   INFECTIVE ENDOCARDITIS: REMOTE EMBOLIC EFFECTS

Embolization of infected vegetations is a serious complication of IE. Small thromboemboli lead to **petechial hemorrhages** in the skin and internal organs. Larger infected thomboemboli, which result from inflammatory damage to the vessel wall, produce mycotic (mushroomlike) aneurysms. Intraluminal obstruction produces infarcts of the tissue supplied by an end artery. With highly virulent organisms, the affected tissue develops an abscess (infected infarct). Infected emboli to one or more coronary arteries can lead to myocardial infarction or to the formation of myocardial abscesses.

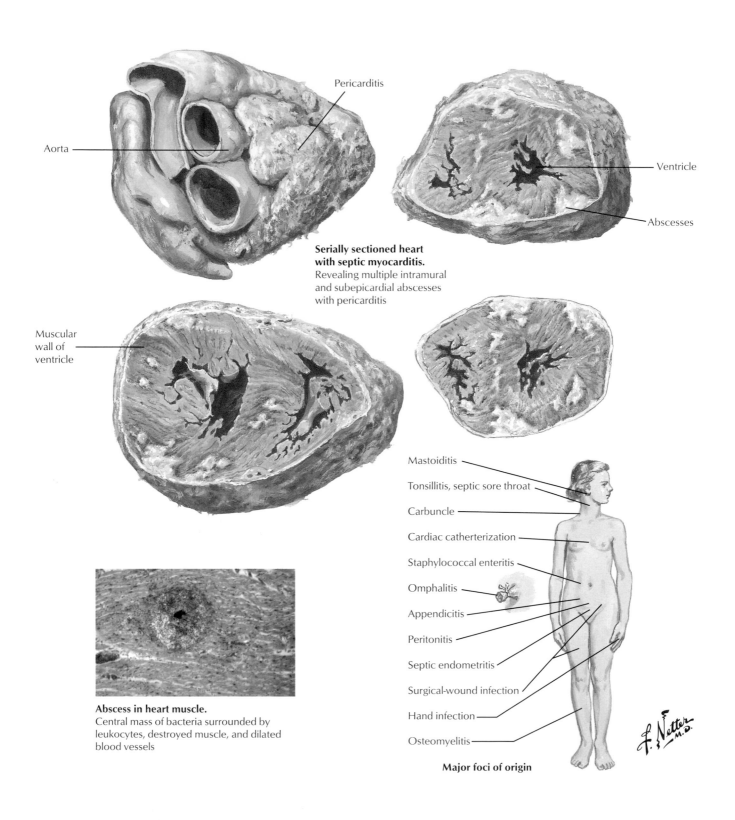

Aorta

Pericarditis

Ventricle

Abscesses

Serially sectioned heart with septic myocarditis.
Revealing multiple intramural and subepicardial abscesses with pericarditis

Muscular wall of ventricle

Abscess in heart muscle.
Central mass of bacteria surrounded by leukocytes, destroyed muscle, and dilated blood vessels

Mastoiditis

Tonsillitis, septic sore throat

Carbuncle

Cardiac catheterization

Staphylococcal enteritis

Omphalitis

Appendicitis

Peritonitis

Septic endometritis

Surgical-wound infection

Hand infection

Osteomyelitis

Major foci of origin

FIGURE 2-39 SEPTIC MYOCARDITIS

Some infections that originate in the skin or an internal organ can give rise to bacteremia or fungemia. Cardiac involvement, which includes **fibrinopurulent pericarditis** and **multifocal suppurative myocarditis** with abscess formation, can occur in the absence of valvular involvement, or the valves may show lesions of marantic endocarditis (with potential for the development of IE). Systemic fungal infections tend to occur in immunosuppressed patients, and the lesions show much diminished inflammatory cellular infiltrates. The heart may also be involved with various protozoal infections, such as **Chagas disease**.

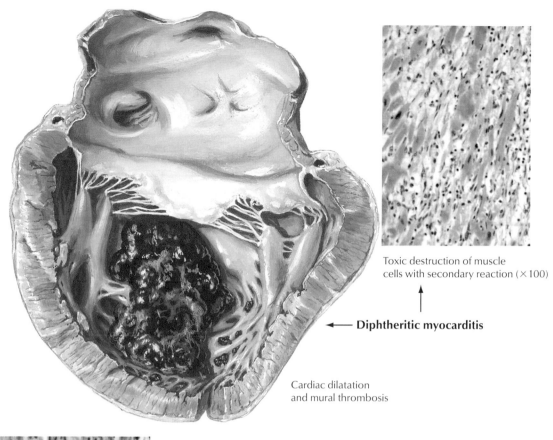

Toxic destruction of muscle
cells with secondary reaction (×100)

← **Diphtheritic myocarditis**

Cardiac dilatation
and mural thrombosis

Viral myocarditis

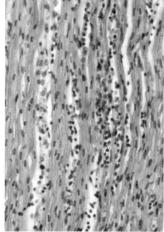

Coxsackie group B virus infection.
Diffuse and patchy interstitial edema;
cellular infiltration with only moderate
muscle-fiber destruction (×100)

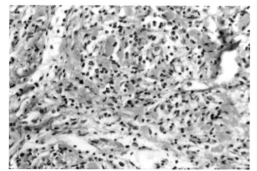

Diffuse cellular infiltration of bundle of His
and right and left bundle branches (×100)

FIGURE 2-40   DIPHTHERITIC AND VIRAL MYOCARDITIS

Microorganisms (viruses, rickettsiae, bacteria, fungi, and protozoa) or their toxins can produce a pattern of **myocarditis** or myopericarditis that is distinctive but not generally microorganism specific. Pericardial involvement consists of a fibrinous exudate often accompanied by a serous effusion. The type of inflammatory cellular infiltrate provides information about the underlying cause (neutrophils with bacterial infection, lympho-

cytes with viral infections, eosinophils with allergic reactions). Viral myocarditis is characterized by multifocal infiltration of the interstitium with lymphocytes and some macrophages (histiocytes) and by variable amounts of myocardial necrosis. The extent of inflammatory cellular infiltrate exceeds the amount of necrosis.

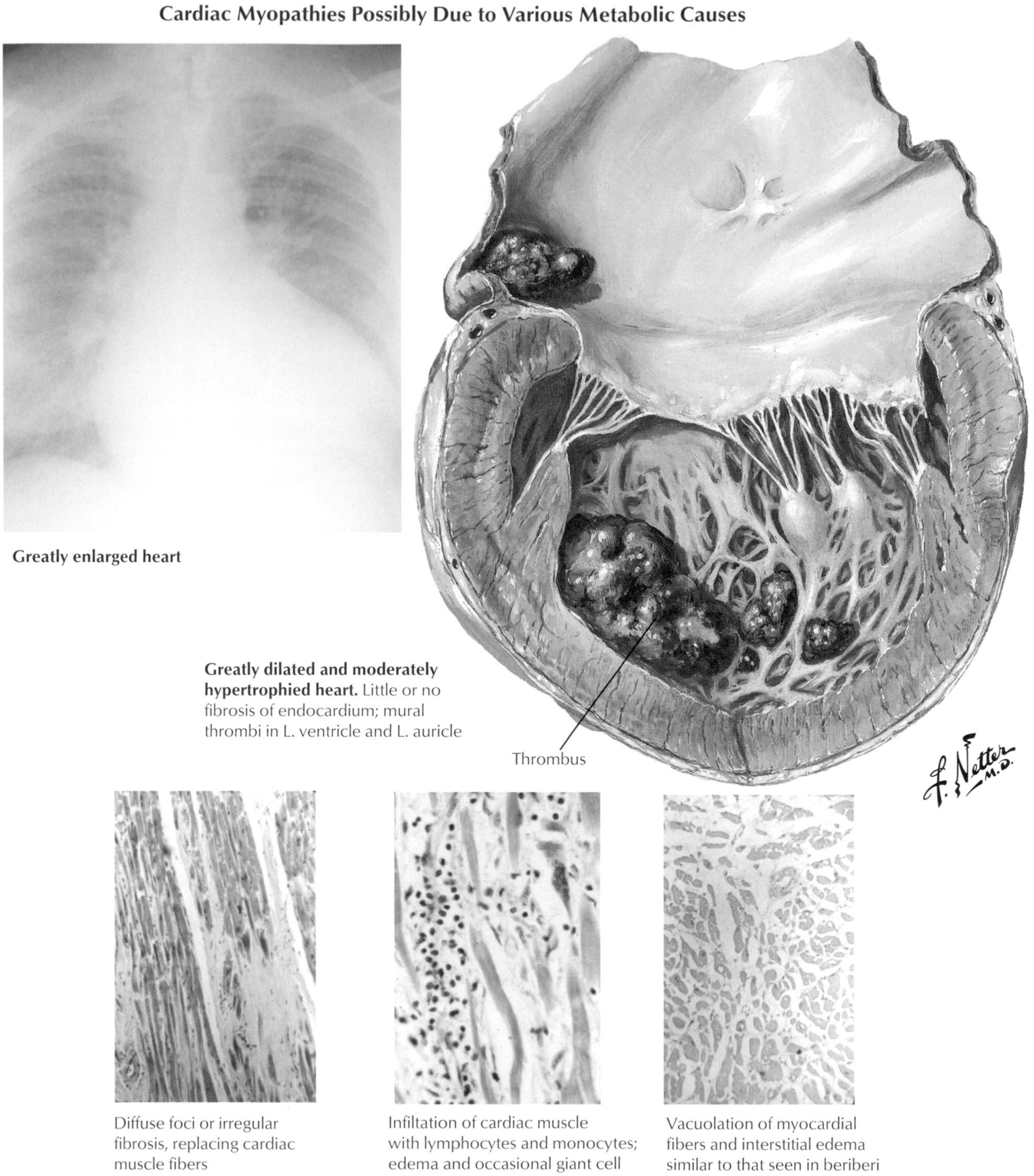

Cardiac Myopathies Possibly Due to Various Metabolic Causes

Greatly enlarged heart

Greatly dilated and moderately hypertrophied heart. Little or no fibrosis of endocardium; mural thrombi in L. ventricle and L. auricle

Thrombus

F. Netter M.D.

Diffuse foci or irregular fibrosis, replacing cardiac muscle fibers

Infiltation of cardiac muscle with lymphocytes and monocytes; edema and occasional giant cell

Vacuolation of myocardial fibers and interstitial edema similar to that seen in beriberi

FIGURE 2-41   DILATED (CONGESTIVE) CARDIOMYOPATHY

Primary (idiopathic) cardiomyopathies develop independently. Secondary cardiomyopathies occur as a component of cardiac disease (not originating in the myocardium) or systemic disease with cardiac involvement. **Dilated (congestive) cardiomyopathy**, the most common type, is characterized by the progressive development of cardiomegaly, CHF, and often arrhythmias. Pathologically, there is symmetrical hypertrophy and dilatation of the 4 cardiac chambers in the absence of significant coronary,

valvular, or congenital cardiac lesions or prominent arteriolone-phrosclerosis. Atrial or ventricular mural thrombi or both may form as a result of poor contractile function. The myocardium frequently shows nonspecific degeneration and fibrosis and, occasionally, some inflammatory infiltrates. The likely causes for this disease include previous myocarditis, chronic alcoholism, and genetic mutations often associated with familial disease.

Frontal Section of Heart With Hypertrophic Subaortic Stenosis

Superior vena cava

Right auricle

Left atrium

Aortic valve

Membranous septum
(interventricular part)

Mitral valve

Intraventricular septum

Anterior papillary muscle

f. Netter
M.D.

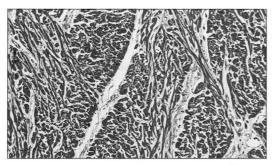

Disordered arrangement of myocardium
(low magnification)

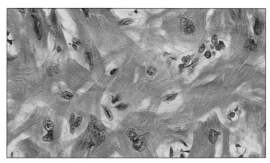

Abnormal shape and arrangement of cardiac myocytes
(higher magnification)

FIGURE 2-42   IDIOPATHIC HYPERTROPHIC SUBAORTIC STENOSIS: HYPERTROPHIC CARDIOMYOPATHY _____

Hypertrophic cardiomyopathy includes the classic IHSS, a condition that produces obstruction of the LVOT at the subvalvular, valvular, or supravalvular level. IHSS is characterized pathologically by asymmetrical ventricular septal hypertrophy (the interventricular septum is at least 1.3 times the thickness of the left ventricular free wall, and, initially, left and right ventricular chambers are small). Myocytes in the affected myocardium have a disorganized, "herringbone" arrangement rather than the normal parallel pattern within muscle bundles. The abnormal pattern of contraction leads to the paradoxical systolic anterior motion of the anterior mitral leaflet toward the bulging interventricular septum, thereby producing functional LVOT obstruction (functional aortic stenosis) and mitral regurgitation. The IHSS phenotype is caused by a variety of genetic mutations of actin, myosin, and other contractile proteins.

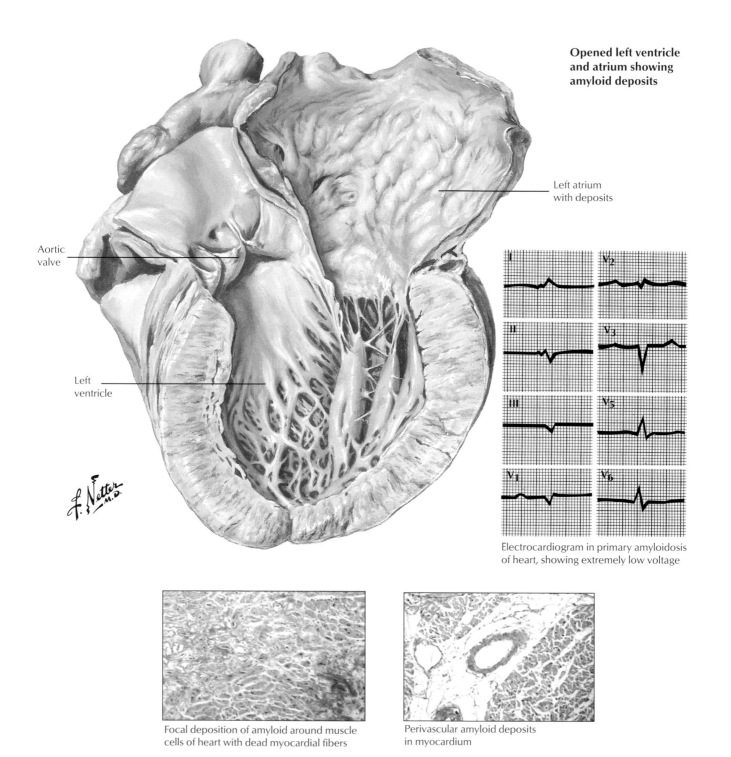

Opened left ventricle and atrium showing amyloid deposits

Left atrium with deposits

Aortic valve

Left ventricle

Electrocardiogram in primary amyloidosis of heart, showing extremely low voltage

Focal deposition of amyloid around muscle cells of heart with dead myocardial fibers

Perivascular amyloid deposits in myocardium

FIGURE 2-43 CARDIAC INVOLVEMENT IN AMYLOIDOSIS: RESTRICTIVE CARDIOMYOPATHY

Cardiac involvement occurs most frequently in **primary systemic amyloidosis** and **senile cardiac amyloidosis**. Myocardial degeneration results from deposits of infiltrative amyloid, which surround the myocytes and cause the classic pattern of low voltage on the ECG. Cardiac amyloidosis and severe fibrosis (collagen deposition) of any cause can produce a restrictive cardiomyopathy. Endomyocardial biopsy is used to distinguish the two conditions and make the diagnosis of amyloidosis. Patients with restrictive cardiomyopathy typically present with symptoms of CHF dominated by those of right-sided failure and a normal-sized heart, which mimic constructive pericarditis on radiographic examination.

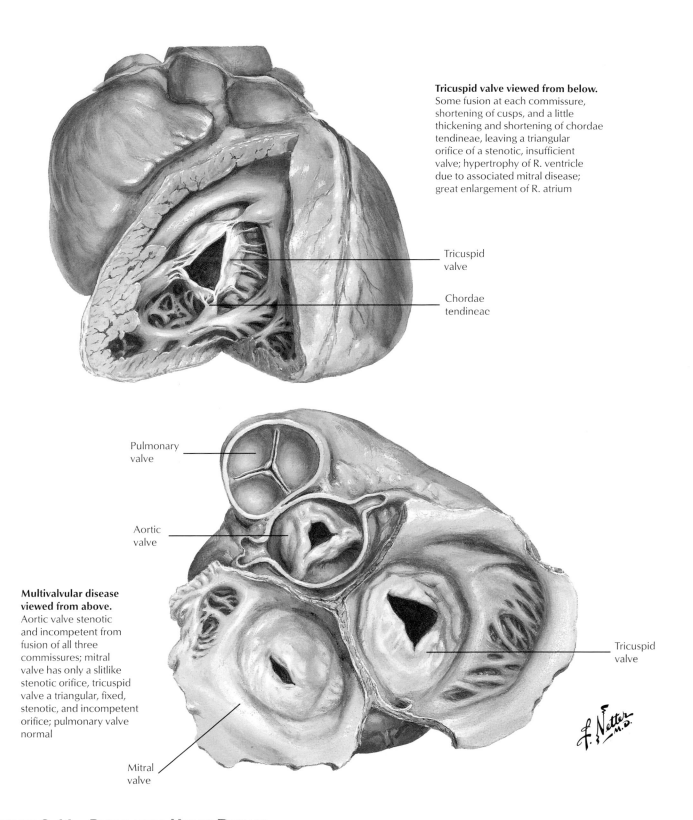

Tricuspid valve viewed from below. Some fusion at each commissure, shortening of cusps, and a little thickening and shortening of chordae tendineae, leaving a triangular orifice of a stenotic, insufficient valve; hypertrophy of R. ventricle due to associated mitral disease; great enlargement of R. atrium

Tricuspid valve

Chordae tendineae

Pulmonary valve

Aortic valve

Multivalvular disease viewed from above. Aortic valve stenotic and incompetent from fusion of all three commissures; mitral valve has only a slitlike stenotic orifice, tricuspid valve a triangular, fixed, stenotic, and incompetent orifice; pulmonary valve normal

Tricuspid valve

Mitral valve

FIGURE 2-44   RHEUMATIC HEART DISEASE

This illustration shows multivalvular disease involving the aortic, mitral, and tricuspid valves produced by chronic RHD. The diffuse fibrosis and variable commissural fusion result in dysfunction dominated by incompetence (insufficiency, regurgitation) or stenosis. **Chronic RHD** results in clinically significant pathology of the mitral valve alone in approximately 40% of cases, the mitral and aortic valves in another 40%, and the aortic valve alone in approximately 20%. Significant rheumatic lesions affect the tricuspid valve in a small percentage of cases, whereas the pulmonic valve is virtually never involved. RHD is only one of a number of diseases that produce significant valvular pathology, which results in incompetence, stenosis, or both of one or more of the valves.

Types of aortic valve stenosis

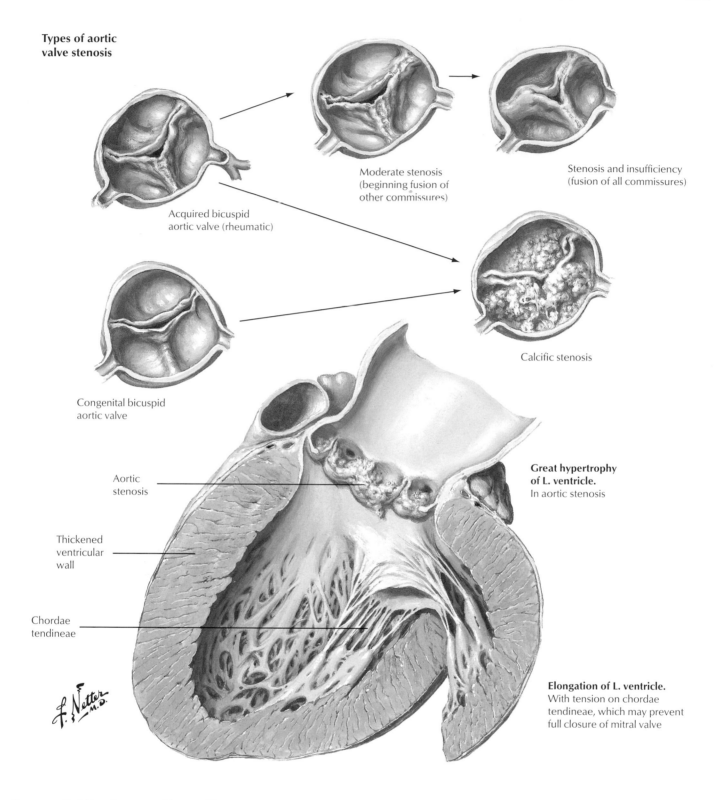

Acquired bicuspid aortic valve (rheumatic)

Moderate stenosis (beginning fusion of other commissures)

Stenosis and insufficiency (fusion of all commissures)

Congenital bicuspid aortic valve

Calcific stenosis

Aortic stenosis

Thickened ventricular wall

Chordae tendineae

Great hypertrophy of L. ventricle. In aortic stenosis

Elongation of L. ventricle. With tension on chordae tendineae, which may prevent full closure of mitral valve

FIGURE 2-45   AORTIC VALVE DISEASE

Valvular heart disease may result from congenital cardiac defects or from immunologic, inflammatory, infectious, or degenerative diseases of the heart. In the United States, nonrheumatic causes are responsible for most valvular heart disease necessitating surgical intervention. **Stenosis of a congenital bicuspid aortic valve** in a middle-aged individual and **stenosis due to senile sclerosis (Mönckeberg) of a tricuspid aortic valve** in an older individual are the conditions that lead most commonly to severe isolated aortic valve disease. RHD can produce **aortic stenosis**, which includes the formation of an acquired bicuspid valve due to fusion of one of the 3 commissures. Patients with valvular aortic stenosis experience left ventricular hypertrophy. They present with symptoms of fatigue and angina pectoris and exhibit a systolic ejection murmur along the right sternal border accompanied by diminished carotid pulsations.

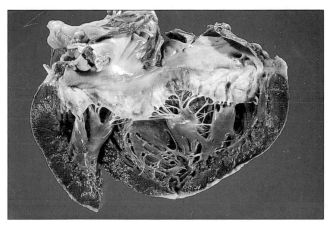

The mitral valve leaflets are thickened and elongated due to myxomatous degeneration

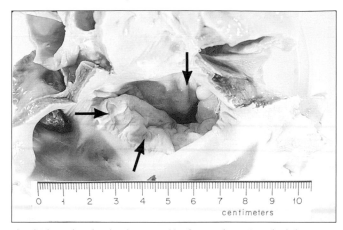

The thickened and redundant mitral leaflets prolapse into the left atrium

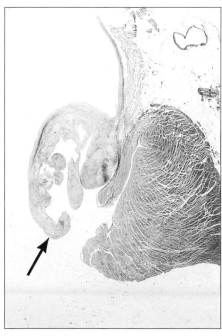

The mitral leaflet is thickened and elongated (low magnification)

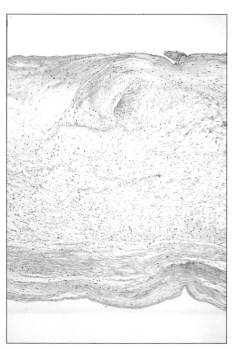

The thickened mitral leaflet is composed of loose myxomatous connective tissue and the normal dense fibrosa is lost (high magnification)

FIGURE 2-46 MITRAL VALVE PROLAPSE

Myxomatous degeneration of the mitral valve gives rise to a redundant valve composed of white, glistening **myxomatous tissue**. Histologically, the normal fibrosa is replaced with myxomatous tissue. The redundant valve prolapses into the left atrium with each systole, which gives rise to mid to late systolic clicks and a short systolic murmur heard at the cardiac apex. The prolapse is readily detected by echocardiography. Some degree of mitral valve prolapse occurs in approximately 2% of the population, with higher frequency in females than in males. The cause is obscure, but there is some evidence that autonomic dysfunction gives rise to an abnormal pattern of cardiac contraction and secondary degenerative change of the mitral valve. A similar lesion is seen with **Marfan syndrome**. Progression of the mitral degeneration can give rise to progressive mitral regurgitation. Rupture of a chordae tendineae, either spontaneously or due to infection, can give rise to acute severe mitral regurgitation.

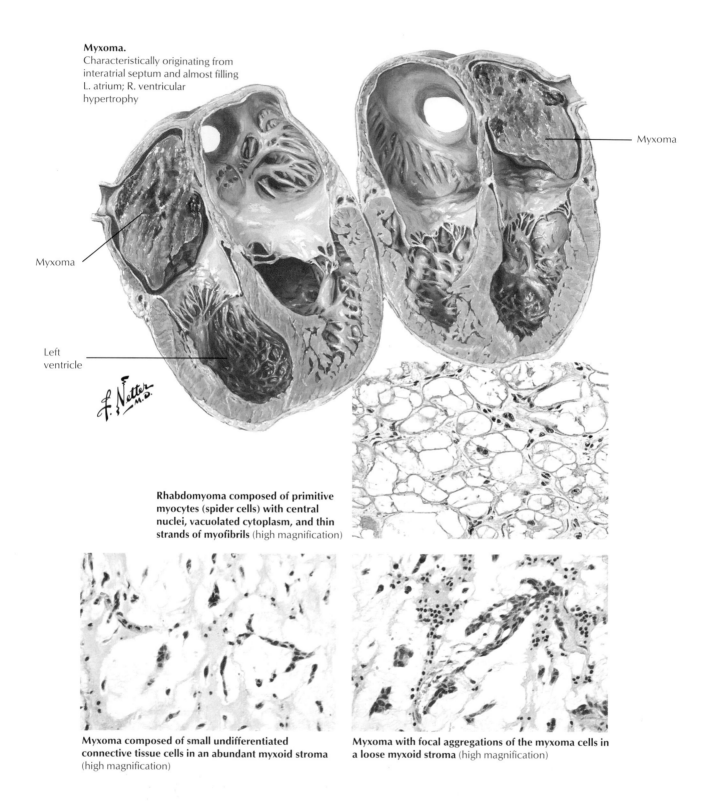

Myxoma.
Characteristically originating from interatrial septum and almost filling L. atrium; R. ventricular hypertrophy

Myxoma

Myxoma

Left ventricle

Rhabdomyoma composed of primitive myocytes (spider cells) with central nuclei, vacuolated cytoplasm, and thin strands of myofibrils (high magnification)

Myxoma composed of small undifferentiated connective tissue cells in an abundant myxoid stroma (high magnification)

Myxoma with focal aggregations of the myxoma cells in a loose myxoid stroma (high magnification)

FIGURE 2-47 PRIMARY HEART TUMORS

Primary tumors of the heart, most of which are benign, occur much less frequently than metastatic tumors of the heart but more often than the rare primary sarcomas of the heart. The most common primary tumor in adults is the **myxoma**, which consists of nondifferentiated small mesenchymal cells in an abundant myxoid stroma. It occurs most commonly in the left atrium and presents with symptoms mimicking mitral stenosis. In infants and children, the **rhabdomyoma** is most common. These tumors may be single or multiple and have a subendocardial, intramural, or subepicardial location. The lesions are composed of primitive myocytes (spider cells). The rhabdomyomas may occur as part of the tuberous sclerosis complex.

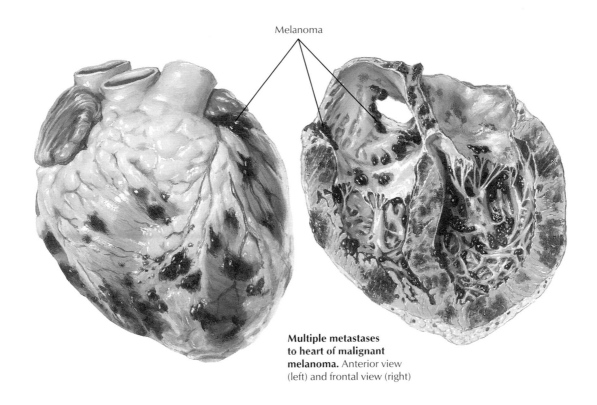

Melanoma

**Multiple metastases
to heart of malignant
melanoma.** Anterior view
(left) and frontal view (right)

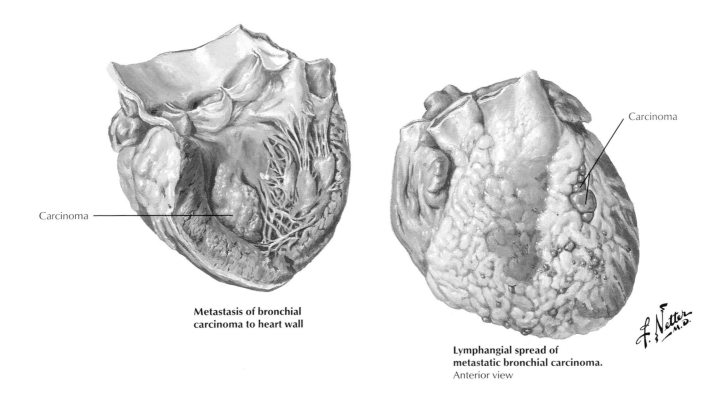

Carcinoma

Carcinoma

**Metastasis of bronchial
carcinoma to heart wall**

**Lymphangial spread of
metastatic bronchial carcinoma.**
Anterior view

FIGURE 2-48   METASTATIC HEART TUMORS

Metastatic cardiac tumors can arise from a number of different malignant neoplasms, including multiple myeloma, bronchogenic carcinoma, breast carcinoma, lymphomas, and leukemias.

Various patterns of metastases, including large masses and lymphangitic spread of tumor, are illustrated.

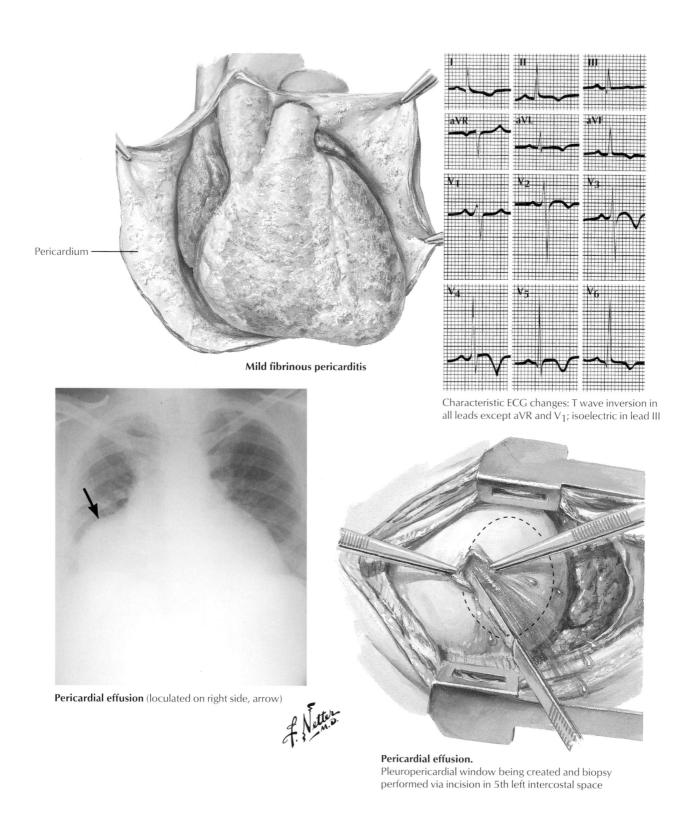

Mild fibrinous pericarditis

Characteristic ECG changes: T wave inversion in all leads except aVR and V_1; isoelectric in lead III

Pericardial effusion (loculated on right side, arrow)

Pericardial effusion.
Pleuropericardial window being created and biopsy performed via incision in 5th left intercostal space

FIGURE 2-49   DISEASES OF THE PERICARDIUM

Congestive heart failure produces pericardial effusion consisting of clear fluid with low protein content (a transudate). **Viral infections**, **renal failure (uremia)**, and **noninfectious immunologic diseases** result in fibrinous pericarditis that is often accompanied by pericardial effusion. **Bacterial infections** produce purulent pericarditis. **Tuberculosis** produces granulomatous pericarditis. Pericardial disease also can result from **metastatic tumors**. Fluid accumulation in the pericardium can result in impaired cardiac function depending on the rapidity and amount of fluid accumulation. Treatment may involve percutaneous pericardiocentesis or a surgically produced pericardial window.

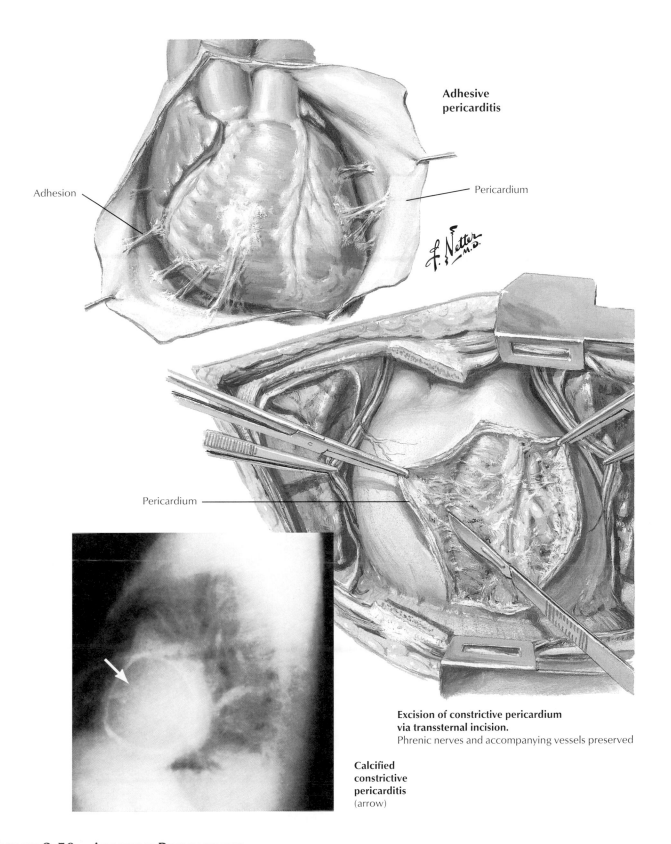

Adhesive pericarditis

Adhesion

Pericardium

Pericardium

Excision of constrictive pericardium via transsternal incision.
Phrenic nerves and accompanying vessels preserved

Calcified constrictive pericarditis
(arrow)

FIGURE 2-50 ADHESIVE PERICARDITIS

Healing of acute pericarditis, particularly with abundant fibrinous exudates or hemorrhage, gives rise to adhesive pericarditis. Adhesions may be severe and may be accompanied by calcification. Severe adhesive pericarditis can produce the clinical syndrome of constrictive pericarditis, which necessitates surgical relief. Previously, tuberculous pericarditis was the leading cause of constrictive pericarditis, but currently, most cases are idiopathic. In the age of hemodialysis, chronic renal disease is a relatively common cause of adhesive pericarditis.

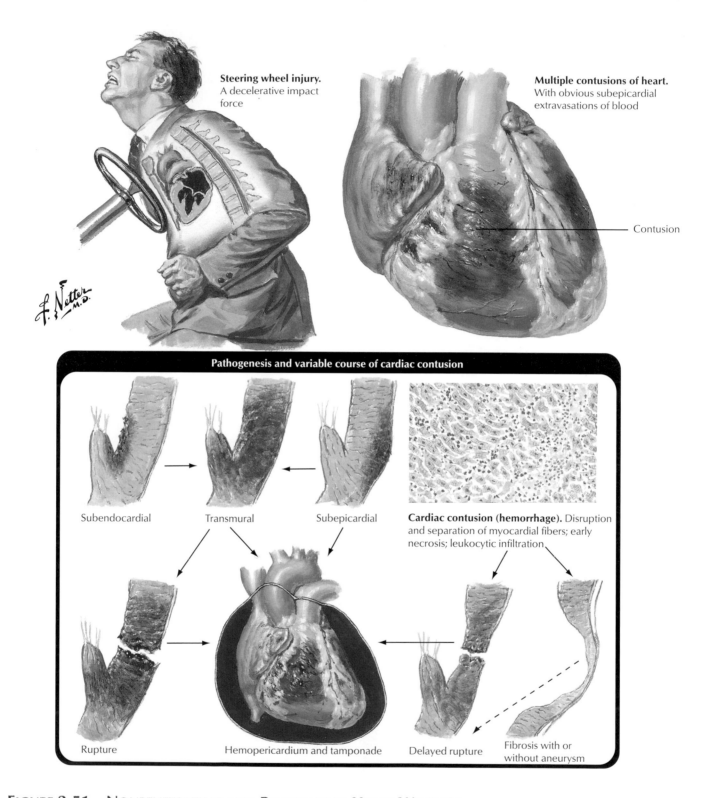

Steering wheel injury.
A decelerative impact force

Multiple contusions of heart.
With obvious subepicardial extravasations of blood

Contusion

Pathogenesis and variable course of cardiac contusion

Subendocardial

Transmural

Subepicardial

Cardiac contusion (hemorrhage). Disruption and separation of myocardial fibers; early necrosis; leukocytic infiltration

Rupture

Hemopericardium and tamponade

Delayed rupture

Fibrosis with or without aneurysm

FIGURE 2-51   NONPENETRATING AND PENETRATING HEART WOUNDS

Severe crush injury of the chest can result in traumatic damage to the heart muscle known as a **cardiac contusion**. The lesions show hemorrhagic necrosis of the myocardium. The lesion can be transmural and result in cardiac rupture and cardiac tamponade due to hemopericardium. The lesions can heal with aneurysm formation. Other traumatic lesions include rupture of the interventricular septum, rupture of a papillary muscle, or rupture of a valve cusp. All of these lesions can produce acute cardiac decompensation. Gunshot or stab wounds of the chest can produce lacerations or perforations of various parts of the heart. This leads to severe bleeding into the pericardium and early or delayed cardiac tamponade due to hemopericardium. This life-threatening condition necessitates rapid evacuation of the hemopericardium.

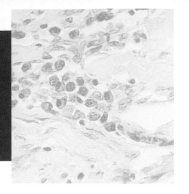

CHAPTER 3
RESPIRATORY SYSTEM

Five major disease categories are presented in this chapter: obstructive and restrictive disorders of gas exchange, vascular diseases of the lung, infectious and inflammatory diseases, and tumors of lungs and pleura.

OBSTRUCTIVE LUNG DISEASES

Chronic obstructive pulmonary disease (COPD) is characterized by a reduction of pulmonary air flow as determined by spirometric function tests with normal or increased total lung capacity (TLC) and forced vital capacity (FVC) in combination with decreased forced expiratory volume (FEV). COPD follows either increased resistance to airflow (e.g., by luminal narrowing of air ducts) or the loss of elastic recoil (by passive widening of air spaces). It can be caused by a number of different respiratory diseases, including chronic bronchitis, bronchiolitis and asthma, cystic fibrosis (CF), bronchiectasis, or α1-antitrypsin deficiency. COPD may lead to progressive and destructive emphysema and, eventually, cor pulmonale, characterized by reduced intrapulmonary blood flow, pulmonary hypertension, and right heart insufficiency.

RESTRICTIVE LUNG DISEASES

In restrictive lung diseases (RLDs), the lungs have a limited potential to expand, and therefore, compliance is reduced. Although extrapulmonary disorders such as chest abnormalities, intraabdominal masses, and neuromuscular diseases also can limit lung expansion, the term *RLD* is generally reserved for intrapulmonary parenchymatous diseases. In these cases, spirometric tests show a reduced FVC with normal or proportionately reduced FEV. RLD occurs in acute and chronic forms. Classic examples of acute RLD are the adult respiratory distress syndrome (ARDS) and acute hypersensitivity pneumonitis. Chronic forms include such pathogenetically different entities as idiopathic pulmonary fibroses (fibrosing alveolitis), chronic interstitial pneumonitis in collagen-vascular diseases, pneumoconioses, and sarcoidosis. Only patients in early stages of acute RLD may recover completely; later stages and especially the chronic forms of RLD remit to scarring or progress to extensive interstitial pulmonary fibrosis with honeycombing, pulmonary hypertension, and development of cor pulmonale. Recurrent superimposed infections further complicate the course of RLD.

VASCULAR LUNG DISEASES

Most common vascular lung diseases fall into 2 major categories: clotting disorders with secondary vascular occlusion and primary structural diseases of blood vessels. Clotting disorders may cause occlusion of pulmonary vessels by embolization or by in situ thrombosis (e.g., after contraceptive medication with high estrogen content or after clotting disorders in pancreatic carcinoma). In situ pulmonary thrombosis also may be a consequence of primary structural diseases of lung vasculature.

PULMONARY INFECTIOUS DISEASES

Infections of the lung present with different pathologic patterns and are classified as bacterial pneumonias, atypical and viral pneumonias, or parasitic (e.g., *Pneumocystis carinii* pneumonia) or fungal pneumonitis. Most bacterial and viral pneumonias initially are acute inflammatory diseases and, with adequate treatment, may resolve completely. However, pneumonias caused by intracellular bacteria (e.g., *Mycobacterium tuberculosis*), parasites, or fungi run a protracted and chronic course entailing an immune response and incomplete resolution. They heal with focal or diffuse scarring and the risk of chronic restrictive pulmonary disease.

TUMORS IN THE LUNGS AND THE PLEURA

As in other organs, tumors of the lung are identified as *carcinomas* (e.g., of bronchial epithelium, bronchial glands, or alveolar lining cells) or as *sarcomas*. They are classified according to their cell of origin (squamous cell carcinoma [SCC], adenocarcinoma [AC], small-cell carcinoma [oat cell carcinoma]) and to their degree of differentiation. Their local extension and metastatic spread determine their prognosis. Consequently, both tumor classification and documentation of its spread (grading and staging) are important responsibilities of diagnostic pathology and form the basis for determining therapeutic intervention. In addition, the lungs are frequent sites of metastases from other locations (e.g., breast, pancreas, testes, bone, malignant melanoma of the skin, and others), which must be distinguished from primary lung tumors.

Pulmonary Function in Obstructive Disease

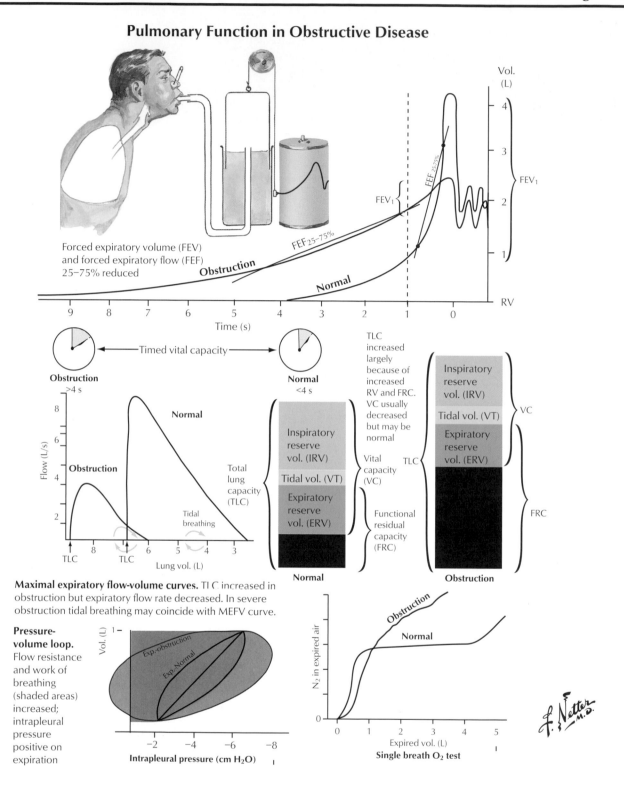

Forced expiratory volume (FEV) and forced expiratory flow (FEF) 25–75% reduced

Maximal expiratory flow-volume curves. TLC increased in obstruction but expiratory flow rate decreased. In severe obstruction tidal breathing may coincide with MEFV curve.

Pressure-volume loop. Flow resistance and work of breathing (shaded areas) increased; intrapleural pressure positive on expiration

TLC increased largely because of increased RV and FRC. VC usually decreased but may be normal

Single breath O_2 test

FIGURE 3-1   CHRONIC OBSTRUCTIVE PULMONARY DISEASE

Chronic obstructive pulmonary disease (COPD) is characterized by reduced pulmonary airflow with normal or increased TLC and FVC combined with decreased FEV as determined by spirometric function tests. COPD follows increased resistance to airflow (by luminal narrowing of air ducts) or loss of elastic recoil (and by passive widening of air spaces). COPD is caused by a number of respiratory diseases, including chronic bronchitis, bronchiolitis and asthma, CF, bronchiectasis, and α1-antitrypsin deficiency. COPD results in a progressive and destructive **emphysema** and reduced intrapulmonary blood flow, pulmonary hypertension, and right heart insufficiency (cor pulmonale).

Bronchiectasis

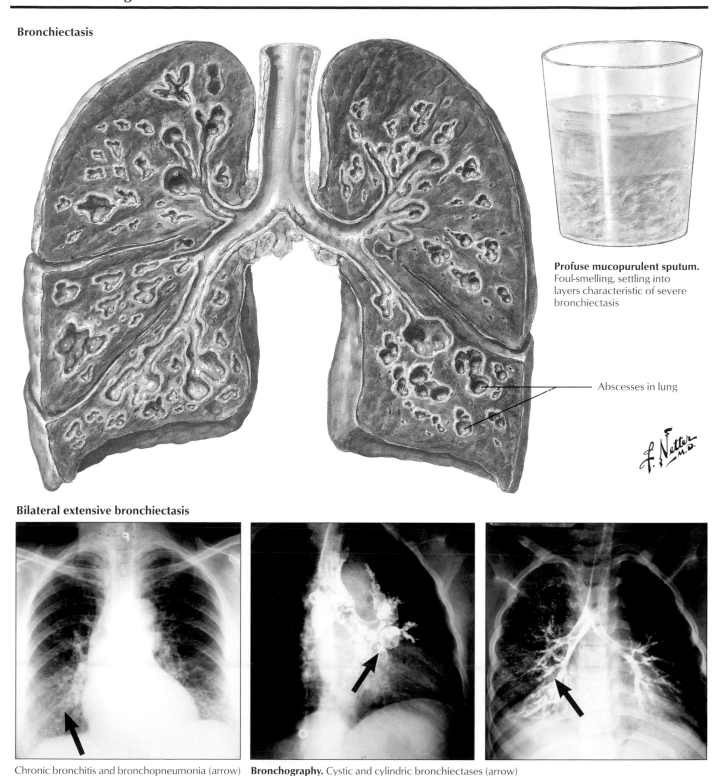

Profuse mucopurulent sputum.
Foul-smelling, settling into
layers characteristic of severe
bronchiectasis

Abscesses in lung

Bilateral extensive bronchiectasis

Chronic bronchitis and bronchopneumonia (arrow)   **Bronchography.** Cystic and cylindric bronchiectases (arrow)

FIGURE 3-2   CHRONIC BRONCHITIS

Chronic bronchitis with persistent and productive cough afflicts up to 25% of persons older than 40 years in smog-ridden cities and up to 15% in smokers. It is accompanied by repeated nonspecific infections, mucosal atrophy with mucoid metaplasia (1 goblet cell per 7 columnar cells changes to 1 goblet cell per 1

columnar cell), reduced dust clearance, and inflammatory destruction of elastic lamellae in the bronchial wall with reactive muscular hypertrophy. Finally, there is degeneration and cylindric **bronchiectases**, transient fibrotic narrowing of bronchioles (small airway disease), and emphysema.

Pathogenesis of Cystic Fibrosis

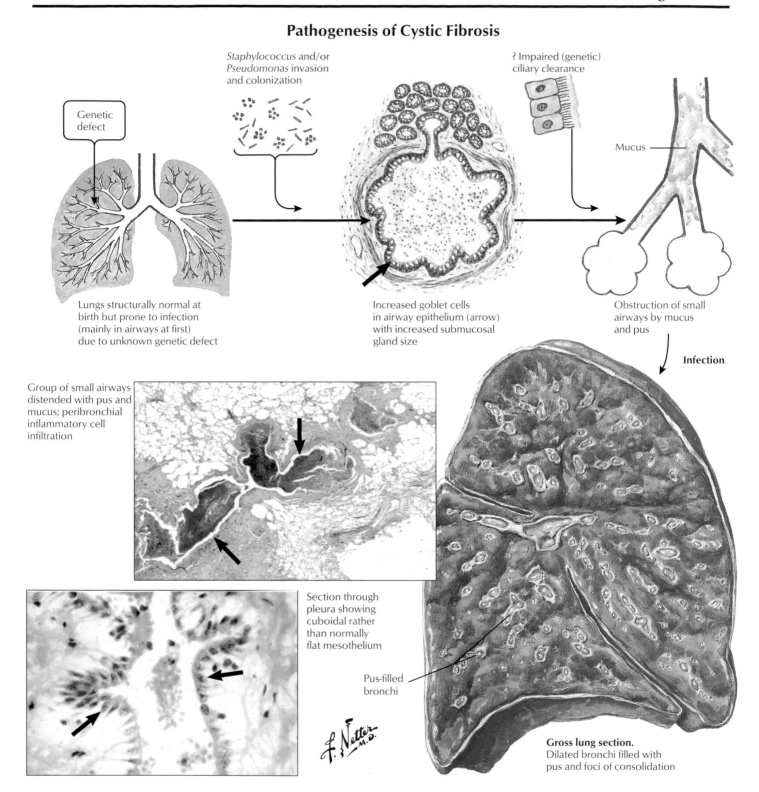

Staphylococcus and/or *Pseudomonas* invasion and colonization

? Impaired (genetic) ciliary clearance

Genetic defect

Mucus

Lungs structurally normal at birth but prone to infection (mainly in airways at first) due to unknown genetic defect

Increased goblet cells in airway epithelium (arrow) with increased submucosal gland size

Obstruction of small airways by mucus and pus

Infection

Group of small airways distended with pus and mucus; peribronchial inflammatory cell infiltration

Section through pleura showing cuboidal rather than normally flat mesothelium

Pus-filled bronchi

f. Netter M.D.

Gross lung section. Dilated bronchi filled with pus and foci of consolidation

FIGURE 3-3   CYSTIC FIBROSIS

In **cystic fibrosis** (CF) (**mucoviscidosis**), a primary defect in chloride ion transport across epithelia results in the secretion of abnormally viscid mucus in all secretory glands, including the bronchial glands. Mucus inspissation blocks the airways, causing **bronchiectasis** and **emphysema**. Chronic abscess formation, which results from recurrent superinfections (*Staphylococcus* and *Pseudomonas* species) can complicate the course of CF. Although CF affects other organs, COPD is the cause of death in 80% to 90% of cases.

Roentgenograms in Chronic Obstructive Pulmonary Disease

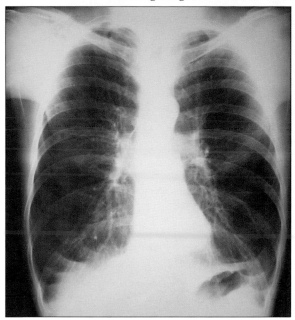

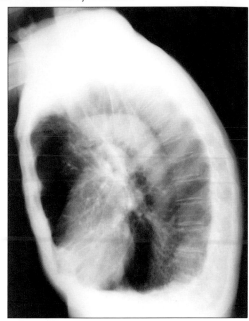

Hyperinflation of lungs; depression of diaphragm with its insertion to ribs evident; peripheral attenuation of pulmonary vessels; heart shadow small relative to lungs. Corresponds to "pink puffer."

Lateral projection of same case as in **left**. Diaphragm not only depressed but actually concave downward. Retrosternal clear space greatly enlarged.

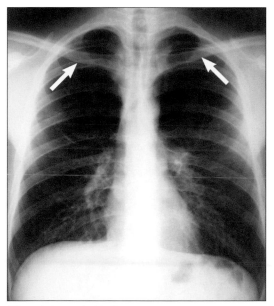

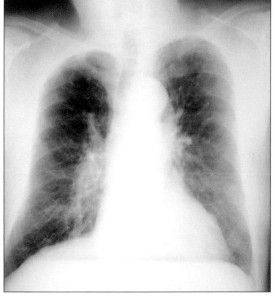

Bilateral giant apical bullae

No hyperinflation; increased bronchovascular markings, especially at bases; diaphragm well rounded. Patient had chronic CO_2 retention, cor pulmonale, and multiple previous episodes of respiratory failure. Corresponds to "blue bloater."

FIGURE 3-4   EMPHYSEMA

In **emphysema**, overinflation of the alveoli located distal to the terminal bronchioles is caused by the destruction of alveolar walls. The pathogenesis is thought to be an imbalance between increased (inflammatory) elastolysis and decreased antiprotease activity (e.g., in α1-antitrypsin deficiency). Emphysema is classified by anatomical nature and location in the lobule: **centrilobular (centriacinar) emphysema** affects the upper part of lungs after inhalation of toxic materials; **panlobular (panacinar) emphysema** is commonly found in the lower part of lungs, such as in α1-antitrypsin deficiency; **paraseptal (distal acinar) emphysema** frequently occurs subpleurally, adjacent to fibrosis; **bullous emphysema** results from enhanced focal destruction of air space walls with confluence of multiple air spaces. **Interstitial emphysema** expands in interstitial septae after acute overinflation of the lungs with rupture and perforation of air spaces into fibrous septae. It may spread to the mediastinum and subcutaneous tissues of the neck.

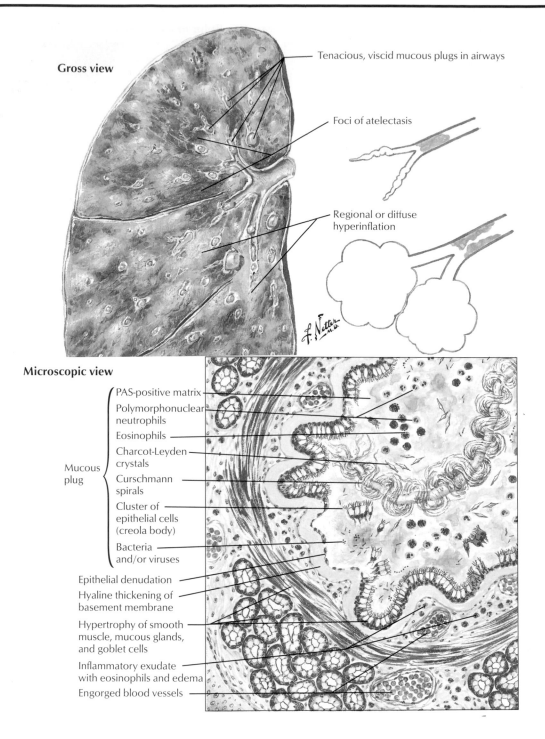

Gross view

Tenacious, viscid mucous plugs in airways

Foci of atelectasis

Regional or diffuse hyperinflation

Microscopic view

Mucous plug {
- PAS-positive matrix
- Polymorphonuclear neutrophils
- Eosinophils
- Charcot-Leyden crystals
- Curschmann spirals
- Cluster of epithelial cells (creola body)
- Bacteria and/or viruses

Epithelial denudation

Hyaline thickening of basement membrane

Hypertrophy of smooth muscle, mucous glands, and goblet cells

Inflammatory exudate with eosinophils and edema

Engorged blood vessels

FIGURE 3-5 ASTHMA

Asthma bronchiale is caused by an enhanced bronchoconstrictor response to type I (allergic) immune reaction to extrinsic or intrinsic stimuli. The etiology and pathogenesis is multifactorial and includes genetic conditions, psychologic stress, and allergic and infectious stimuli. Severe coughing with expectoration of a characteristic mucoid sputum with masses of eosinophils and their breakdown products (**Charcot-Leyden crystals**), gyrate mucus clumps (**Curschmann spirals**), and clusters of epithelial cells (**Creola bodies**) follows the acute phase of the attack. Histologically, **asthmatic bronchitis** appears as a mucoid metaplasia of bronchial epithelium, eosinophilic infiltration, hyaline thickening of the basement membrane, and muscular and glandular hypertrophy. Bronchial lumina are often occluded by mucous plugs. **Status asthmaticus** is a severe persistent broncho-constriction that does not respond to treatment. It leads to severe hypoxia, acidosis, and hypercapnia and may be fatal.

Hyaline membrane disease

Type I pneumocyte (alveolar cell)

Type II pneumocyte (alveolar cell)

Alveolus (air space)

Normal production of surfactant (output greatly increases in fetus near term)

Capillary

Lamellar bodies

P

$\text{Glucose} \xrightarrow{\text{TPNH}} \text{Gycerophosphate}$

De novo synthesis

$\text{Palmitic acid} \rightarrow \text{Dipalmitoyl lecithin}$

Glucose

Palmitic and other fatty acids (plus albumin)

Other lipids

Apoprotein

Ribosomes

Glucocorticoids promote maturation of lung and production of surfactant

Surface-active layer of phospholipid (lecithin) protein complex (surfactant). Deficiency leads to hyaline membrane disease (I IMD).

TABLE 3-1 CONDITIONS THAT CAN CAUSE ARDS/DAD*

Conditions	Causes
Infectious diseases	Septicemia with DAD and DIC (especially gram negative), diffuse pneumonitis by virus, mycoplasma, pneumocystis, tuberculosis (certain forms, e.g., typhobacillosis Landouzy)
Chemical injury and inhalants	Oxygen, irritant gases and inhaled chemicals, barbiturate overdose, salicylic acid, paraquat, heroin or methadone overdose, cytotoxic drugs, uremic pneumonitis, gastric aspiration
Physical injury	Trauma to lungs (contusion), head injury, fat embolism of various causes, air embolism, burns, ionizing radiation
Other	Shock of any cause, acute pancreatitis, near drowning aspiration

*ARDS indicates adult respiratory distress syndrome; DAD, diffuse alveolar damage; DIC, disseminated intravascular coagulation.

Pathology of hyaline membrane disease

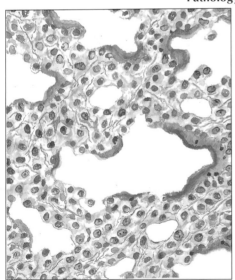

Atelectasis. With eosinophilic hyaline membrane partially lining most peripheral air space

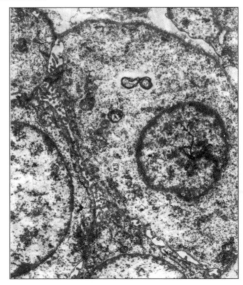

Electron photomicrograph. Type II pneumocyte practically devoid of lamellar bodies

FIGURE 3-6   ADULT RESPIRATORY DISTRESS SYNDROME

Adult respiratory distress syndrome is defined by reduced arterial oxygenation, decreased lung compliance, and diffuse noncardiogenic pulmonary infiltrates. The morphology is represented by **diffuse alveolar damage (DAD)**. Alveolar and interstitial edema develops subsequent to diffuse alveolar epithelial and vascular endothelial injury with capillary congestion. **Alveolar cell necrosis** may occur with focal hemorrhage and capillary microthrombosis. The formation of hyaline membranes composed of plasma proteins, cellular debris, and fibrin precipitates is characteristic in **ARDS**. The decrease in functioning surfactant factor leads to a loss of type I alveolar cells and a reactive proliferation of type II alveolar cells. Progressive fibroblast proliferation leads to fibrosis. The etiology of ARDS/DAD is diverse and often cannot be identified from the morphologic substrate. Causes of ARDS/DAD are summarized in Table 3-1.

Hypersensitivity Pneumonitis

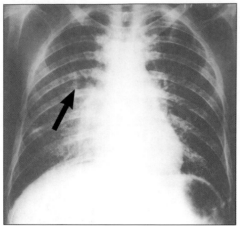

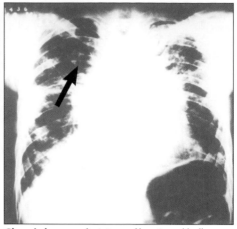

Acute bagassosis. Small nodular and miliary densities (arrow) throughout both lungs. Deposits may be more hazy and homogeneous in some cases.

Chronic bagassosis. Intense fibrosis and bullous emphysema after many episodes of respiratory illness during 9 years of industrial exposure.

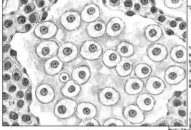

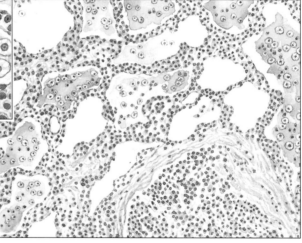

Tissue reaction in bagassosis. Alveolar walls thickened with infiltrate of plasma cells and lymphocytes. Some alveolar spaces contain edema fluid and desquamated histiocytes with vacuolated cytoplasm. High-power section inset above shows macrophages with vacuolated cytoplasm filling alveolar space.

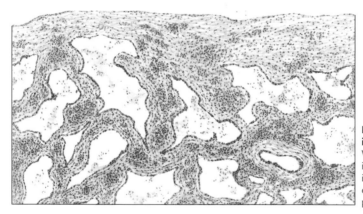

Extensive subpleural and interalveolar fibrosis. With inflammatory cell infiltration characteristic of advanced stage of farmer's lung (low-power section)

FIGURE 3-7 EXTRINSIC ALLERGIC ALVEOLITIS

Hypersensitivity pneumonitis (extrinsic allergic alveolitis [EAA]), an acute immunologic reaction of the lung to inhaled antigens, is typically caused by occupational exposure to organic dusts (e.g., **farmer's disease** bagassosis). Although EAA is classified as an acute RLD, its appearance is distinct from that of ARDS/DAD. EAA may run an acute or a chronic course with lymphoplasma-cytic and monocytic interstitial infiltration (rarely eosinophils),

mild alveolar exudate, and reactive alveolar cell proliferation (catarrh). There are noncaseating granulomas in approximately one third of cases. EAA is characterized by progressive fibroblast proliferation with interstitial and intraalveolar budding fibrosis and obliterative bronchiolitis. Inflammatory infiltrates usually recede in end-stage disease, leaving the nonspecific scenario of usual interstitial pneumonitis or fibrosis.

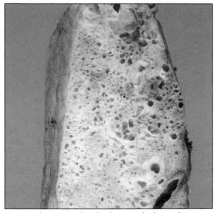

Gross photograph of advanced idiopathic pulmonary fibrosis (IPF), also called usual interstitial pneumonitis (UIP). Normal air spaces are replaced by extensive fibrosis and cyst formation (honeycombing)

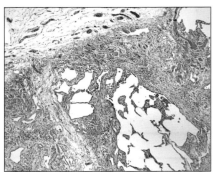

Subpleural region showing extensive subpleural and interalveolar fibrosis with focal inflammatory cell infiltration (low-power section)

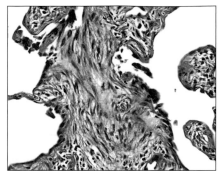

Markedly thickened alveolar wall containing fibroblasts and inflammatory cells (high power section)

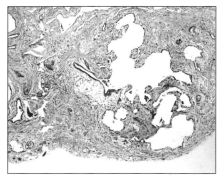

Subpleural region stained for collagen (green) showing similar changes with marked fibrosis and honeycomb cysts (low-power section)

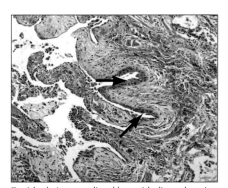

Residual air space lined by epithelium showing squamous metaplasia (arrows) and thick fibrotic wall containing inflammatory cells (medium power section)

TABLE 3-2   CLASSIFICATION OF IDIOPATHIC PULMONARY FIBROSIS*

Feature	NSIP	UIP	DIP	AIP	LIP	COP
Interstitial inflammation	Prominent	Scant	Scant	Scant	Prominent	Scant
Interstitial fibrosis						
Collagen	Variable, diffuse	Patchy	Variable, diffuse	No	Some areas	No
Fibroblast foci	Occasional	No	No	Yes, diffuse	No	No
BOOP	Occasional, focal	Occasional, focal	No	Occasional, focal	No	Prominent
Intraalveolar macrophages	Occasional, patchy	Occasional, patchy	Yes, diffuse	No	Patchy	No
Hyaline membranes	No	No	No	Yes, focal	No	No
Honeycombing	Rare	Yes	No	No	Sometimes	No

*AIP indicates acute interstitial pneumonitis; BOOP, bronchiolitis obliterans organizing pneumonitis; DIP, desquamative interstitial pneumonitis; NSIP, nonspecific interstitial pneumonitis; UIP, usual interstitial pneumonitis, LIP lymphocytic interstitial pneumonitis, COP cryptogenic organizing pneumonitis.
From Leslie KO, Wick MR. *Practical Pulmonary Pathology*. Philadelphia, 2005, Churchill Livingstone.

FIGURE 3-8   IDIOPATHIC PULMONARY FIBROSIS (IDIOPATHIC INTERSTITIAL PNEUMONIA)

Idiopathic pulmonary fibrosis (IPF) refers to a poorly understood chronic inflammatory and progressive fibrosing disorder of the lung. It is not a single entity but a mixture of pathogenetically variable diseases, which may progress in part from an acute RLD (e.g., EAA). **Hamman-Rich syndrome** is the classic description of IPF. The etiology of IPF and its subtypes is often unclear. Potential causes include postinfectious syndromes (e.g., postadenovirus, parainfluenza virus, and influenza B virus infections). The pathogenesis seems to be (auto)immune because the bronchoalveolar lavage contains increased numbers of neutrophils, macrophages, T lymphocytes, and occasionally eosinophils. Tissue biopsy shows expression of major histocompatibility complex (MHC) II antigens in alveolar epithelial cells. Infiltrating lymphocytes show a predominance of CD4+ and CD8+ T cells. Classifications of IPF are shown in Table 3-2.

Rheumatoid arthritis.
Nodular and streaklike infiltrations (arrows)

Rheumatoid arthritis: Lung involvement

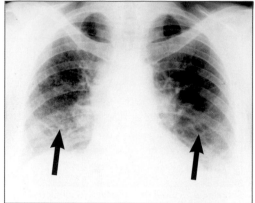

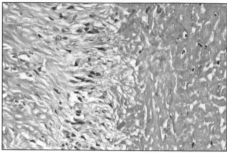

Portion of rheumatic nodule. Fibrinoid necrosis on right, palisading epithelial cells in middle, dense collagen on left

Progressive systemic sclerosis (scleroderma): Lung involvement

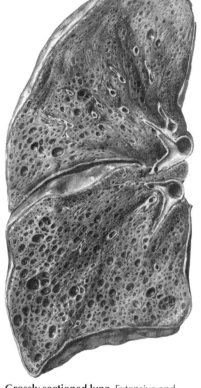

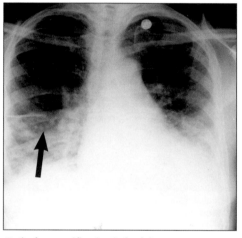

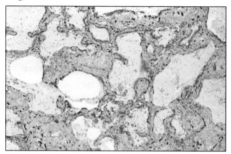

Microscopic section of lung. Fibrosis with formation of microcysts, many of which represent dilated bronchioles

Reticular opacification in both lungs. Small radiolucencies interspersed (arrow)

Grossly sectioned lung. Extensive and multitudinous small cysts. Visceral pleura thickened but not adherent to chest wall

Systemic lupus erythematosus: Lung involvement

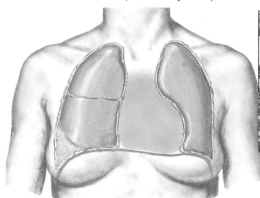

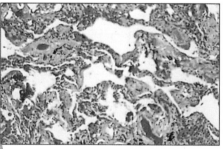

Reticular fibrosis of alveolar septa in SLE. Scattered anthracotic and iron deposits also present

Bilateral pleural thickening with small effusion outside of right lung. Globular cardiac silhouette suggests pericardial or cardiac involvement

FIGURE 3-9   COLLAGEN-VASCULAR DISEASE: LUNG INVOLVEMENT

Restrictive pulmonary disease is evident in up to 70% of patients with **systemic lupus erythematosus** (**SLE**), approximately 50% of patients with progressive systemic sclerosis (PSS), and up to 20% of patients with rheumatoid arthritis (RA). Lung involvement in RA is characterized by diffuse interstitial fibrosis (fibrosing alveolitis), bronchiolitis obliterans, sclerosing granulomas and necrotizing nodules, and isolated fibrinous pleuritis. In SLE, characteristic pulmonary changes are DAD, nonspecific interstitial pneumonitis with focal atelectasis, nonspecific infections, leukocytoclastic vasculitis, and focal pulmonary hemorrhage. PSS presents as an IPF (cryptogenic fibrosing alveolitis) with vascular involvement and pleurisy.

Polyarteritis Nodosa, Wegener Granulomatosis, and Allergic Granulomatosis

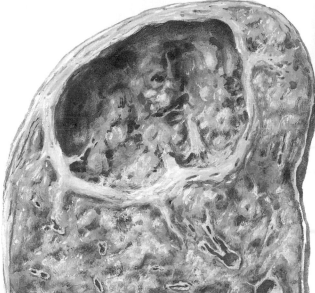

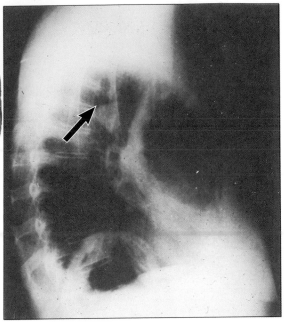

Wegener granulomatosis. Cavity in upper lobe of right lung lined with necrotic material

Wegener granulomatosis of lungs. With cavitation (arrow). Lateral view

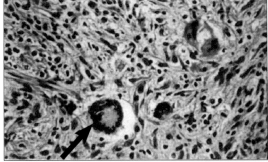

Wegener granuloma. With giant cells (arrow)

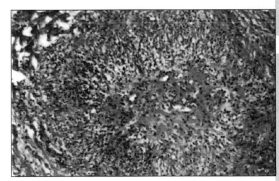

Severe arteritis. With destruction of vessel wall in Wegener granulomatosis

Clinical manifestations of Wegener granulomatosis

Upper respiratory involvement
Ulcerative lesions of nose, sinuses, mouth, pharynx

Lower respiratory involvement
Necrotic areas and cavitation in lungs; cough; dyspnea; hemoptysis; chest pain

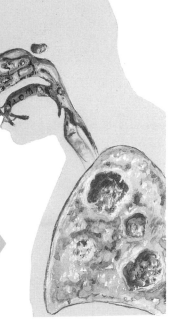

FIGURE 3-10 SYSTEMIC VASCULITIS: WEGENER DISEASE

Several of the systemic vasculitis syndromes affect the lungs regularly or incidentally. The classic example is **Wegener granulomatosis**, which is characterized by necrotizing granulomatous lesions in the upper and lower respiratory tract accompanied by systemic vasculitis involving arteries and veins and focal necrotizing glomerulitis. Radiographs of the lungs reveal irregular and frequently multiple densities with or without cavitation, which may resemble metastatic disease. Bronchial disease may cause pulmonary atelectases.

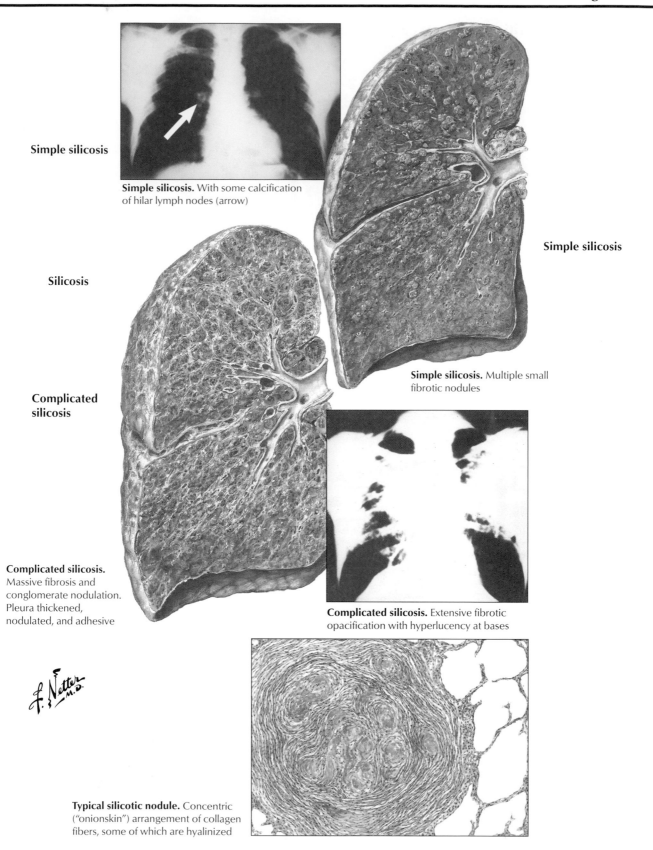

Simple silicosis

Simple silicosis. With some calcification of hilar lymph nodes (arrow)

Silicosis

Simple silicosis

Complicated silicosis

Simple silicosis. Multiple small fibrotic nodules

Complicated silicosis. Massive fibrosis and conglomerate nodulation. Pleura thickened, nodulated, and adhesive

Complicated silicosis. Extensive fibrotic opacification with hyperlucency at bases

Typical silicotic nodule. Concentric ("onionskin") arrangement of collagen fibers, some of which are hyalinized

FIGURE 3-11   PNEUMOCONIOSIS

Pneumoconiosis describes a group of chronic RLDs that are caused by inhalation of mineral dusts. The most common forms of these occupational diseases are caused by coal dust, quartz, asbestos, and beryllium. Pneumoconioses are characterized by progressive pulmonary fibrosis, which reflects the dose, particle size, and fibroblastic potential of the individual dust. The dose is a function of dust concentration and duration of exposure. **Silicosis,** which is caused by inhalation of silica dust, is an example of a common pneumoconiosis. Characteristics of the more common pneumoconioses are shown in Table 3-3.

TABLE 3-3 CLINICAL AND PATHOLOGIC FEATURES OF PNEUMOCONIOSES*

Entity	Clinical Appearance	Pathologic Changes
Coal miner's lung	Black lung disease	Diffusely distributed, small focal anthracosilicosis, initially centriacinar and peribronchiolar with many carbon-laden macrophages and perifocal emphysema; extent of fibrosis depends on admixture of quartz
Silicosis	Acute silicosis (uncommon)	Alveolar lipoproteinosis and progressive diffuse interstitial fibrosis secondary to inhalation of small particulate silica crystals (e.g., after sand blasting)
	Nodular silicosis (common)	Multiple growing silicotic nodules, usually 2 mm to 1 cm in diameter: fibrosing granulomas with concentric fibrous layering, some anthracotic pigment, small slitlike spaces, and needle-shaped crystalline spicules on polarization; perifocal emphysema
	Progressive massive silicosis	Multiple silicotic granulomas up to 10 cm in diameter, both lungs involved, massive and rapidly progressive fibrosis
Asbestosis and asbestosrelated diseases	Asbestosis per se	Alveolitis with progressive interstitial fibrosis, deposition of asbestos bodies (golden-brown beaded rods consisting of asbestos fibers coated by ferroproteinaceous material); final stage: honeycombing lung
	Pleural plaques and rounded atelectasis	Recurrent pleural fibrinous effusions, pleural fibrosis and pleural plaques ("sugar coating"), focal atelectasis secondary to pleural fibrosis
	Neoplasms	Malignant mesothelioma ($\uparrow$ risk of bronchogenic carcinoma)
Berylliosis	Berylliosis per se	Acute and recurrent pneumonitis, systemic sarcoidlike and fibrosing granulomas
Talcosis	Talcosis per se	Foreign body granulomas with birefringent talcum deposits, micronodular and diffuse interstitial fibrosis

*Caplan syndrome occurs in patients with rheumatoid arthritis and some form of nodular silicosis. Deposition of microparticulate iron causes siderotic macrophage response with secondary focal or diffuse interstitial fibrosis.

FIGURE 3-11 PNEUMOCONIOSIS (CONTINUED)

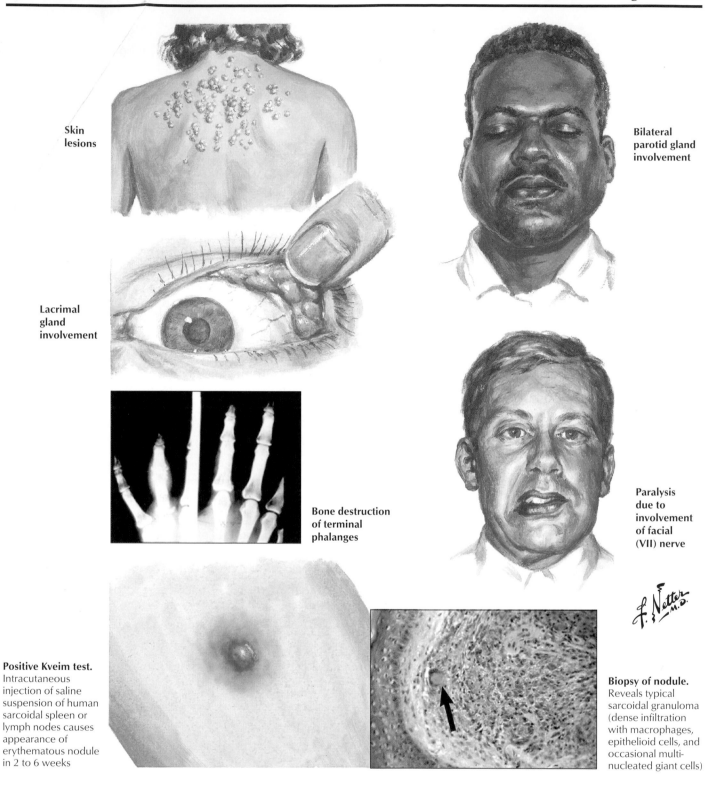

Skin lesions

Lacrimal gland involvement

Bilateral parotid gland involvement

Bone destruction of terminal phalanges

Paralysis due to involvement of facial (VII) nerve

Positive Kveim test. Intracutaneous injection of saline suspension of human sarcoidal spleen or lymph nodes causes appearance of erythematous nodule in 2 to 6 weeks

Biopsy of nodule. Reveals typical sarcoidal granuloma (dense infiltration with macrophages, epithelioid cells, and occasional multi-nucleated giant cells)

FIGURE 3-12   SARCOIDOSIS

Sarcoidosis is a systemic disease of unknown origin characterized by the development of noncaseating epithelioid cell (EC) granulomas with subsequent fibrosis. On radiographs, **pulmonary sarcoidosis** shows a typical reticulonodular infiltrate with hilar lymphadenopathy. Histologically, multiple noncaseating granulomas are found in the bronchial or bronchiolar submucosa, along intralobular septae or the pleura. Granulomas undergo peripheral and "reticulated" fibrosis with final scarring. Multi-

nucleated giant cells similar to Langhans cells may show intracytoplasmic star-shaped or laminar calcified inclusions (**asteroid bodies**, **Schaumann bodies**). The course may be acute or chronic persistent or progressive. Approximately one third of cases are complicated by sarcoid vasculitis. Approximately 20% of patients experience repeated recurrences and pulmonary dysfunction; 10% progress to pulmonary fibrosis and cor pulmonale.

Embolism of Lesser Degree Without Infarction

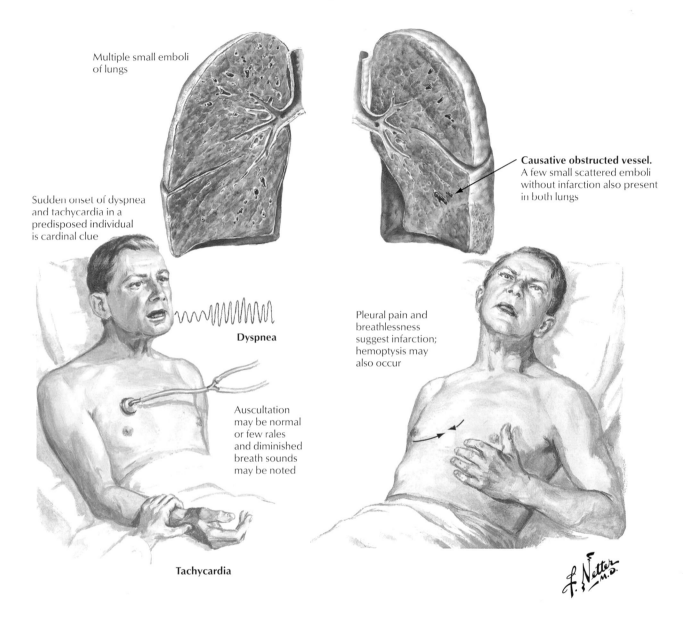

Multiple small emboli of lungs

Sudden onset of dyspnea and tachycardia in a predisposed individual is cardinal clue

Causative obstructed vessel.
A few small scattered emboli without infarction also present in both lungs

Dyspnea

Auscultation may be normal or few rales and diminished breath sounds may be noted

Pleural pain and breathlessness suggest infarction; hemoptysis may also occur

Tachycardia

FIGURE 3-13 PULMONARY EMBOLISM

More than 90% of emboli in the pulmonary arteries arise from venous thromboses of the lower extremities. Approximately 60% to 80% of **pulmonary embolisms** (PEs) remain silent, presumably because of the small size of the thrombi. **PE without infarction** occurs without preexisting circulatory insufficiency. The tissue framework and collateral circulation remain intact because the dual arterial blood supply (pulmonary and bronchial arteries) prevents the thrombosis from occluding the pulmonary artery. The lung parenchyma shows severe congestions, with eventual intraalveolar hemorrhage. **PE with pulmonary infarction** occurs when blood supplied to the lung via the bronchial artery is insufficient, such as in chronic congestive heart failure (CHF) or in chronic pulmonary diseases with reduced vascularization. This hemorrhagic pulmonary infarction causes ischemic necrosis of lung tissue in addition to severe congestion. The infarction appears as a wedge-shaped, dark purple lung lesion with the base pointing toward the pleura and the occluded pulmonary artery at the tip.

TABLE 3-4   INFECTIOUS AGENTS CAUSING PNEUMONIA

Class	Etiologic Agent	Type of Pneumonia
Bacteria	*Streptococcus pneumoniae* *Streptococcus pyogenes* *Staphylococcus aureus* *Klebsiella pneumoniae* *Pseudomonas aeruginosa* *Escherichia coli* *Yersinia pestis* *Legionella pneumophila* *Peptostreptococcus, Peptococcus* *Bacteroides* *Fusobacterium* *Veillonella*	Legionnaires disease Aspiration (anaerobic) pneumonia Bacterial pneumonias
Actinomycetes	*Actinomyces israelii* *Nocardia asteroides*	Pulmonary nocardiosis Pulmonary actinomycosis
Fungi	*Coccidioides immitis* *Histoplasma capsulatum* *Blastomyces dermatitidis* *Aspergillus* *Phycomycetes*	Coccidioidomycosis Histoplasmosis Blastomycosis Aspergillosis Mucormycosis
Rickettsia	*Coxiella burnetii*	Q fever
Chlamydia	*Chlamydia psittaci*	Psittacosis Ornithosis
Mycoplasma	Mycoplasma pneumoniae	Mycoplasmal pneumonia
Viruses	Influenza virus, adenovirus, respiratory syncytial virus, etc.	Viral pneumonia
Protozoa	*Pneumocystis carinii*	*Pneumocystis* pneumonia (plasma cell pneumonia)

Infection of the lungs cause **pneumonia** (also "pneumonitis"). Following the rules of general inflammation (Chapter 1: Figures 1-5 to 1-8), pulmonary inflammation presents itself as **alveolar pneumonia** (common bacterial), **interstitial lymphocytic pneumonitis** (viral, immunological), **granulomatous pneumonitis** (Tb, allergic) or mixtures of the latter (certain viruses, protozoal, immunological). Table 3-4 summarizes common infectious agents causing pneumonia. Figures 3-14, 3-15, 3-16, and 3-17 present representative examples. Figures 3-5, 3-7, and 3-8 show examples of immunologic forms of pneumonitis. The prognosis of pneumonia depends upon the type of inflammatory reaction in the lungs: acute alveolar pneumonia (serofibrinous, neutrophilic) or pure interstitial lymphocytic pneumonitis (common cold virus) may resolve with complete recovery. Structural damage (e.g., abscess formation) or chronic infiltrative diseases (e.g., tuberculosis) always results in scarring, the extent of which will determine the persistence of clinical symptoms.

Pneumococcal pneumonia

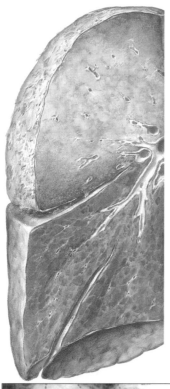

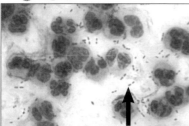

Purulent sputum with pneumococci
(diplococci) (Gram stain)

***Klebsiella* (Friedländer) pneumonia**

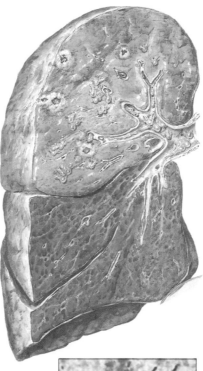

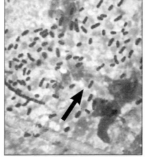

Gram stain of sputum containing
Klebsiella pneumoniae organisms
with mucoid capsule

Staphylococcal pneumonia

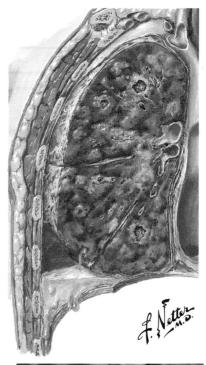

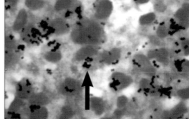

Staphylococci and polymorphonuclear
leukocytes in sputum (Gram stain)

FIGURE 3-14 BACTERIAL PNEUMONIAS

Bacterial pneumonias (Table 3-4) are caused by aerogenic infection (***bronchopneumonia,*** BP) or hematogenous spread of infectious organisms (***hematogenous pneumonia,*** HP). BP starts focally in one lobe with centrifugal spread (pneumococcal or *Klebsiella* BP), while HP affects both lungs in the peripheral **mantle zone** with centripetal spread. BP is accompanied by infectious bronchitis, HP rather by infectious (septic) vasculitis. The inflammatory reaction and its extent depend on the nature (toxicity) of the infectious organism and on the host defense

status. Necrotizing or hemorrhagic reactions are caused by bacterial exo or endotoxins. Increased coagulation of the exudate may favor abscess formation (staphylococci) and decreased coagulation rapid spread (pneumococci). Segmental pneumonia indicates some defense deficiency. Lobar pneumonia is complicated by a local hypersensitivity reaction. Location, composition, and spread of the inflammatory reaction in pneumonia thus may permit some conclusion of nature and source of the infectious agent.

Varicella Pneumonia

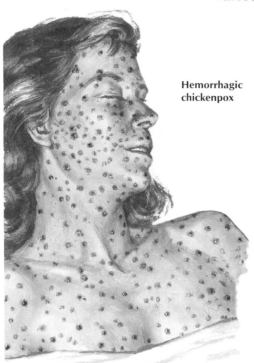

Hemorrhagic chickenpox

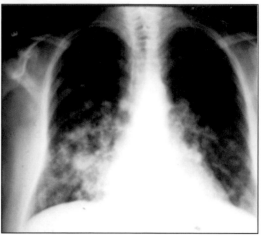

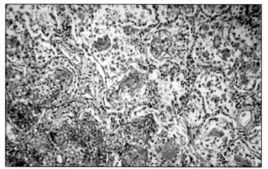

Varicella pneumonia. Nodular infiltrates in both lower lobes, more marked and coalescing on right side

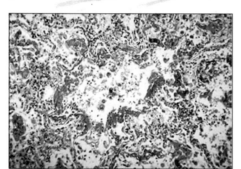

Mononuclear infiltrate in interstitium and fibrin lining alveoli. High power

Pulmonary histology. Low power. Alveoli filled with fibrin, fluid, and cellular exudate

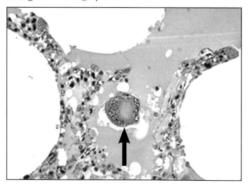

Multinucleated giant cell (arrow) with much fluid in alveolus

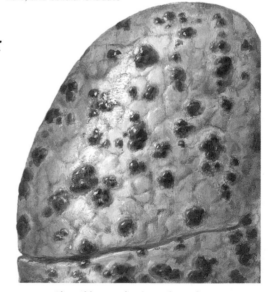

Pleural hemorrhagic pocks on lung

FIGURE 3-15   VIRAL PNEUMONIAS

Viral pneumonitis is characterized by interstitial lymphocytic infiltration (nonspecific interstitial pneumonitis) combined with variable signs of DAD. Some cases are complicated by bronchiolitis obliterans (influenza virus, respiratory syncytial virus) or by focal necroses and eventual hemorrhage (herpes simplex virus [HSV], varicella-zoster and respiratory syncytial viruses, measles,

influenza). Viruses that cause diagnostic cytopathic effects during some stages of infection include measles virus (**Warthin-Finkeldey** multinucleated giant cells), cytomegalovirus (giant cells with **Cowdry** type A intranuclear inclusions), other HSVs, and adenoviruses. **Varicella pneumonia**, a typical viral pneumonia, is caused by the varicella zoster virus.

TABLE 3-5   PULMONARY FUNGAL INFECTIONS IN IMMUNOCOMPROMISED PATIENTS

Organism	Pathologic Lesion
Candida albicans tropicalis	Participation of the lungs in systemic candidiasis: a. Hematogenous miliary candida abscesses with associated necrotizing focal pneumonitis b. Bronchogenic pneumonia with abscess formation (e.g., after aspiration)
Aspergillus fumigatus niger flavus	Necrotizing bronchopneumonia with eventual hemorrhagic infarcts
Mucor (phycomycosis)	Necrotizing bronchopneumonia with prominent vascular invasion and hemorrhagic infarction and hemoptysis
Cryptococcus neoformans	Alveolar mucoid exudate with organisms and mild foreign body (occasionally tuberculoid) granulomatous reaction
Histoplasma capsulatum	Tuberculoid granulomatous and necrotizing bronchopneumonia
Blastomyces dermatitidis	Puriform and bronchopneumonia with abscess formation, chronic cavernous bronchopneumonia

(A) *P. carinii* pneumonia

(B) PAS stain (periodic acid-Fuchsin) of pneumocystis organisms

(C) *P. carinii* (arrow). Methenamine-silver stain of pneumocystis organisms

(D) Lung in CMV disease with typical fleshy appearance

(E) Cytomegalovirus pneumonia. Cytomegalic cells (arrow)

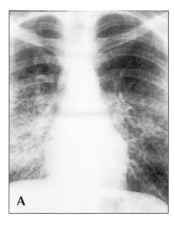

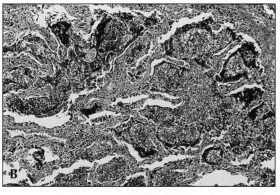

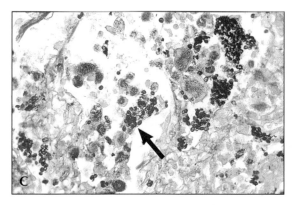

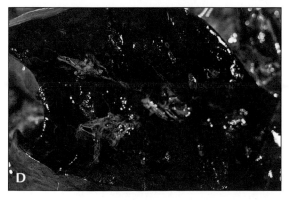

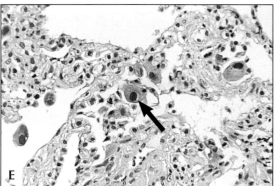

FIGURE 3-16   OPPORTUNISTIC PNEUMONIAS

Fungal infections are a major cause for opportunistic pneumonitis in immunodeficient patients (Table 3-5). The most common lesions appear grossly as irregular yellowish-gray infiltrates with a granular dry and firm cut surface. Hemorrhage and occasional regional infarcts may occur in certain infections secondary to vascular involvement (e.g., in mucor mycosis). Some forms closely resemble tuberculosis (TB) (e.g., histoplasma capsulatum infections). Besides cytomegalovirus and various fungi, *P carinii* organisms are frequently isolated from "opportunistic" pneumonitis. Pathologic changes in ***P. carinii* pneumonia** show an interstitial plasmacellular (lymphoplasmacytic) pneumonia with alveolar foamy exudate, proliferating type II alveolar cells, and silver-stainable organisms. Certain fungal lung infections that occur in previously healthy persons may be accompanied by severe allergic reactions (e.g., allergic aspergillosis with bronchopulmonary infiltrates, eosinophilia, developing bronchiectasis, and eventual aspergilloma).

Evolution of Tubercle

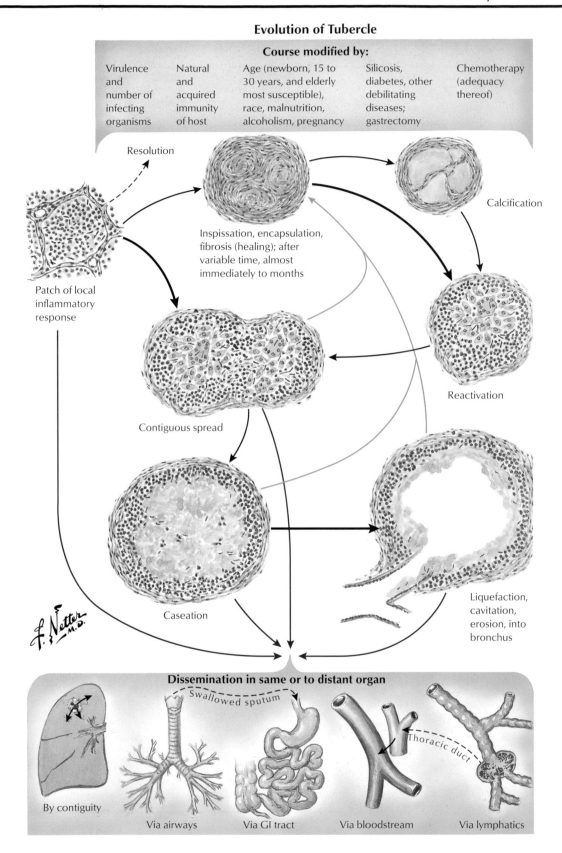

Course modified by:

| Virulence and number of infecting organisms | Natural and acquired immunity of host | Age (newborn, 15 to 30 years, and elderly most susceptible), race, malnutrition, alcoholism, pregnancy | Silicosis, diabetes, other debilitating diseases; gastrectomy | Chemotherapy (adequacy thereof) |

Resolution

Inspissation, encapsulation, fibrosis (healing); after variable time, almost immediately to months

Calcification

Patch of local inflammatory response

Reactivation

Contiguous spread

Caseation

Liquefaction, cavitation, erosion, into bronchus

Dissemination in same or to distant organ

Swallowed sputum

Thoracic duct

By contiguity

Via airways

Via GI tract

Via bloodstream

Via lymphatics

FIGURE 3-17   PULMONARY TUBERCULOSIS

Pulmonary tuberculosis (TB) usually results from aerogenic infection with *M. tuberculosis, typus humanus*. The tuberculous granuloma is a classic epitheloid cell (EC) granuloma with palisading of EC around a central caseous necrosis. The EC layer contains multinucleated giant cells with peripherally located nuclei in a "string of pearls" pattern (**Langhans-giant cells**) surrounded by accumulations of lymphocytes. Tissue reaction to the state of immune reactivity forms for staging the clinicopathologic features of TB (Table 3-6). Infection in immunodeficient patients such as in human immunodeficiency virus (HIV) does not

TABLE 3-6   FORMS AND FEATURES OF PULMONARY TUBERCULOSIS*

Stage	Immune Reactivity	Clinicopathologic Features
Stage I (primary)		
a. Initial infection	No immunity	Clinically inapparent nonspecific alveolitis
b. Initial infection	Developing immunity	Ghon's primary affection: isolated granulomatous reaction, most commonly in right upper lobe
c. Primary lymphatic spread	Developing immunity	Lymphatic spread of infection to regional lymph nodes with respective granulomas: Ranke's primary complex
Stage II (early postprimary generalization)		
a. Lymphatic spread	Good	Isolated subpleural caseous granuloma, upper segments of right upper lobe
b. Bronchogenic spread	Intermediate	Acinar-nodular pulmonary tuberculosis with progressive caseous granulomas
	Poor	Progressive caseous pneumonia without prominent granulomatous reaction
c. Hematogenous spread	Intermediate	Systemic hematogenous caseous granulomas of different sizes (i.e., different ages)
(late postprimary generalization)		
d. Hematogenous spread	Nonimmune → reactive	Miliary tuberculosis with systemic granulomas of uniform size (and age)
e. Hematogenous spread (also in early postprimary spread)	A-reactive	Miliary systemic necroses, tuberculosepsis acutissima, typhobacillosis Landouzy
Stage III (isolated organ tuberculosis)	High	Limited spread in isolated organs: cavernous pulmonary of renal tuberculosis, isolated tuberculomas (granulomas) in brain, spine, and other organs
Late generalization	High → low	Local or systemic spread of isolated organ tuberculosis (lymphatic, bronchogenic, or hematogenous)

*The degree of immune reactivity (not resistance to disease) can be monitored by tuberculin skin testing; toxicity of tubercle bacteria is partly determined by "cord factor."

FIGURE 3-17   PULMONARY TUBERCULOSIS *(CONTINUED)*

lead to typical tuberculous granulomas but to a nonspecific accumulation of macrophages at the sites of bacterial deposition (**mycobacterial histiocytosis**). Severe defense deficiencies cause tuberculosepsis acutissima (**typhobacillosis Landouzy**), a rapidly progressive and systemic form of TB with extensive caseous pneumonia in the lungs.

Classification of Bronchogenic Carcinoma (= 95% of All Lung Carcinoma)

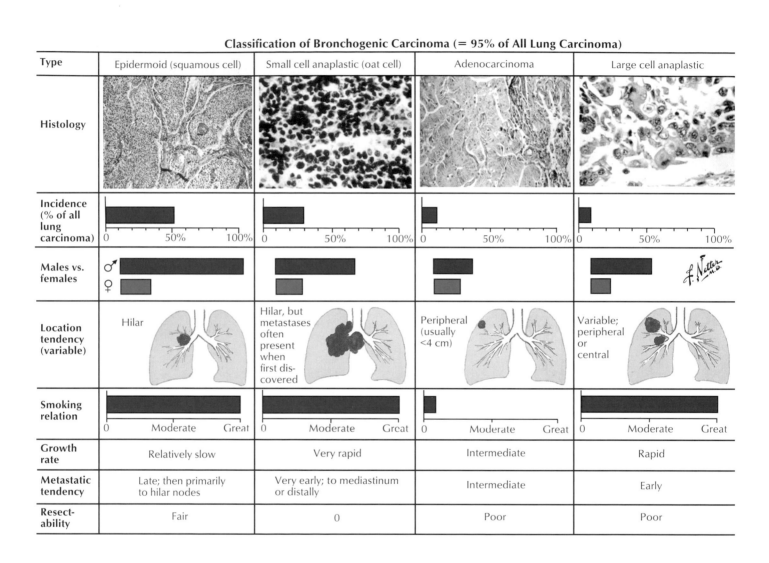

Type	Epidermoid (squamous cell)	Small cell anaplastic (oat cell)	Adenocarcinoma	Large cell anaplastic
Histology				
Incidence (% of all lung carcinoma)				
Males vs. females	♂ / ♀			
Location tendency (variable)	Hilar	Hilar, but metastases often present when first discovered	Peripheral (usually <4 cm)	Variable; peripheral or central
Smoking relation				
Growth rate	Relatively slow	Very rapid	Intermediate	Rapid
Metastatic tendency	Late; then primarily to hilar nodes	Very early; to mediastinum or distally	Intermediate	Early
Resect-ability	Fair	0	Poor	Poor

FIGURE 3-18   LUNG CANCER

Carcinoma of the lung is the most frequent cause of cancer death worldwide (32% of cancer deaths in males, 25% in females). Bronchogenic carcinoma is classified into **small-cell lung carcinoma** ([SCLC] oat cell) and **non–small-cell lung carcinoma** (NSCLC), which includes **squamous cell carcinoma** (SCC),

large-cell anaplastic carcinoma (LC), and **adenocarcinoma** (AC). Lung carcinomas vary in their primary location, spread, and overall biologic behavior. They frequently metastasize to regional lymph nodes (hilar, mediastinal) and to extralymphatic sites such as adrenal glands, brain, bone, and liver.

Small Cell Lung Carcinoma (Oat Cell Carcinoma)

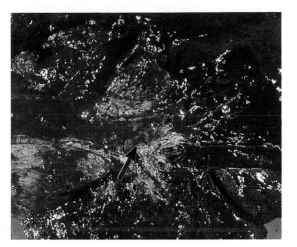

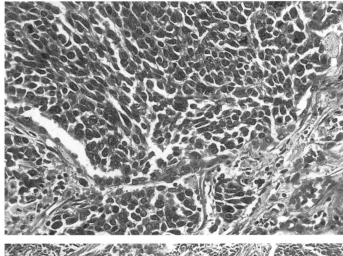

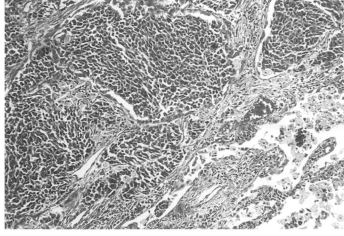

FIGURE 3-19   SMALL-CELL LUNG CANCER

Small-cell lung cancer accounts for 20% of all lung cancers, with a male predominance and relation to cigarette smoking. It presents as a rapidly growing and metastasizing central lung mass occasionally accompanied by a **paraneoplastic syndrome** (myasthenia of **Eaton-Lambert syndrome**, ectopic corticotropin production, diabetes insipidus). The tumor consists histologically of sheets of small round or spindle cells with high mitotic index and scattered necroses. SCLC is essentially more sensitive to chemotherapy and therefore separated from all other lung cancers. However, it has the poorest 5-year survival rate (approximately 5%).

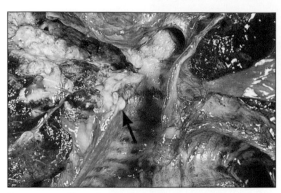
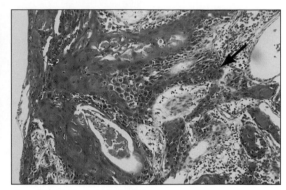

Squamous cell carcinoma (SCC). Arrow points to gross lung section (**left**), microscopic (**right**)

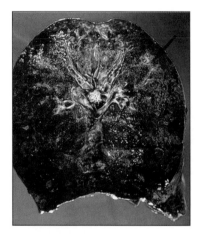
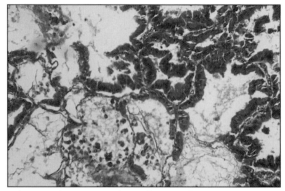

Adenocarcinoma (AC) shown here, (pulmonary adenomatosis) (arrow). Gross lung section (**left**). Note the pneumonia-like infiltration, microscopic (**right**) with alveolar lining of tumor cells

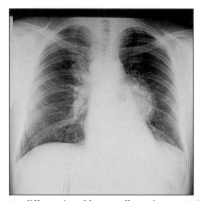
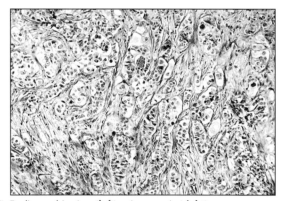

Undifferentiated large cell carcinoma (LC). Radiographic view (**left**), microscopic (**right**)

FIGURE 3-20   NON–SMALL-CELL LUNG CANCER

Squamous cell carcinoma (SCC), accounts for 30% of all lung cancers and is related to chemical carcinogens and cigarette smoking. SCC usually presents as a central lung mass invading the bronchial wall with rapid spread to local lymph nodes, brain, bone, and liver. Pancoast tumor is a variant of SCC in the apex of the lung that extends into adjacent thoracic and cervical nerves. Microscopically, tumor cells growing in sheets show variable degrees of squamous differentiation with keratinization. **Adeno-carcinoma** (AC) accounts for another 30% of invasive lung

cancers. It has a rather peripheral location and early lymphatic spread. There are several histologic subtypes (acinar, papillary bronchioloalveolar) and mixtures of these with variable degrees of differentiation (e.g., large-cell poorly differentiated AC). **Large cell carcinoma** (LC) accounts for approximately 10% of all lung cancers and may show features of squamous or glandular differentiation or both and pleomorphic or spindle cell variants. LC has the poorest 5-year survival rate of all NSCLCs (approximately 10%).

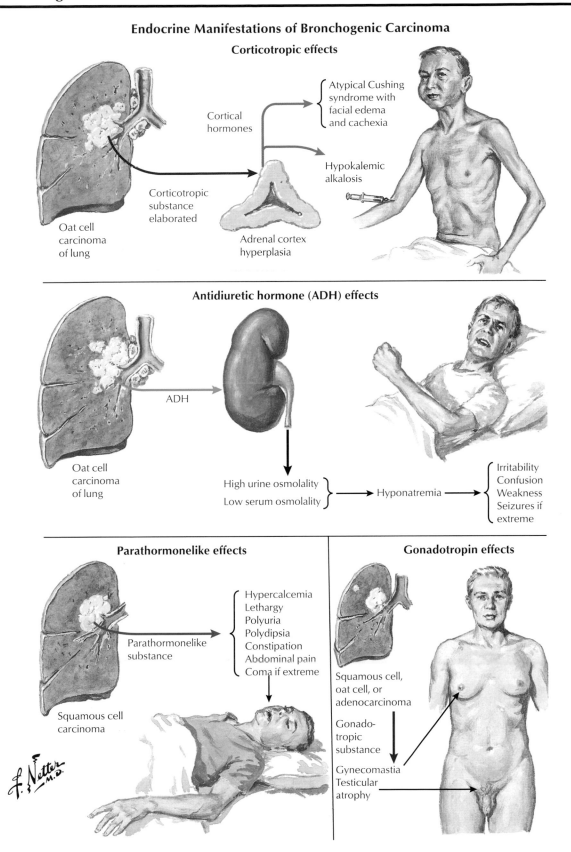

Endocrine Manifestations of Bronchogenic Carcinoma

Corticotropic effects

Cortical hormones

Atypical Cushing syndrome with facial edema and cachexia

Hypokalemic alkalosis

Corticotropic substance elaborated

Adrenal cortex hyperplasia

Oat cell carcinoma of lung

Antidiuretic hormone (ADH) effects

ADH

Oat cell carcinoma of lung

High urine osmolality
Low serum osmolality
} → Hyponatremia →
Irritability
Confusion
Weakness
Seizures if extreme

Parathormonelike effects

Parathormonelike substance

Hypercalcemia
Lethargy
Polyuria
Polydipsia
Constipation
Abdominal pain
Coma if extreme

Squamous cell carcinoma

Gonadotropin effects

Squamous cell, oat cell, or adenocarcinoma

Gonadotropic substance

Gynecomastia
Testicular atrophy

FIGURE 3-21   LUNG CANCER: EXTRAPULMONARY MANIFESTATIONS

There are several nonmetastatic extrapulmonary manifestations of primary **lung carcinoma**, which are summarized as **paraneoplastic syndromes**. In addition to those pictured, these include skin changes, such as acanthosis nigricans, dermatomyositis/polymyositis, and myasthenia. Progressive multifocal leukoencephalopathy, occasionally also described as paraneoplastic

syndrome, results from reactivation of latent polyomavirus infection (JC virus), and progressive focal demyelination in the central nervous system as can also be seen in other cases of immune deficiency (e.g., in HIV/acquired immunodeficiency virus [AIDS] and in certain cases of chronic lymphocytic leukemia).

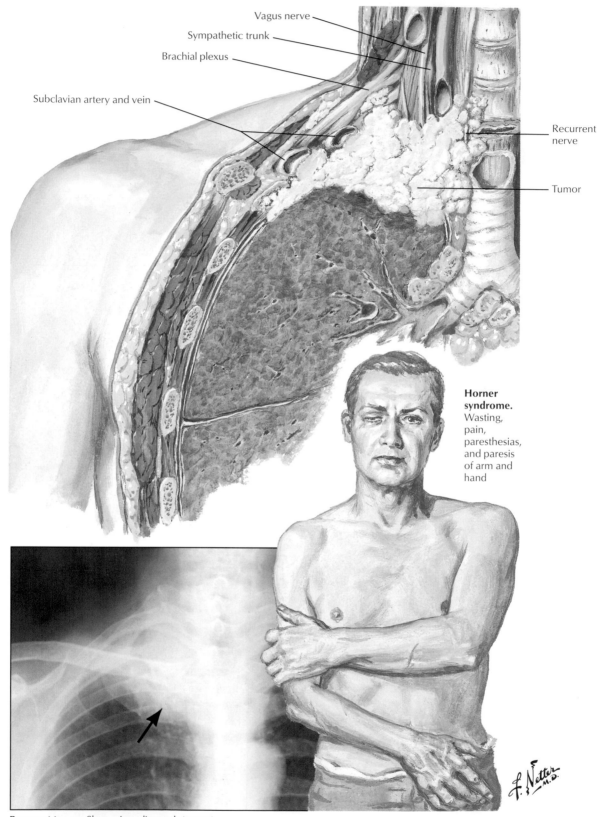

Vagus nerve

Sympathetic trunk

Brachial plexus

Subclavian artery and vein

Recurrent nerve

Tumor

Horner syndrome. Wasting, pain, paresthesias, and paresis of arm and hand

Pancoast tumor. Shown in radiograph (arrow)

FIGURE 3-22   PANCOAST TUMOR

Pancoast tumor characterizes a special growth pattern of bronchogenic carcinoma with early invasion of homolateral soft tissues of the lower neck. The tumor subsequently grows into regional nerves (arm plexus, sympathicus, parasympathicus) and vessels, causing the clinical **Horner syndrome**: enophthalmos, ptosis, miosis, and anhydrosis (sunken-in eyeball, lowering of upper eyelid, narrowing of pupil, and loss of sweating).

Mesothelioma of Pleura

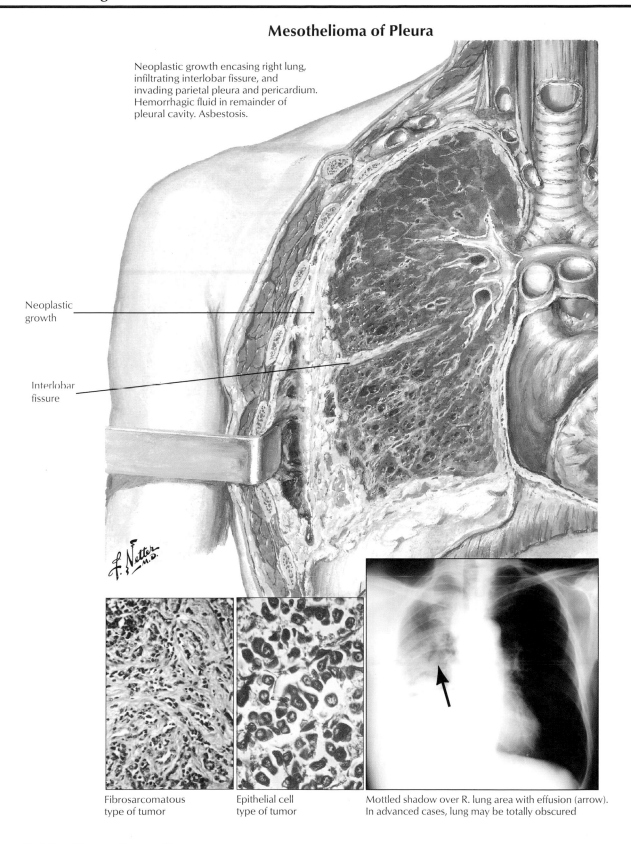

Neoplastic growth encasing right lung, infiltrating interlobar fissure, and invading parietal pleura and pericardium. Hemorrhagic fluid in remainder of pleural cavity. Asbestosis.

Neoplastic growth

Interlobar fissure

Fibrosarcomatous type of tumor

Epithelial cell type of tumor

Mottled shadow over R. lung area with effusion (arrow). In advanced cases, lung may be totally obscured

FIGURE 3-23   OTHER LUNG TUMORS

Other primary tumors of the lungs include **carcinoids** (a neuroendocrine tumor), **mucoepidermoid** and **adenoid cystic carcinoma** (counterparts to salivary gland tumors of bronchial glands), **pulmonary blastoma**, **angiosarcoma** and **hemangioendothelioma**, and **malignant lymphoma**. **Malignant mesothelioma**, a pleural fibrous tumor with adenoid mesothelial structures, may compli-cate pulmonary asbestosis. This firm tumor encases and compresses the lung (or both lungs) with limited direct invasion of peripheral lung parenchyma. Lymph nodes are rarely affected. The tumor extends locally within the thoracic cavity and along the mediastinum into bones, peritoneum, liver, and adrenals.

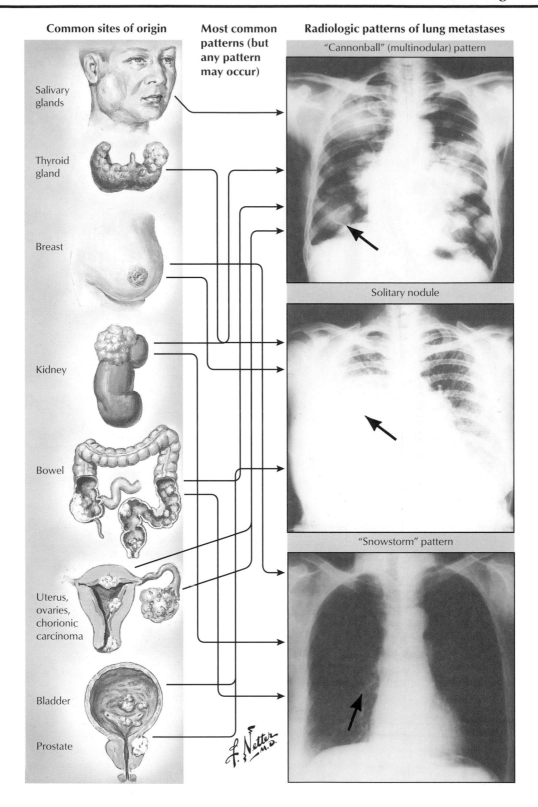

Common sites of origin

Salivary glands

Thyroid gland

Breast

Kidney

Bowel

Uterus, ovaries, chorionic carcinoma

Bladder

Prostate

Most common patterns (but any pattern may occur)

Radiologic patterns of lung metastases

"Cannonball" (multinodular) pattern

Solitary nodule

"Snowstorm" pattern

FIGURE 3-24   METASTATIC MALIGNANCY TO THE LUNG

Metastases to the lungs occur in approximately 30% of all extrapulmonary malignant tumors. In the absence of a known primary tumor, clinical differential diagnosis may pose a problem. In contrast to a primary lung tumor, (hematogenous) metastases usually occur at multiple sites in both lungs. They are usually well-circumscribed foci, and cavitations occur rarely.

Certain tumors, such as carcinoma of the pancreas and stomach, may show lymphangitic spread in the lungs, giving a characteristic appearance of fine-nodular and linear (reticulonodular) infiltrations. Diagnosis and search for the primary tumor is usually guided by biopsy of a lung metastasis with histologic and immunocytochemical investigation.

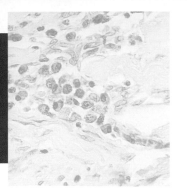

CHAPTER 4
GASTROINTESTINAL SYSTEM

Common diseases of the esophagus, the stomach, and the small and large intestines include functional disorders, inflammation, infections, and tumors.

DISEASES OF THE ESOPHAGUS

Esophageal diseases of various kinds are characterized by fairly uniform clinical symptoms of dysphagia (swallowing difficulties), heartburn (retrosternal pain), and vomiting (with or without blood). The most frequent causes are inflammatory or neoplastic diseases. Other esophageal problems that should be considered in differential diagnosis include diverticula and fistulas, atresia in the newborn, motility changes (e.g., achalasia), and a number of diseases that affect the esophagus secondarily (e.g., Mallory-Weiss lacerations in alcoholism, varices in hepatic cirrhosis, esophageal sclerosis in primary systemic sclerosis, and bulemia).

DISEASES OF THE STOMACH

Congenital diseases of the stomach, such as congenital pyloric stenosis, congenital hernias, diverticula, and cysts, are rare. The 2 most frequent disorders affecting large numbers of patients are inflammation of the stomach (gastritis) and epithelial tumors (carcinoma). These are discussed in more detail here, in addition to the frequent adult hernias, a common cause of reflux esophagitis and, potentially, esophageal cancer.

NONTUMOROUS DISEASES OF THE SMALL AND LARGE INTESTINES

Congenital disorders of the intestines are uncommon and are discussed in Table 4-1 and malabsorption syndromes in Table 4-4.

Infectious enterocolitis (IEC) and food poisoning are diseases of worldwide prevalence characterized by diarrhea and (gastro)intestinal inflammation with increased intestinal secretion and reduced absorption. Mucosal necrosis, hemorrhage, and ulceration develop according to local or systemic toxic influences of the causative agent. Loss of fluid and toxic side effects are especially dangerous for children and the elderly. Etiologic agents frequently identified in acute IEC are viruses (rotavirus, Norwalk agent) and bacteria (enterotoxic *Escherichia coli*); however, in up to 50% of cases, no organism is identified. In the United States, the most common causative agents in fatal IEC, in order of frequency, are *Salmonellae, Listeria, Toxoplasma,* Norwalk agent, *E. coli,* and *Campylobacter.*

TABLE 4-1   DEVELOPMENTAL INTESTINAL DISEASES

Disease	Features
Small intestine	
Atresia	Complete occlusion of intestinal lumen secondary to intraluminal diaphragm or disconnected blind ends (occurs in fetuses of mothers with polyhydramnios)
Stenosis	Partial occlusion (stricture) of the intestinal lumen secondary to incomplete intraluminal diaphragm, external adhesions (e.g., secondary to [transient] volvulus)
Duplications	Tubular or cystic structures (enteric cysts) that may communicate with the intestinal lumen (most common in ilium; may contain gastric mucosa and cause peptic ulcer similar to Meckel diverticulum)
Meckel diverticulum	Partial persistence of the vitelline duct, 60–100 cm before the ileocecal valve, with all layers of intestinal or gastric mucosa
Large intestine	
Malrotation	Abnormal positioning of colon in abdominal cavity (e.g., cecum in left upper quadrant); may give rise to volvulus
Hirschsprung disease	Congenital megacolon secondary to aganglionic segment (lack of Auerbach and Meissner plexus preferentially in sigmoid colon and rectum)

The most common vascular lesions of the small and large bowel are phlebectases (hemorrhoids) and ischemic and thrombotic disorders; less common are local vasculitis accompanying systemic vasculitis and collagen-vascular diseases as well as angiodysplasia.

TUMORS OF THE SMALL AND LARGE INTESTINES

Benign tumors of the intestines are most often epithelial in nature and are referred to clinically as *polyps*. They usually are rare in the small intestine but frequent in the large intestine (colonic polyps increase in frequency from approximately 20% before the age of 40 years to 50% beyond the age of 60 years). The clinical entity *polyp* is subclassified pathologically into polyps as such (i.e., reactive lesions, such as hyperplastic, hamartomatous, or inflammatory polyps) and adenomas (i.e., benign neoplastic lesions, such as tubular or villous adenomas). The pathologic entity *polyp* does not possess malignant potential, whereas adenomas (also referred to as *adenomatous polyps*) do. Depending on their size, there is a 10% to 15% risk of cancer development within 5 years in tubular adenomas and a 30% to 40% risk in villous adenomas. The risk of malignancy increases with the number of adenomas; especially prone for malignant change are familial polyposis syndromes (e.g., Gardner syndrome) in which the occurrence of cancer approaches 100% by midlife.

Other more infrequent benign lesions of the intestines are lipomas, leiomyomas, neurofibroma, and hemangioma, which may also impress clinically as *polyps* and rather rarely may cause complications (e.g., erosion, bleeding and anemia, obstruction, or intussusception).

Malignant tumors of the small intestine account for less than 0.1% of tumors diagnosed at autopsy, or less than 5% of all gastrointestinal (GI) tumors. They consist primarily of adenocarcinomas, malignant lymphomas, and carcinoid tumors (CTs). Even less frequent are stromal tumors, such as leiomyosarcoma and gastrointestinal stromal tumors (GIST). By contrast, adenocarcinomas of the colon and the rectum are among the most common malignant tumors in the Western world, accounting for approximately 15% of all cancer deaths in the United States (approximately 150,000 new cases diagnosed every year, with a peak incidence at the age of 60-70 years). Other malignant tumors of the large bowel include CTs and, rarely, malignant lymphomas and (anal) melanomas. As in the small intestine, stromal tumors occasionally occur.

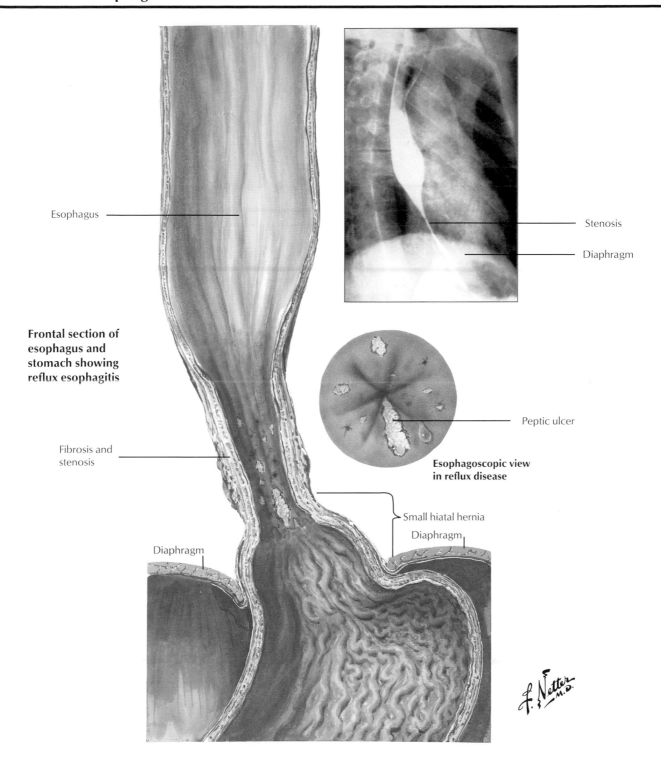

Esophagus

Stenosis

Diaphragm

Frontal section of esophagus and stomach showing reflux esophagitis

Peptic ulcer

Esophagoscopic view in reflux disease

Fibrosis and stenosis

Small hiatal hernia

Diaphragm

Diaphragm

FIGURE 4-1 ESOPHAGITIS

Esophagitis, which affects up to 20% of people in developed countries, is usually caused by gastric reflux (**reflux esophagitis**). Reflux esophagitis follows a "chemical" irritation by gastric fluids containing acid and pepsin (**peptic esophagitis**), which is secondary to improper closure of the lower esophageal sphincter. The tonus of the lower esophageal sphincter may be decreased by hiatal hernia of the stomach; voluminous intake of fatty foods; increased chocolate, alcohol, or nicotine consumption; hormonal factors (estrogen therapy, pregnancy); or treatment with central nervous system (CNS) depressants such as diazepam or opiates. Pathologically, acute reflux esophagitis shows hyperemia and mild degenerative changes such as ballooning of epithelial cells, occasional mild superficial erosion, and occasionally eosinophilic (rarely neutrophilic) infiltration. Chronic disease results in fibrosis and stenosis.

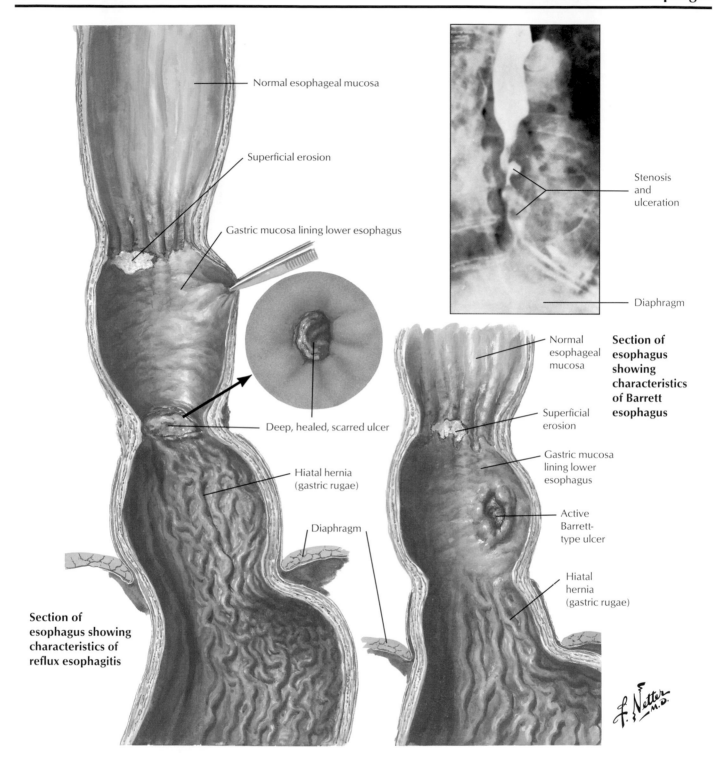

Normal esophageal mucosa

Superficial erosion

Gastric mucosa lining lower esophagus

Stenosis and ulceration

Diaphragm

Deep, healed, scarred ulcer

Hiatal hernia (gastric rugae)

Diaphragm

Section of esophagus showing characteristics of reflux esophagitis

Normal esophageal mucosa

Section of esophagus showing characteristics of Barrett esophagus

Superficial erosion

Gastric mucosa lining lower esophagus

Active Barrett-type ulcer

Hiatal hernia (gastric rugae)

FIGURE 4-2   CHRONIC REFLUX ESOPHAGITIS AND BARRETT ESOPHAGUS

Chronic reflux esophagitis is classified into stages of severity. Stage I is characterized by epithelial hyperplasia and keratosis (clinical finding: leukoplakia) with sparse submucosal lymphocytic infiltrate. Stage II resembles stage I, with the addition of superficial erosion and neutrophilic infiltration. Stage III resembles stage II, with epithelial ulceration and more pronounced epithelial regeneration (elongated epithelial papillae). Complications of chronic reflux esophagitis include fibrous scarring and stenosis, mucosal metaplasia, and cancer. **Barrett esophagus** (BE) is the focal replacement of stratified squamous epithelium by metaplastic columnar epithelium with goblet cells. BE appears grossly as velvety, pink islands of mucosa in the lower third of the esophagus. Besides the intestinal-type mucosa, gastric mucosal elements (cardia- or fundus-type glands, including parietal and chief cells) are frequent. BE is associated with a greatly increased incidence of adenocarcinoma.

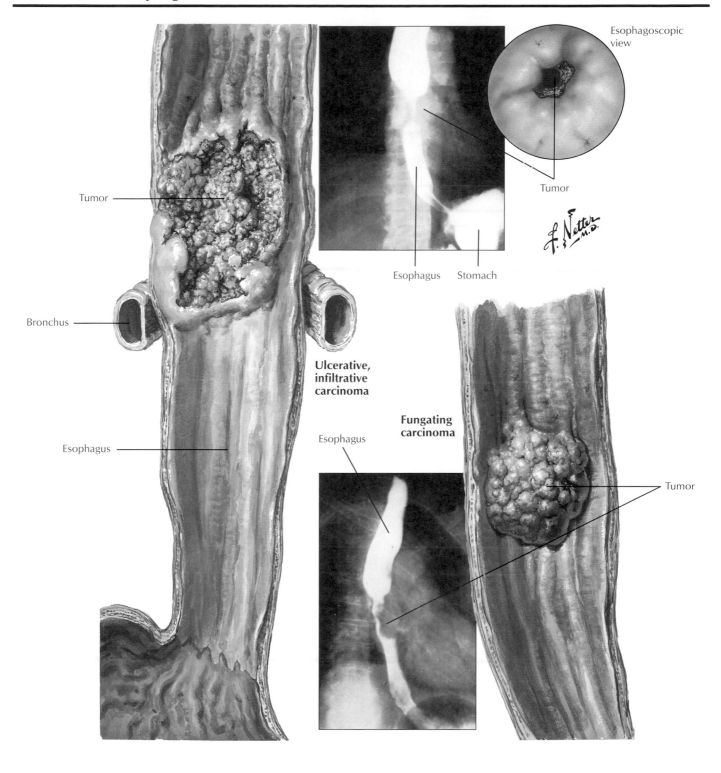

Tumor

Esophagoscopic view

Tumor

Esophagus   Stomach

Bronchus

Ulcerative, infiltrative carcinoma

Esophagus

Fungating carcinoma

Esophagus

Tumor

FIGURE 4-3   ESOPHAGEAL CANCER: SQUAMOUS CELL CARCINOMA

Malignant neoplasms of the esophagus account for up to 2% of cancer deaths in the United States annually. Certain ill-defined genetic predispositions, exposure to food carcinogens (e.g., nitrosamines), tobacco smoke, chronic alcoholism, and chronic esophagitis (especially with BE) seem to be important pathogenetic factors. Loss of p53 tumor suppressor gene function is one of the most frequently observed molecular changes in esophageal cancer. **Squamous cell carcinoma** usually impresses as a

plaquelike or fungating white lesion in the upper or medial part of the esophagus. The tumor infiltrates the esophageal wall deeply, penetrates into the mediastinum, and spreads via lymphatic channels. Invasion of the bronchial tree may occur with fistulation. Severe dysphagia and anorexia cause pronounced cachexia. The 5-year survival rate is 10% for patients with squamous cell carcinoma.

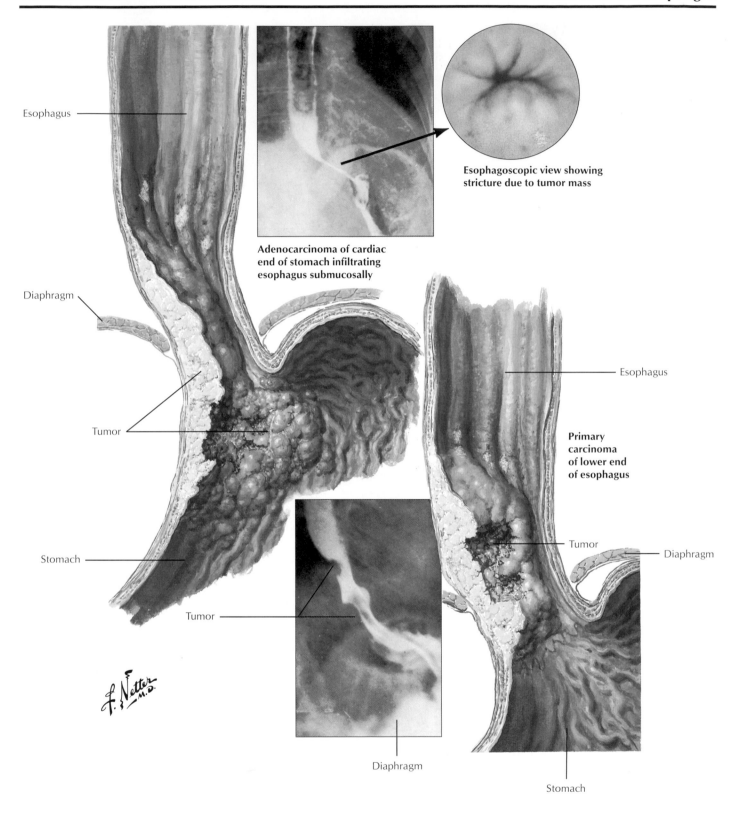

Esophagus

Esophagoscopic view showing
stricture due to tumor mass

Adenocarcinoma of cardiac
end of stomach infiltrating
esophagus submucosally

Diaphragm

Esophagus

Tumor

Primary
carcinoma
of lower end
of esophagus

Tumor

Diaphragm

Stomach

Tumor

Diaphragm

Stomach

FIGURE 4-4   ESOPHAGEAL CANCER: ADENOCARCINOMA

Adenocarcinomas, which account for 25% of cases of esophageal cancer, are pinkish elevated or ulcerative lesions in the lower third of the esophagus. Ulcerative lesions may appear as direct extensions of lesions in the gastric cardia. Onset is usually insidious, and tumors develop slowly. Dysphagia, weight loss, anorexia, and fatigue are the most common symptoms. Surgical removal of the tumor is frequently incomplete because of the early and extensive local metastases within the gastroesophageal wall and into the mediastinum. Even with surgery, the 5-year survival rate is 20% for patients with adenocarcinoma.

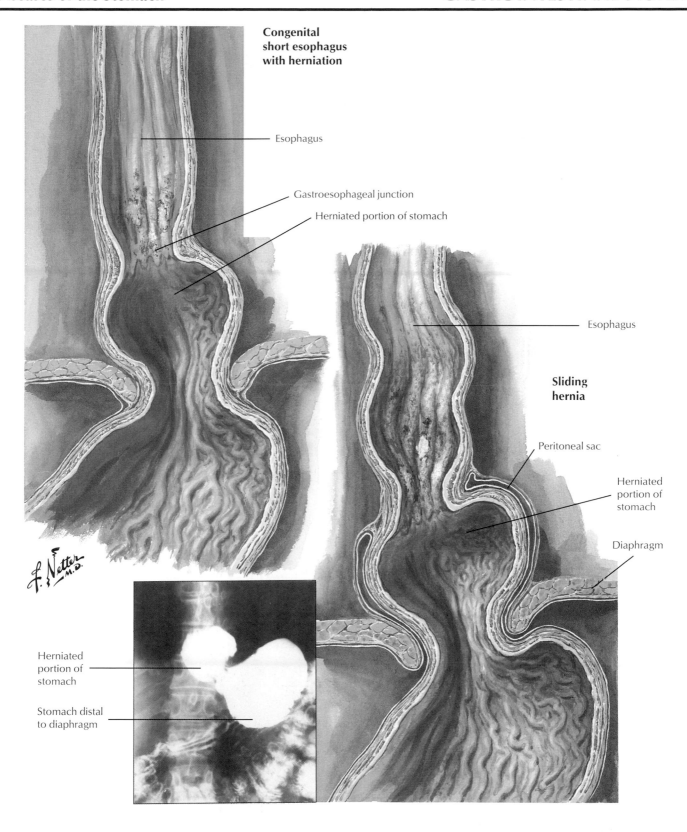

Congenital
short esophagus
with herniation

Esophagus

Gastroesophageal junction

Herniated portion of stomach

Esophagus

Sliding
hernia

Peritoneal sac

Herniated
portion of
stomach

Diaphragm

Herniated
portion of
stomach

Stomach distal
to diaphragm

FIGURE 4-5 GASTRIC HERNIA

There are 2 types of gastric herniation (**hiatal hernia**) into the thoracic space: sliding (axial) hernias and paraesophageal (nonaxial) hernias. **Sliding hernia** constitutes approximately 95% of hiatal hernias. Systematic radiologic studies reveal sliding hernias in up to 20% of the population, only approximately half of which are symptomatic. Symptoms consist of heartburn and regurgitation of gastric contents and subsequent reflux esophagitis. **Paraesophageal hernia** causes strangulation of parts or all of the stomach incarcerated above the diaphragm. Surgical correction should be considered for both types of hernia.

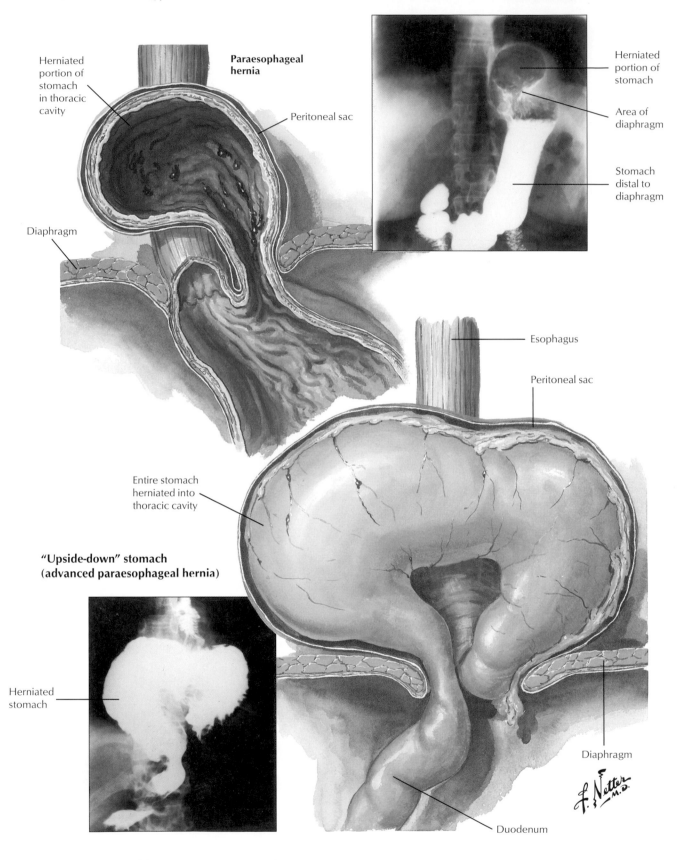

Paraesophageal hernia

Herniated portion of stomach in thoracic cavity

Peritoneal sac

Diaphragm

Herniated portion of stomach

Area of diaphragm

Stomach distal to diaphragm

Esophagus

Peritoneal sac

Entire stomach herniated into thoracic cavity

"Upside-down" stomach (advanced paraesophageal hernia)

Herniated stomach

Diaphragm

Duodenum

FIGURE 4-5 GASTRIC HERNIA (CONTINUED)

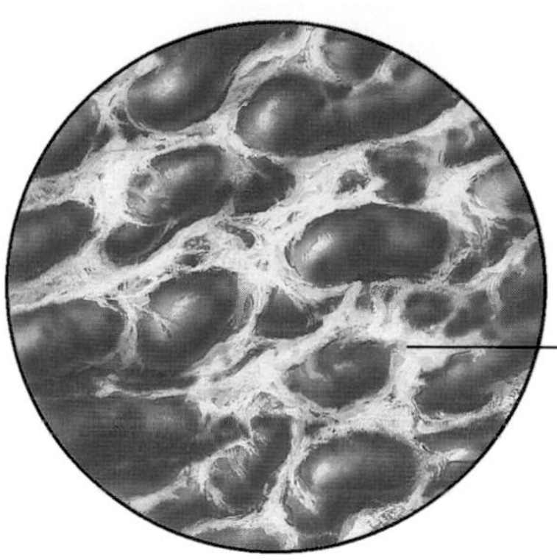

Acute gastritis
(gastroscopic view)

Superficial erosions

TABLE 4-2   HISTOLOGIC CLASSIFICATION OF GASTRITIS

Type of Gastritis	Histologic Features	Course
Common acute gastritis	Mucosal edema Neutrophilic infiltration with or without erosions Petechiae with or without mild lymphoplasmacytic infiltration Epithelial regeneration in neck region of glands	Usually transient
Eosinophilic gastritis	Eosinophilic infiltrates of all layers, frequently with muscular hypertrophy	Incidental or recurrent (may be related to allergies or ingestion of chemical irritants)
Chronic type B gastritis (more common)	Superficial lymphoplasmacellular infiltrate Neutrophils if erosive, with or without lymph follicles Colonization by *Helicobacter pylori* Elongation of glandular necks with epithelial regeneration Intestinal metaplasia in late phase	Chronic persistent or recurrent May predispose to carcinoma or lymphoma
Chronic type A gastritis	Patchy lymphocytic infiltrate with invasion of crypt epithelia and epithelial degeneration Loss of acidophilic cells Intestinal metaplasia	Chronic aggressive Decreased vitamin B_{12} resorption may predispose to cancer*

*Decreased vitamin B_{12} resorption is followed by various B_{12} deficiency diseases, such as pernicious anemia, spinal cord demyelination, and others.

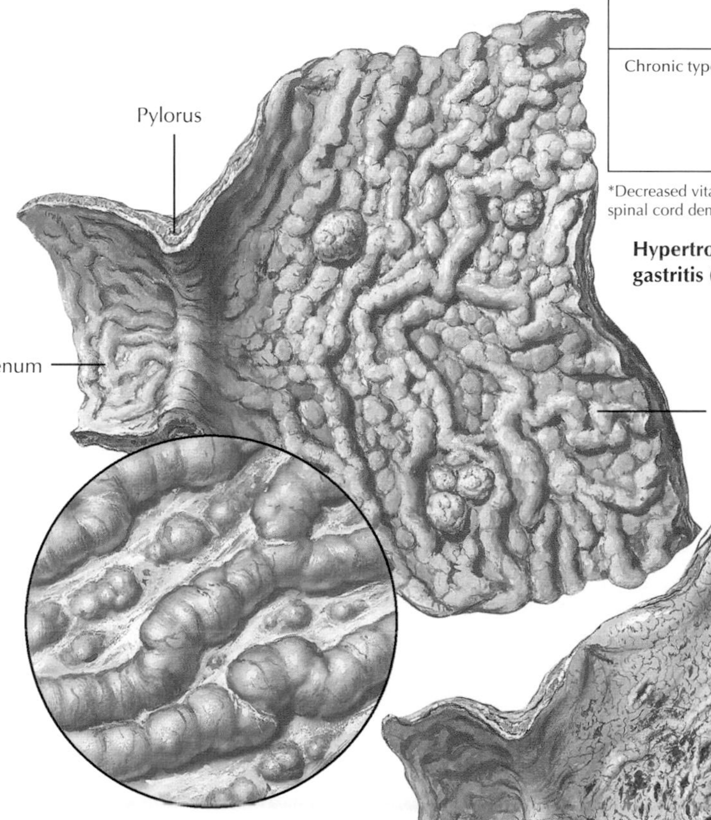

Pylorus

Duodenum

Hypertrophic gastritis (e.g., in alcoholism)

Stomach

Gastroscopic view

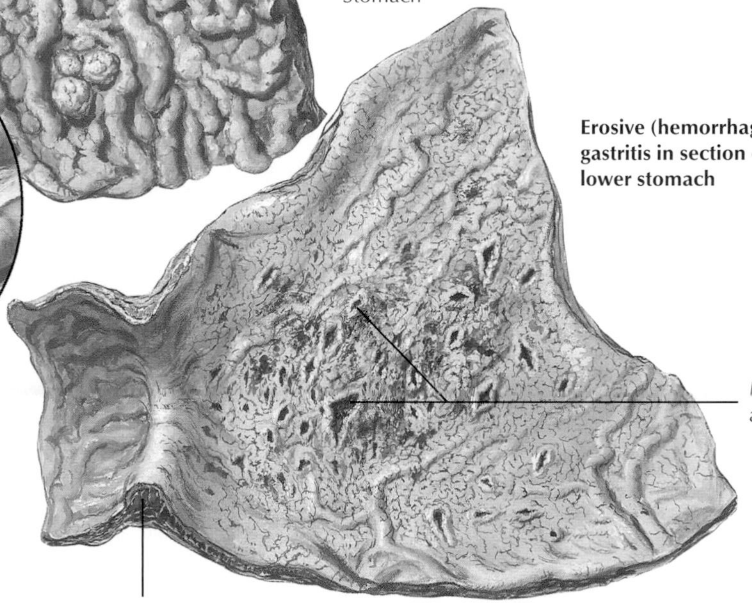

Erosive (hemorrhagic) gastritis in section of lower stomach

Multiple erosions and stress ulcers

Pylorus

FIGURE 4-6   GASTRITIS

Gastritis is the most common cause of upper abdominal pain in adults. Gastroscopy differentiates the gross features of acute gastritis, erosive gastritis, hypertrophic gastritis, and chronic (atrophic) gastritis. Biopsy and pathologic investigation offer a more exact classification of pathogenesis and prognosis (Table 4-2). Acute gastritis is usually caused by chemical irritation by alcohol, cigarette smoke, or drugs (e.g., aspirin, nonsteroidal antiinflammatory drugs, chemotherapeutics), uremia, or suicidal ingestion of acids or alkali. Severe stress can cause acute gastritis with erosion and ulceration (**"stress ulcer"**). Systemic infections, shock involving the stomach, loss of pyloric function (e.g., after surgery) or duodenobiliary reflux can initiate acute gastritis. Infection with *Helicobacter pylori* accounts for 50% to 80% of cases of chronic type B gastritis. Chronic type A gastritis, an autoimmune gastritis, may occur alone or accompany other autoimmune disorders (thyroiditis, insulin-dependent diabetes mellitus, Addison disease).

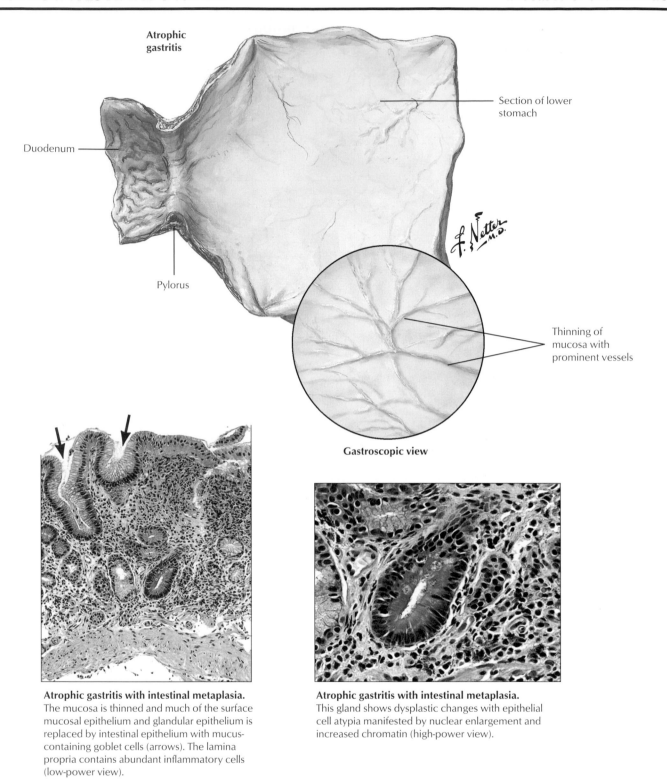

Atrophic
gastritis

Section of lower
stomach

Duodenum

Pylorus

Thinning of
mucosa with
prominent vessels

Gastroscopic view

Atrophic gastritis with intestinal metaplasia.
The mucosa is thinned and much of the surface
mucosal epithelium and glandular epithelium is
replaced by intestinal epithelium with mucus-
containing goblet cells (arrows). The lamina
propria contains abundant inflammatory cells
(low-power view).

Atrophic gastritis with intestinal metaplasia.
This gland shows dysplastic changes with epithelial
cell atypia manifested by nuclear enlargement and
increased chromatin (high-power view).

FIGURE 4-7 ATROPHIC GASTRITIS

The pathologic term **atrophic gastritis** is reserved for chronic
gastritis with intestinal metaplasia (i.e., specific crypts of the
gastric corpus are replaced by intestinal glands with goblet cells).
Glandular necks are markedly elongated with extended epithelial
regeneration involving surface epithelia and increasing amounts

of dysplastic glands and epithelial atypia. Patients with atrophic
gastritis have the highest risk of developing gastric cancer. Table
4-2 summarizes the histologic features and the courses of various
types of gastritis.

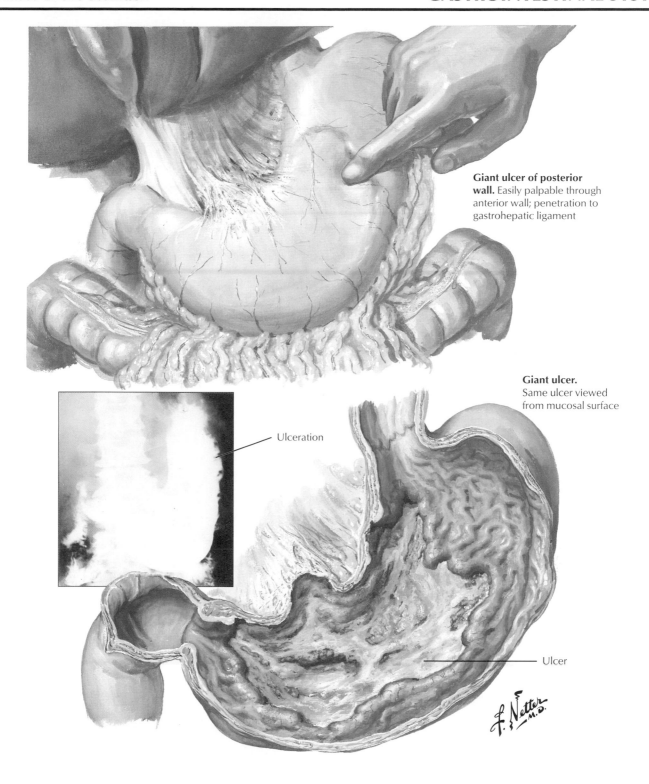

Giant ulcer of posterior wall. Easily palpable through anterior wall; penetration to gastrohepatic ligament

Giant ulcer. Same ulcer viewed from mucosal surface

Ulceration

Ulcer

FIGURE 4-8   PEPTIC ULCERS

Peptic ulcers (PUs) of the stomach or duodenum represent approximately 98% of ulcerations in this region. PUs are usually chronic, whereas the less common "stress ulcers," which may accompany extensive burns, severe trauma, or other situations of excessive stress or the administration of certain drugs (corticosteroids), are acute. The pathogenesis of PU includes excessive action of gastric acid and pepsin, reduced mucosal defense mechanisms (e.g., reduced mucus production, reduced epithelial regeneration such as in tobacco smoking), and, frequently, infection with *H pylori*. PUs require treatment because of the possibility of complications, including acute or chronic hemorrhage and anemia, perforation, chronic scarring and stenosis (e.g., in pyloric or postpyloric ulcers), penetration into adjacent organs (e.g., into the pancreas with subsequent pancreatitis), and development of carcinoma within the regenerating mucosa adjacent to the ulcer.

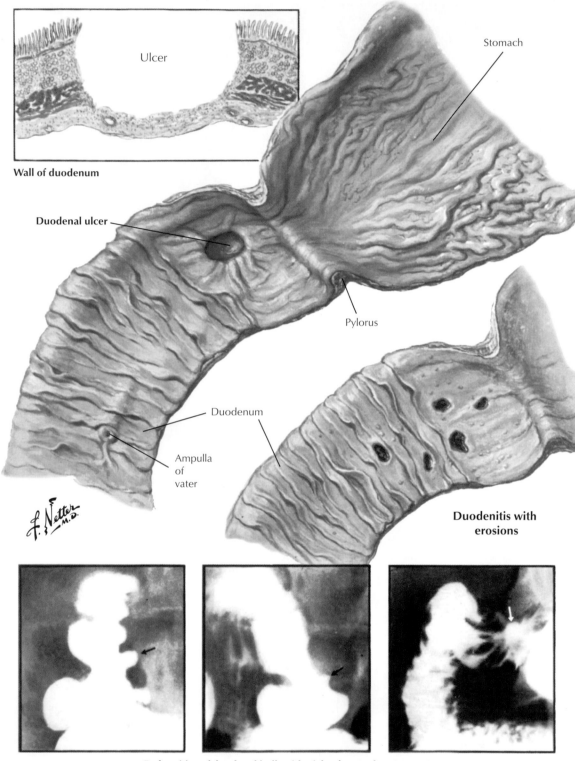

Ulcer

Wall of duodenum

Stomach

Duodenal ulcer

Pylorus

Duodenum

Ampulla of vater

Duodenitis with erosions

Deformities of duodenal bulb with niche due to ulcer (arrows)

FIGURE 4-9   DUODENAL ULCERS

Duodenal ulcers are usually located in the anterior or posterior wall of the bulbus and occur secondary to hyperacidification. The mucosa in this area is especially sensitive to acid juices. The pathogenesis and complications of duodenal ulcers resemble those of stomach ulcers, although malignant transformation to cancer is rare.

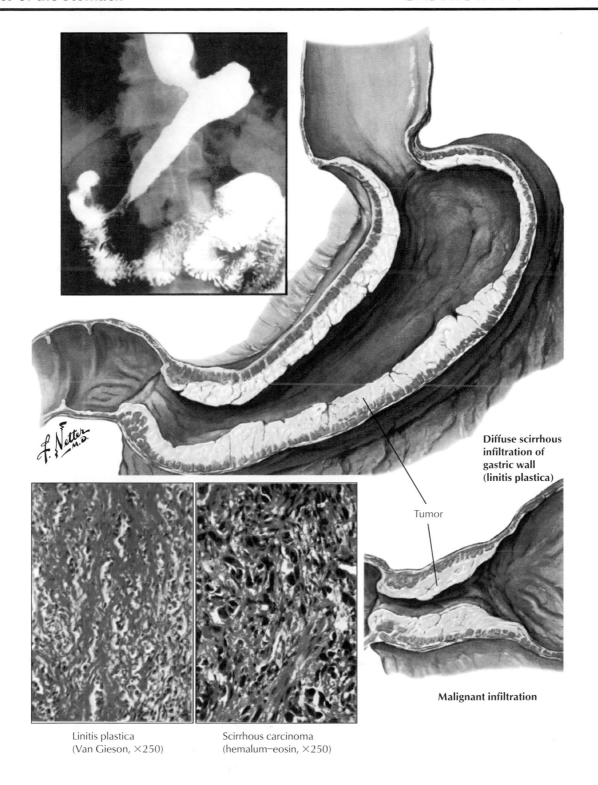

Diffuse scirrhous infiltration of gastric wall (linitis plastica)

Tumor

Malignant infiltration

Linitis plastica
(Van Gieson, ×250)

Scirrhous carcinoma
(hemalum–eosin, ×250)

FIGURE 4-10 CARCINOMAS OF THE STOMACH

Carcinomas of the stomach are among the most common tumors in the Western world and Japan. Approximately 50% develop in the antrum or pyloric region, approximately 25% develop in the corpus, and 25% develop in the fundus. Most tumors are located in the lesser curvature. Their gross features vary from mucosal flattening and thickening with erosions to diffuse thickening of the gastric wall (**linitis plastica**), to large ulcers or polypoid-fungating masses. Stomach carcinomas are classified as type I: protruding nodular or polypoid lesion; type II: slightly elevated or depressed flat lesion; and type III: excavated or ulcerated lesion. There are 2 main histologic types of classic carcinoma of the stomach: the intestinal type with tubular glands, which simulates atypical intestinal mucosa, and the diffuse type with extensive mucus production by signet ring cells (signet ring cell carcinoma and linitis plastica including also less mature cells). Polypoid adenocarcinomas are found in the cardia and in rare preexistent adenomas.

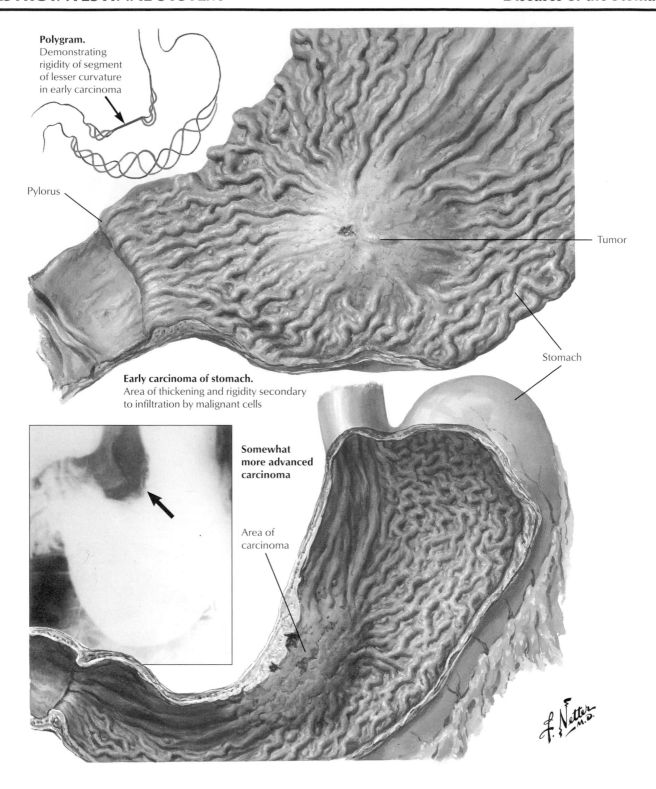

Polygram. Demonstrating rigidity of segment of lesser curvature in early carcinoma

Pylorus

Tumor

Stomach

Early carcinoma of stomach. Area of thickening and rigidity secondary to infiltration by malignant cells

Somewhat more advanced carcinoma

Area of carcinoma

FIGURE 4-11   EARLY GASTRIC CANCER

Early gastric cancer is a pathologic term for a tumor confined to mucosa or submucosa. It is generally asymptomatic and is detected only by chance. Patients with this tumor have a 10-year survival rate of 95% after surgical intervention; patients with other stomach tumors have a combined survival rate of only 20%. Advanced gastric cancer also may be clinically occult except for undefined abdominal discomfort and weight loss. Large tumors in the prepyloric area may cause obstruction. Acute massive bleeding, even in ulcerated tumors, is uncommon, whereas chronic bleeding with significant anemia is frequently observed.

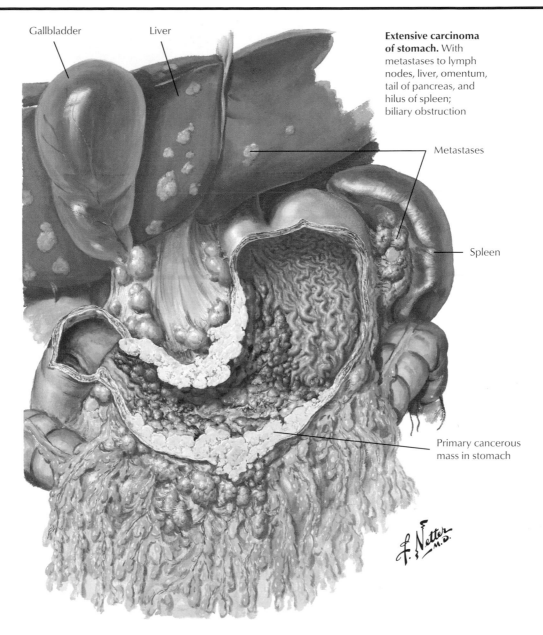

Extensive carcinoma of stomach. With metastases to lymph nodes, liver, omentum, tail of pancreas, and hilus of spleen; biliary obstruction

Gallbladder — Liver

Metastases

Spleen

Primary cancerous mass in stomach

TABLE 4-3   PATHOGENESIS OF CARCINOMA OF THE STOMACH

Factors	Prevalence and Examples
Nutritional factors	Apparently account for geographic variations in cancer incidence: large amounts of smoked fish, pickled vegetables, highly salted foods; diets low in fruits and vegetables (i.e., in protective antioxidants) Identified carcinogens: nitrosamines, benzpyrene
Infections	Chronic *Helicobacter pylori* infection as cofactor (see above)
Genetic factors	Approximately half of cancer patients possess blood group A No clearcut genetic traits identified Changes in tumor suppressor gene activity (e.g., p53), germline mutations, and genetic mismatch repair similar to cancer of the colon (see there)
Other factors	Low socioeconomic status (probably related to nutritional factors and infection)

FIGURE 4-12   SPREAD OF GASTRIC CARCINOMAS

All **gastric carcinomas** spread by direct extension to nearby organs or metastasize via lymphatic channels and the bloodstream. Even in early cancer, there is a 5% risk of regional lymphatic metastases at the time of initial tumor diagnosis. The most common sites of metastasis are lymph nodes at the lesser or greater curvature of the stomach, in the subpyloric region, and in the porta hepatis. More distant metastases involve the left supraclavicular lymph nodes (**Virchow node**), the lungs, the bone marrow, and the ovaries (**Krukenberg tumor**). The etiology and pathogenesis of gastric cancer are reviewed in Table 4-3.

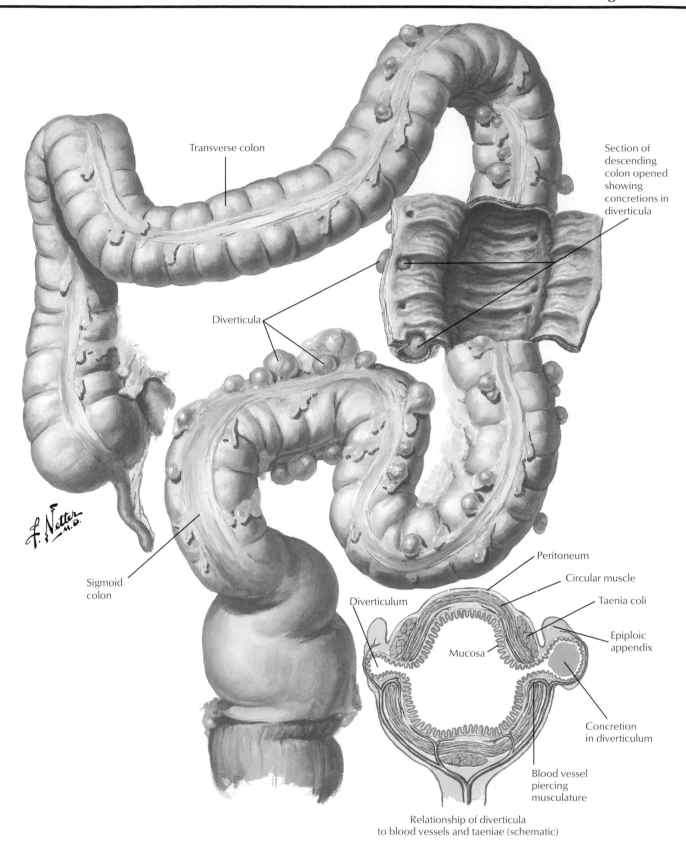

Transverse colon

Section of descending colon opened showing concretions in diverticula

Diverticula

Sigmoid colon

Peritoneum

Circular muscle

Taenia coli

Diverticulum

Epiploic appendix

Mucosa

Concretion in diverticulum

Blood vessel piercing musculature

Relationship of diverticula to blood vessels and taeniae (schematic)

FIGURE 4-13   DIVERTICULOSIS OF THE COLON

Diverticulosis of the colon is a herniation of the colonic mucosa and submucosa through the intestinal muscular wall, with cystic expansion in the adventitial tissue. In Western countries, it affects up to half of persons older than 60 years. Diverticulosis is found most often in the sigmoid colon, although it may affect any part of the intestine. **Diverticula**, which develop at sites of weakness in the muscle wall of the intestine (sites of vascular and nerve penetrations), are secondary to increased colon pressure

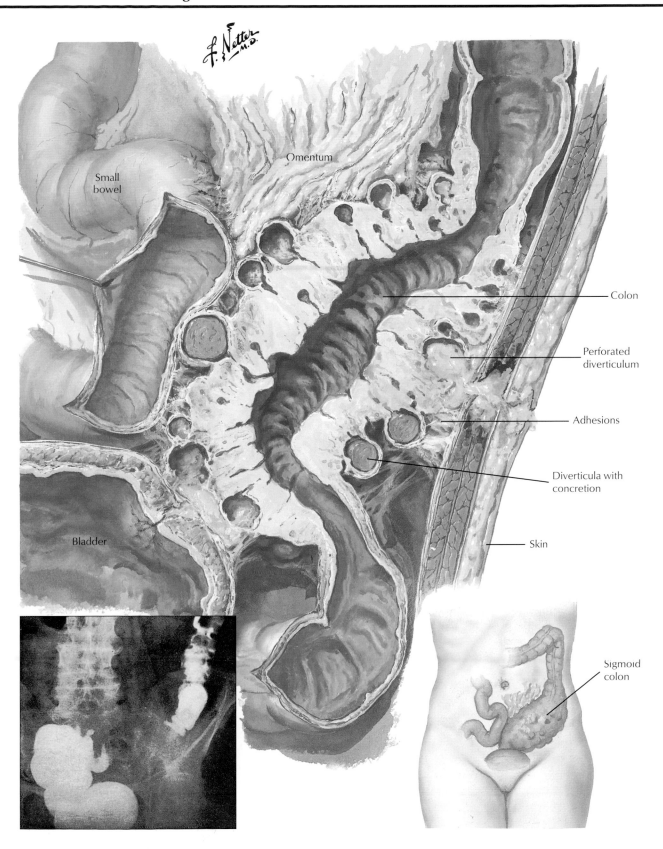

FIGURE 4-13   DIVERTICULOSIS OF THE COLON *(CONTINUED)*

(enhanced peristaltic contractions) induced by a low-fiber diet. Gross bleeding or subclinical chronic bleeding from the diverticula may occur, especially in elderly persons. Stasis of feces in the diverticula is followed by recurrent inflammation (**diverticuli-** **tis**) with adhesions, occasional intestinal distortion, and obstruction. Inflamed diverticula can perforate and induce life-threatening fecal peritonitis. In advanced cases, surgical correction may be necessary.

TABLE 4-4 PATHOGENESIS OF MALABSORPTION SYNDROMES*

Major Cause of MAS	Specific Disturbance
Defective intraluminal digestion	Deficiency in bile or pancreaticenzymes or both
	Inactivation of pancreatic enzymes by excess gastric acid
	Disturbed resorption by bacterial overgrowth
Defective intestinal digestion	Deficiency in hydrolytic enzymes and peptidases secondary to bacterial overgrowth with mucosal atrophy
Defective transepithelial transport	Abetalipoproteinemia
Reduction in resorptive surface	Gluten-sensitive enteropathy (celiac sprue)
	Crohn disease
	After surgery (gastrectomy, bypass, short bowel)
Specific infections	Whipple disease
	Tropical sprue
	Parasitic infestations
	Tuberculosis
Malignancies	Intestinal lymphoma (IPSID)

*IPSID indicates immunoproliferative small intestinal disease; MAS, malabsorption syndrome.

Physical Findings

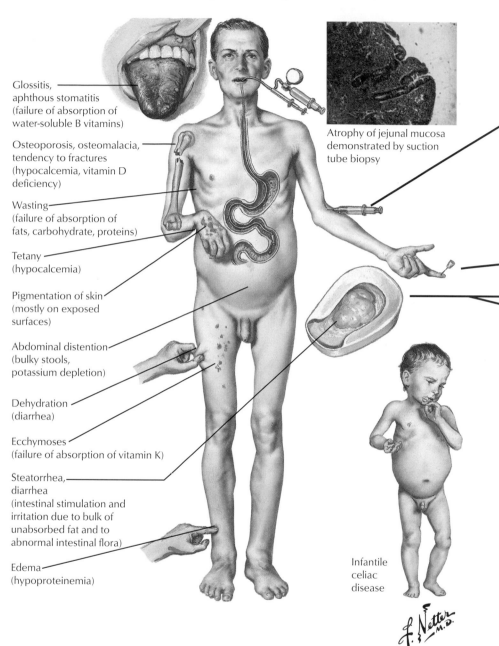

Glossitis, aphthous stomatitis (failure of absorption of water-soluble B vitamins)

Osteoporosis, osteomalacia, tendency to fractures (hypocalcemia, vitamin D deficiency)

Wasting (failure of absorption of fats, carbohydrate, proteins)

Tetany (hypocalcemia)

Pigmentation of skin (mostly on exposed surfaces)

Abdominal distention (bulky stools, potassium depletion)

Dehydration (diarrhea)

Ecchymoses (failure of absorption of vitamin K)

Steatorrhea, diarrhea (intestinal stimulation and irritation due to bulk of unabsorbed fat and to abnormal intestinal flora)

Edema (hypoproteinemia)

Atrophy of jejunal mucosa demonstrated by suction tube biopsy

Infantile celiac disease

FIGURE 4-14 MALABSORPTION SYNDROME

Malabsorption syndrome (MAS) is characterized by the failure of the intestinal mucosa to absorb nutrients from food. It results from insufficient digestion (luminal and intestinal phases) or transepithelial transport. MAS is a heterogeneous syndrome that can result from a variety of disorders (Table 4-4). Most commonly, MAS results from chronic pancreatitis, **Crohn disease**, or celiac sprue. Histologically, **celiac sprue** appears as villous atrophy in the upper small intestine with elongation and arborization of glandular crypts, atrophic and regenerative epithelial changes, mild neutrophilic infiltration, and an increase in immunoglobulin (Ig) G– or IgM-containing plasma cells or both. **Whipple disease**, in which the intestinal mucosa contains large accumulations of periodic acid-Schiff (PAS) reaction–positive macrophages packed with rod-shaped bacilli, is also associated with clinical

Laboratory Findings

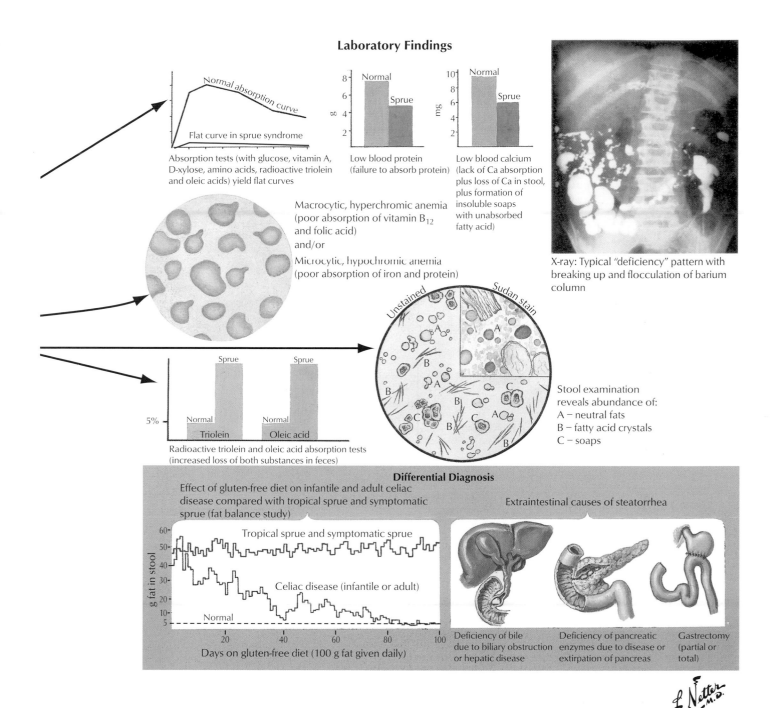

Absorption tests (with glucose, vitamin A, D-xylose, amino acids, radioactive triolein and oleic acids) yield flat curves

Low blood protein (failure to absorb protein)

Low blood calcium (lack of Ca absorption plus loss of Ca in stool, plus formation of insoluble soaps with unabsorbed fatty acid)

Macrocytic, hyperchromic anemia (poor absorption of vitamin B$_{12}$ and folic acid) and/or

Microcytic, hypochromic anemia (poor absorption of iron and protein)

X-ray: Typical "deficiency" pattern with breaking up and flocculation of barium column

Radioactive triolein and oleic acid absorption tests (increased loss of both substances in feces)

Stool examination reveals abundance of:
A – neutral fats
B – fatty acid crystals
C – soaps

Differential Diagnosis

Effect of gluten-free diet on infantile and adult celiac disease compared with tropical sprue and symptomatic sprue (fat balance study)

Days on gluten-free diet (100 g fat given daily)

Extraintestinal causes of steatorrhea

Deficiency of bile due to biliary obstruction or hepatic disease

Deficiency of pancreatic enzymes due to disease or extirpation of pancreas

Gastrectomy (partial or total)

FIGURE 4-14   MALABSORPTION SYNDROME *(CONTINUED)*

malabsorption. The presentation of MAS is determined by the deficits in nonabsorbed nutrients. General symptoms of weight loss, anorexia, and abdominal distention are combined with specific deficiencies of nutrients such as vitamin B$_{12}$ or folic acid (megaloblastic anemia), vitamin K deficiency (bleeding with petechiae), vitamin D and calcium deficiency (osteomalacia,

tetany), vitamin A deficiency (hyperkeratoses and dermatitis), protein deficiencies (edema, malnutrition), and zinc deficiency (dermatitis and immune defects). Stools are bulky, yellowish gray, and greasy. Treatment, clinical course, and prognosis are based on the primary disorder.

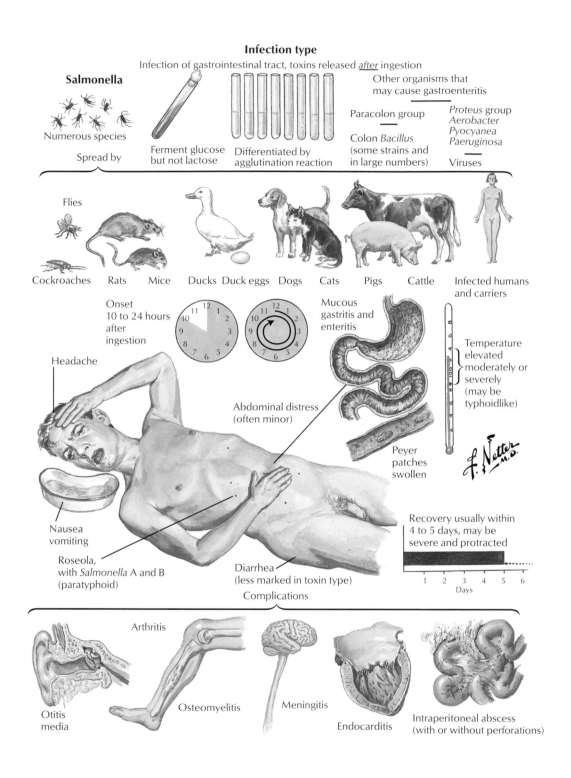

Infection type

Infection of gastrointestinal tract, toxins released *after* ingestion

Salmonella

Numerous species

Spread by

Ferment glucose but not lactose

Differentiated by agglutination reaction

Other organisms that may cause gastroenteritis

Paracolon group

Colon *Bacillus* (some strains and in large numbers)

Proteus group
Aerobacter
Pyocyanea
Paeruginosa

Viruses

Flies

Cockroaches   Rats   Mice   Ducks   Duck eggs   Dogs   Cats   Pigs   Cattle   Infected humans and carriers

Onset 10 to 24 hours after ingestion

Headache

Mucous gastritis and enteritis

Abdominal distress (often minor)

Temperature elevated moderately or severely (may be typhoidlike)

Peyer patches swollen

Nausea vomiting

Roseola, with *Salmonella* A and B (paratyphoid)

Diarrhea (less marked in toxin type)

Recovery usually within 4 to 5 days, may be severe and protracted

1 2 3 4 5 6
Days

Complications

Otitis media

Arthritis

Osteomyelitis

Meningitis

Endocarditis

Intraperitoneal abscess (with or without perforations)

FIGURE 4-15   FOOD POISONING

Food poisoning is an acute diarrheal GI disease that follows the ingestion of contaminated food. It is caused by colonization of the GI tract with pathogenic organisms released after ingestion of contaminated food (infection type), by toxins produced in food

before ingestion (toxin type), or by a combination of both. The infection type affects the small intestine preferentially. Most cases of food poisoning resolve in 1 to 5 days, except for those caused by *Clostridium botulinum,* which is frequently lethal within 5

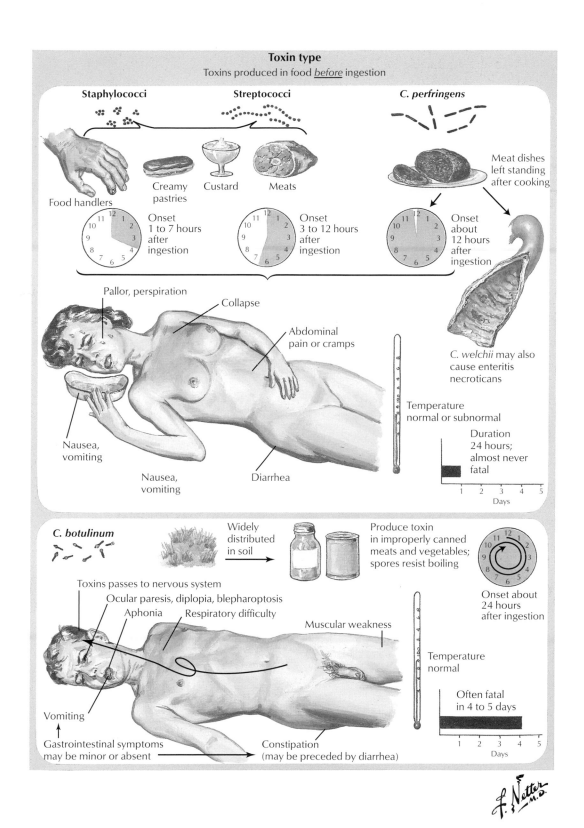

FIGURE 4-15 FOOD POISONING (CONTINUED)

days. Infection with enterotoxic *E. coli* and with *Salmonella* species (especially in older persons) may cause more frequent deaths. *Salmonella* organisms may persist in asymptomatic carriers after resolution of the acute enteric disease and become the source of future food poisoning cases.

Bacillary Dysentery (Shigellosis)

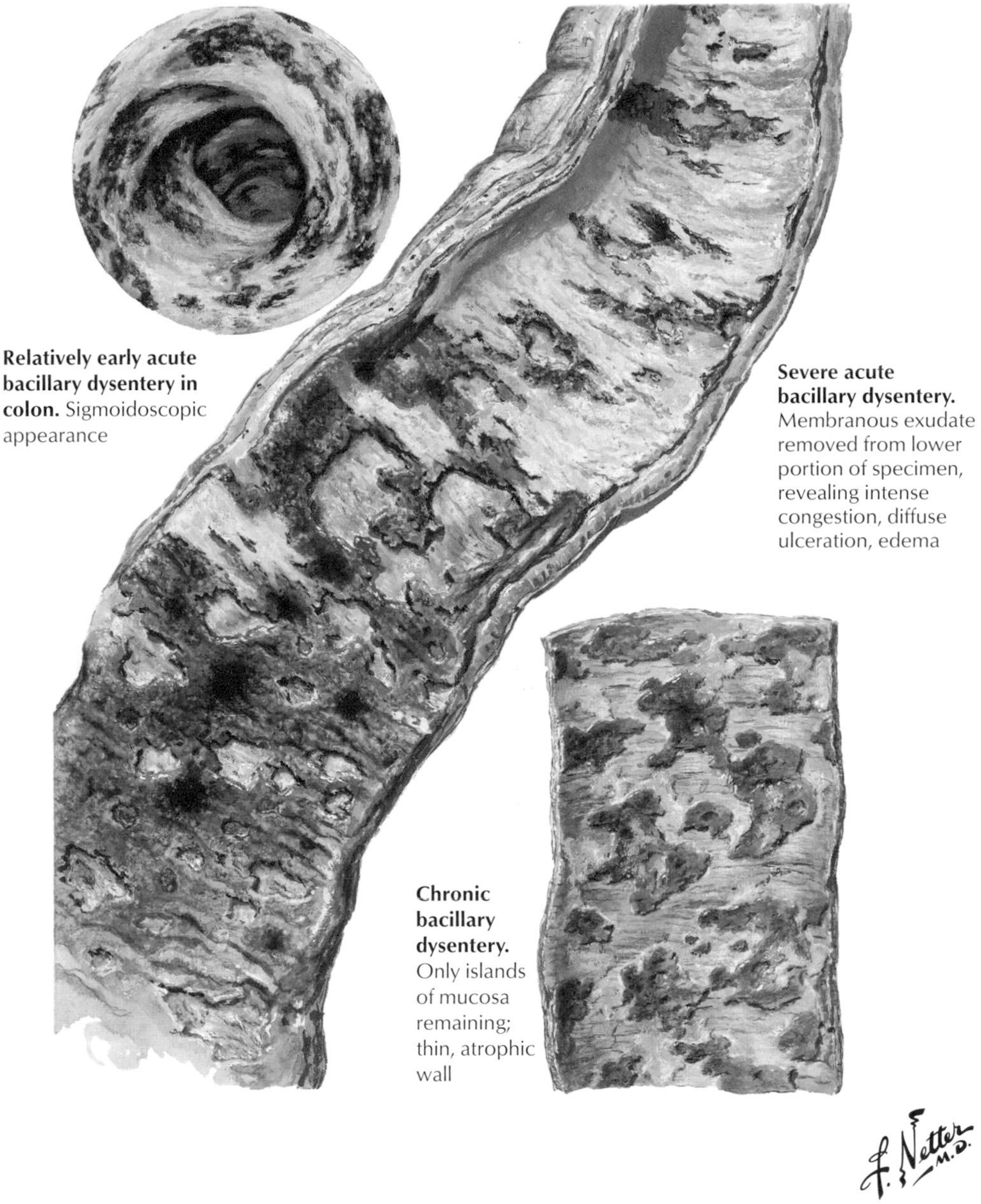

Relatively early acute bacillary dysentery in colon. Sigmoidoscopic appearance

Severe acute bacillary dysentery. Membranous exudate removed from lower portion of specimen, revealing intense congestion, diffuse ulceration, edema

Chronic bacillary dysentery. Only islands of mucosa remaining; thin, atrophic wall

FIGURE 4-16   SHIGELLOSIS

Shigellosis, an **enterocolitis**, is caused by infection with *Shigella* organisms. These organisms produce either potent exotoxins, which cause acute disease (*S. kruse*) or endotoxins, which cause insidious onset of chronic disease (*S. flexner, S. sonnei*). The incubation period is usually short (2–4 days). Pathologic lesions in the large intestine consist of irregular patchy pseudomembranous colitis (i.e., fibrinopurulent inflammation with superficial erosions and eventual ulceration) within a markedly hyperemic mucosa and increased mucus production. Clinical symptoms include frequent bowel movements and diarrhea, colicky pains, and, eventually, bloody stools with mucoid streaks. Prognosis is good when fever and fluid loss are promptly controlled and specific antibiotic/sulfonamide therapy is administered. Occasionally, fulminating toxic and lethal conditions may arise in small children and in the elderly.

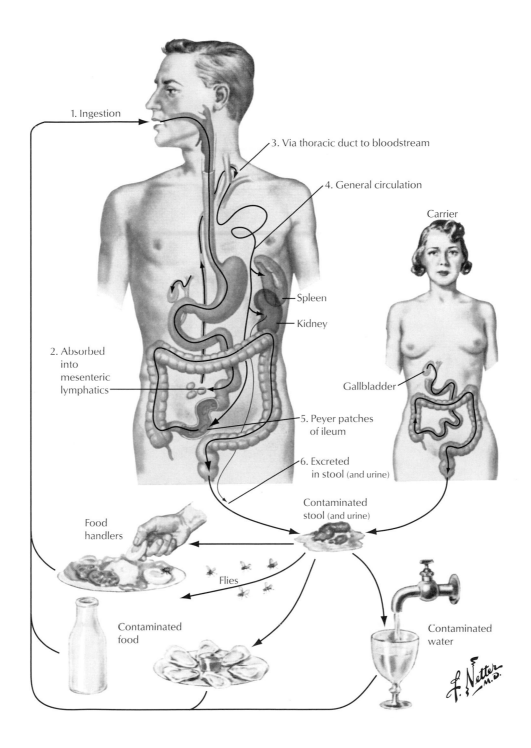

FIGURE 4-17   TYPHOID FEVER

Typhoid fever (TF), which is prevalent in underdeveloped countries but rare in the Western world, is caused by *Salmonella typhi Eberthi*. The common source of infection is bacteria from contaminated meat, milk, or eggs. A brief transient febrile illness with abdominal discomfort ensues, during which the organisms settle in macrophages and lymphoid tissues with respective stimulation of the immune system. The **cyclic infectious disease** phase of TF starts after a latent period of 10 days to 3 weeks, during which bacteria spread via lymphatics and blood and

immunity is established. Bacteria accumulate in intestinal lymphatic tissues, especially in the Peyer patches, which become inflamed and ulcerated. Transient pseudomembranes shaped like Peyer patches cover these ulcers. TF evolves into a systemic infection through the hematogenous spread of organisms. Immunologically induced granulomas develop at the sites of bacterial colonization such as in the spleen, the liver, the bone marrow, and the spine, and hepatosplenomegaly ensues.

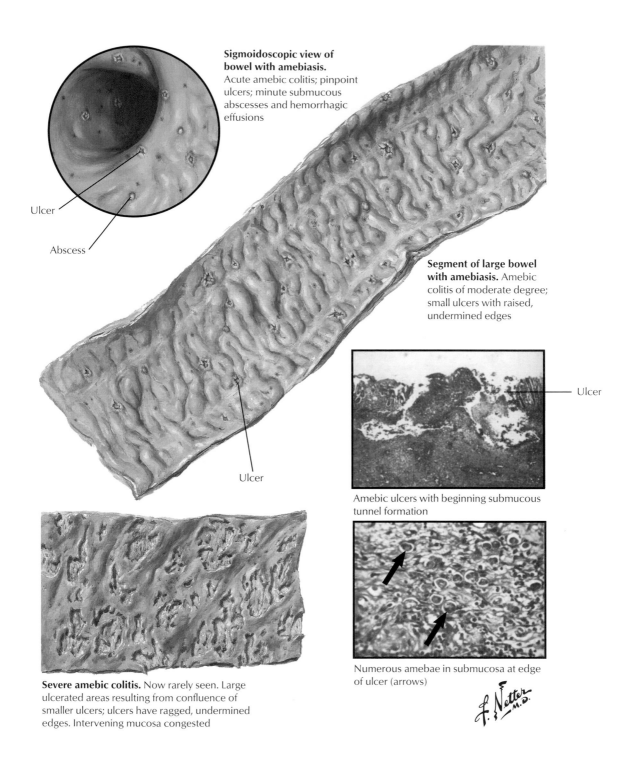

Sigmoidoscopic view of bowel with amebiasis. Acute amebic colitis; pinpoint ulcers; minute submucous abscesses and hemorrhagic effusions

Ulcer

Abscess

Segment of large bowel with amebiasis. Amebic colitis of moderate degree; small ulcers with raised, undermined edges

Ulcer

Ulcer

Ulcer

Amebic ulcers with beginning submucous tunnel formation

Numerous amebae in submucosa at edge of ulcer (arrows)

Severe amebic colitis. Now rarely seen. Large ulcerated areas resulting from confluence of smaller ulcers; ulcers have ragged, undermined edges. Intervening mucosa congested

---

FIGURE 4-18   AMEBIASIS

Protozoal infection by *Entamoeba histolytica* (amebiasis) causes up to 10% of human intestinal infections. Ingestion of cysts in food or drink contaminated by human fecal materials, including manure-fertilized vegetables, causes the infection. Flies and other insects that feed on human feces transfer the protozoa to foods. **Amebiasis** is marked by ulcerating proctosigmoiditis and **colitis**. Typical colonic ulcers contain many amebae with neutrophilic

reaction and undermining edges. Infection may cause extensive ulcerating lesions with mucoid and puriform, partially bloody discharges, fever, abdominal pain, and severe tenesmus, or it may remain clinically inapparent for a long period. Rarely, the spread of infection via lymph or blood may cause localized abscesses in the liver, in the lung, or in the brain.

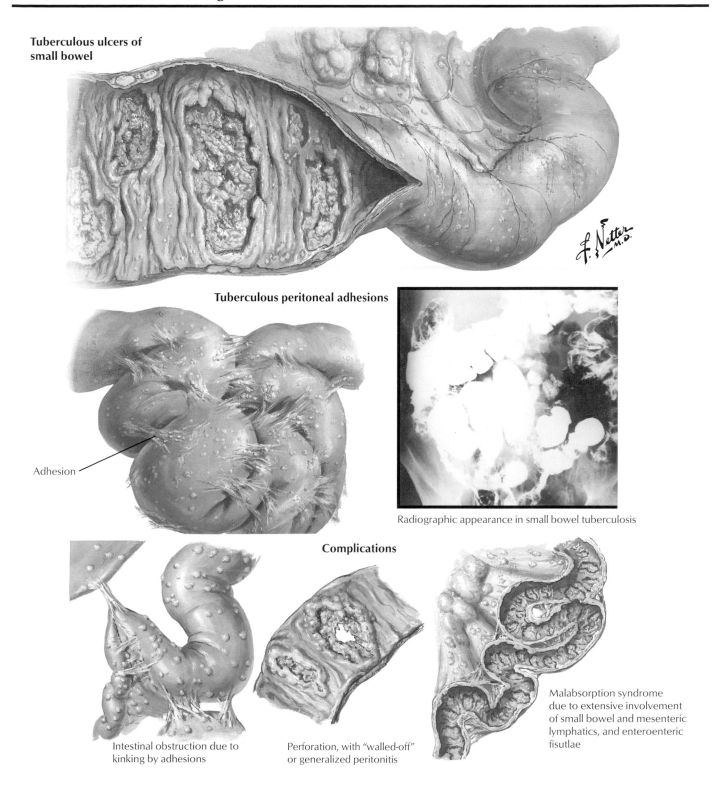

Tuberculous ulcers of small bowel

Tuberculous peritoneal adhesions

Adhesion

Radiographic appearance in small bowel tuberculosis

Complications

Intestinal obstruction due to kinking by adhesions

Perforation, with "walled-off" or generalized peritonitis

Malabsorption syndrome due to extensive involvement of small bowel and mesenteric lymphatics, and enteroenteric fisutlae

FIGURE 4-19   GASTROINTESTINAL TUBERCULOSIS

Gastrointestinal tuberculosis, which follows primary infection of the GI tract with *M. tuberculosis bovinum*, is rare in Western countries. Endoscopy reveals typical tuberculous ulcers (granulomas with caseous necrosis and ulceration) perpendicular to the intestinal axis. Bacterial superinfection with puriform ulcers may blur the characteristic features. Intestinal tuberculosis is accompanied by prominent focal peritoneal fibrosis with subsequent adhesions, shrinkage, bowel obstruction, fecal stasis, and perforation. Lymphatic spread of the infection is followed by multiple small peritoneal granulomas, which add to the peritoneal fibrotic process. Occlusion of intramural and mesenteric lymphatic channels may cause malabsorption. Treatment is a combination of tuberculostatic chemotherapy and surgery.

Oxyuriasis (Pinworm)

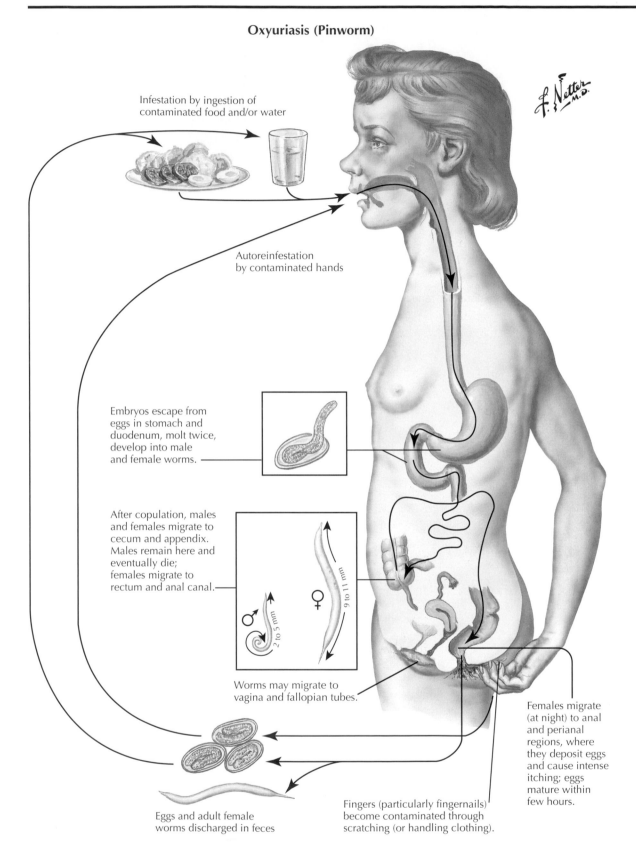

Infestation by ingestion of contaminated food and/or water

Autoreinfestation by contaminated hands

Embryos escape from eggs in stomach and duodenum, molt twice, develop into male and female worms.

After copulation, males and females migrate to cecum and appendix. Males remain here and eventually die; females migrate to rectum and anal canal.

Worms may migrate to vagina and fallopian tubes.

Females migrate (at night) to anal and perianal regions, where they deposit eggs and cause intense itching; eggs mature within few hours.

Fingers (particularly fingernails) become contaminated through scratching (or handling clothing).

Eggs and adult female worms discharged in feces

FIGURE 4-20 PARASITIC DISEASE OF THE GASTROINTESTINAL TRACT

Parasitic disease of the GI tract follows infestation with various worms, including human **whipworm** (*Trichocephalus trichuris*), **intestinal roundworm** (*Ascaris lumbricoides*), **human pinworm** (*Oxyuris vermicularis*), **beef tapeworm** (*Taenia saginata*), and **pork**

tapeworm (*Taenia solium*). The source of infection is contaminated foods with or without an intermediate animal host. **Oxyuriasis** and **cysticercosis** are shown here. Oxyuriasis occurs in children and can be the cause of poor growth and

Cysticercosis (Tapeworm)

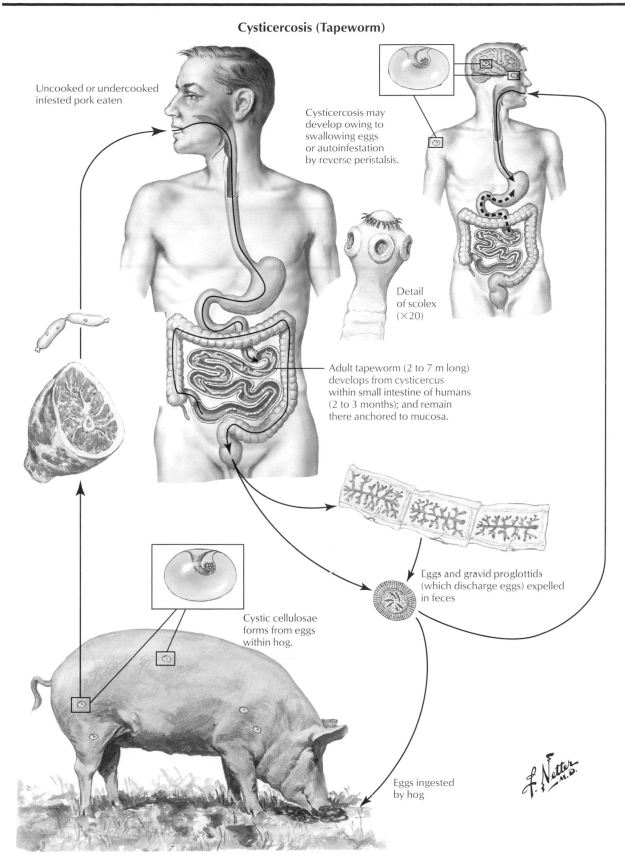

Uncooked or undercooked infested pork eaten

Cysticercosis may develop owing to swallowing eggs or autoinfestation by reverse peristalsis.

Detail of scolex (×20)

Adult tapeworm (2 to 7 m long) develops from cysticercus within small intestine of humans (2 to 3 months); and remain there anchored to mucosa.

Eggs and gravid proglottids (which discharge eggs) expelled in feces

Cystic cellulosae forms from eggs within hog.

Eggs ingested by hog

FIGURE 4-20   PARASITIC DISEASE OF THE GASTROINTESTINAL TRACT (CONTINUED)

development. Pruritus ani (caused by worms leaving the anus) with frequent scratching, eczema, erosions, and eventual superinfection is a common symptom. Cysticercosis is caused by consumption of infested pork meat. Eggs from tapeworms in the small intestine develop into multiple cystic larvae (*Cysticercus cellulosae*) in organs and tissues, including muscle and the brain. Such isolated cysts may contain multiple "embryos," which may promote further infestation and should be removed surgically.

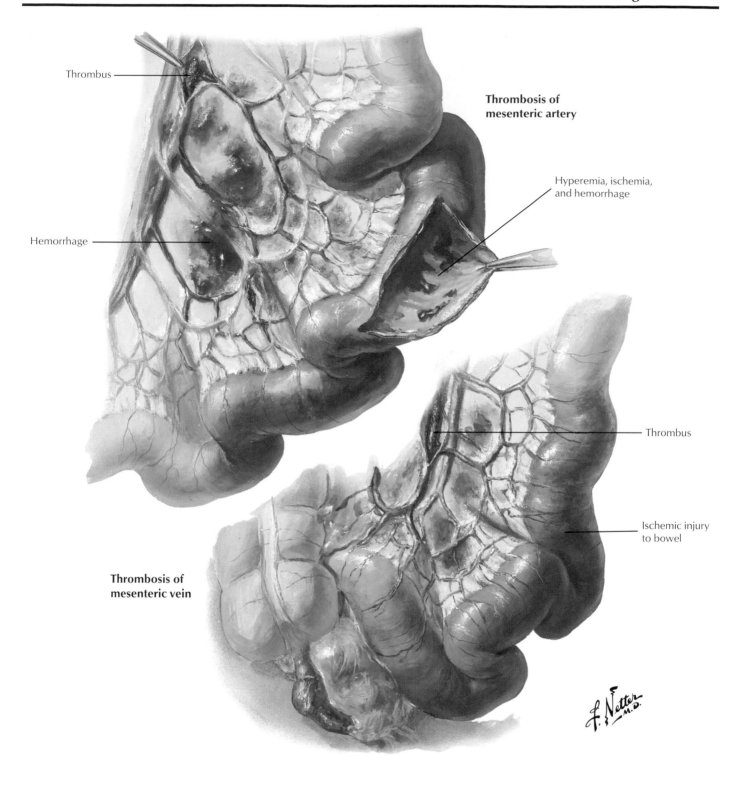

Thrombus

Thrombosis of
mesenteric artery

Hyperemia, ischemia,
and hemorrhage

Hemorrhage

Thrombus

Ischemic injury
to bowel

Thrombosis of
mesenteric vein

FIGURE 4-21   MESENTERIC VASCULAR OCCLUSION

Mesenteric artery thrombosis or **thromboembolism** and **venous thrombosis** produce hemorrhagic infarction of the intestines because of overlapping vascularization. Arterial thrombosis may follow severe arteriosclerosis, systemic vasculitis, or a dissecting aneurysm. Left cardiac ventricular thrombi secondary to myocardial infarction, cardiac fibrillation, or endocarditis are the common sources of the thromboembolism. Venous thrombosis can follow abdominal trauma or surgery, sepsis, or hypercoagulation states. Whether the infarction is mural or transmural depends on the extent and duration of the vascular occlusion. There is massive hyperemia, hemorrhage, and progressive necrobiosis of tissue components (ischemic injury starts approximately 18 hours after occlusion). Bacteria migrating into the intestinal wall cause severe gangrenous enteritis and peritonitis and eventually perforation of the bowel. Early surgical resection of the infarcted area is the only lifesaving procedure.

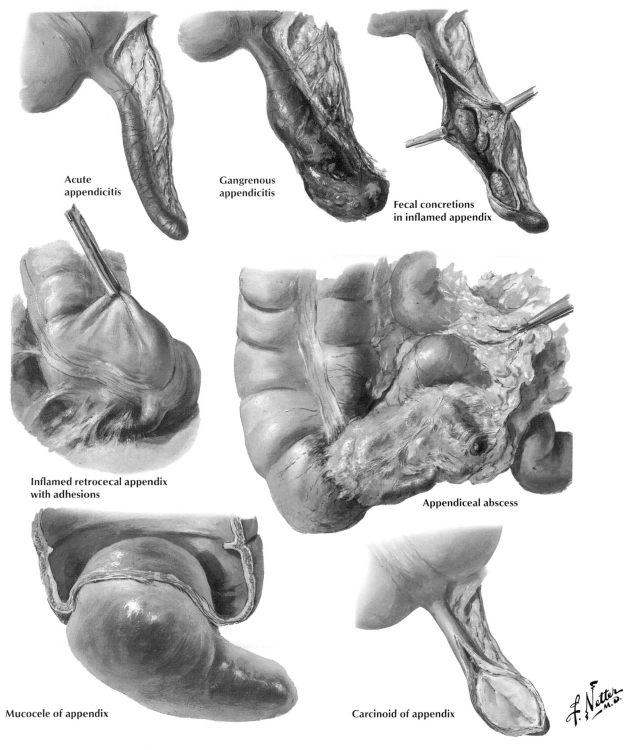

Acute
appendicitis

Gangrenous
appendicitis

Fecal concretions
in inflamed appendix

Inflamed retrocecal appendix
with adhesions

Appendiceal abscess

Mucocele of appendix

Carcinoid of appendix

Note: Mucocele, i.e., mucus and debris accumulation secondary to cicatricial occlusion of appendiceal orifice.
Carcinoid, i.e., endocrine tumor (see also Figure 4-31).

FIGURE 4-22   ACUTE APPENDICITIS

Acute appendicitis (AA) (i.e., acute catarrhal or puriform inflammation of the appendix vermiformis) is the most frequent reason for laparotomy. AA is commonly caused by bacterial infections, sometimes after fecal stasis or oxyuriasis (pinworm infection). Acute pain in the right lower quadrant of the abdomen is often accompanied by fever, nausea, vomiting, constipation, or diarrhea. A circumscribed tenderness in the right lower quadrant on palpation and increased blood leukocyte counts complete clinical diagnosis. Surgical removal of the appendix to avoid complications such as penetration of infection and perityphlitic abscess, perforation and generalized peritonitis, and, more rarely, puriform endophlebitis and liver abscesses is the treatment of choice.

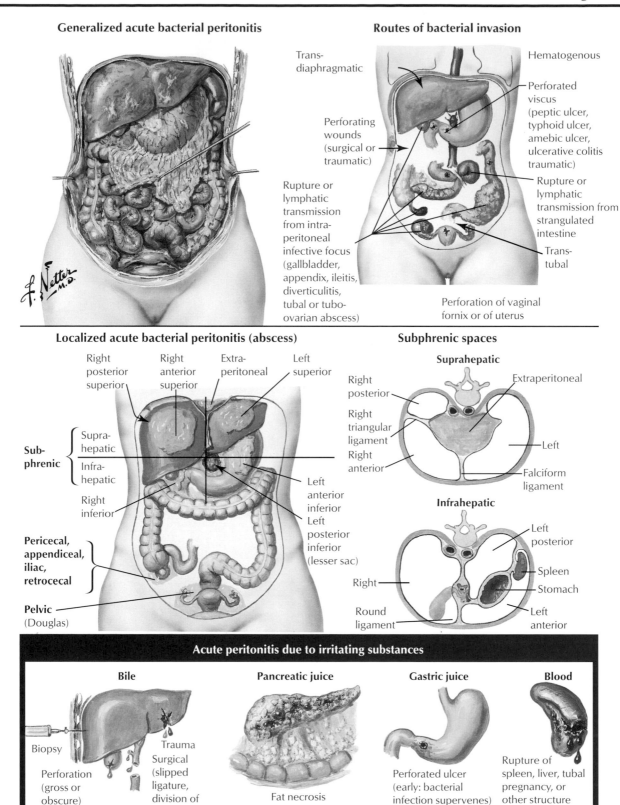

Generalized acute bacterial peritonitis

Routes of bacterial invasion

Trans-diaphragmatic

Hematogenous

Perforating wounds (surgical or traumatic)

Perforated viscus (peptic ulcer, typhoid ulcer, amebic ulcer, ulcerative colitis traumatic)

Rupture or lymphatic transmission from intra-peritoneal infective focus (gallbladder, appendix, ileitis, diverticulitis, tubal or tubo-ovarian abscess)

Rupture or lymphatic transmission from strangulated intestine

Trans-tubal

Perforation of vaginal fornix or of uterus

Localized acute bacterial peritonitis (abscess)

Subphrenic spaces

Right posterior superior

Right anterior superior

Extra-peritoneal

Left superior

Sub-phrenic { Supra-hepatic / Infra-hepatic }

Right inferior

Pericecal, appendiceal, iliac, retrocecal

Pelvic (Douglas)

Left anterior inferior

Left posterior inferior (lesser sac)

Suprahepatic

Right posterior

Right triangular ligament

Right anterior

Extraperitoneal

Left

Falciform ligament

Infrahepatic

Left posterior

Spleen

Stomach

Right

Round ligament

Left anterior

Acute peritonitis due to irritating substances

Bile

Biopsy

Perforation (gross or obscure)

Trauma Surgical (slipped ligature, division of common duct)

Pancreatic juice

Fat necrosis

Gastric juice

Perforated ulcer (early: bacterial infection supervenes)

Blood

Rupture of spleen, liver, tubal pregnancy, or other structure

FIGURE 4-23   ACUTE PERITONITIS

Acute peritonitis, an inflammation of the peritoneum, is caused by bacterial invasion or chemical irritation. It is usually a complication of perforation of the intraabdominal organs (ruptured appendix, perforated ulcer, diverticula), abdominal surgery, or peritoneal dialysis. Pathologic changes are those of a typical fibrinopurulent, gangrenous, or fecal inflammation with fibrous adhesions and concretions of bowel loops. Symptoms include those of acute abdomen (nausea, vomiting, diffuse abdominal tenderness and pain, abdominal distention, reduction of intestinal motility, or paralytic ileus, with ensuing high fever and septic shock). Treatment consists of antibiotics, surgical drainage, and/or debridement and supportive measures.

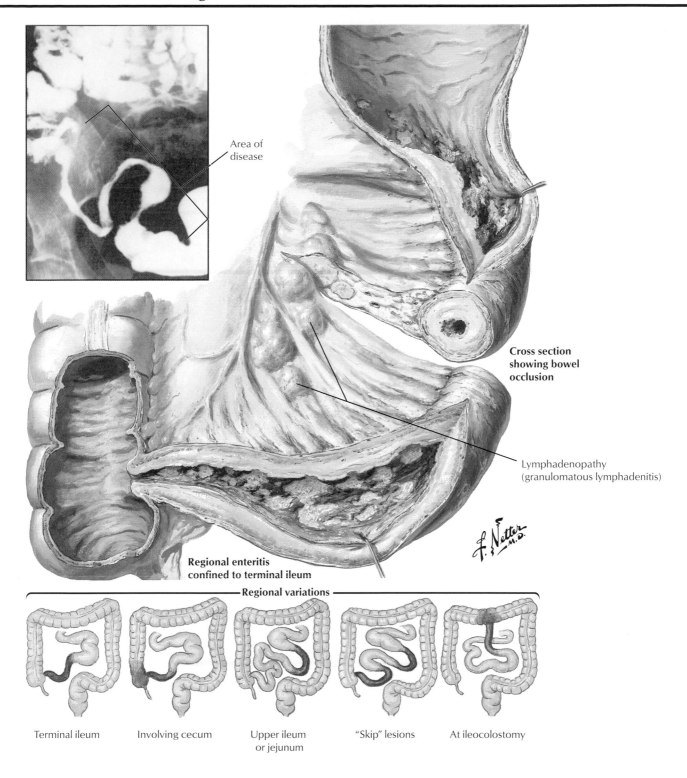

Area of disease

Cross section showing bowel occlusion

Lymphadenopathy (granulomatous lymphadenitis)

Regional enteritis confined to terminal ileum

Regional variations

Terminal ileum   Involving cecum   Upper ileum or jejunum   "Skip" lesions   At ileocolostomy

FIGURE 4-24 CROHN'S DISEASE

Crohn's disease (**enteritis regionalis**) is a chronic granulomatous disease of the GI tract, mainly of the terminal ileum. It affects approximately 5 per 100,000 persons per year, with young adults of European ancestry affected most prominently. The etiology remains unknown, although family studies suggest a genetic susceptibility. Characteristic histologic changes are transmural edema (with subsequent fibrosis), nodular and follicular lympho-

cytic infiltrates, epithelioid cell granulomas, and fistulation. Inflammatory infiltrates are patchy with unchanged intestinum in between ("skip lesions") and extend to involve the adventitial fat tissue ("creeping fat") and regional lymph nodes. Symptoms include diffuse abdominal pain, diarrhea, and recurrent fever and malabsorption. Intestinal obstruction and fistulation may necessitate surgery.

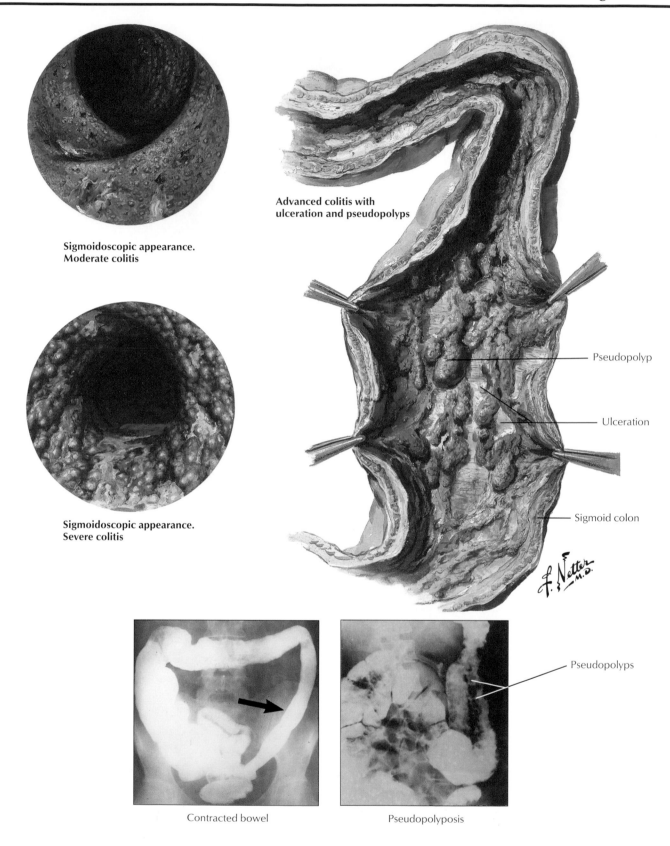

Sigmoidoscopic appearance.
Moderate colitis

Advanced colitis with
ulceration and pseudopolyps

Sigmoidoscopic appearance.
Severe colitis

Pseudopolyp

Ulceration

Sigmoid colon

Contracted bowel

Pseudopolyposis

Pseudopolyps

FIGURE 4-25   ULCERATIVE COLITIS

Ulcerative colitis (UC) is a chronic inflammatory bowel disease of unknown etiology. Systemic complications may affect the liver, the joints, the heart, the oral mucosa, and the eyes. The tendency of UC to run in families suggests a genetic predisposition. The association of UC with autoimmune disorders (e.g., sclerosing cholangitis, migratory polyarthritis) suggests an immune component to the disease. Histologic investigation reveals a mucosal, erosive, and ulcerative colitis with neutrophilic infiltration

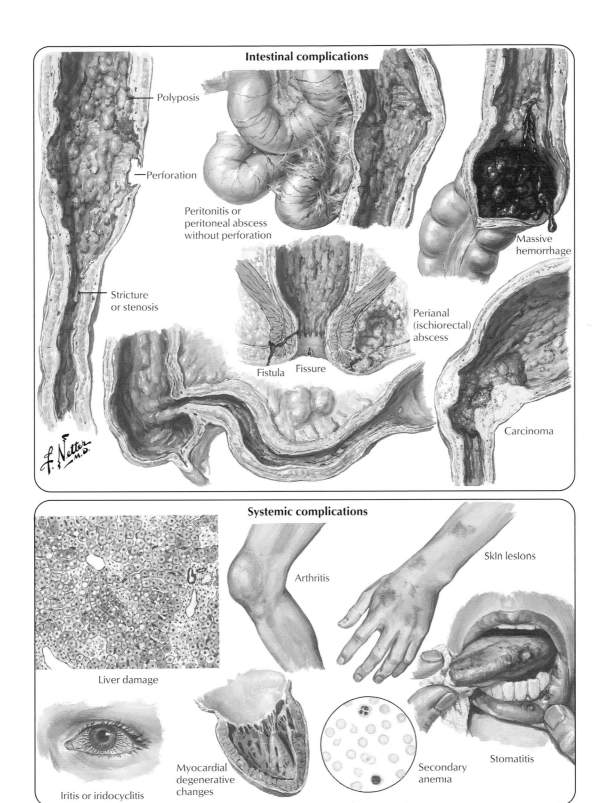

Intestinal complications

Polyposis

Perforation

Stricture or stenosis

Peritonitis or peritoneal abscess without perforation

Massive hemorrhage

Perianal (ischiorectal) abscess

Fistula   Fissure

Carcinoma

Systemic complications

Liver damage

Arthritis

Skin lesions

Iritis or iridocyclitis

Myocardial degenerative changes

Secondary anemia

Stomatitis

FIGURE 4-25   ULCERATIVE COLITIS *(CONTINUED)*

(neutrophils in glands: **cryptal abscesses**), epithelial regenerative changes with elongation of neck area of crypts, and spreading of regenerating cells to the mucosal surface. Increasing epithelial atypia in prolonged disease may lead to adenocarcinoma. In late stages of the disease, epithelial regeneration and formation of pseudopolyps cause a "cobblestone appearance" of the mucosa between ulcerations.

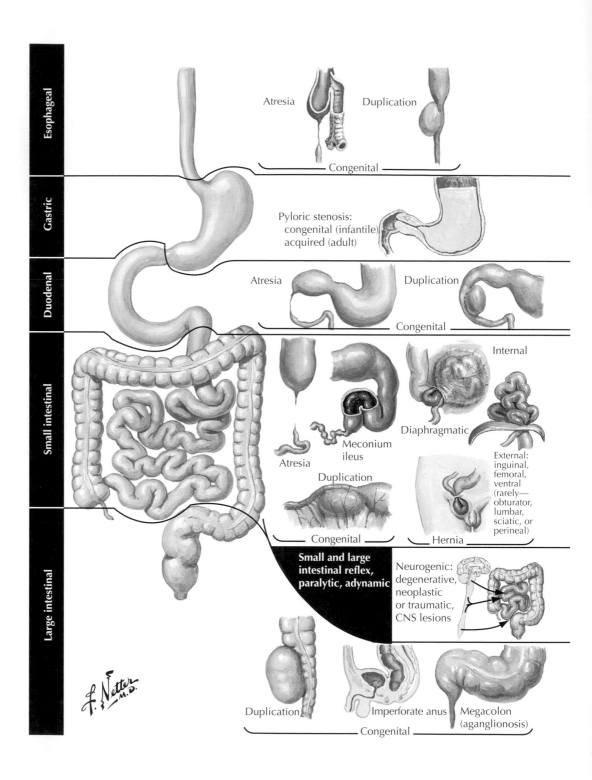

Esophageal

Atresia   Duplication

Congenital

Gastric

Pyloric stenosis:
congenital (infantile)
acquired (adult)

Duodenal

Atresia   Duplication

Congenital

Small intestinal

Internal

Diaphragmatic

Atresia   Meconium
ileus

External:
inguinal,
femoral,
ventral
(rarely—
obturator,
lumbar,
sciatic, or
perineal)

Duplication

Congenital   Hernia

**Small and large
intestinal reflex,
paralytic, adynamic**

Neurogenic:
degenerative,
neoplastic
or traumatic,
CNS lesions

Large intestinal

Duplication   Imperforate anus   Megacolon
(aganglionosis)

Congenital

FIGURE 4-26   OBSTRUCTION OF THE BOWEL

Obstruction of the bowel (OB) is any mechanical or functional impediment of the normal propulsion of bowel contents. In newborns, congenital abnormalities, including atresias (esophagus, gastral, intestinal, anal), malrotation and volvulus, and aganglionic segments (colon), may cause OB. Mechanical obstruction by **meconium** (meconium ileus) or, at later age, by hernia, incarceration, and volvulus (peritoneal bands) must be considered. In adults, OB may result from ingested materials, spastic or cicatricial occlusion, compression from the outside (hernia, intussusception, volvulus, tumors), and chronic inflammatory diseases. When OB results in intestinal ileus, no bowel movement sounds are heard on auscultation ("silent abdomen").

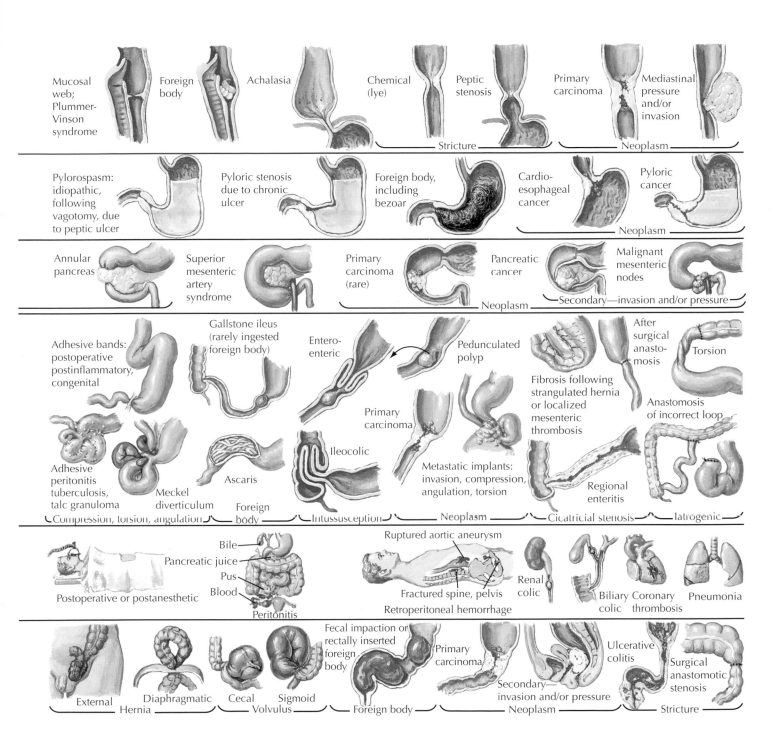

FIGURE 4-26   OBSTRUCTION OF THE BOWEL (CONTINUED)

Abdominal radiography shows distended small or large intestinal parts or both with accumulation of gas and fluids. Complications include paralytic ileus, infarction, invasion of the intestinal wall by enterobacteria and peritonitis, perforation, fecal peritonitis, and (septic) shock.

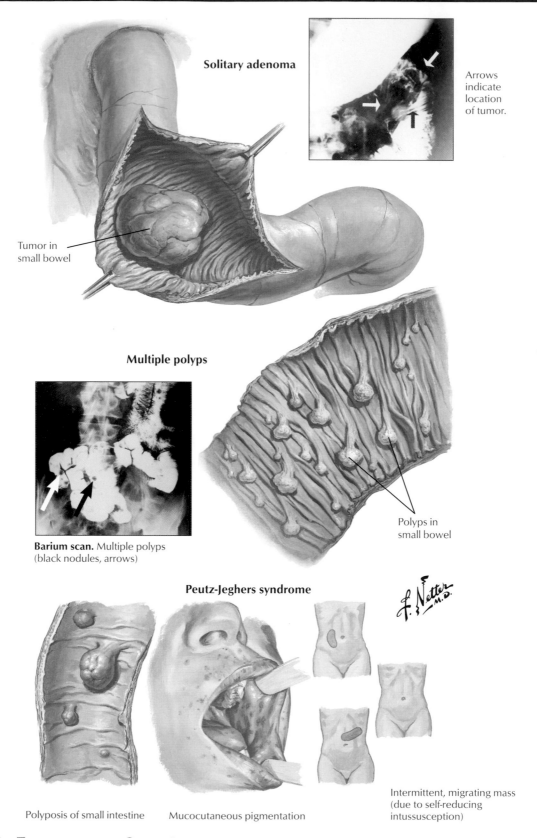

Solitary adenoma

Arrows indicate location of tumor.

Tumor in small bowel

Multiple polyps

Barium scan. Multiple polyps (black nodules, arrows)

Polyps in small bowel

Peutz-Jeghers syndrome

Polyposis of small intestine

Mucocutaneous pigmentation

Intermittent, migrating mass (due to self-reducing intussusception)

FIGURE 4-27 TUMORS OF THE SMALL INTESTINE

Most **polyps** and **adenomas** in the small intestine are benign sessile or pedunculated intraluminal tumors, which cause irregularly arranged intestinal glands and increased mucus production. Solitary tumors are rare. **Peutz-Jeghers syndrome** (PJS), a heritable small bowel polyposis, consists of multiple hamartomatous polyps in combination with abnormal mucocuta-

neous (perioral, buccal, perianal) pigmentation. PJS is associated with mutational inactivation of a protein kinase encoded on chromosome 19p (gene *LKB1*). Bleeding, anemia, and intussusception are common complications. Tumor development is very rare, and it does not necessarily occur within the polyps. (See also Fig. 1-10.)

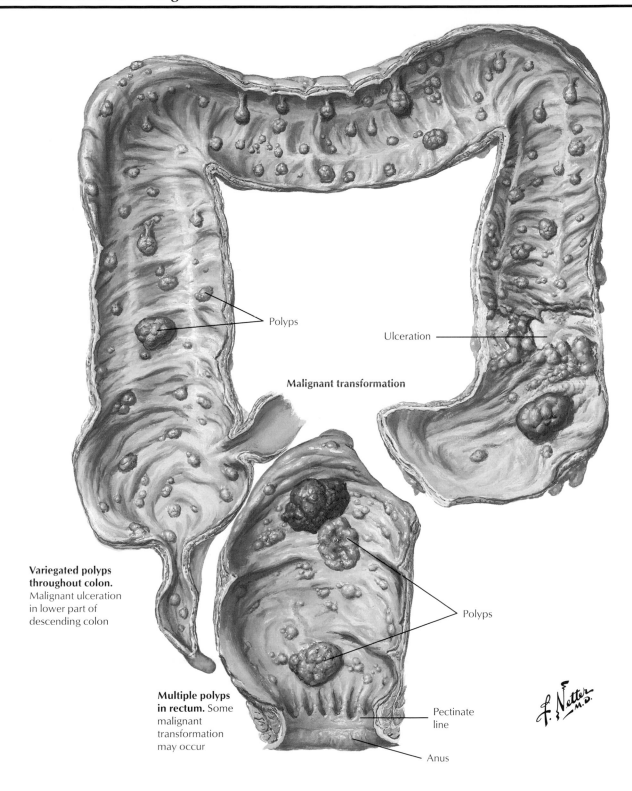

Polyps

Ulceration

Malignant transformation

**Variegated polyps
throughout colon.**
Malignant ulceration
in lower part of
descending colon

Polyps

**Multiple polyps
in rectum.** Some
malignant
transformation
may occur

Pectinate
line

Anus

FIGURE 4-28   FAMILIAL POLYPOSIS OF THE LARGE INTESTINE

Familial polyposis of the large intestine is an autosomal dominant inherited disease, which, in contrast to PJS, consists of true adenomas (**familial adenomatous polyposis**) scattered throughout the large bowel. The risk of malignant transformation as early as the age of 40 years approaches 100%. Many adenomas are tubular adenomas; others are tubulovillous or villous adenomas.

The disease is characterized by a germline mutation of chromosome 5 (5q21). **Gardner syndrome** combines a familial polyposis syndrome with extraintestinal lesions such as soft tissue and bone tumors. **Turcot syndrome** describes familial polyposis syndrome in combination with malignant tumors of the CNS.

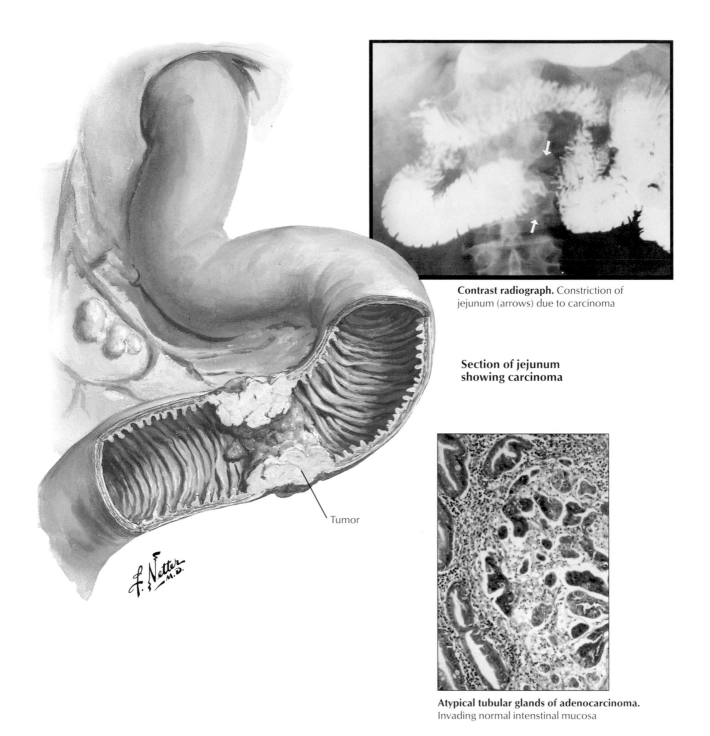

Contrast radiograph. Constriction of jejunum (arrows) due to carcinoma

Section of jejunum showing carcinoma

Tumor

Atypical tubular glands of adenocarcinoma. Invading normal intenstinal mucosa

FIGURE 4-29   CANCER OF THE SMALL INTESTINE: ADENOCARCINOMAS

Malignant tumors of the small intestine, which consist of **adenocarcinoma**, **malignant lymphomas**, and CTs, constitute approximately 5% of all GI tumors. Adenocarcinoma presents as a circular constricting mass or as an intraluminal polypoid mass. Most adenocarcinomas are located in the duodenum and the jejunum. They are classified as glandular/acinar types, medullary carcinomas, or undifferentiated types based on their histologic characteristics. Chronic inflammatory diseases are a risk factor for the development of adenocarcinoma in the small bowel. Adenocarcinomas in the duodenum are frequently located within the ampulla vater (ampullary carcinoma) and cause obstructive jaundice or pancreatitis or both.

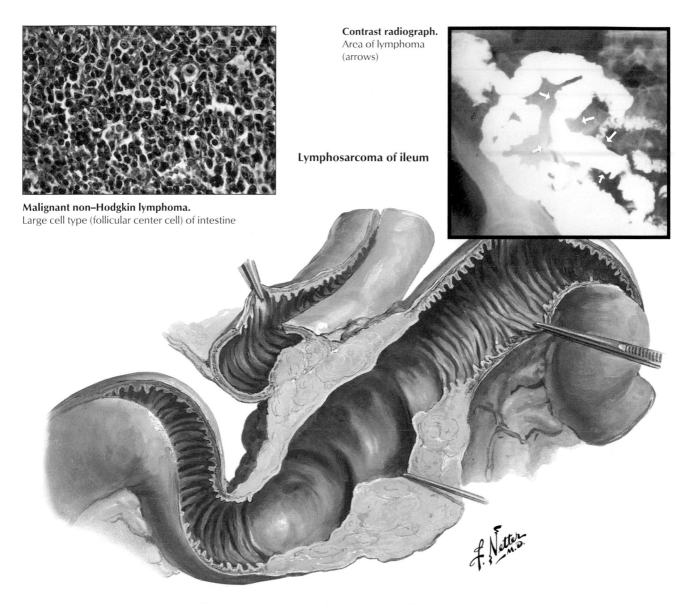

Contrast radiograph. Area of lymphoma (arrows)

Lymphosarcoma of ileum

Malignant non–Hodgkin lymphoma. Large cell type (follicular center cell) of intestine

Lymphoma. Infiltrating two separate portions of small bowel

FIGURE 4-30   CANCER OF THE SMALL INTESTINE: LYMPHOMAS

Primary **malignant non-Hodgkin lymphoma** (NHL) is a common tumor in the small intestine. It occurs in 2 major forms: Mediterranean-type lymphoma (**immunoproliferative small intestinal disease** [IPSID]), and Western-type malignant NHL. IPSID, with higher incidences in underdeveloped populations, appears infection-related and consists of progressive proliferation of IgA secreting plasmacytoid B lymphocytes (**alpha chain disease**) with signs of malabsorption. The terminal stage consists of an overt immunoblastic NHL. Western-type NHL tends to develop in the ilium as tumorous plaquelike infiltrates or intraluminal fungating masses, which result in bleeding, obstruction, and occasional intussusception. Histologically, these tumor cells, which consist of the **mucosa-associated lymphoid tissue** (MALT), are referred to as MALT lymphomas. Follicular center cell lymphomas and other types may also be found.

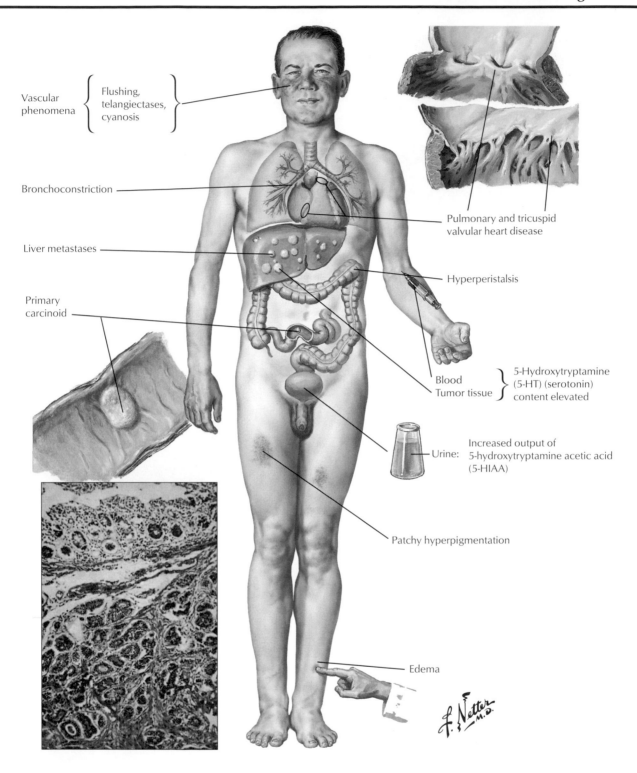

FIGURE 4-31   CANCER OF THE SMALL INTESTINE: CARCINOID TUMORS

Carcinoid tumors (CCTs), which account for approximately 20% of small intestine tumors, can occur in other organs, including the intestines, the stomach, the liver, and the lungs. CTs are derived from argentaffine endocrine cells (enterochromaffin cells or **Kulchitsky cells**). CTs can occur as multiple isolated tumors or as part of a systemic disease (multiple endocrine neoplasia [MEN], type I). CTs less than 1 cm in diameter rarely behave malignantly and usually do not metastasize, whereas 50% or more of tumors

1 cm or larger with the same gross and histologic features metastasize. The tumor spreads most frequently to the liver. Carcinoid syndrome (diarrhea, flushing, bronchospasm, cyanosis, and skin telangiectases) is caused by episodic massive serotonin production by tumor cells. The 5-hydroxyindolacetic acid (5-HIAA) test, which measures 5-HIAA in the urine, is the diagnostic test of choice.

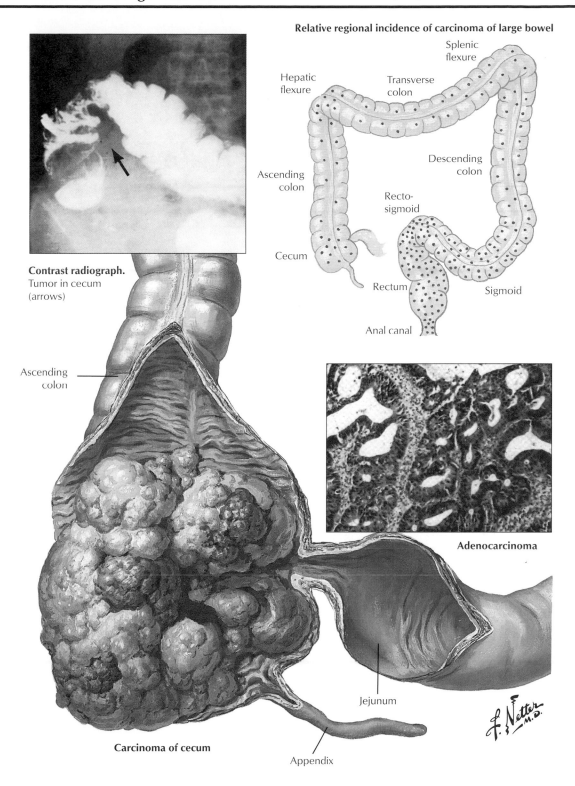

Relative regional incidence of carcinoma of large bowel

Splenic flexure

Hepatic flexure

Transverse colon

Ascending colon

Descending colon

Recto-sigmoid

Cecum

Rectum

Sigmoid

Anal canal

Contrast radiograph.
Tumor in cecum
(arrows)

Ascending
colon

Adenocarcinoma

Carcinoma of cecum

Jejunum

Appendix

FIGURE 4-32 COLON CANCER

Adenocarcinomas account for 98% of all carcinomas in the colon and the rectum. They may develop de novo or from preexisting adenomas. Adenocarcinomas are located most often in the sigmoid colon and the rectum, followed by the descending colon. They are less frequent in the transverse colon and rare in the ascending colon. The gross appearance of adenocarcinomas of the colon and the rectum is polypoid and ulcerating. Some are plaquelike, infiltrating, and circularly constricting; others are flat but deeply infiltrating and inconspicuous endoscopically. Most

tumors are well-differentiated adenocarcinomas with some mucus secretion; a few are mucinous adenocarcinomas or signet ring cell carcinomas. The degree of differentiation influences spread and prognosis. Colonic adenocarcinomas spread by direct extension through the intestinal layers, to regional lymph nodes by invasion of lymph vessels, and to the liver through the portal vein. Tumors in the deep sigmoid colon and rectum spread to the lungs hematogenously via tributaries of the vena cava inferior.

CHAPTER 5

LIVER, GALLBLADDER, AND PANCREAS

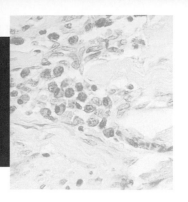

The liver maintains the physiologic and metabolic balance of the body. Therefore, disease of the liver may have numerous effects throughout the body: it may cause disturbances in carbohydrate, lipid, amino acid, and vitamin metabolism and interfere with protein synthesis, blood clotting, and detoxification of endogenous and exogenous substances (Table 5-1).

INFLAMMATORY DISEASES OF THE LIVER

Viral hepatitis is an acute inflammation of the liver, usually caused by the hepatitis viruses (HAV-HGV), rarely by such other viruses as enteroviruses and herpesviruses (CMV, EBV, HHV-6, or HSV). Symptoms do not develop until the onset of immune reactions against the virus or

TABLE 5-1 CLINICAL FEATURES OF LIVER FAILURE

Clinical Feature	Pathogenesis
Jaundice	a. Intracellular retention of bilirubin (hepatocyte failure) b. Intercellular and canalicular (bile stasis)
Malabsorption, weight loss, bleeding tendency, muscle wasting	Bile, enzyme, and vitamin deficiency
Edema, muscle wasting	Decreased protein (albumin) synthesis
Spider nevi, palmar erythema, gynecomastia	Disturbed hormone metabolism
Ascites, splenomegaly, varices (gastroesophageal)	Portal hypertension
Hepatic encephalopathy	Toxic metabolites (acetoin, acyloin, ammonia)
Hepatorenal syndrome	Cause unknown (renal vasoconstriction?)

TABLE 5-2 CHARACTERISTICS OF PRIMARY AUTOIMMUNE DISORDERS OF THE LIVER*

Features	AIH	PBC	PSC
Serology (autoantibodies)	Antinuclear (ANA) Anti–smooth muscle (ASMA) Anti–liver/kidney membrane (LKM) Antiliver (LSP)	Anti–native DNA Antiribosomal Antimitochondrial (AMA) ASMA Anti–bile proteins Antithyroid LSP	ANA Antineutrophils (ANCA) Anti–bile duct epithelia
Genetics	Nonspecific	Female predominance	Male predominance Increased expression: HLA-DR3, HLA-DRW52a, HLA-B8 (DR2,4, DRb12)
Associated diseases	Rheumatoid arthritis Pernicious anemia Cryoglobulinemia Peripheral neuropathy Hemolytic anemia	Raynaud syndrome Thyroid dysfunction Seronegative arthritis Scleroderma Keratoconjunctivitis	Ulcerative colitis Riedel thyroiditis Retroperitoneal fibrosis Orbital pseudotumor (may be complicated by cholangiocarcinoma)

*AIH indicates autoimmune hepatitis; PBC, primary biliary cirrhosis; PSC, primary sclerosing cholangitis.
Overlap syndromes combine features of cholestatic and chronic hepatitic forms of diseases, e.g., AIH + PBC, PBC + PSC, or PBC + sarcoidosis.

virus-infected cells, 2 to 26 weeks after infection (**incubation period**). Bacteria, fungi, and parasites also may cause hepatitis.

Noninfectious causes of liver inflammation include toxic and immunologic disorders of the liver (see Table 5-2). These are discussed together because certain forms of toxic hepatitis may mimic autoimmune disorders or may be mediated through hypersensitivity reactions. A large variety of substances can cause liver damage, and they are associated with an equally large variety of lesions. A selection is shown in Table 5-3.

There are 3 major groups of autoimmune disorders affecting the liver: primary hepatic autoimmune diseases (Table 5-3), liver diseases with secondary autoimmune component, and systemic autoimmune diseases involving the liver.

METABOLIC DISEASES INVOLVING THE LIVER

A number of metabolic disorders affect the liver, some of which are consequences of **inborn errors of metabolism**. Major forms discussed in this chapter are hemochromatosis, Wilson disease (WD), and amyloidosis.

PRIMARY TUMORS OF THE LIVER

The most frequent tumors in the liver are metastases, often from the gastrointestinal (GI) tract, the lungs, or the mammary glands. Primary tumors originating in the liver consist of benign hepatic hamartomas and adenomas, bile duct angiomas, and cavernous hemangiomas. Two benign lesions must be distinguished from well-differentiated hepatocellular carcinoma (HCC): hepatocellular adenoma and focal nodular hyperplasia (FNH) of the liver. Adenomas (single or multiple) are well-circumscribed, yellowish masses of liver tissue with a fibrous capsule and histologically lobular architecture devoid of central vein, portal triads, and bile ductules. They occur preferentially in women of reproductive age and seem to be related to the use of oral contraceptives. FNHs, which occur equally in the two sexes, are solitary masses of hypertrophic hepatocellular nodules divided by fibrous septae, with prominent central scarring, large central nutritive ves-

sels, bile ductules and cholestasis, and a pseudocapsule. The most frequent malignant tumors of the liver are HCC and cholangiocarcinoma (CAC). Less frequent are hepatoblastoma (in small children) and hemangiosarcoma.

CHOLELITHIASIS AND CHOLECYSTITIS

Cholelithiasis (CHL) is the formation of stones in the gallbladder and large bile ducts, usually in extrahepatic locations. CHL occurs in up to 20% of the Western population, approximately four fifths of whom have no symptoms (**silent CHL**). The prevalence of gallstones increases with age, with most patients being older than 40 years. Females experience CHL approximately twice as often as males, suggesting that a role is played by the endocrine system (increased estrogens, oral contraceptives, obesity, and hypercholesterolemia). Additional risk factors are hyperlipidemia, rapid weight loss, inborn errors of bile acid metabolism, and GI diseases such as Crohn ileitis, pancreatic insufficiency, and mucoviscidosis.

TUMORS OF THE GALLBLADDER AND THE BILE DUCTS

Papillomas, adenomas, and adenomyomas of deeper (submucosal) glands may occur in the gallbladder. Most remain clinically inapparent except when they cause obstruction (e.g., papillomas in bile ducts or papilla of Vater). The majority of malignant tumors in the gallbladder are adenocarcinomas, which are found in approximately 2% of resected gallbladders. Approximately 5% of malignant tumors in this organ are squamous cell carcinomas.

ACUTE AND CHRONIC PANCREATITIS

Inflammation of the pancreas, usually caused by CHL or alcoholism, is characterized by massive activation of pancreatic enzymes, which, in acute cases, may cause life-threatening **autodigestion** and shock. Chronic cases cause extensive destruction of pancreatic parenchyma with fibrosis and loss of enzymatic activities.

TABLE 5-3   TOXIC HEPATITIS AND ITS LESIONS

Mechanism	Lesion	Exemplary Substances
Direct and indirect toxicity	Hepatocellular necrosis and steatosis	Alcohol, CCl_4, phosphorus methyl-DOPA, tetracyclines
Cholestatic	Hepatocanalicular cholestasis	Steroids
Hypersensitivity	Hepatocellular and hepatocanalicular, necrosis, cholestasis, granulomatous	Erythromycin, chlorpromazine phenytoin
	Vasculitis (panarteritis nodosa type)	Penicillin, allopurinol, sulfathiazole chlorpromazide, diphenylhydantoin, chlorothiazide, methamphetamine
	Sclerosing cholangitis type	Floxuridine
Metabolic	Hepatocellular and hepatocanalicular	Isoniazid, halothane

CYSTIC FIBROSIS (MUCOVISCIDOSIS)

Cystic fibrosis (CF) is the most common autosomal recessively inherited disease in children and young adults, with an incidence in Western populations of 1 in 2000 live births. It is caused by variable mutations of the CF gene on chromosome 7 (7q31-32). The primary defect caused by these mutations is in chloride ion channels, which transport chloride ions across epithelial barriers. Deficient chloride ion transport interferes with sodium and water secretion in exocrine glands, resulting in the production of a viscous mucoid material that obstructs glandular ducts in salivary glands, bronchial glands, the pancreas, and others. (See also Fig. 3-3.)

NEOPLASMS OF THE PANCREAS

Benign tumors of the exocrine pancreas are rare and consist essentially of ductal serous or mucinous cystadenomas. They must be distinguished clinically from inflammatory pseudocysts rather than from carcinoma. Carcinoma of the pancreas is the fourth most common tumor in the Western world, is even more frequent in the Pacific region, and is increasing in incidence. Approximately 23,000 new cases are diagnosed every year in the United States; only approximately 1% of these patients survive 5 years. No clear cause of human pancreatic cancer has been identified. Chronic pancreatitis is a recognized risk factor for carcinoma of the pancreas. Dietary factors, such as high fat and meat intake, may be contributory.

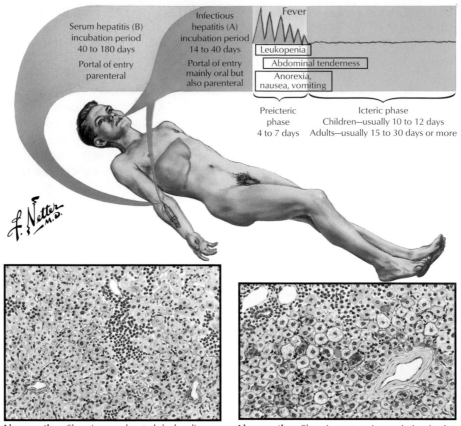

Liver section. Showing moderate lobular disarray; shrunken and swollen cells and nuclei; circumscribed replacement of liver cells with round cells

Liver section. Showing extensive variation in size and shape of liver cells; binucleate cells; thickening of central vein; circumscribed inflammatory infiltrations

TABLE 5-4   MEMBERS AND CHARACTERISTICS OF THE HEPATITIS VIRUSES*

Name (Molecule)	Family	Transmission	Incubation, weeks	Disease	Carrier	Chronic	Cancer
HAV (ssRNA)	Picorna	Enteral	2–6	Hepatitis, fulminant hepatitis	0	0	0
HBV (dsDNA)	Hepadna	Parenteral	4–26	Hepatitis, fulminant hepatitis, cirrhosis	–1%	–10%	Yes
HCV (ssRNA)	Flavivirus	Parenteral	2–26	Hepatitis, cirrhosis, extrahepatic disorders	–1%	–50%	Yes
HDV (ssRNA)	Subviral satellite (HBV helper)	Parenteral	4–7 (super-infection)	Hepatitis, fulminant hepatitis	–10%	–5%	0
HEV (ssRNA)	Calicivirus	Enteral	2–8	Hepatitis	?	0	0
HGV (ssRNA)	Flavivirus	Parenteral	?	Hepatitis, extrahepatic disorders in drug addicts	–2%	0	?

*ds indicates double-stranded; ss, single-stranded.

FIGURE 5-1   ACUTE VIRAL HEPATITIS

Acute viral hepatitis, an inflammatory disease of the hepatic parenchyma, is caused most frequently by the hepatitis viruses (HVs) and less frequently by other viruses (Table 5-4). In the Western world, HBV and HBC are most prevalent. Disease symptoms develop between 2 and 26 weeks after the onset of immune reactions against virus/virus-infected cells. The pathogenesis of liver injury in viral hepatitis is not completely clear, although a cytotoxic T-lymphocyte reaction against hepatocytes presenting viral antigens seems to be the key reaction. Histology shows many lymphocytes invading the liver parenchyma from portal triads, which causes adjacent hepatocellular necroses (**piecemeal necroses**). Infected hepatocytes change to a **ground-glass** appearance. In more severe disease, infected hepatocytes show ballooning degeneration. In addition, there are single or multiple hepatocellular coagulation necroses of virus-infected hepatocytes (**Councilman bodies**) or lytic necroses (**dropout necroses**).

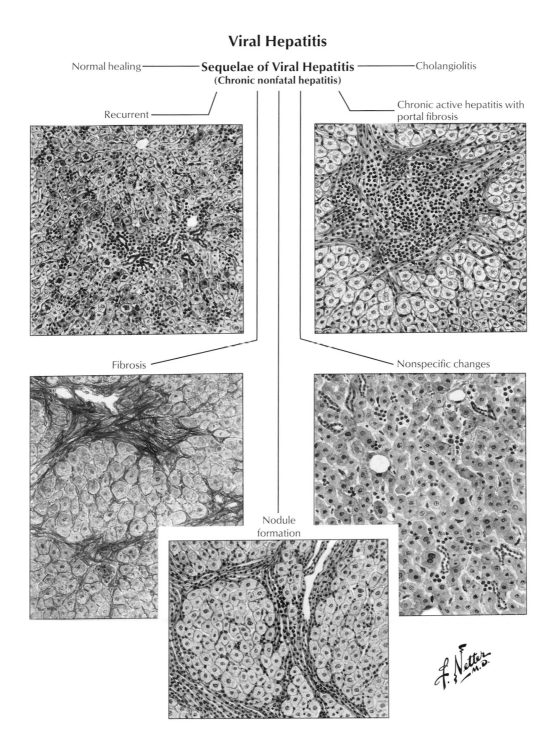

Viral Hepatitis

Normal healing ——— **Sequelae of Viral Hepatitis** ——— Cholangiolitis
(**Chronic nonfatal hepatitis**)

Recurrent ———

Chronic active hepatitis with portal fibrosis

Fibrosis ———　　　　　　　　　　　——— Nonspecific changes

Nodule formation

FIGURE 5-2　CHRONIC HEPATITIS

The onset of **chronic hepatitis** is characterized by **reticular fibrosis**, which surrounds necrobiotic hepatocytes and frequently precedes the formation of collagen fibrils. **Collagenous fibrosis** replaces damaged liver parenchyma, starting from a simple portal fibrosis and progressing to formation of fibrous septae (septal fibrosis) and final invasion and disruption of the acinus (pseudo-acinus formation). The final stage of this fibrotic process is the development of hepatic cirrhosis with diffuse fine-nodular

change. The general outcome of infections with HBV and HCV is usually the following: (1) symptomatic acute hepatitis (35% in HBV, 10% in HCV); (2) development of chronic hepatitis (10% in HBV, 50-70% in HCV); (3) development of cirrhosis (10-30% in HBV, at least 35% in HCV); (4) development of HCC (roughly estimated at 5-10% in both HBV and HCV). An additional threat is the high incidence of an asymptomatic carrier state in 70% to 90% of patients.

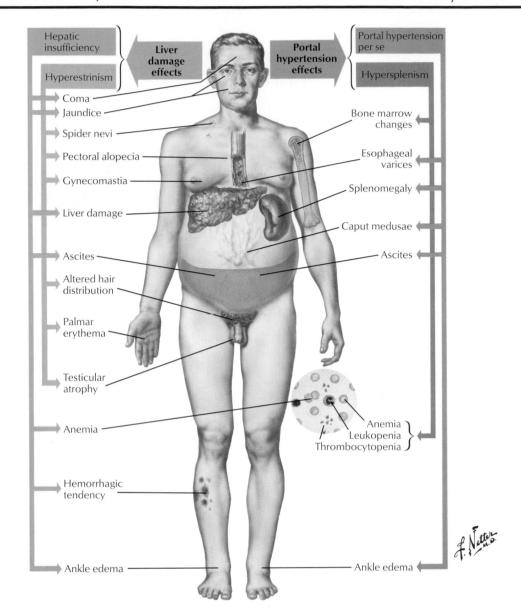

TABLE 5-5   GROSS FEATURES AS RELATED TO THE PATHOGENESIS OF LIVER CIRRHOSIS*

Gross Appearance	Pathogenesis
Diffuse, finely nodular (classic Laennec type: with atrophy)	Post–hepatitis virus cirrhosis
Same with or without fatty infiltration	Post–alcoholic cirrhosis
Diffuse, medium-sized nodular, dark purple (classic Hanot type with hypertrophy)	Chronic congestive (practically only seen in constrictive pericarditis)
Same with severe jaundice (green liver)	Primary biliary cirrhosis or chronic sclerosing cholangitis
Same with "dirty" gray-brown appearance (and similarly pigmented pancreas)	Hemochromatosis, Wilson disease
Diffuse, irregularly nodular, preferentially small- to medium-sized nodular	Autoimmune hepatitis and cirrhosis
Irregular, medium- to large-sized nodular, with jaundice (green liver)	Secondary biliary cirrhosis (i.e., extrahepatic bile duct obstruction)
Same with regular color or with fatty infiltration	"Postnecrotic" cirrhosis of variable etiology (e.g., post-HSV + alcoholic or other toxic influences)

*HSV indicates herpes simplex virus.

FIGURE 5-3   CIRRHOSIS OF THE LIVER

Cirrhosis of the liver with its extensive scarring and structural and functional alterations constitutes the end stage of various chronic inflammatory liver diseases. Histologically, it is defined by the triad of fibrosis, **umbau** (reconstruction with pseudoacini), and excess regeneration (hepatocellular nodules, bile duct proliferation). Pseudoacini (pseudolobules) originate from collagen fibers that invade the hepatic acinus, causing it to split. The sections that separate from the hepatic acinus do not contain a central vein and cannot function adequately. This scenario is further complicated by regenerative liver nodules. In the Western world, alcoholic liver cirrhoses constitute approximately 60% to 70% of all cases. Approximately 10% of cases are HV-induced cirrhoses, and 5% to 10% are primary and secondary biliary cirrhoses. Diagnostic gross features of different types of liver cirrhoses are outlined in Table 5-5.

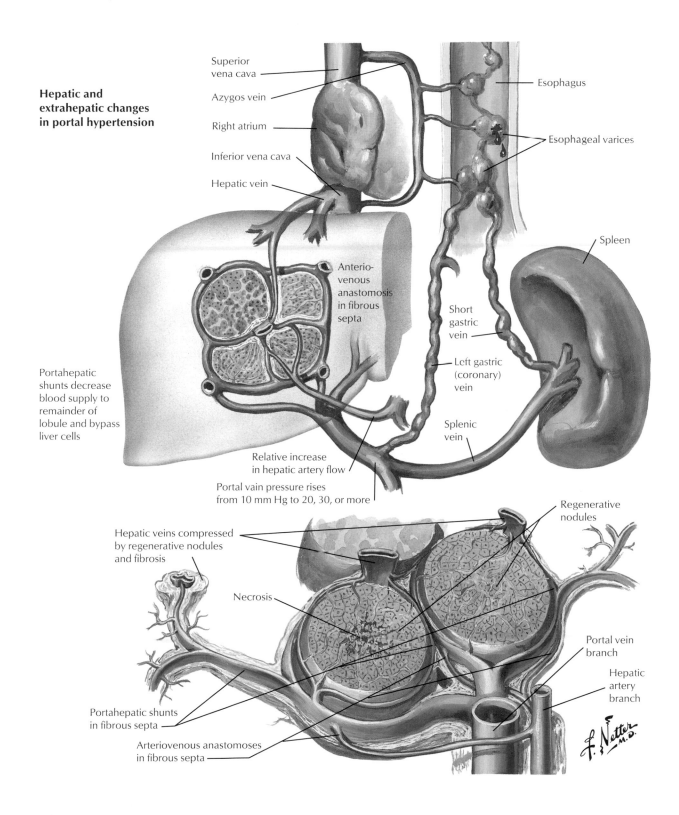

Hepatic and extrahepatic changes in portal hypertension

Superior vena cava

Azygos vein

Right atrium

Inferior vena cava

Hepatic vein

Esophagus

Esophageal varices

Spleen

Anterio-venous anastomosis in fibrous septa

Short gastric vein

Left gastric (coronary) vein

Splenic vein

Portahepatic shunts decrease blood supply to remainder of lobule and bypass liver cells

Relative increase in hepatic artery flow

Portal vain pressure rises from 10 mm Hg to 20, 30, or more

Regenerative nodules

Hepatic veins compressed by regenerative nodules and fibrosis

Necrosis

Portal vein branch

Hepatic artery branch

Portahepatic shunts in fibrous septa

Arteriovenous anastomoses in fibrous septa

FIGURE 5-4 PORTAL HYPERTENSION

Fibrosis and **umbau** cause severe obstruction of intrahepatic blood flow with portal hypertension. Other causes of portal hypertension include thrombosis of major hepatic veins (**Budd-Chiari syndrome**) and of the portal vein. Symptoms of portal hypertension are splenomegaly, ascites, and gastroesophageal varices. **Ascites** is usually the result of increased venous pressure, hypoalbuminemia (secondary to hepatocellular damage with reduced protein synthesis), and sodium retention (secondary by hepatocellular damage with diminished inactivation of antidiuretic hormone [ADH] and aldosterone). Bleeding from esophageal varices is a major cause of death in patients with liver cirrhosis and portal hypertension.

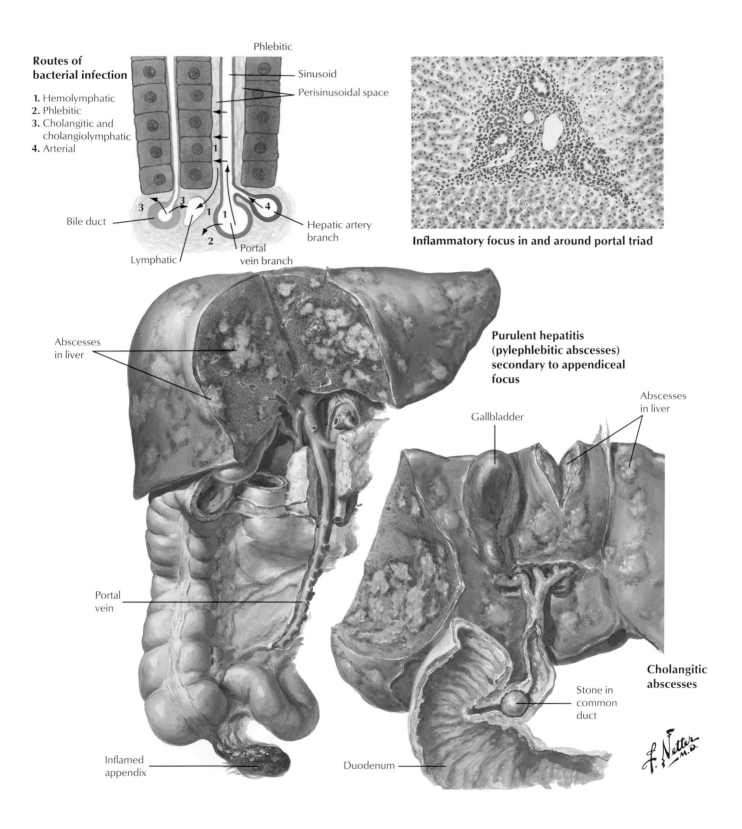

Routes of bacterial infection

1. Hemolymphatic
2. Phlebitic
3. Cholangitic and cholangiolymphatic
4. Arterial

Phlebitic

Sinusoid

Perisinusoidal space

Bile duct

Hepatic artery branch

Lymphatic

Portal vein branch

Inflammatory focus in and around portal triad

Abscesses in liver

Purulent hepatitis (pylephlebitic abscesses) secondary to appendiceal focus

Gallbladder

Abscesses in liver

Portal vein

Inflamed appendix

Duodenum

Cholangitic abscesses

Stone in common duct

FIGURE 5-5 BACTERIAL INFECTIONS OF THE LIVER

Bacterial infections of the liver frequently occur as part of a systemic infection (**septic abscesses**) or through lymphatic (**lymphangitis**) or venous (**pylephlebitis**) spread from infections of adjacent organs such as appendicitis, infectious cholangitis, diverticulitis, or pancreatitis. Microorganisms entering the liver are taken up by sinusoidal **Kupffer cells**, which proliferate to form small Kupffer cell nodules intermixed with hematogenous polymorphonuclear leukocytes (neutrophils). The neutrophils are even more pronounced in and around lymph channels and veins. A more toxic inflammatory reaction produces circumscribed necroses and abscesses in the liver.

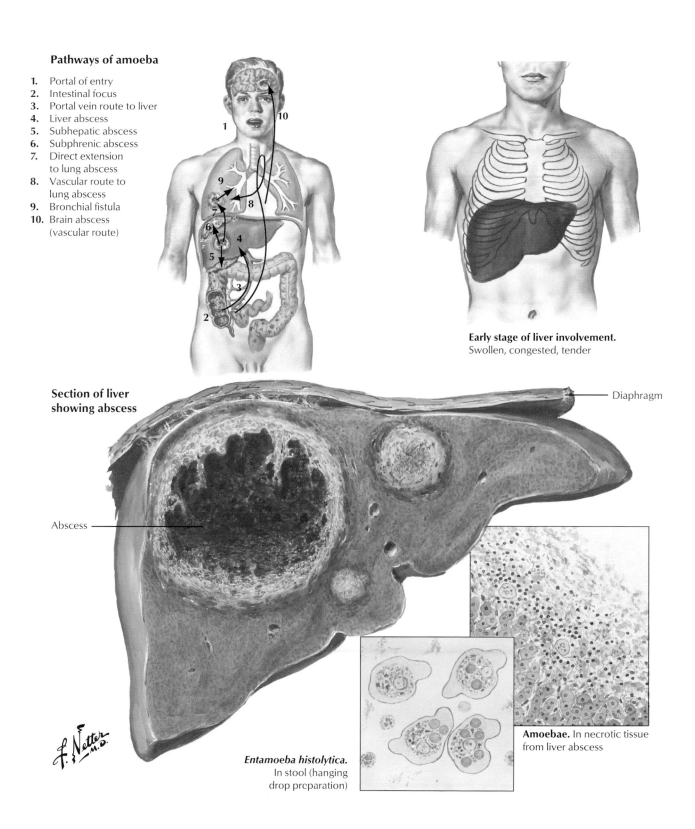

Pathways of amoeba

1. Portal of entry
2. Intestinal focus
3. Portal vein route to liver
4. Liver abscess
5. Subhepatic abscess
6. Subphrenic abscess
7. Direct extension to lung abscess
8. Vascular route to lung abscess
9. Bronchial fistula
10. Brain abscess (vascular route)

Early stage of liver involvement. Swollen, congested, tender

Section of liver showing abscess

Diaphragm

Abscess

Entamoeba histolytica. In stool (hanging drop preparation)

Amoebae. In necrotic tissue from liver abscess

FIGURE 5-6   LIVER ABSCESSES

Liver abscesses are the most common extraintestinal complication of **amebiasis**. They occur infrequently in the average US population but are more prevalent in homosexual men and especially in populations of tropical and subtropical zones (**tropical abscesses**). Abscesses impress as large well-circumscribed masses in the liver, which empty a dirty brownish material onto a cut surface. **Amebic trophozoites** accumulate in the border zone of abscess and viable liver parenchyma. Bacterial superinfection is frequent. Complications are rupture of the abscess into the peritoneal cavity or hematogenous spread of amebae with development of multiple lung and brain abscesses. Mortality in this stage is high (up to 40%).

147

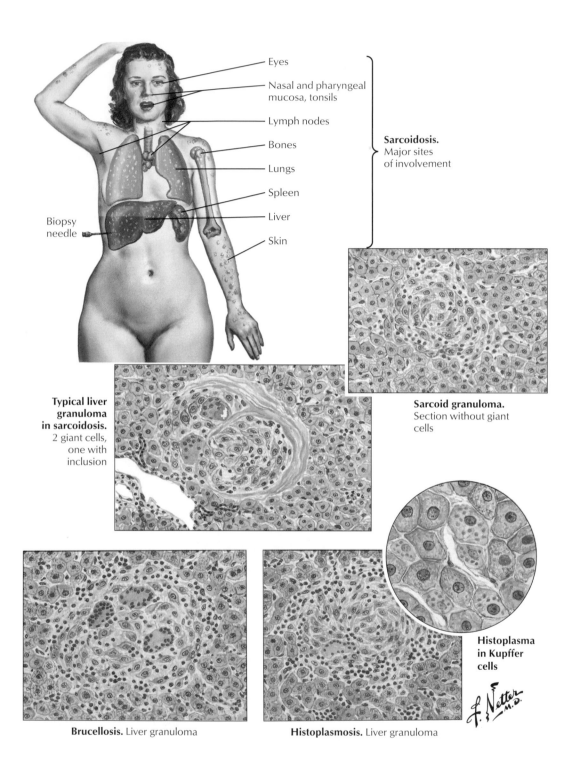

Sarcoidosis. Major sites of involvement

- Eyes
- Nasal and pharyngeal mucosa, tonsils
- Lymph nodes
- Bones
- Lungs
- Spleen
- Liver
- Skin

Biopsy needle

Typical liver granuloma in sarcoidosis. 2 giant cells, one with inclusion

Sarcoid granuloma. Section without giant cells

Histoplasma in Kupffer cells

Brucellosis. Liver granuloma

Histoplasmosis. Liver granuloma

FIGURE 5-7   GRANULOMATOUS HEPATITIS

Granulomatous hepatitis is associated with systemic infections such as tuberculosis, typhoid fever, and sarcoidosis. In addition, *brucellosis* (Mediterranean fever, undulant fever) is a zoonosis caused by microorganisms of the genus *Brucella* (*B abortus Bang, B melitensis, B suis, B canis*). Infection follows direct contact with infected animals or foods. Bacteria invade through the alimentary tract, the lungs, or skin abrasions and localize in cells of the reticuloendothelial tissues. Liver biopsy results reveal a mild nonspecific hepatitis with or without noncaseating granulomas, which are sometimes suppurative and calcifying. **Histoplasmosis** is a systemic soil-borne fungal infection caused by inhalation of *Histoplasma capsulatum*. Systemic histoplasmosis affects the liver with epithelioid cell granulomas with or without caseation.

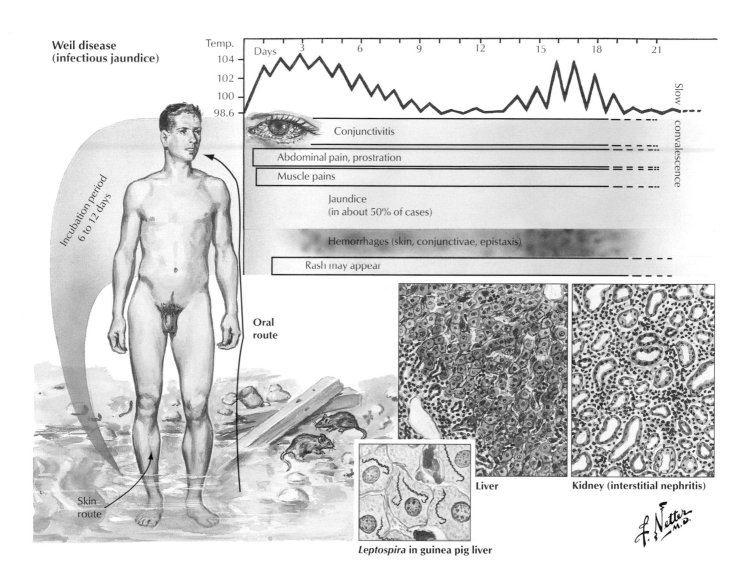

Weil disease
(infectious jaundice)

Incubation period
6 to 12 days

Skin
route

Oral
route

Conjunctivitis

Abdominal pain, prostration

Muscle pains

Jaundice
(in about 50% of cases)

Hemorrhages (skin, conjunctivae, epistaxis)

Rash may appear

Slow convalescence

Liver

Kidney (interstitial nephritis)

Leptospira in guinea pig liver

FIGURE 5-8   WEIL DISEASE

Spirochetal infections of the liver include **Weil disease** and **syphilis**. Weil disease (infectious jaundice) is caused by the spirochete *Leptospira,* a widespread zoonotic inhabitant in wild rats and mice. Liver involvement occurs in 50% of cases with noncharacteristic centrilobular and midzone necroses, Council-man bodies and ballooning degeneration of hepatocytes with signs of regeneration (anisonucleosis, multinucleated cells, mitotic figures), portal inflammation, and Kupffer cell hyperplasia.

The liver appears grossly yellow-green because of combined hepatocellular degeneration, hemolysis, and cholestasis. Lepto-spires can be identified microscopically in Kupffer cells and especially in renal tubular cells in approximately 65% of patients. Severe disease may be fatal. Syphilitic lesions occur in 2 forms: congenital syphilis, with mild triaditis, mild hepatocellular necrosis, and diffuse fibrosis, and tertiary syphilis, characterized by multiple granulomas (gummas) and scarring.

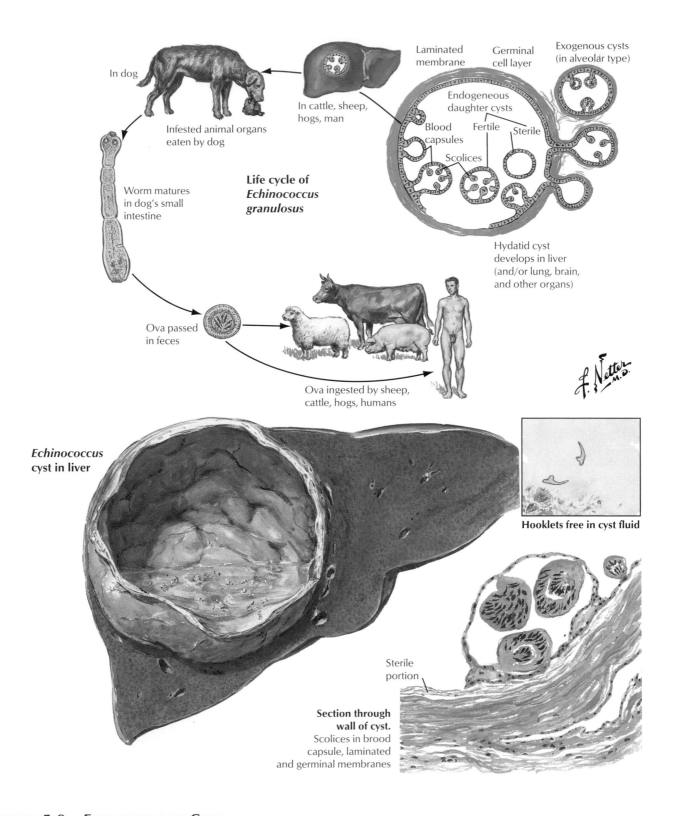

Laminated membrane

Germinal cell layer

Exogenous cysts (in alveolar type)

In dog

In cattle, sheep, hogs, man

Endogeneous daughter cysts

Blood capsules

Fertile

Sterile

Scolices

Infested animal organs eaten by dog

Life cycle of Echinococcus granulosus

Worm matures in dog's small intestine

Hydatid cyst develops in liver (and/or lung, brain, and other organs)

Ova passed in feces

Ova ingested by sheep, cattle, hogs, humans

Echinococcus cyst in liver

Hooklets free in cyst fluid

Sterile portion

Section through wall of cyst. Scolices in brood capsule, laminated and germinal membranes

FIGURE 5-9 *ECHINOCOCCUS* CYST

Parasitic diseases of the liver include infestations by tapeworms of *Echinococcus* species. ***Echinococcus* infection** is common in the Mediterranean, southern South America, the Middle East, central Asia, and Africa. Incidence is low in the United States. Humans become infected through ingestion of eggs in contaminated food. Approximately 60% of cysts develop in the liver, where they usually remain asymptomatic. Other sites that can be involved are the lungs, the brain, the kidneys, soft tissues, and bone. When cysts grow larger than 10 cm in diameter, they may cause compression of liver tissue with jaundice, portal hypertension, and cholangitis. Resorption of fluid materials from cysts causes immunologic sensitization of patients with secondary arthritis and membranous glomerulonephritis. Rupture of cysts in such conditions can lead to anaphylactic shock.

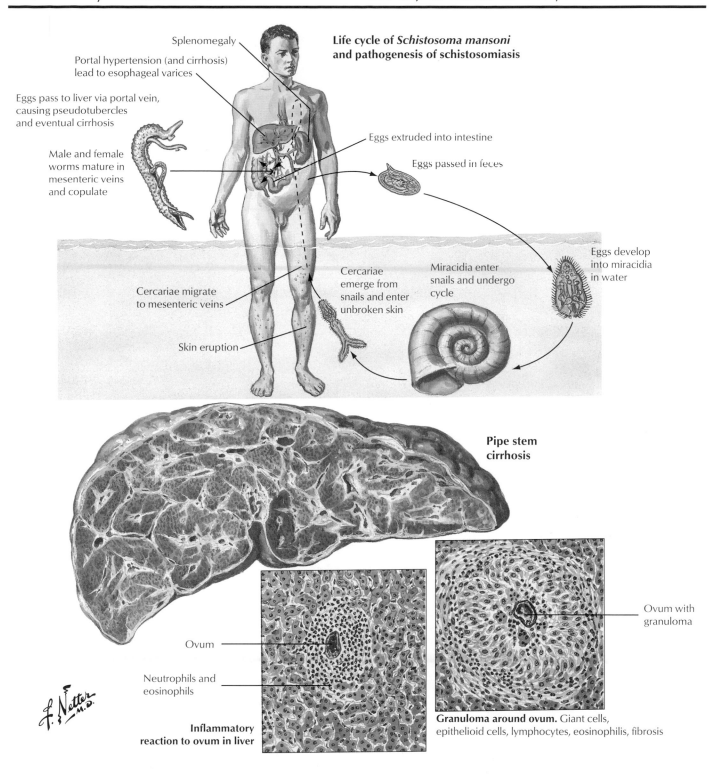

Life cycle of *Schistosoma mansoni* and pathogenesis of schistosomiasis

Splenomegaly

Portal hypertension (and cirrhosis) lead to esophageal varices

Eggs pass to liver via portal vein, causing pseudotubercles and eventual cirrhosis

Male and female worms mature in mesenteric veins and copulate

Eggs extruded into intestine

Eggs passed in feces

Cercariae migrate to mesenteric veins

Cercariae emerge from snails and enter unbroken skin

Miracidia enter snails and undergo cycle

Eggs develop into miracidia in water

Skin eruption

Pipe stem cirrhosis

Ovum

Neutrophils and eosinophils

Ovum with granuloma

Inflammatory reaction to ovum in liver

Granuloma around ovum. Giant cells, epithelioid cells, lymphocytes, eosinophilis, fibrosis

FIGURE 5-10   SCHISTOSOMIASIS

Schistosomiasis is caused by trematodes of the *Schistosoma* genus. It is endemic in large parts of Africa, the Americas, and the Far East. Humans are the principle hosts for the adult worms, which reside in the intestines, the urinary bladder, and the venous system. Sexual reproduction of worms produces eggs, which infest water and develop into a ciliated intermedia, the **miracidia**. Miracidia penetrate into a snail where they reproduce asexually within 4 to 6 weeks to produce hundreds of **cercariae**, which enter humans through the skin when they bathe in infected waters. The cercariae migrate to the lungs and mature into adult worms, which travel via blood vessels (veins) to distant organs. Up to 10% of patients in endemic regions develop schistosomiasis of the liver, which consists of granulomatous hepatitis (around schistosomal eggs) with eosinophils and portal fibrosis. Progression to cirrhosis is exceptional.

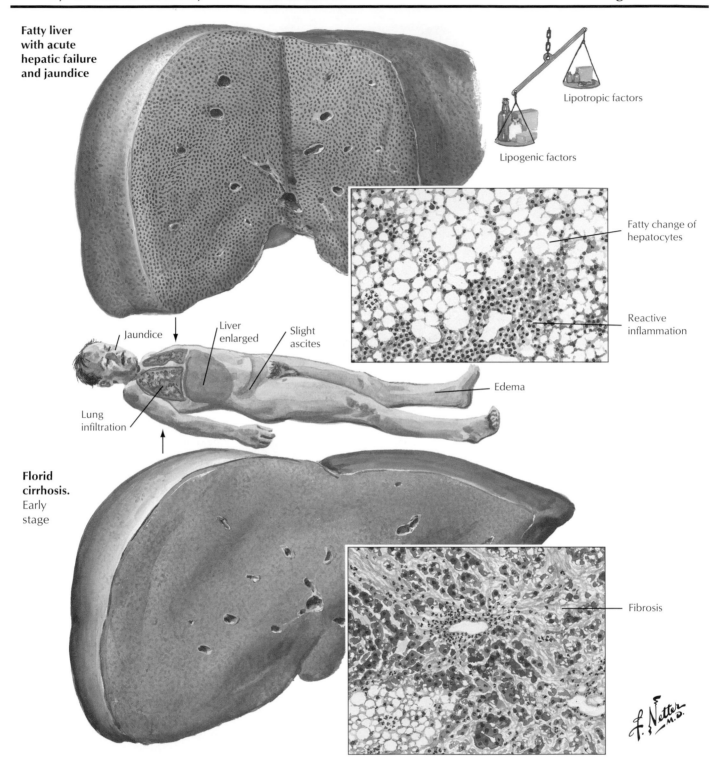

Fatty liver with acute hepatic failure and jaundice

Lipotropic factors

Lipogenic factors

Fatty change of hepatocytes

Reactive inflammation

Jaundice

Liver enlarged

Slight ascites

Edema

Lung infiltration

Florid cirrhosis. Early stage

Fibrosis

FIGURE 5-11   ALCOHOLISM

In Western countries, **alcoholism** is the most frequent cause of fatty liver (**hepatic steatosis**) and "toxic" hepatitis. Seventy percent of liver cirrhoses (Table 5-3) are alcoholic cirrhoses. Chronic daily intake of 80 to 160 g ethanol increases peripheral lipolysis and causes influx of fatty acids into the liver, enhances intrahepatic fatty acid and triglyceride synthesis, and reduces fatty acid oxidation and the release of lipoproteins. Hepatic steatosis develops in 3 stages: **stage I fatty liver** (**simple steatosis**): 50% or

more of hepatocytes show fatty infiltration; **stage II fatty liver hepatitis** (**alcoholic hepatitis**): steatosis, focal hepatocellular necrosis/degeneration (fatty and ballooning degeneration of hepatocytes with **alcoholic** hyaline [**Mallory bodies**]), and reactive-type hepatitis with or without reticular and septal fibrosis; **stage III fatty liver cirrhosis** (**alcoholic cirrhosis**): steatosis (may be absent in later stages) with diffuse micronodular cirrhosis.

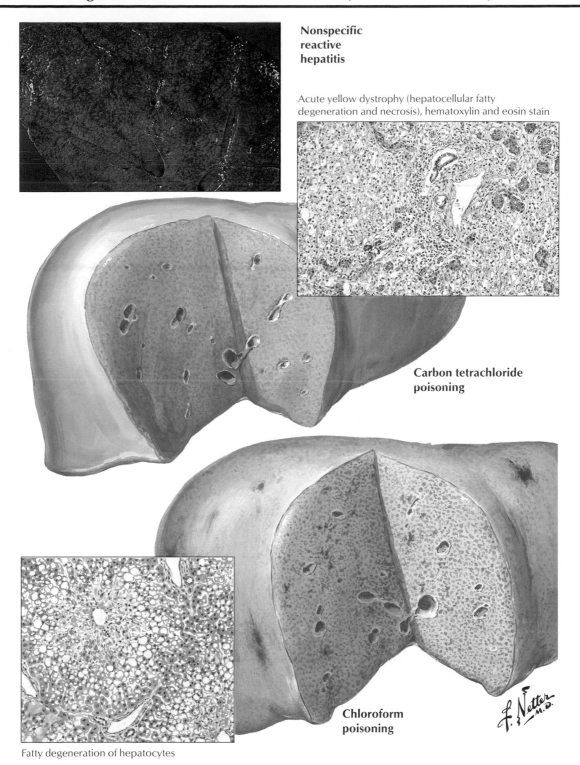

Nonspecific
reactive
hepatitis

Acute yellow dystrophy (hepatocellular fatty
degeneration and necrosis), hematoxylin and eosin stain

Carbon tetrachloride
poisoning

Chloroform
poisoning

Fatty degeneration of hepatocytes

FIGURE 5-12　TOXIC INJURIES

Significant fatty infiltration and necrosis result from fungus poisoning (especially with *Amanita muscaria*) or exposure to organic solvents (chloroform) or phosphorus, all of which cause rapidly progressive liver failure and death in **liver coma**. Other toxic injuries to the liver—with or without steatosis—are outlined in Table 5-3. Another toxic condition with extensive hemorrhagic necroses in the liver is eclampsia (**toxemia of pregnancy**), a hypertensive disorder of pregnancy with edema, proteinuria, vascular endothelial injury, and coagulation abnormalities. The latter causes **disseminated intravascular coagulation**, with the most prominent lesions in the liver, the brain, and the kidneys. Patients usually die of cerebral hemorrhages and symptoms of coma and convulsions.

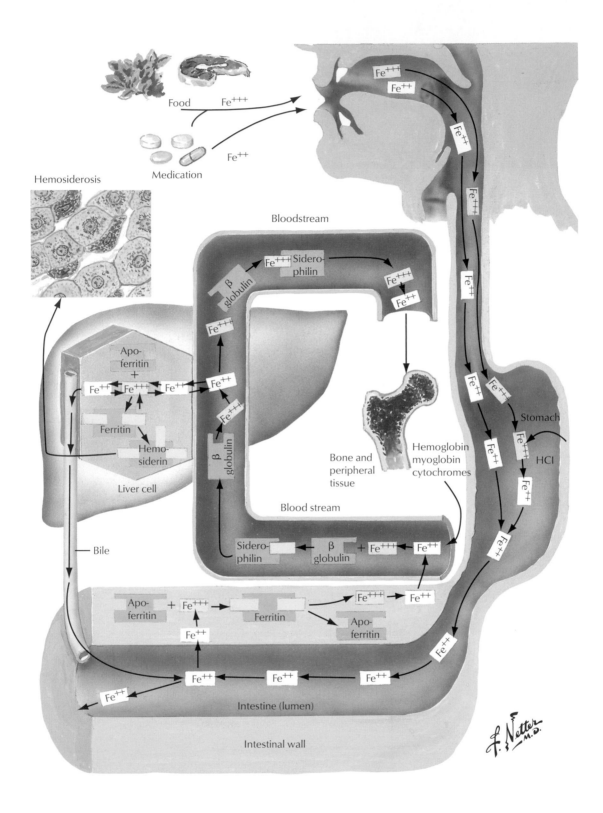

FIGURE 5-13 HEMOCHROMATOSIS

Hemochromatosis, a common autosomal recessive disorder, is characterized by iron accumulation in the liver, the heart, the pancreas, and other organs. It affects men 10 times more frequently than women and is based on a genetic change on chromosome 6, gene HLA-H (HFE gene), which controls iron absorption. Iron accumulates in the liver and other organs at a rate of up to 1 g/y; clinical symptoms occur when the body iron stores exceed 20 g (normal, 3–4 g). Liver tissue contains 6000 to 18,000 µg/g dry weight iron as compared with the normal storage of 300 to 1400 µg/g. **Hemosiderosis** (secondary exogenous hemochromatosis) represents a secondary iron overload syndrome, usually after hypertransfusion with blood.

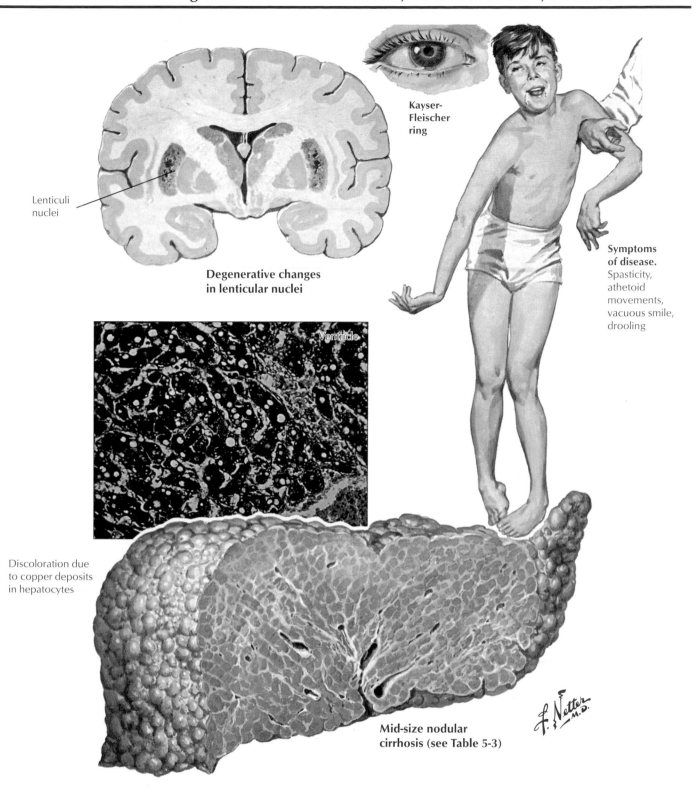

Kayser-
Fleischer
ring

Lenticuli
nuclei

**Degenerative changes
in lenticular nuclei**

Ventricle

**Symptoms
of disease.**
Spasticity,
athetoid
movements,
vacuous smile,
drooling

Discoloration due
to copper deposits
in hepatocytes

F. Netter
M.D.

**Mid-size nodular
cirrhosis (see Table 5-3)**

FIGURE 5-14　WILSON DISEASE

Wilson disease (WD; **hepatolenticular degeneration**) is an autosomal recessive disorder of hepatobiliary copper excretion with progressive accumulation of the toxic metal in the liver, the brain, the eyes, and many other organs. The genetic disturbance is located on chromosome 13. The incidence of WD is 1:30,000. First symptoms are usually noted during the second decade of life. Liver pathology shows acute (necrotizing) hepatitis, chronic active hepatitis with cholestasis, or cirrhosis with or without copper deposition (copper usually in excess of 250 µg/g dry weight). Hepatic changes without excess copper are indistinguishable from viral hepatitis and cirrhosis. Of diagnostic value are copper deposits in the corneal limbus, which impress on inspection as brown-greenish rings (**Kaiser–Fleischer rings**). WD runs a progressive downhill course until copper is reduced by chelating agents, except for rare cases of fulminant hepatitis, which have an unfavorable prognosis.

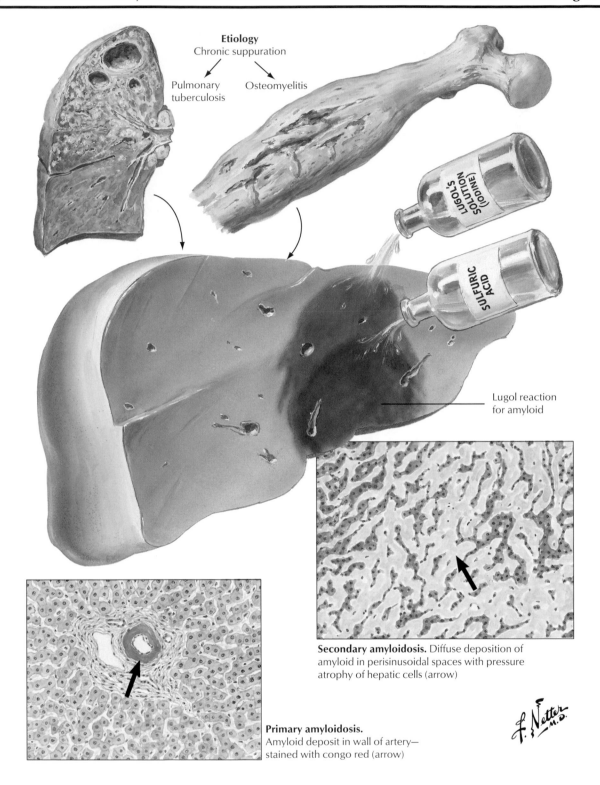

Etiology
Chronic suppuration

Pulmonary
tuberculosis

Osteomyelitis

Lugol reaction
for amyloid

Secondary amyloidosis. Diffuse deposition of
amyloid in perisinusoidal spaces with pressure
atrophy of hepatic cells (arrow)

Primary amyloidosis.
Amyloid deposit in wall of artery—
stained with congo red (arrow)

FIGURE 5-15   AMYLOIDOSIS OF THE LIVER

Amyloidosis of the liver occurs in 2 forms: diffuse perisinusoidal amyloidosis (secondary amyloidosis) after chronic infections, and focal vascular (portal) amyloidosis (primary amyloidosis). **Secondary amyloidosis** causes enlargement of the liver with effacement of the gross lobular structure. The cut surface is smooth and rubbery and of yellowish-brown color. **Primary amyloidosis**, which is not associated with inflammatory diseases of other organs, frequently follows abnormal protein production by plasma cells (**plasma cell dyscrasia**). Therefore, it is frequently accompanied by diffuse plasmacytosis or malignant plasmacytoma. Vascular (primary) amyloidosis typically involves mesenchymal tissues of other organs such as the myocardium, skeletal muscle, the tongue, the skin, the kidneys, and the spleen. Both forms of liver amyloidosis are part of a systemic process, and involvement of other organs may determine the outcome (e.g., cardiac or renal failure).

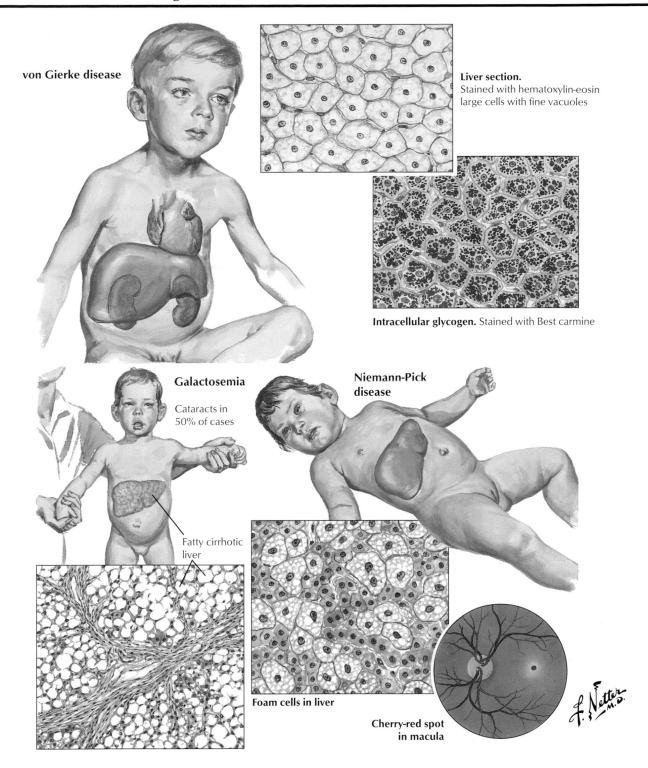

von Gierke disease

Liver section. Stained with hematoxylin-eosin large cells with fine vacuoles

Intracellular glycogen. Stained with Best carmine

Galactosemia

Cataracts in 50% of cases

Fatty cirrhotic liver

Niemann-Pick disease

Foam cells in liver

Cherry-red spot in macula

FIGURE 5-16 STORAGE DISEASES

Storage diseases (**thesaurismoses**) affect children preferentially and cause hepatomegaly. Most common are **glycogen storage diseases** (**von Gierke disease** and others) and **sphingolipidoses** (**Niemann-Pick, Tay-Sachs,** and **Gaucher diseases**). Nonmetabolized substances accumulate because of genetic mutations of lysosomal hydrolytic enzymes. Glycogen preferentially accumulates in hepatocytes in the liver, whereas other substances are taken up more intensely by cells of the reticulohistiocytic (phagocytic) series (Kupffer cells) in the liver. These cells are greatly enlarged, leading to compression and atrophy of hepatocytes. **Galactosemia** results from deficiency of a transferase that converts galactose into glucose, resulting in deposition of galactose in several organs, such as the liver, the spleen, the kidneys, the central nervous system (CNS), and the eyes. Malnutrition in these infants contributes to diffuse fatty degeneration of hepatocytes with development of liver cirrhosis and portal hypertension.

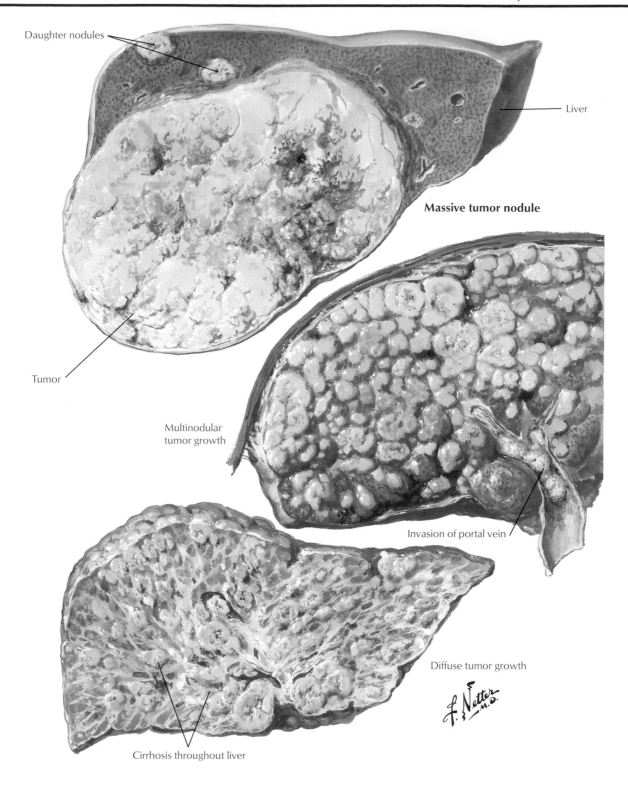

Daughter nodules

Liver

Massive tumor nodule

Tumor

Multinodular
tumor growth

Invasion of portal vein

Diffuse tumor growth

Cirrhosis throughout liver

FIGURE 5-17   HEPATOCELLULAR CARCINOMA

Hepatocellular carcinoma, which occurs in adults with cirrhotic livers (in children it is seen without cirrhosis), is associated with persistent infection by HBV and HCV, including asymptomatic carriers (i.e., patients with occult liver cirrhosis). Other patients with liver cirrhosis who are at risk for developing HCC are those with hemochromatosis and α1-antitrypsin deficiency. Most patients with alcoholic cirrhosis and HCC are also infected with HCV or HBV. The gross picture of HCC is that of one or several irregular soft yellowish-green nodules in a cirrhotic liver with intrahepatic (parenchymatous, intravascular) spread. The histologic appearance varies from a trabecular and acinar pattern of well-differentiated hepatocytes to a poorly differentiated fibrolamellar tumor or a tumor with cholangiocellular features. The ascites color may change to bloody. Serum levels of α-fetoprotein increase dramatically (400–4000 ng/mL).

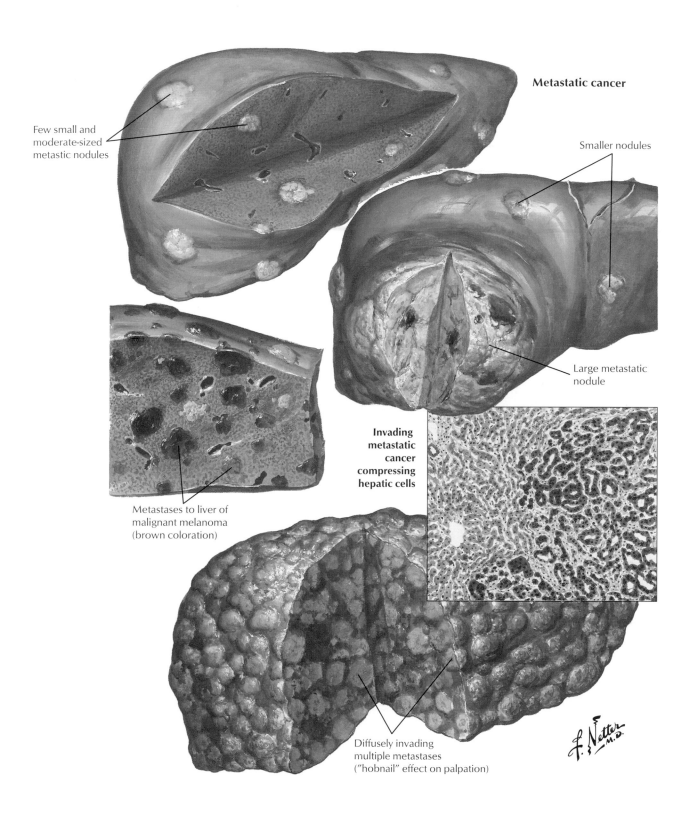

Metastatic cancer

Few small and moderate-sized metastic nodules

Smaller nodules

Large metastatic nodule

Invading metastatic cancer compressing hepatic cells

Metastases to liver of malignant melanoma (brown coloration)

Diffusely invading multiple metastases ("hobnail" effect on palpation)

f. Netter M.D.

FIGURE 5-18   INTRAHEPATIC CHOLANGIOCARCINOMA

Although more rare than HCC, intrahepatic (peripheral) CAC also is associated with cirrhosis. It is derived from small **intrahepatic bile canaliculi** with lymphatic spread to portal lymph nodes (less frequently than HCC via hepatic vessels). The tumor is usually well differentiated with clearly defined tubular structures and pronounced desmoplasia (tumor fibrosis). Bile pigment is absent.

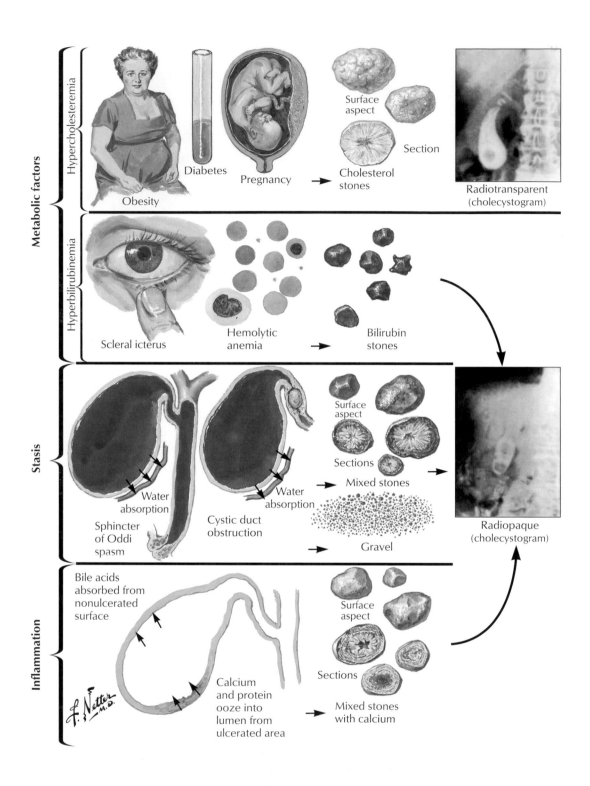

FIGURE 5-19   CHOLELITHIASIS

Cholelithiasis (CL) results from the formation of stones in the gallbladder and in large bile ducts. Bile stones are composed of bile (bile acids, bile pigments, and cholesterol) with various amounts of calcium. Stones are classified as cholesterol stones, pigment stones, and mixed stones according to the prevalent component. More than half of stones are **cholesterol stones**, which consist of precipitated cholesterol (nutritional hypercholes-

terolemia, reduced solubilization by bile acids) with crystal formation. **Pigment stones** are usually smaller and consist of blood pigments (calcium bilirubinate is contained in bilirubin stones). They occur most frequently in patients with some form of hemolytic anemia (e.g., thalassemia, sickle cell anemia) but also occur in patients with infections of the biliary tract. **Mixed stones** usually result from inflammation and bile stasis.

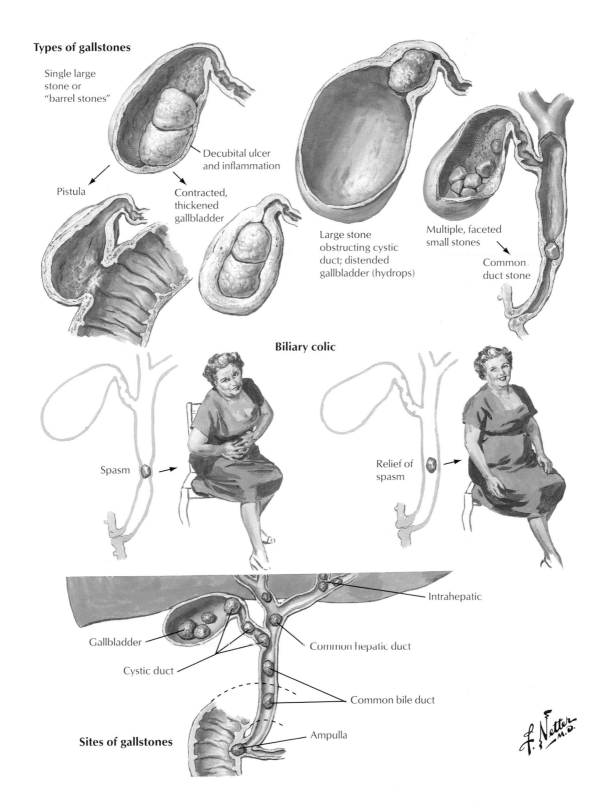

Types of gallstones

Single large stone or "barrel stones"

Decubital ulcer and inflammation

Pistula

Contracted, thickened gallbladder

Large stone obstructing cystic duct; distended gallbladder (hydrops)

Multiple, faceted small stones

Common duct stone

Biliary colic

Spasm

Relief of spasm

Sites of gallstones

Gallbladder

Cystic duct

Intrahepatic

Common hepatic duct

Common bile duct

Ampulla

FIGURE 5-20   CHOLELITHIASIS: COMPLICATIONS

Only 20% of patients with CHL become clinically symptomatic. Complications usually arise from obstruction of bile passageways by stones, which results in acute severe pain (**biliary colic**) and inflammation. Obstruction by stones may occur at various sites from the cystic duct to the choledochus and the papilla. Papillary obstruction causes acute pancreatitis in cases of coincident obstruction of the pancreatic duct. Complications of chronic CHL are bile stasis, superinfection with pus accumulation in the bladder (**empyema**), perforation of a stone into the peritoneum with resultant peritonitis or into the intestines with eventual obstruction (**gallstone ileus**), and fibrous obstruction of the cystic duct with resorption of bile, which leaves a mucoid intraluminal fluid (**mucocele**). Stones in the common bile duct or in the major intrahepatic ducts cause obstructive cholestasis in the liver.

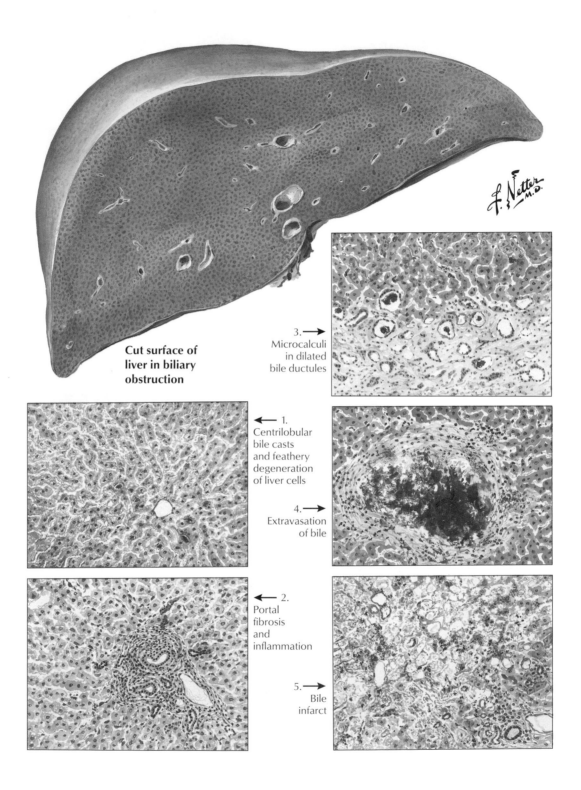

Cut surface of liver in biliary obstruction

3. → Microcalculi in dilated bile ductules

← 1. Centrilobular bile casts and feathery degeneration of liver cells

4. → Extravasation of bile

← 2. Portal fibrosis and inflammation

5. → Bile infarct

FIGURE 5-21 CHOLESTASIS: EXTRAHEPATIC AND INTRAHEPATIC

Extrahepatic biliary obstruction causes bile casts, which are most prominent in the peripheral part of the lobule. They are usually accompanied by secondary hepatocellular degeneration (**feathery degeneration**, see Figure 1-1, top right), portal inflammation (neutrophilic and lymphoplasmacytic), and portal and septal fibrosis. The liver is enlarged and dark green but rarely cirrhotic. **Intrahepatic cholestasis** shows portal and centrilobular bile stasis without major hepatocellular degeneration. Prominent reparative

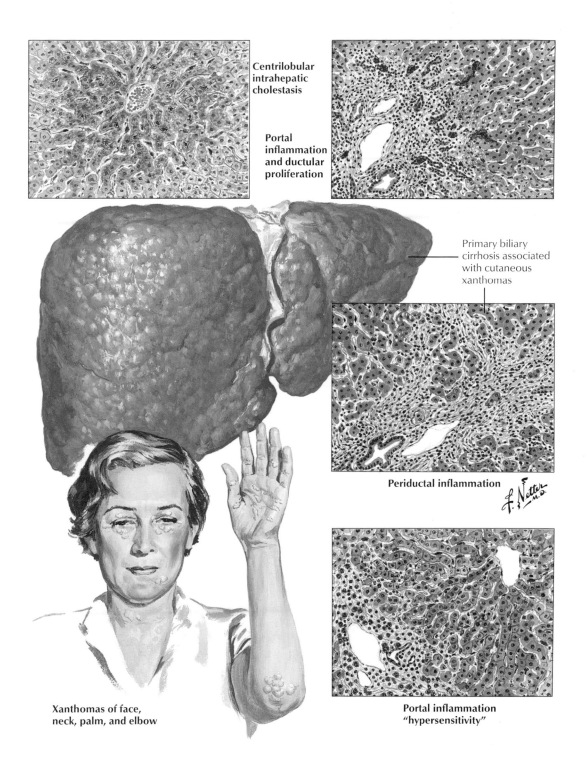

Centrilobular intrahepatic cholestasis

Portal inflammation and ductular proliferation

Primary biliary cirrhosis associated with cutaneous xanthomas

Periductal inflammation

Xanthomas of face, neck, palm, and elbow

Portal inflammation "hypersensitivity"

FIGURE 5-21 CHOLESTASIS: EXTRAHEPATIC AND INTRAHEPATIC (CONTINUED)

bile duct proliferation occurs in portal triads with chronic inflammation, progressive fibrosis, and, finally, cirrhosis. Intrahepatic cholestasis usually accompanies other liver diseases, such as viral or toxic hepatitis, but its etiology can remain obscure. In later stages, hepatocytes show ballooning degeneration, and chronic portal inflammation leads to portal and septal fibrosis with regenerative proliferation of bile ducts.

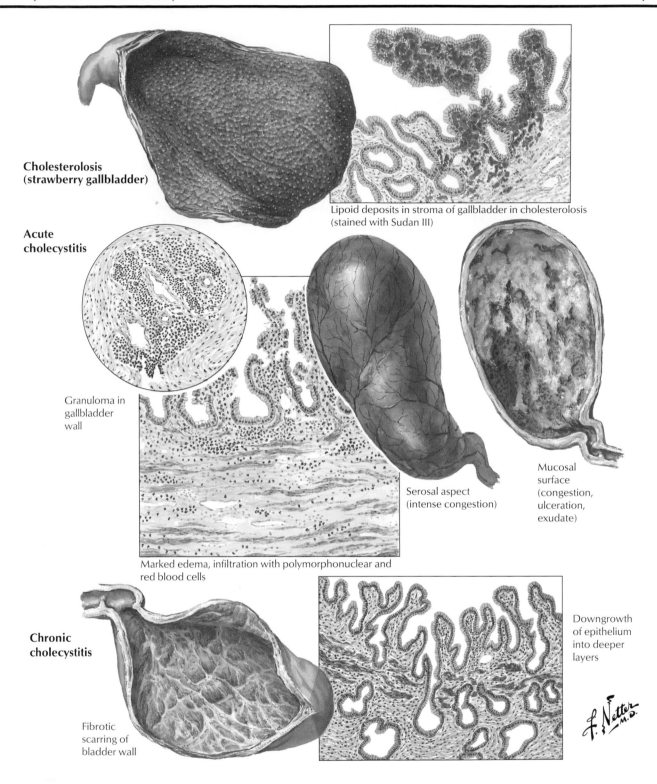

Cholesterolosis (strawberry gallbladder)

Lipoid deposits in stroma of gallbladder in cholesterolosis (stained with Sudan III)

Acute cholecystitis

Granuloma in gallbladder wall

Marked edema, infiltration with polymorphonuclear and red blood cells

Serosal aspect (intense congestion)

Mucosal surface (congestion, ulceration, exudate)

Chronic cholecystitis

Fibrotic scarring of bladder wall

Downgrowth of epithelium into deeper layers

FIGURE 5-22 CHOLECYSTITIS

Acute and chronic cholecystitis, diffuse inflammations of the gallbladder wall, are most frequently caused by CHL. They can occur with or without lipid deposits in mucosal macrophages, causing typical foam cells. Cholecystitis not associated with CHL may be seen in infections (sepsis, salmonella), in autoimmune vasculitis (e.g., panarteritis nodosa), or secondary to trauma. **Acute cholecystitis** is characterized by edematous thickening of the bladder wall with neutrophilic infiltration and eventual hemorrhage. Cholesterol resorption may cause occasional foreign body granulomas (giant cells with cholesterol clefts). Empyema and perforation are possible complications. **Chronic cholecystitis** shows mucosal atrophy, fibrous thickening of the bladder wall, and hypertrophy and hyperplasia of deeper glands. There may be extensive adhesions of the gallbladder to adjacent organs (e.g., the large intestine).

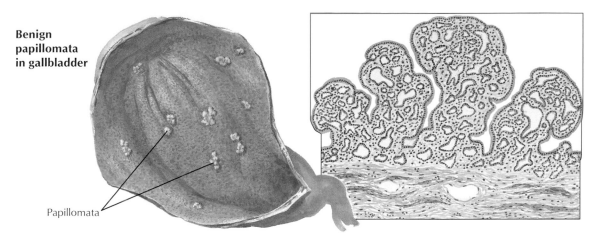

Benign papillomata in gallbladder

Papillomata

Polypoid hyperplasia of mucosa

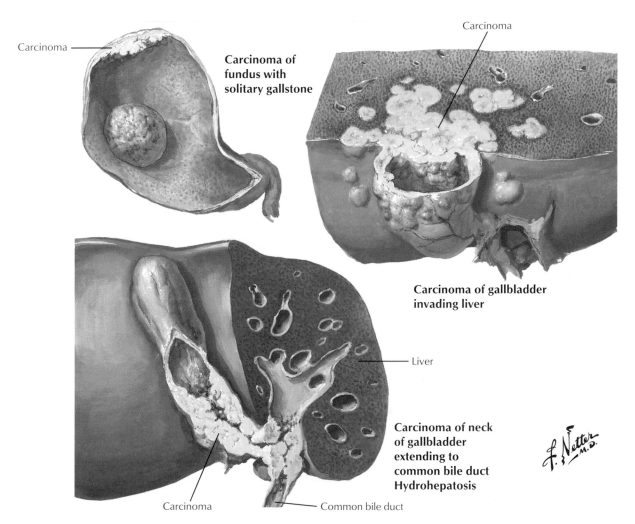

Carcinoma

Carcinoma of fundus with solitary gallstone

Carcinoma

Carcinoma of gallbladder invading liver

Liver

Carcinoma of neck of gallbladder extending to common bile duct Hydrohepatosis

Carcinoma

Common bile duct

FIGURE 5-23 CANCER OF THE GALLBLADDER

Adenocarcinoma of the gallbladder, the fifth most common tumor in the GI tract, usually occurs later in life. There are 2 major types: (1) a flat, scirrhous, and infiltrating form (not well differentiated) and (2) a polypoid-fungating form (well differentiated). More than 60% of these cancers are associated with CHL. Nearly all have spread to liver and peribiliary fat tissue at the time of the initial diagnosis so that the mean 5-year survival is only approximately 1%. Biliary adenocarcinoma metastasizes preferentially within the peritoneal cavity to regional lymph nodes and other organs of the GI tract. It spreads to the lungs less frequently.

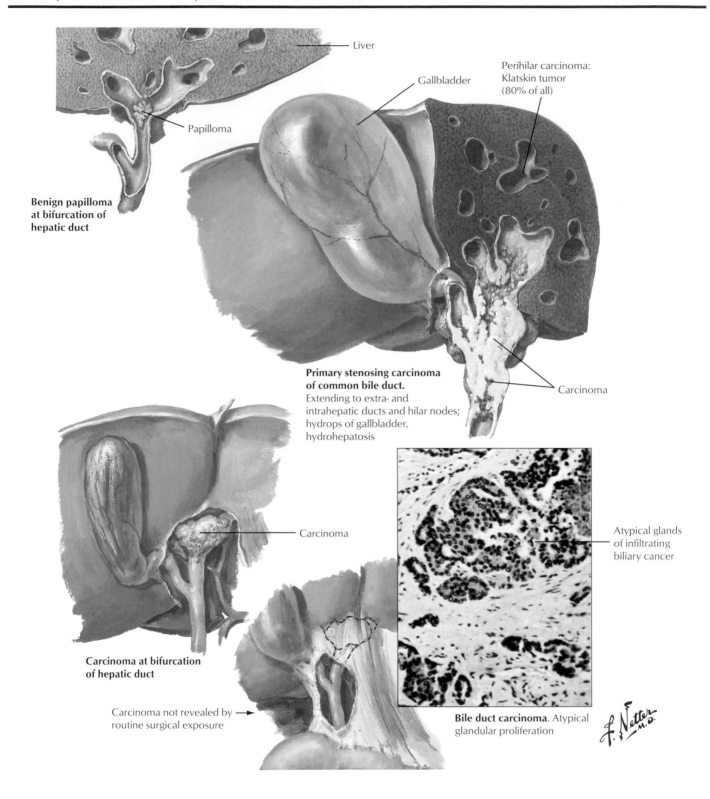

Benign papilloma
at bifurcation of
hepatic duct

Papilloma

Liver

Gallbladder

Perihilar carcinoma:
Klatskin tumor
(80% of all)

Primary stenosing carcinoma
of common bile duct.
Extending to extra- and
intrahepatic ducts and hilar nodes;
hydrops of gallbladder,
hydrohepatosis

Carcinoma

Carcinoma at bifurcation
of hepatic duct

Carcinoma not revealed by
routine surgical exposure

Carcinoma

Atypical glands
of infiltrating
biliary cancer

Bile duct carcinoma. Atypical
glandular proliferation

FIGURE 5-24 CANCER OF THE BILE DUCTS AND THE AMPULLARY REGION

Adenocarcinoma of extrahepatic bile ducts and of the ampullary region occurs in older patients. It is not usually related to bile stones and is more frequent in areas where infestation with the fluke *Clonorchis sinensis* is endemic. Hepatic pathology secondary to obstruction and bile stasis causes liver enzymes to increase, especially alkaline phosphatase. Early detection while tumors are still small may result in a more favorable prognosis than in cancer of the gallbladder, with a mean 35% five-year survival for patients with ampullary cancers. Common adenocarcinoma of the bile ducts has usually spread at the time of diagnosis, rendering surgical resections incomplete and resulting in an average survival of 18 months.

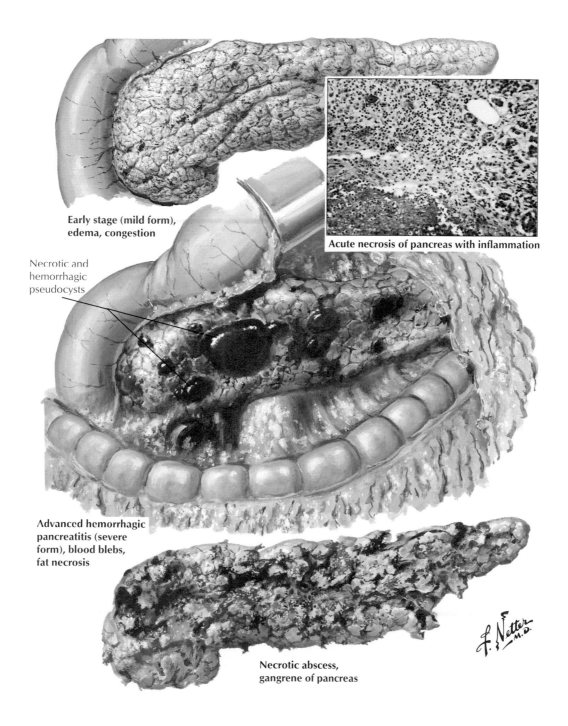

Early stage (mild form), edema, congestion

Acute necrosis of pancreas with inflammation

Necrotic and hemorrhagic pseudocysts

Advanced hemorrhagic pancreatitis (severe form), blood blebs, fat necrosis

Necrotic abscess, gangrene of pancreas

FIGURE 5-25   ACUTE PANCREATITIS

Acute pancreatitis presents in 3 forms: (1) a mild, self-limited disease with little destruction of acinar cells; (2) a recurrent inflammation, which progresses to chronic pancreatitis; or (3) a life-threatening disease with gross necrosis of pancreatic and fat tissue. The **mild form** is characterized by interstitial edema with neutrophilic infiltration and occasional acinar cell degeneration. **Virally induced pancreatitis** occurs as acute or chronic recurrent pancreatitis with a lymphocytic infiltrate, some epithelial necrosis (ductal and acinar), and occasional cytopathic changes (cytome-

galic **owl eye cells**). In the **severe form**, massive enzymatic digestion by proteases causes extensive necroses and hemorrhage secondary to necrotic blood vessels. Lipases cause extensive necrosis of fat tissue (lipolytic necroses) with precipitation of calcium salts. Fatty acids and calcium form insoluble salts at the site of fatty necroses with a characteristic soapy appearance. There are few neutrophils and, eventually, granulation tissue. Massive necrosis may cause pancreatic pseudocysts on resorption of the necrotic debris.

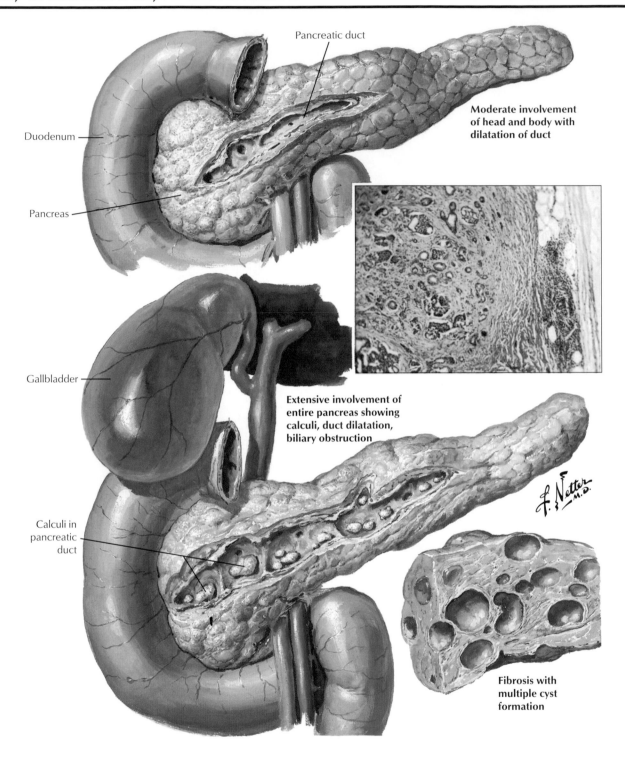

Pancreatic duct

Moderate involvement
of head and body with
dilatation of duct

Duodenum

Pancreas

Gallbladder

Extensive involvement of
entire pancreas showing
calculi, duct dilatation,
biliary obstruction

Calculi in
pancreatic
duct

Fibrosis with
multiple cyst
formation

FIGURE 5-26   CHRONIC PANCREATITIS

Chronic pancreatitis with progressive destruction of the parenchyma and fibrosis results from recurrent acute pancreatitis. Various lymphoplasmacytic infiltrates invade disrupted exocrine glandular acini. In end-stage disease, only pancreatic ducts and some islets may remain in the extensive scar tissue. In disease caused by long-term alcohol abuse, there is additional mucus plugging of major pancreatic ducts with secondary calcification

(**chronic calcifying pancreatitis**). Other causes of chronic pancreatitis are mucoviscidosis (CF), which is also characterized by mucus plugging of ducts (**chronic obstructive pancreatitis**); WD; hemochromatosis; rare forms of hereditary pancreatitis (in childhood); and idiopathic forms. Chronic pancreatitis usually runs a long, debilitating course with a cumulative mortality of 50% in approximately 20 years.

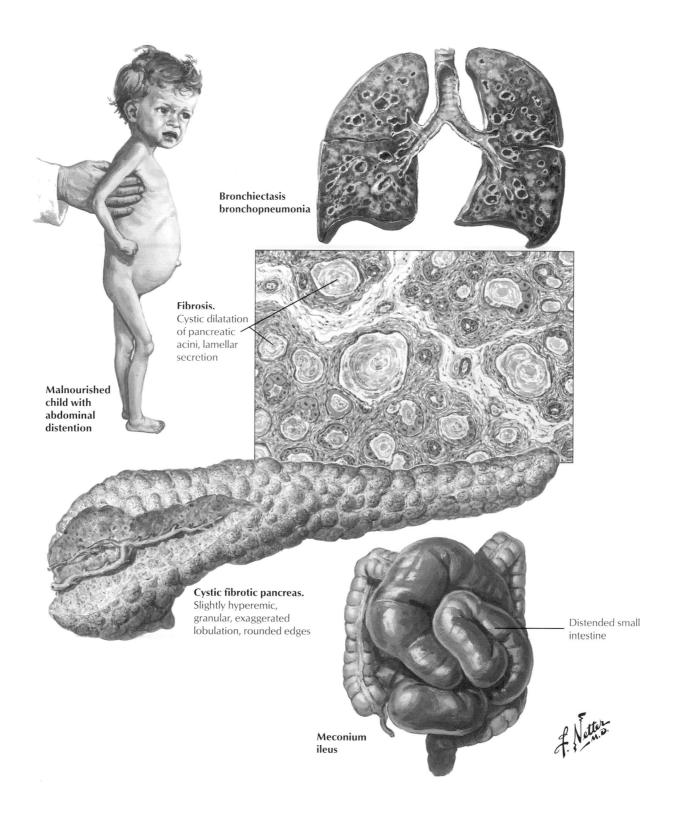

Bronchiectasis bronchopneumonia

Fibrosis. Cystic dilatation of pancreatic acini, lamellar secretion

Malnourished child with abdominal distention

Cystic fibrotic pancreas. Slightly hyperemic, granular, exaggerated lobulation, rounded edges

Distended small intestine

Meconium ileus

FIGURE 5-27 CYSTIC FIBROSIS (see also Figure 3-3)

More than 80% of patients with **CF** (**mucoviscidosis**) have visible secretory abnormalities of the pancreas, which cause mucus inspissation in major ducts and secondary atrophy of exocrine glands. Dilated and plugged ducts may cause multiple cysts, and degrading (sometimes superinfected) mucus leads to chronic resorptive inflammation with lymphoplasmacytic and phagocytic infiltration and progressive collagenous fibrosis. Ductal epithelia may undergo squamous metaplasia (supported by deficient vitamin A resorption). Clinical features are those of malabsorption with abdominal distention, bulky foul stools, and a failure to thrive.

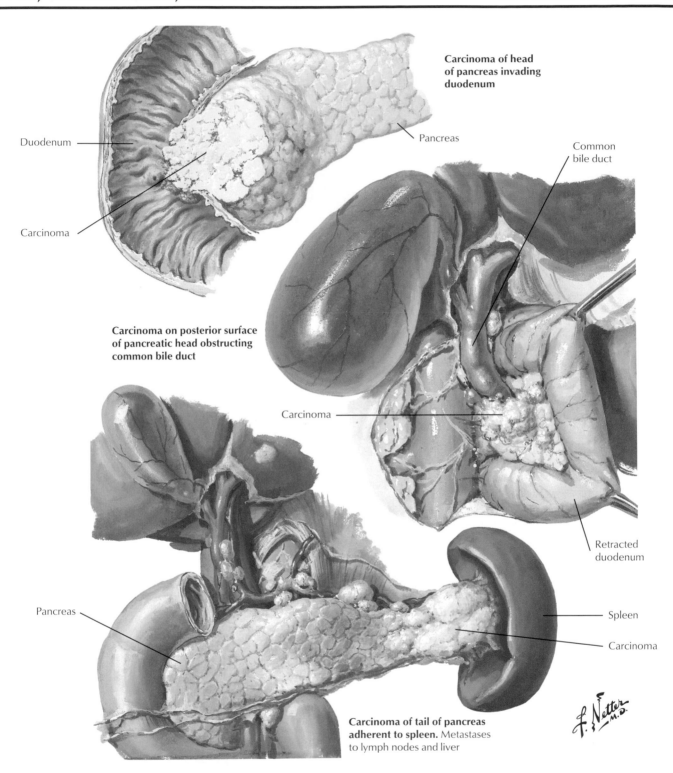

Carcinoma of head
of pancreas invading
duodenum

Duodenum

Pancreas

Common
bile duct

Carcinoma

Carcinoma on posterior surface
of pancreatic head obstructing
common bile duct

Carcinoma

Retracted
duodenum

Pancreas

Spleen

Carcinoma

Carcinoma of tail of pancreas
adherent to spleen. Metastases
to lymph nodes and liver

FIGURE 5-28 PANCREATIC CANCER

Carcinoma of the pancreas develops from ductal epithelial cells. Approximately 60% of pancreatic cancers are located in the head of the organ, 10% are located in the body, and 5% are located in the tail. The residual tumors show diffuse organ involvement without indication of their initial site. Usually, the tumor has already metastasized at the time of diagnosis. On gross inspection, the carcinoma of pancreas appears as poorly demarcated, white scarred or nodular areas with or without involvement of the common duct, the papilla, or the duodenum. Obstruction of the common bile duct may cause a characteristic dilatation of the gallbladder with jaundice (**Courvoisier sign**). An important complication of pancreatic cancer is a variable and migrating thrombosis (**migratory thrombophlebitis**), which may bring patients to clinical attention for multiple pulmonary thromboses and infarcts of unknown origin.

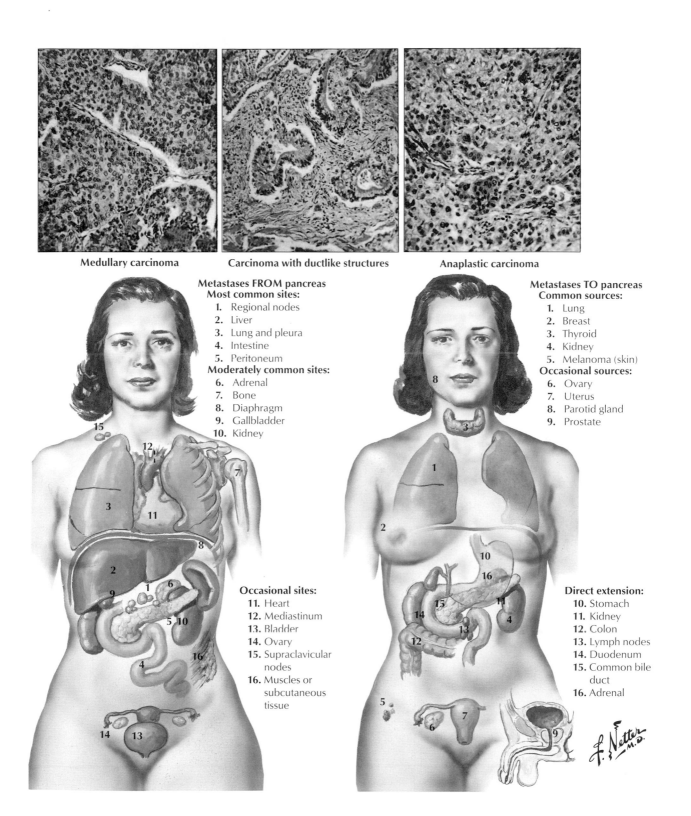

Medullary carcinoma

Carcinoma with ductlike structures

Anaplastic carcinoma

Metastases FROM pancreas
Most common sites:
1. Regional nodes
2. Liver
3. Lung and pleura
4. Intestine
5. Peritoneum

Moderately common sites:
6. Adrenal
7. Bone
8. Diaphragm
9. Gallbladder
10. Kidney

Occasional sites:
11. Heart
12. Mediastinum
13. Bladder
14. Ovary
15. Supraclavicular nodes
16. Muscles or subcutaneous tissue

Metastases TO pancreas
Common sources:
1. Lung
2. Breast
3. Thyroid
4. Kidney
5. Melanoma (skin)

Occasional sources:
6. Ovary
7. Uterus
8. Parotid gland
9. Prostate

Direct extension:
10. Stomach
11. Kidney
12. Colon
13. Lymph nodes
14. Duodenum
15. Common bile duct
16. Adrenal

FIGURE 5-29   TUMORS OF THE PANCREAS: METASTASES

Tumors of the pancreas grow into the adjacent peritoneum and organs (duodenum, stomach, liver, colon, spleen) by direct extension and metastasize most commonly to regional lymph nodes and the liver. Lymphangitic metastases to the lungs and hematogenous spread to the bone marrow (occasionally with fatty necroses) are also found. Most tumors are well-differentiated tubular adenocarcinomas with or without mucin secretion and associated fibrosis (**desmoplastic tubular carcinoma**).

CHAPTER 6

KIDNEYS, URETERS, AND URINARY BLADDER

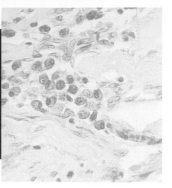

The organ system examined in this chapter is the site of numerous diverse conditions, including congenital and hereditary diseases of the kidney, primary disease of the kidney, systemic diseases affecting the kidney, and diseases of the urinary system.

The kidneys are the primary regulators of the internal environment, particularly the volume, tonicity, and compartmental distribution of body fluids. They perform this function by exchanging and excreting water, minerals, and nonmetabolized solutes from the daily diet and end products of nitrogen metabolism (**urea** and **creatinine**). To accomplish this task, the kidneys produce an ultrafiltrate of plasma amounting to 180 L per day, reabsorbing more than 99% of it to produce an average of 1.5 L urine per day. Normal kidney function requires well-regulated blood flow through the kidneys, amounting to approximately 20% of the cardiac output, even though both kidneys comprise only approximately 1% of total body weight. Thus, even minor changes in renal structure can cause major functional disturbances and diseases. Consequently, microscopic investigations of the kidneys (e.g., by biopsy) are valuable for the diagnosis and classification of renal diseases.

PRIMARY DISEASES OF THE KIDNEY

Acute renal failure (ARF), which occurs in approximately 5% of hospitalized patients, is defined as an increase in serum creatinine of 0.5 to 1.0 mg/dL. *Chronic renal failure* (CRF) is a long-standing and usually irreversible impairment of renal function with reduction of the filtration rate, azotemia, and uremia. Common causes of ARF and CRF, as discussed in this chapter, are diverse, and both renal and extrarenal diseases must be considered in differential diagnosis.

The etiopathogenesis of glomerular and tubuloglomerular diseases (e.g., **glomerulonephritis** and **nephrotic syndrome**) is also highly diverse, as reflected in the difficulty in their classification. Many cases follow an autoimmune disorder; therefore, it is necessary to supplement the usual biopsy histology for staging and grading of the disease with immunohistologic procedures, occasionally including serology. Consequently, although the primary manifestation of an autoimmune renal disease may be the kidney, virtually all these conditions should be considered systemic processes (as in postinfectious autoimmune glomerulonephritis). Some, such as **anaphylactoid purpura, lupus nephritis**, and **Wegener syndrome** (see below), show systemic organ involvement from the beginning.

THE KIDNEY AND SYSTEMIC DISEASES

Many primary systemic diseases affect the kidney, including diabetes mellitus (DM), essential hypertension, various renovascular diseases, and several toxic and metabolic disorders. Progressive renal disease (**diabetic nephrosclerosis, Kimmelstiel-Wilson disease**) is a common complication of DM (see chapter 12) and is responsible for renal failure in 30% to 40% of patients with insulin-dependent DM and 20% of those with non–insulin-dependent DM. Benign and malignant nephrosclerosis are the renal manifestations of **essential hypertension** and must be distinguished from

TABLE 6-1 SUMMARY OF SYSTEMIC VASCULITIS SYNDROMES (PRIMARY AND SECONDARY)

Affected Vessel	Entity	Clinical Features
Small	Wegener disease Microscopic polyangiitis Henoch-Schönlein purpura Leukocytoclastic vasculitis Postinfectious vasculitis (eg, viral)	Microhematuria, purpura, hemoptyses, perimyocarditis, episcleritis, vertigo, polyneuritis, melena
Medium	Pan(poly)arteritis nodosa Churg-Strauss disease Lupus erythematosus Rheumatoid arthritis Progressive systemic sclerosis	Infarction in various organs including kidneys, hemorrhage from ruptured microaneurysms, hypertension, renal failure
Large	Giant cell arteritis Takayasu arteritis	Arterial stenoses, phlebothromboses, aortic arch syndrome, subclavian steal syndrome

renovascular hypertension, the consequence of renal artery stenosis. Hypertensive vascular diseases affect approximately 20% of the population and, with the complications of myocardial infarction, renal failure, and stroke, constitute a major health hazard. (The cause and pathogenesis of hypertension are discussed in chapter 2.) Systemic vasculitis syndromes frequently affect renal vessels or glomeruli or both (Table 6-1). **Toxic nephropathy** encompasses a large variety of diseases of different origins causing pathologic changes including cortical necrosis, tubular necrosis, focal hemorrhage, interstitial nephritis, and papillary necrosis. Causative toxins may be exogenous (e.g., drugs, plant toxins, allergens) or endogenic (e.g., **toxemia of pregnancy**), and the pathogenesis may include immune mechanisms (e.g., **Shwartzman-Sanarelli syndrome**). Metabolic disturbances such as amyloidosis and hypokalemic and calcium nephropathy also are associated with renal pathology.

DISEASES OF THE URINARY SYSTEM

Common diseases of the urinary system include pyelonephritis, obstructive uropathy, infections (e.g., tuberculosis, parasitic infections, cystitis) nephrolithiasis, some malformations (cystic disease, diverticula), neurogenic bladder, and neoplastic diseases. **Obstructive nephropathy** and **hydronephrosis** result from mechanical impediment of urine flow with renal dysfunction, dilatation of the collecting system, and frequent infections. Causes include intraluminal calculi (urolithiasis) and tumors (papilloma), compression (prostatic hypertrophy, pregnancy, retroperitoneal fibromatosis or tumors) and ureteral dysfunctions (amyloidosis, malformations, neurogenic conditions). Infections resulting from such functional disturbances are frequent causes of **pyelonephritis**, a bacterial infection of the renal parenchyma calyces and pelvis.

Other frequent and important diseases discussed in this chapter are malignant tumors such as **adenocarcinoma** and **nephroblastoma** of the kidney and **transitional carcinoma** of the urinary tract and bladder. Adenocarcinoma (renal cell carcinoma [RCC]) constitutes approximately 90% of renal malignancies; it occurs in more than 10,000 persons per year in the United States, and its annual incidence is increasing. A few cases occur as hereditary tumors and may be part of a cancer syndrome (e.g., **von Hippel-Lindau syndrome**). Clinical features are hematuria, pain, and an abdominal mass, which may lead to diagnosis and treatment by surgical resection. The 5-year survival rate of RCC is 40%. Urothelial cell (transitional cell) carcinoma (UCC) of the renal pelvis represents 5% to 10% of all kidney tumors. UCCs are more frequent in the urinary tract and account for 80% of neoplasms in the bladder. As long as the disease is confined to the bladder, as it is in approximately 85% of cases at initial presentation, survival after surgery amounts to 57% and 35% for low-grade and high-grade malignancy tumors, respectively. Nephroblastoma (**Wilms tumor** [WT]) constitutes the most frequent solid abdominal tumor in children. WTs may develop bilaterally and may accompany various congenital syndromes (e.g., **Beckwith-Wiedemann syndrome**). Karyotypic analysis reveals characteristic chromosomal changes in sporadic and congenital WTs such as alterations of the tumor suppressor gene *WT1* or the susceptibility gene *WT2*. These changes apparently support the unrestricted growth of the nephrogenic blastoma, resulting in a tumor composed of blastemal, stromal, and epithelial elements. Early diagnosis before the age of 2 years with surgical removal of the tumor, radiation therapy, and chemotherapy may result in long-term survival of up to 90%.

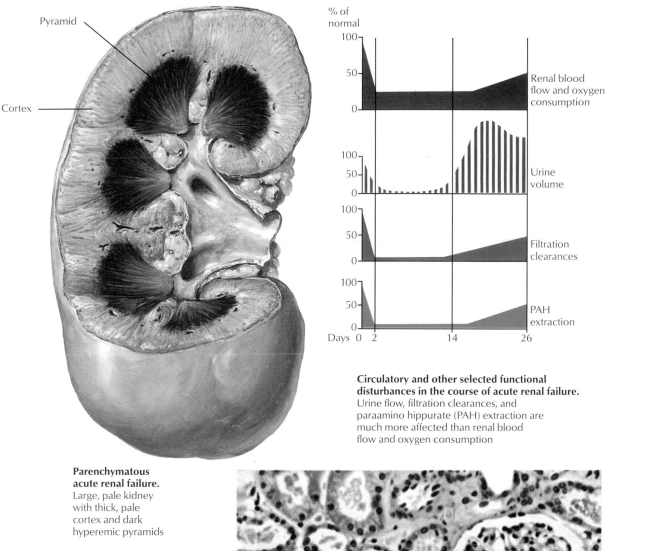

Pyramid

Cortex

% of normal

Renal blood flow and oxygen consumption

Urine volume

Filtration clearances

PAH extraction

Days 0 2   14   26

Circulatory and other selected functional disturbances in the course of acute renal failure. Urine flow, filtration clearances, and paraamino hippurate (PAH) extraction are much more affected than renal blood flow and oxygen consumption

Parenchymatous acute renal failure. Large, pale kidney with thick, pale cortex and dark hyperemic pyramids

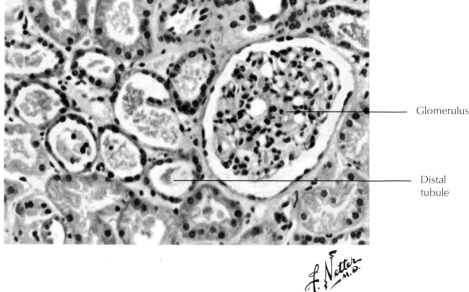

Glomerulus

Distal tubule

Biopsy section. Glomerulus normal; distal convoluted tubules dilated, with flattened epithelium, "pretzel-like" distortion, and containing heme cast (H and E stain)

FIGURE 6-1 ACUTE RENAL FAILURE I

Acute renal failure is a sudden reduction in renal function with accompanying oliguria or anuria and potentially fatal outcome. There are 3 types of ARF: prerenal, renal (parenchymal), and postrenal. In **prerenal** failure, which is reversible, renal function is reduced by factors extrinsic to the kidney, such as hypotension, salt depletion, dehydration, or an obstruction in the urinary tract. **Renal (parenchymal)** failure follows malfunction of the nephrons in a wide variety of diseases, including acute glomerulonephritis,

acute pyelonephritis, toxic nephropathy, and severe circulatory impairments, with the latter resulting in acute tubulointerstitial nephropathy or "shock kidney." The pathophysiologic derangements in ARF are complex but include reduced and maldistributed cortical blood flow with resulting local ischemia while total blood flow is partially preserved. **Postrenal** causes of ARF are various forms of urinary tract obstruction.

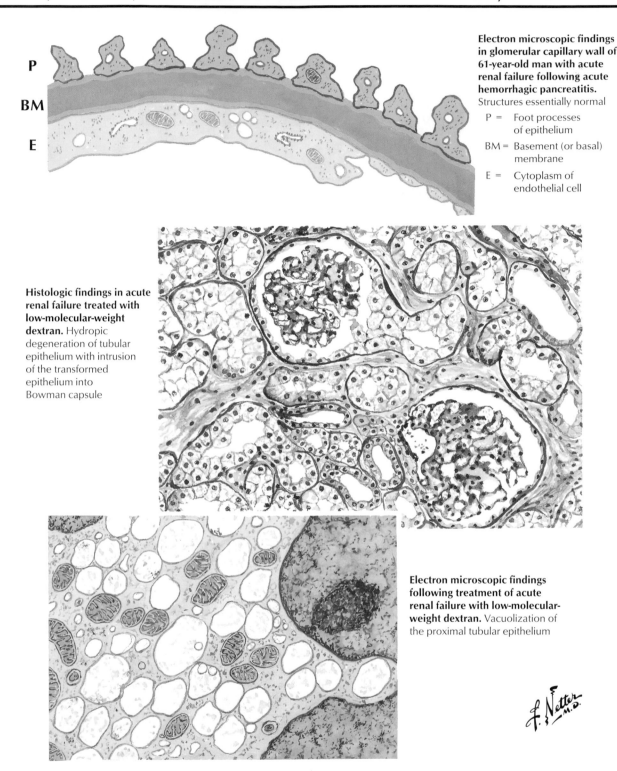

P

BM

E

Electron microscopic findings in glomerular capillary wall of 61-year-old man with acute renal failure following acute hemorrhagic pancreatitis. Structures essentially normal

P = Foot processes of epithelium

BM = Basement (or basal) membrane

E = Cytoplasm of endothelial cell

Histologic findings in acute renal failure treated with low-molecular-weight dextran. Hydropic degeneration of tubular epithelium with intrusion of the transformed epithelium into Bowman capsule

Electron microscopic findings following treatment of acute renal failure with low-molecular-weight dextran. Vacuolization of the proximal tubular epithelium

FIGURE 6-2 ACUTE RENAL FAILURE II

The kidneys of patients with **acute renal failure** (ARF) are large and pale, with a pale cortex and a dark, hyperemic medulla. Histologically, the hallmark of the condition is multifocal dilation with epithelial flattening of the distal convoluted tubules and, to some extent, the proximal convoluted tubules. The glomeruli are normal. Tubular epithelial cells exhibit degenerative and hydropic changes. Interstitial edema and focal collections of lymphocytes may be present. Electron microscopy confirms the normal

structure of the glomeruli and reveals subcellular degenerative changes of organelles. There is a progressive decrease in urine output and a progressive increase in azotemia, metabolic acidosis, and serum potassium levels. Renal function returns if the underlying disease process is contained and the renal-induced metabolic and electrolyte abnormalities are treated successfully.

1. Primarily glomerular disease

Acute glomerulonephritis

Anti–glomerular basement membrane disease

Chronic glomerulonephritis

Focal glomerulonephritis

Goodpasture syndrome

Intercapillary glomerulosclerosis

Rapidly progressive glomerulonephritis

2. Primarily tubular disease

Chronic hypercalcemia

Chronic potassium depletion

Fanconi syndrome and variants

Heavy metal poisoning
(lead, cadmium, etc.)

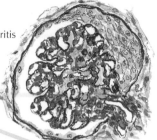

3. Vascular disease

Ischemic disease of kidneys,
congenital or acquired bilateral
renal artery stenosis; bilateral
fibromuscular hyperplasia

Malignant phase of
essential hypertension

Nephrosclerosis

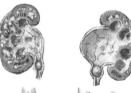

8. Congenital anomalies of kidney

Hypoplastic kidneys

Medullary cystic disease

Polycystic kidneys

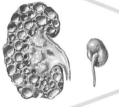

**Etiology
of chronic
renal failure**

4. Infections

Chronic pyelonephritis

Tuberculosis

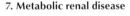

7. Metabolic renal disease

Amyloidosis

Chronic phenacetin
overdosage

Gout with hyperuricemic
nephropathy

Primary hyperparathyroidism

Milk-alkali syndrome

Sarcoidosis

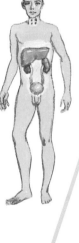

6. Collagen disease

Diffuse systemic sclerosis
(scleroderma)

Disseminated (systemic)
lupus erythematosus

Polyarteritis nodosa

5. Obstructive disease

Upper
   Calculi

   Neoplasms

   Retroperitoneal fibrosis
Lower
   Congenital anomalies
   of bladder neck and/or
   or urethra

   Prostatic enlargement

   Urethral stricture

F. Netter M.D.

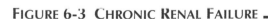

FIGURE 6-3 CHRONIC RENAL FAILURE

Chronic renal failure (CRF) is a marked impairment in renal homeostatic function coupled with abnormalities in composition of body fluids. The most common causes of CRF are various types of glomerulonephritis and other nephritides. The functional and structural consequences of ischemia—obstruction with increased intra-pelvic pressure, infection with microorganisms, or deposition of antigen-antibody-complement complexes—may also result in CRF. Renal insufficiency is characterized by impaired renal adaptive function without major alterations in body fluid composition. Further loss in function results in CRF and culminates in uremia. Changes induced by CRF include secondary hyperparathyroidism and metabolic bone disease. In humans, the common structural basis for renal failure is thought to be a progressive reduction in the number of functioning nephrons, while the remaining nephrons develop hypertrophy and increased work per nephron, until these nephrons also are lost.

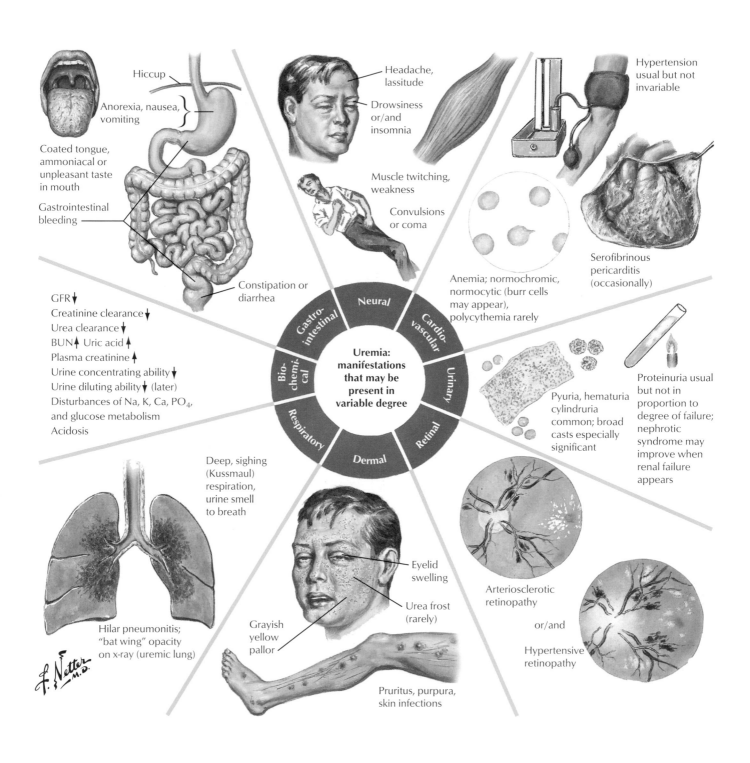

Hiccup

Anorexia, nausea, vomiting

Coated tongue, ammoniacal or unpleasant taste in mouth

Gastrointestinal bleeding

Headache, lassitude

Drowsiness or/and insomnia

Muscle twitching, weakness

Convulsions or coma

Hypertension usual but not invariable

Serofibrinous pericarditis (occasionally)

Anemia; normochromic, normocytic (burr cells may appear), polycythemia rarely

Constipation or diarrhea

GFR↓
Creatinine clearance↓
Urea clearance↓
BUN↑ Uric acid↑
Plasma creatinine↑
Urine concentrating ability↓
Urine diluting ability↓ (later)
Disturbances of Na, K, Ca, PO₄, and glucose metabolism
Acidosis

Pyuria, hematuria cylindruria common; broad casts especially significant

Proteinuria usual but not in proportion to degree of failure; nephrotic syndrome may improve when renal failure appears

Uremia: manifestations that may be present in variable degree

Gastro-intestinal · Neural · Cardio-vascular · Urinary · Retinal · Dermal · Respiratory · Bio-chemi-cal

Deep, sighing (Kussmaul) respiration, urine smell to breath

Hilar pneumonitis; "bat wing" opacity on x-ray (uremic lung)

Grayish yellow pallor

Eyelid swelling

Urea frost (rarely)

Pruritus, purpura, skin infections

Arteriosclerotic retinopathy

or/and

Hypertensive retinopathy

FIGURE 6-4 UREMIA

Uremia is characterized by multiple clinical and laboratory findings resulting from severe renal failure. **Azotemia,** a hallmark of renal failure, which is characterized by increased concentration of nonprotein nitrogenous compounds in blood, is measured with the blood urea nitrogen (BUN) test. Reduction in glomerular filtration can be measured by the diminution of creatine clearance and resulting increase of creatinine in the blood.

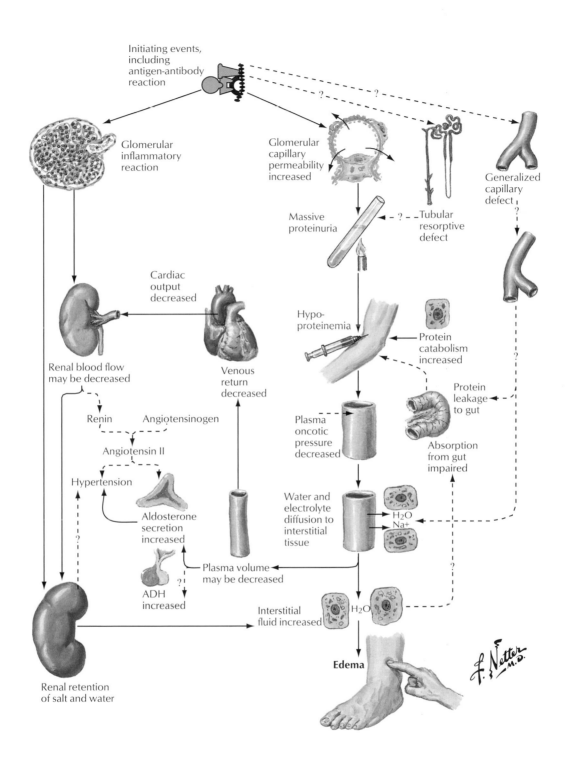

FIGURE 6-5 NEPHROTIC SYNDROME: PATHOPHYSIOLOGY

Nephrotic syndrome may be induced by noninflammatory or inflammatory (glomerulonephritic) conditions. The resultant damage, which may be subtle, produces increased permeability of the glomerular capillaries leading to proteinuria. Clinically, nephrotic syndrome is characterized by proteinuria in excess of 3.5 g/d/1.73 m² body surface area, edema, hypoalbuminemia,

and hyperlipidemia. Prolonged massive proteinuria and resultant hypoproteinemia are the common denominators for all consequent metabolic and nutritional defects. Glomerular inflammation also may lead to a decrease in renal blood flow, which may activate the renin-angiotensin system, increasing production of angiotensin II and causing hypertension.

Minimal disease

Epithelial cell
Basement membrane
Foot processes fused
Subendothelial "fluff"

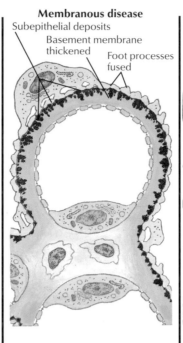

Glomerular capillary lumen

Endothelial cell
Mesangial cell

Electron microscopic findings.
Only fusion of epithelial foot processes and some subendothelial "fluff"

Membranous disease

Subepithelial deposits
Basement membrane thickened
Foot processes fused

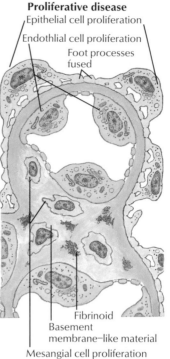

Electron microscopic findings.
Electron-dense deposits beneath epithelial cells, thickening of basement membrane, and fusion of foot processes

Proliferative disease

Epithelial cell proliferation
Endothlial cell proliferation
Foot processes fused

Fibrinoid
Basement membrane–like material
Mesangial cell proliferation

Electron microscopic findings.
Epithelial, endothelial, and mesangial cell proliferation; little or no thickening of basement membrane, but variable amount of basement membrane–like material (mesangial matrix) deposited in mesangium; foot processes fused

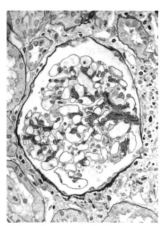

Light microscopic findings.
Glomerulus appears normal; protein may be present in tubule lumina and lipoid droplets in tubule cells (PAS, X250)

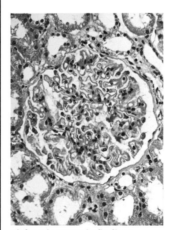

Light microscopic findings.
Basement membrane thickened and eosinophilic; prominence but no numerical increase of epithelial, endothelial, and mesangial cells (H and E, X250)

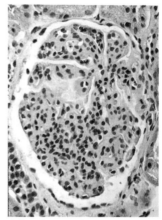

Light microscopic appearance.
Cellular proliferation—epithelial, endothelial, and mesangial; very little, if any, basement membrane thickening (H and E, X250)

FIGURE 6-6 NEPHROTIC SYNDROME: PATHOLOGY

A spectrum of glomerular lesions can produce nephrotic syndrome. Minimal change disease (**lipoid nephrosis**) shows little or no change by light microscopy. Fused epithelial foot processes and occasional immunoglobulin (Ig) M deposits are seen by electron microscopy. If the disease is complicated by focal and segmental sclerosis, fused epithelial foot processes, capillary collapse, or mesangial expansion with γ-globulin deposits, response to immunosuppressive therapy deteriorates. **Membranous nephropathy** is characterized by thickened capillary walls, spikes in the basement membrane due to antigen-antibody complexes beneath the epithelial cells (membranous disease), and diffuse granular deposits of IgG and C₃ (complement). **Mesangioproliferative glomerulonephritis** shows thickening of glomerular capillary walls complicated by mesangial proliferation and sclerosis with subendothelial deposits of C₃ and IgG in a lumpy, nonlinear pattern. Focal segmental inflammatory necrosis and crescent formation signals a poor response to immunosuppressive therapy.

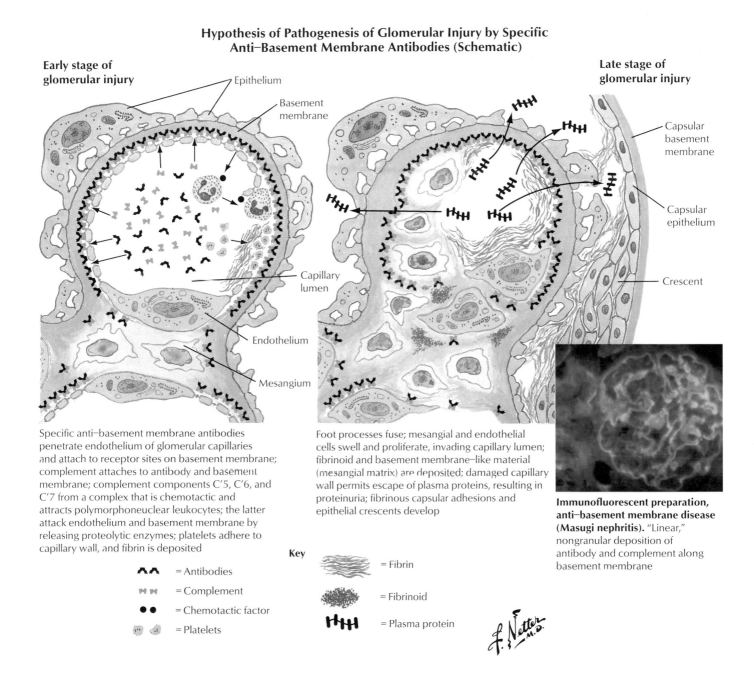

Hypothesis of Pathogenesis of Glomerular Injury by Specific Anti–Basement Membrane Antibodies (Schematic)

Early stage of glomerular injury

Epithelium

Basement membrane

Capillary lumen

Endothelium

Mesangium

Late stage of glomerular injury

Capsular basement membrane

Capsular epithelium

Crescent

Specific anti–basement membrane antibodies penetrate endothelium of glomerular capillaries and attach to receptor sites on basement membrane; complement attaches to antibody and basement membrane; complement components C'5, C'6, and C'7 from a complex that is chemotactic and attracts polymorphoneuclear leukocytes; the latter attack endothelium and basement membrane by releasing proteolytic enzymes; platelets adhere to capillary wall, and fibrin is deposited

Foot processes fuse; mesangial and endothelial cells swell and proliferate, invading capillary lumen; fibrinoid and basement membrane–like material (mesangial matrix) are deposited; damaged capillary wall permits escape of plasma proteins, resulting in proteinuria; fibrinous capsular adhesions and epithelial crescents develop

Immunofluorescent preparation, anti–basement membrane disease (Masugi nephritis). "Linear," nongranular deposition of antibody and complement along basement membrane

Key

∧∧ = Antibodies

= Complement

●● = Chemotactic factor

= Platelets

= Fibrin

= Fibrinoid

= Plasma protein

F. Netter M.D.

FIGURE 6-7 ANTI–GLOMERULAR BASEMENT MEMBRANE DISEASE

In **anti–glomerular basement membrane** (GBM) disease, the antibody is directed against the GBM, the antigen being a normal component of the glomerulus. Anti-GBM disease, whether produced by heterologous antibodies or autoantibodies, has the following features: (1) it is produced by circulating antibodies; (2) the antibodies (γ globulins) and complement are readily detected by immunofluorescence with a distribution along the basement membrane of every glomerulus in a highly distinctive, continuous, linear pattern; and (3) electron microscopy reveals inconspicuous deposits along the endothelial side of the basement membrane. Leukocytes recruited by locally produced chemotactic factors contribute to the glomerular damage. Forms of anti-GBM disease in humans include rapidly progressive, subacute glomerulonephritis and **Goodpasture syndrome**, which is characterized by lung hemorrhage and severe and rapidly progressive glomerulonephritis.

Hypothesis of Pathogenesis of Acute Glomerular Injury by Circulating Immune Complexes (Schematic)

Early stage of glomerular injury

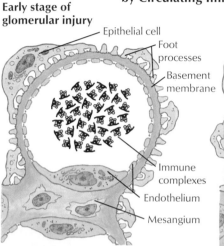

Epithelial cell
Foot processes
Basement membrane
Immune complexes
Endothelium
Mesangium

Circulating immune complexes, formed anywhere in the body, consisting of antigen, antibody, and complement components, arrive at glomerular capillaries in large amounts over a short period of time

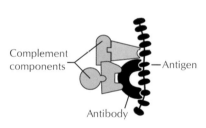

Complement components
Antigen
Antibody

Composition of complexes

Late stage of glomerular injury

Red blood cell
Plasma protein

Complexes penetrate endothelium and basement membrane of glomerular capillaries and form large isolated deposits (humps); foot processes fuse; mesangial and endothelial cells swell and proliferate, invading capillary lumen; fibrillar basement membrane–like material (mesangial matrix) is deposited between cells; increased porosity of capillary walls permits escape of plasma proteins and blood cells, causing proteinuria and hematuria

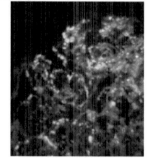

Immunofluorescent preparation, acute glomerulonephritis. Irregular lumpy deposits of γ-globulin (IgG) and complement, resembling experimental acute immune complex disease

FIGURE 6-8 ACUTE AND CHRONIC GLOMERULAR INJURY PRODUCED BY CIRCULATING IMMUNE COMPLEXES

Acute glomerular injury results when large amounts of immune complexes are delivered to the glomerular capillaries over a short period of time; examples are poststreptococcal glomerulonephritis and the glomerulonephritis associated with subacute bacterial endocarditis. The immune complexes form large deposits on the epithelial side of the basement membranes, which are detected by immunofluorescence as irregular lumpy deposits and by electron microscopy as subepithelial humps in the basement membranes.

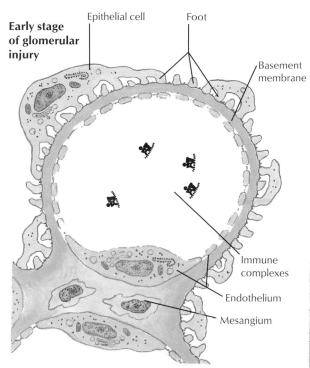

Early stage of glomerular injury

Epithelial cell — Foot — Basement membrane — Immune complexes — Endothelium — Mesangium

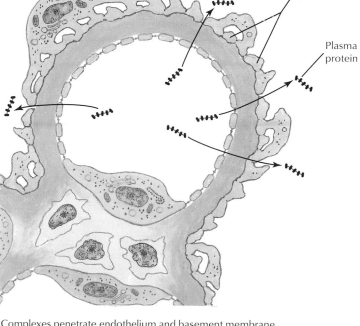

Late stage of glomerular injury

Fused foot processes — Plasma protein

Circulating immune complexes, formed anywhere in the body, consisting of antigen, antibody, and complement components, arrive at glomerular capillaries in small amounts over a prolonged period of time

Complexes penetrate endothelium and basement membrane of glomerular capillaries and form diffuse granular deposits; basement membrane proliferates to encompass deposits; foot processes fuse; little or no endothelial cell or mesangial cell proliferation occurs, but porosity of capillary wall is increased, permitting escape of plasma proteins and causing proteinuria

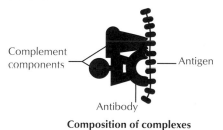

Complement components — Antigen — Antibody

Composition of complexes

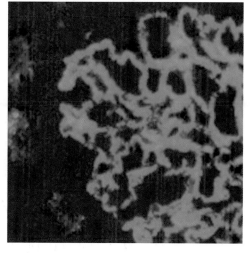

Immunofluorescent preparation, membranous nephropathy. Diffuse granular deposits on basement membrane, resembling findings in experimental chronic serum sickness

---

FIGURE 6-8 ACUTE AND CHRONIC GLOMERULAR INJURY PRODUCED BY CIRCULATING IMMUNE COMPLEXES (CONTINUED)

The immune complexes stimulate an inflammatory response that leads to acute glomerulonephritis. **Chronic glomerular injury** also results when small amounts of immune complexes are delivered to the glomerular capillaries over a prolonged period, as seen in systemic lupus erythematosus. Electron microscopy and immuno-

fluorescence show extensive deposits of immune complexes along the epithelial side of the basement membrane. The glomerular injury may progress to include proliferative and sclerosing changes.

Acute glomerulonephritis: Electron microscopic findings

Epithelial cell swollen

Electron-dense "hump" γ-globulin (IgG) and immune bodies

Basement membrane usually normal

Foot processes only focally fused

Erythrocyte and proteinaceous deposits in urinary (Bowman) space

Polymorphonuclear leukocyte

Swollen endothelial cell bulging into capillary lumen

Mesangial cell proliferation Thickening lobular stalk and narrowing capillary lumen

Mesangial matrix deposited in stalk

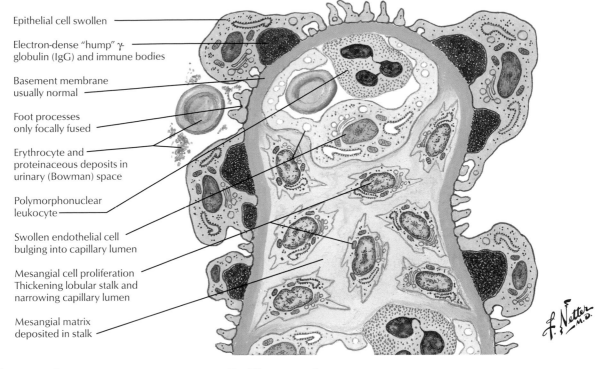

Rapidly progressive glomerulonephritis

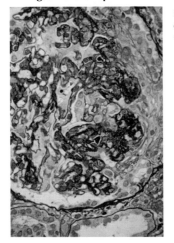

Early crescent

Large crescent compressing glomerular tuft

Rapidly progressive glomerulonephritis

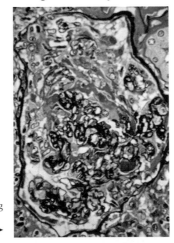

Acute diffuse glomerulonephritis

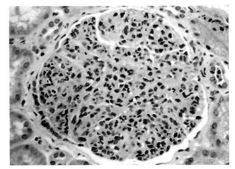

Glomerulus. Greatly increased cellularity and mesangial matrix and almost complete obliteration of capillary lumina. The cells are chiefly mesangial, with some polymorphonuclear leukocytes and a few eosinophils.

FIGURE 6-9 ACUTE GLOMERULONEPHRITIS

The kidneys in **acute diffuse (poststreptococcal) glomerulonephritis** show enlargement and pallor. Abnormally large and cellular glomeruli are seen microscopically; the capillary walls are swollen, and the lumens are narrowed. The hypercellularity is caused by proliferation of mesangial cells with associated increased mesangial matrix. A variable amount of infiltration by polymorphonuclear leukocytes is seen early in the disease. Other changes include casts and erythrocytes in the tubules and interstitial edema and focal inflammation. Electron microscopy reveals swelling of epithelial and endothelial cells and increased numbers of mesangial cells. The presence of semicircular or triangular "humps" (protein deposits) between the basement membrane and epithelial cells are considered to be diagnostic. **Rapidly progressive (extracapillary) glomerulonephritis** is characterized by the presence of many large cellular crescents consisting of proliferated epithelial cells of Bowman capsules, macrophages, and matrix.

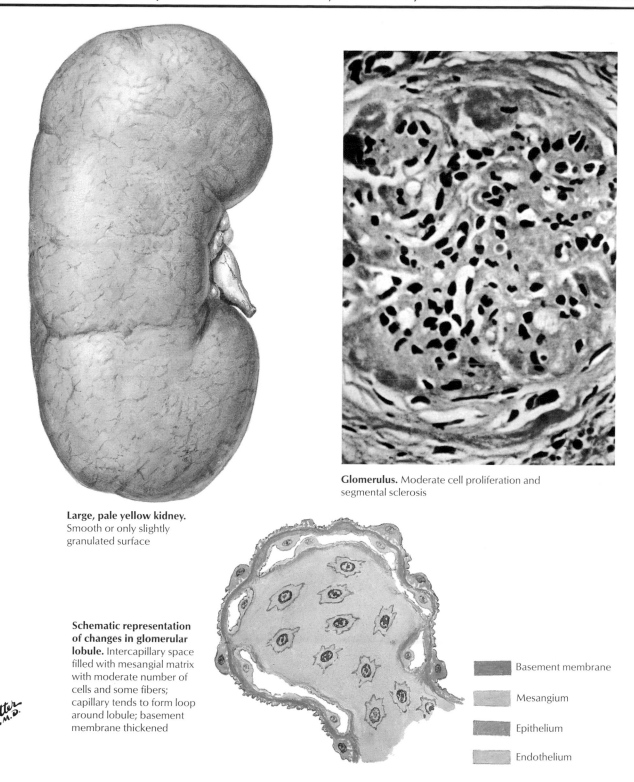

Glomerulus. Moderate cell proliferation and segmental sclerosis

Large, pale yellow kidney. Smooth or only slightly granulated surface

Schematic representation of changes in glomerular lobule. Intercapillary space filled with mesangial matrix with moderate number of cells and some fibers; capillary tends to form loop around lobule; basement membrane thickened

Basement membrane

Mesangium

Epithelium

Endothelium

FIGURE 6-10 CHRONIC GLOMERULONEPHRITIS: EARLY STAGE

Chronic glomerulonephritis is characterized pathologically by sclerosis of many glomeruli and clinically by manifestations of renal insufficiency. The disease progresses because of inflammation leading to sclerosis of glomeruli and scarring. The kidney may be normal or slightly increased or decreased in size and is often pale yellow with smooth or slightly granular surfaces. On cut section, the cortex is often pale and swollen as a result of

lipid in the tubules and interstitial edema. In **proliferative** and **sclerosing glomerulonephritis**, the glomeruli typically exhibit cellular proliferation and deposition of intercellular material with an approximate balance between proliferation of cells and sclerosis. In contrast, in **membranous glomerulonephritis**, cell proliferation and sclerosis are absent, and the histologic changes are limited to the capillary walls, at least in the early stages.

Mesangiocapillary (Membranoproliferative, Lobular, or Hypocomplementemic) Glomerulonephritis

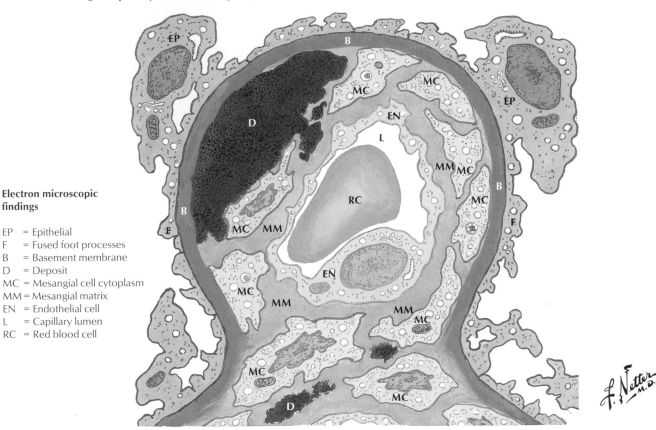

Electron microscopic findings

EP = Epithelial
F = Fused foot processes
B = Basement membrane
D = Deposit
MC = Mesangial cell cytoplasm
MM = Mesangial matrix
EN = Endothelial cell
L = Capillary lumen
RC = Red blood cell

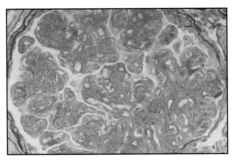

Typical light microscopic findings. Glomerulus enlarged; lobulation prominent; moderate number of cells; much mesangial matrix (stained pink with PAS); capillary walls thickened and lumina narrowed

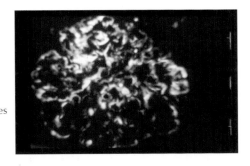

Immunofluorescent preparation stained for complement. Irregular deposition along walls of capillaries

FIGURE 6-11 CHRONIC GLOMERULONEPHRITIS: MESANGIOCAPILLARY GLOMERULONEPHRITIS

Mesangiocapillary glomerulonephritis (membranoproliferative, lobular, or hypocomplementemic glomerulonephritis) occurs most often in children and young adults. Patients present with components of the nephrotic syndrome and, usually, depression of serum complement. Typically, the disease progresses slowly. Histologically, the glomeruli are enlarged and moderately cellular, and the lobular centers are expanded as a result of proliferation of the mesangial cells and matrix. Ingrowth of the mesangium into the capillary wall causes capillary wall thickening, separates the endothelium from the basement membrane, and narrows the lumen. Immunofluorescence reveals deposits of complement (C_3) and small amounts of γ globulin (IgG, IgM) within the mesangial matrix.

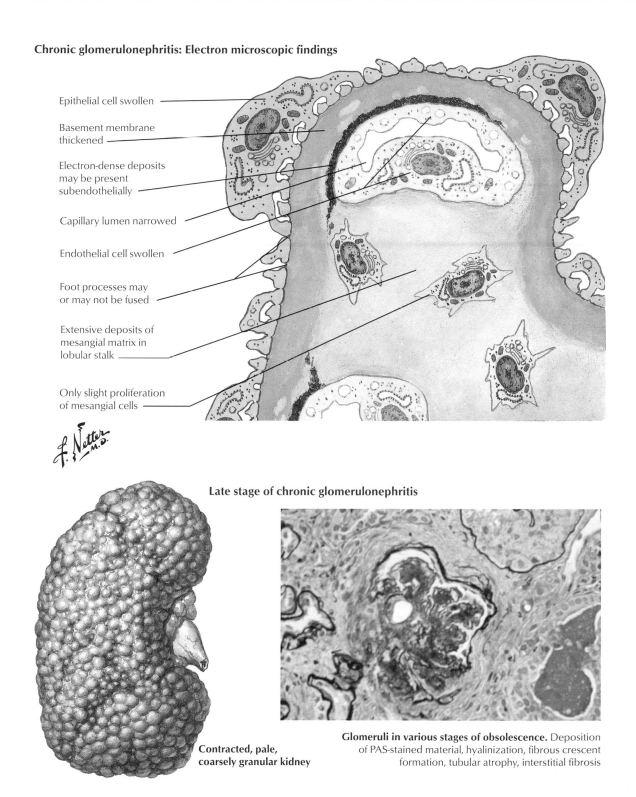

Chronic glomerulonephritis: Electron microscopic findings

Epithelial cell swollen

Basement membrane thickened

Electron-dense deposits may be present subendothelially

Capillary lumen narrowed

Endothelial cell swollen

Foot processes may or may not be fused

Extensive deposits of mesangial matrix in lobular stalk

Only slight proliferation of mesangial cells

Late stage of chronic glomerulonephritis

Contracted, pale, coarsely granular kidney

Glomeruli in various stages of obsolescence. Deposition of PAS-stained material, hyalinization, fibrous crescent formation, tubular atrophy, interstitial fibrosis

FIGURE 6-12 CHRONIC GLOMERULONEPHRITIS: MEMBRANOUS GLOMERULONEPHRITIS

Membranous glomerulonephritis is common in adults but not in children. Characteristic changes in the capillary basement membranes are seen by electron and light microscopy (silver stains). Small, dense protein deposits that contain γ globulin (IgG) and complement are located between the basement membrane and the overlying, fused epithelial cell foot processes

(see Fig. 6-6). The deposits are interrupted by focal thickening or by projections (spikes) of the basement membrane. Late **chronic glomerulonephritis** represents an end-stage common pathway of many glomerular diseases. Pathologically, it is characterized by the predominance of scarring and atrophy of both glomeruli and tubules with secondary arteriolosclerosis.

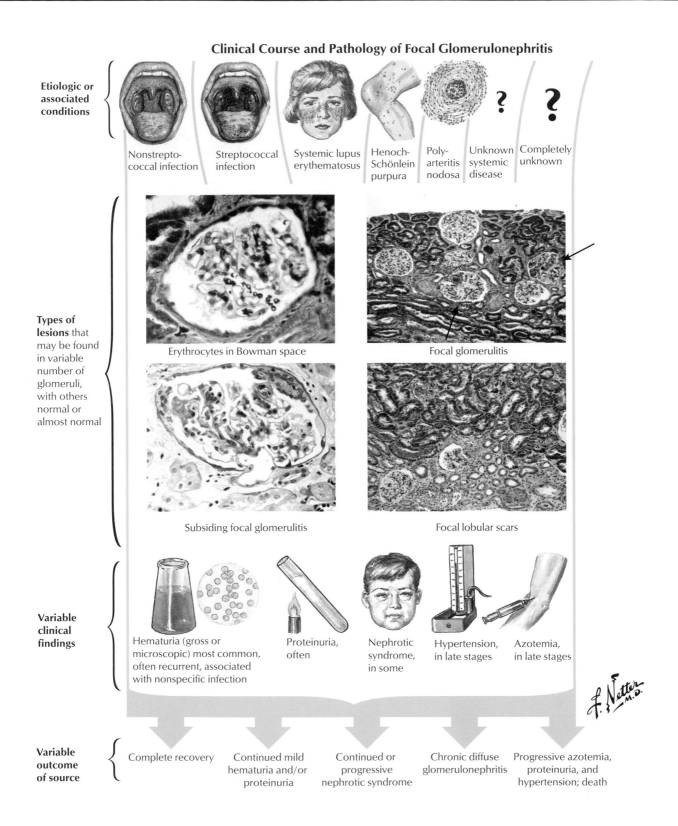

Clinical Course and Pathology of Focal Glomerulonephritis

Etiologic or associated conditions

Nonstrepto-coccal infection | Streptococcal infection | Systemic lupus erythematosus | Henoch-Schönlein purpura | Poly-arteritis nodosa | Unknown systemic disease | Completely unknown

Types of lesions that may be found in variable number of glomeruli, with others normal or almost normal

Erythrocytes in Bowman space

Focal glomerulitis

Subsiding focal glomerulitis

Focal lobular scars

Variable clinical findings

Hematuria (gross or microscopic) most common, often recurrent, associated with nonspecific infection | Proteinuria, often | Nephrotic syndrome, in some | Hypertension, in late stages | Azotemia, in late stages

Variable outcome of source

Complete recovery | Continued mild hematuria and/or proteinuria | Continued or progressive nephrotic syndrome | Chronic diffuse glomerulonephritis | Progressive azotemia, proteinuria, and hypertension; death

FIGURE 6-13 FOCAL SEGMENTAL GLOMERULONEPHRITIS

Focal segmental glomerulonephritis refers to disease processes in which some but not all glomeruli are involved, portions but not the entirety of each glomerulus are involved, or both. Etiologic or associated conditions include streptococcal and nonstreptococcal infections; autoimmune and immunologically mediated diseases, including systemic lupus erythematous and Henoch-Schönlein purpura; and various vasculitides, including polyarteritis nodosa. A variety of pathologic lesions ranging from mild or moderate to severe focal glomerular damage may be found. Clinical findings may include hematoma, azotemia, hypertension, and nephrotic syndrome. The clinical course and outcome range from self-limited disease to death.

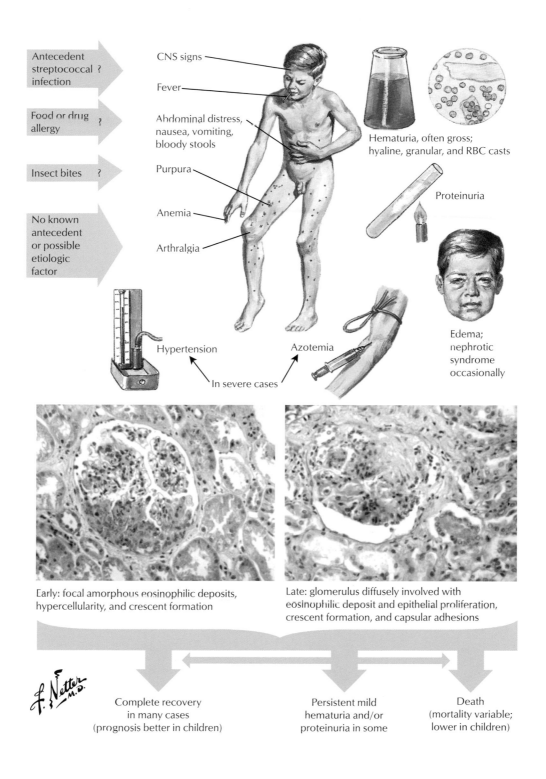

Early: focal amorphous eosinophilic deposits, hypercellularity, and crescent formation

Late: glomerulus diffusely involved with eosinophilic deposit and epithelial proliferation, crescent formation, and capsular adhesions

Complete recovery in many cases (prognosis better in children)

Persistent mild hematuria and/or proteinuria in some

Death (mortality variable; lower in children)

FIGURE 6-14 NEPHROPATHY IN ANAPHYLACTOID PURPURA

Anaphylactoid purpura (Henoch-Schönlein disease), a hypersensitivity disorder with renal involvement, usually affects children. The disorder closely resembles serum sickness in humans and experimental animals. Multiple allergens may be involved. Skin lesions include urticaria, maculopapular rash, petechiae, and purpura. Joints may become inflamed, painful, and swollen. Other features may include central neurologic signs, gastrointesti-nal involvement, and anemia. Renal manifestations are dominated by hematuria and nephrotic syndrome, which in severe cases may be accompanied by hypertension and azotemia. Renal biopsies show variable involvement of most of the glomeruli, with focal changes consisting of proliferation of endothelial and mesangial cells and accumulation of periodic acid-Schiff (PAS) reaction–positive matrix material.

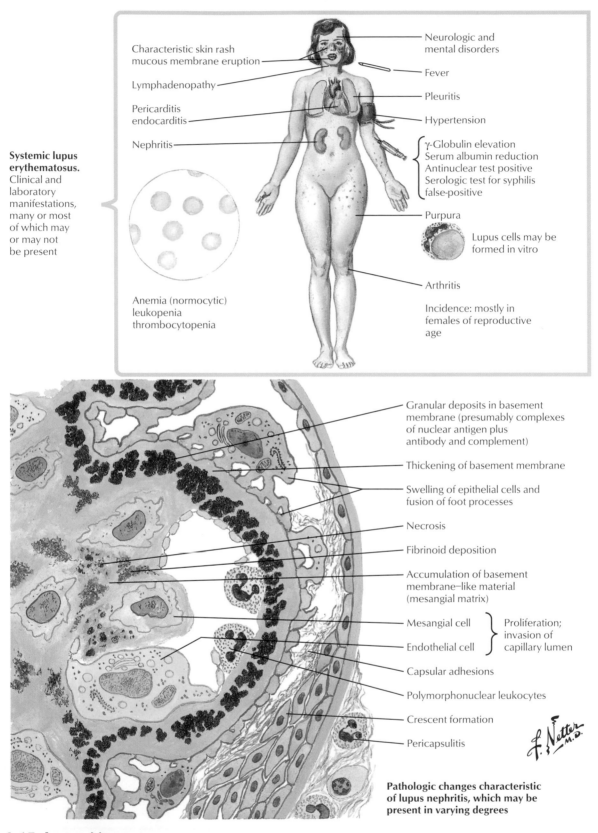

Systemic lupus erythematosus. Clinical and laboratory manifestations, many or most of which may or may not be present

Characteristic skin rash mucous membrane eruption

Lymphadenopathy

Pericarditis endocarditis

Nephritis

Neurologic and mental disorders

Fever

Pleuritis

Hypertension

γ-Globulin elevation
Serum albumin reduction
Antinuclear test positive
Serologic test for syphilis false-positive

Purpura

Lupus cells may be formed in vitro

Arthritis

Incidence: mostly in females of reproductive age

Anemia (normocytic) leukopenia thrombocytopenia

Granular deposits in basement membrane (presumably complexes of nuclear antigen plus antibody and complement)

Thickening of basement membrane

Swelling of epithelial cells and fusion of foot processes

Necrosis

Fibrinoid deposition

Accumulation of basement membrane–like material (mesangial matrix)

Mesangial cell

Endothelial cell

Proliferation; invasion of capillary lumen

Capsular adhesions

Polymorphonuclear leukocytes

Crescent formation

Pericapsulitis

Pathologic changes characteristic of lupus nephritis, which may be present in varying degrees

Figure 6-15 Lupus Nephritis

Systemic lupus erythematosus, an autoimmune disease that occurs predominantly in young women, involves many tissues and organs. Important renal abnormalities involving the glomeruli include swelling and proliferation of endothelial and mesangial cells, fibrinoid necrosis, thrombi, neutrophil infiltration, crescent formation, increased mesangial matrix, and thickening. Deposits of antigen-antibody complexes in the basement membrane often appear as "wire-loop" lesions. **Focal proliferative lupus nephritis** (class III) is characterized by focal involvement of some of the glomeruli, swelling and proliferation of endothelial and mesangial cells, neutrophil accumulation, and necrosis.

Histologic and Clinical Classification of Lupus Nephritis

Focal proliferative	**Diffuse proliferative**	**Membranous**
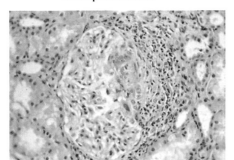	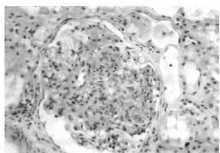	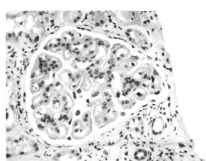

Pathology (findings by light microscopy)

Only ***portions*** (segmental) of ***some*** (focal) glomeruli are affected; the majority appear normal. In affected areas there are swelling and proliferation of mesangial and 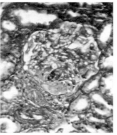 endothelial cells, capsular adhesions, and localized periglomerulitis, as shown in H and E section above. Necrosis, deposits of fibrinoid, and crescent formation may occur, as in the azocarmine section to the right. Occasionally, "wire loops" and intracapillary thrombi may be seen (not illustrated).

Glomerular abnormalities are similar to those of focal proliferative, but ***all or almost all glomeruli are involved***, and larger portions of glomeruli are affected. In H and E section above, there are severe, irregular swelling and proliferation of endothelial and mesangial cells, with obliteration of capillaries, necrosis, and karyorrhexis. Hematoxylin bodies and crescents may sometimes be seen.

Characterized by ***diffuse, fairly uniform thickening of glomerular capillary walls,*** as illustrated in H and E section above. 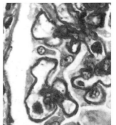 Necrosis, neutrophil infiltration, or crescents are ***not found***, and only mesangial cell proliferation is present. If intracapillary cell proliferation is prominent, the condition is classified as *diffuse proliferation.* In azocarmine section at right, diffuse thickening of capillary wall is seen to be due mainly to deposits of carminophilic material along outer side of basement membrane.

Clinical course

Microscopic hematuria	Gross hematuria	Gross hematuria
Proteinuria, usually slight but occasionally heavy	Heavy proteinemia	Heavy proteinuria
Nephrotic syndrome, rarely	Nephrotic syndrome, usually	Nephrotic syndrome, almost invariably
Moderate hypertension, occasionally	Hypertension, usually	Hypertension, usually
BUN elevation, rarely	Renal insufficiency and azotemia, usually	Renal insufficiency, occasionally
Remission usually complete, either spontaneously or in response to corticosteroid therapy. Relapses respond to treatment except in rare cases of transition to diffuse proliferative type.	Remission may occur but is rarely complete Relapses common Usually does ***not*** respond to treatment	May remit with treatment but usually relapses Usually characterized by heavy proteinuria with little or no renal insufficiency

Prognosis

Patients usually survive for many years Do not ordinarily develop renal insufficiency or nephrotic syndrome	Renal insufficiency and nephrotic syndrome progress Death commonly occurs within 5 years but may come much earlier; death usually due to other aspects of SLE or its complications rather than to uremia	Most patients survive for many years In some, complete remission may be maintained for long periods Death in uremia rare

f. Netter M.D.

FIGURE 6-15 LUPUS NEPHRITIS *(CONTINUED)*

Diffuse proliferative lupus nephritis (class IV) is characterized by involvement of most glomeruli coupled with more prominent accumulation of basement membrane material and more severe and widespread interstitial inflammation. **Diffuse membranous** **lupus nephritis** is characterized by diffuse abnormalities of the basement membranes resembling those of idiopathic membranous nephropathy.

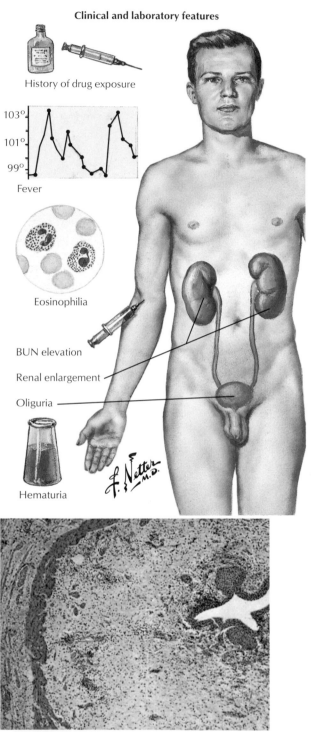

Clinical and laboratory features

History of drug exposure

Fever

Eosinophilia

BUN elevation

Renal enlargement

Oliguria

Hematuria

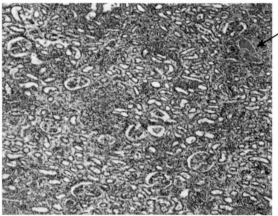

Kidney, low power. Prominence of interstitial tissue due to clustered foci of cells; necrotic tubules in upper right corner (H and E stain)

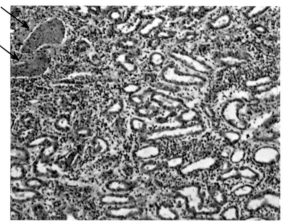

Kidney, medium power. Uniform interstitial edema and cellular infiltration, chiefly of lymphocytes; tubules relatively normal except necrotic tubules at upper left (H and E stain)

Ureter, low power. Extensive edema resulting in marked narrowing of lumen; cellular infiltration in submucosa and in musculature (H and E stain)

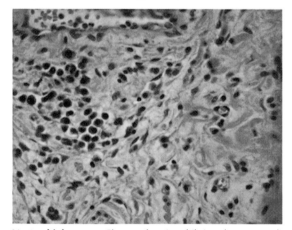

Ureter, high power. Cluster of eosinophils in submucosa adjacent to band of smooth muscle (H and E stain)

FIGURE 6-16 ACUTE DIFFUSE INTERSTITIAL NEPHRITIS

Acute diffuse interstitial nephritis, although uncommon, is an important cause of acute oliguric renal failure. It usually occurs as a manifestation of a hypersensitivity reaction to sulfonamides, penicillins, or other drugs (drug reaction). The characteristic features are fever, rash, eosinophilia, hematuria, oliguria, and azotemia. The kidneys are enlarged and may be 3 times their normal weight. Microscopy reveals pronounced edema and cellular infiltration by lymphocytes, eosinophils, and, occasionally, plasma cells. Parenchymal damage is minimal and is usually limited to focal tubular necrosis.

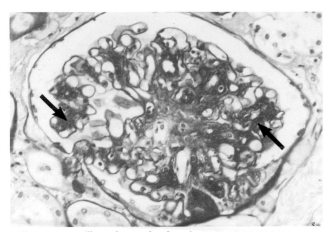

Diffuse intercapillary glomerulosclerosis. PAS stain

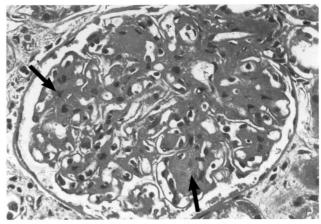

Diffuse intercapillary glomerulosclerosis. H and E stain

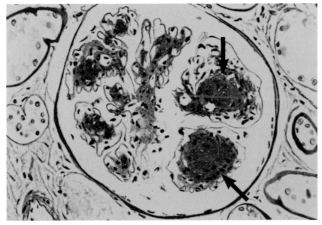

Nodular intercapillary glomerulosclerosis. PAS stain

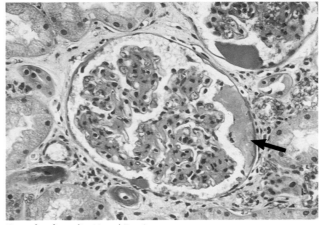

Capsular deposits. H and E stain

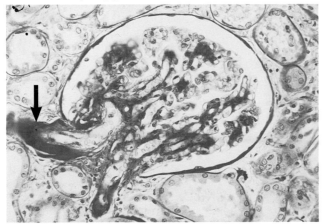

Arteriolosclerosis. Hyalinization of efferent and afferent arteriole; aniline blue stain

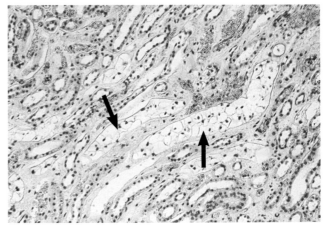

Armanni-Ebstein cells in renal tubules. H and E stain

FIGURE 6-17 DIABETIC NEPHROPATHY: RENAL PATHOLOGY

In **diabetic glomerulosclerosis**, a characteristic lesion occurs in diffuse and nodular (Kimmelstiel-Wilson) forms when increased amounts of PAS basement membrane material accumulate in the mesangium (intercapillary glomerulosclerosis) and the capillary walls. The pathogenesis of the glomerulopathy seems to involve accelerated degeneration and turnover of connective tissue cells coupled with abnormal glycosylation of matrix proteins. The capillary walls, although thickened, become porous, giving rise to nephrotic syndrome. Similar degeneration and accumulation of glycosylated proteins occurs in the walls of the microvasculature, giving rise to hyaline thickening (arteriolosclerosis) of both the afferent and efferent glomerular arterioles. Other lesions include hyaline, lipoproteinaceous deposits in the parietal layer of Bowman capsules, lipohyaline deposits in glomerular capillaries, thickening of the tubular basement membranes, and glycogen-filled epithelial cells in the distal, straight portion of the proximal tubule (the Armanni-Ebstein lesion).

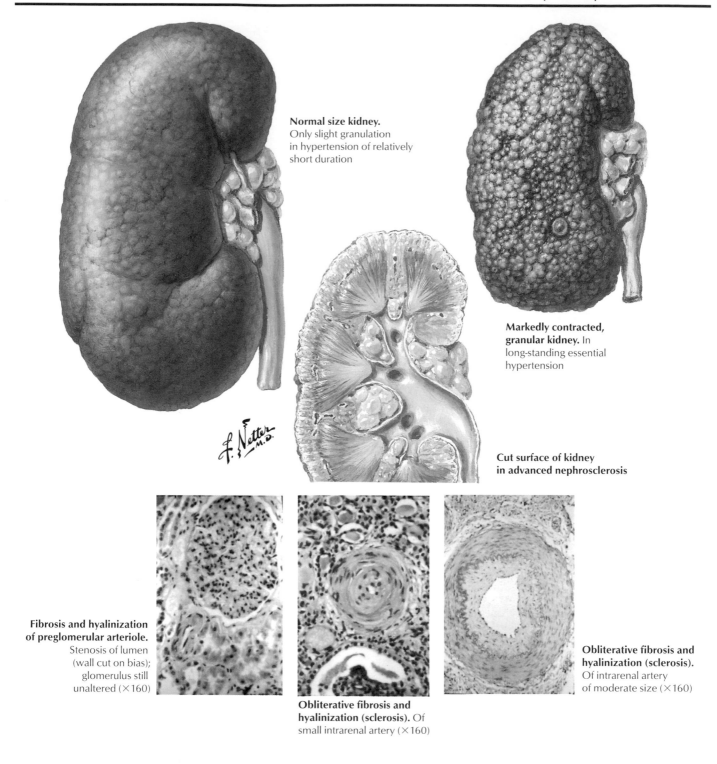

Normal size kidney. Only slight granulation in hypertension of relatively short duration

Markedly contracted, granular kidney. In long-standing essential hypertension

Cut surface of kidney in advanced nephrosclerosis

Fibrosis and hyalinization of preglomerular arteriole. Stenosis of lumen (wall cut on bias); glomerulus still unaltered (×160)

Obliterative fibrosis and hyalinization (sclerosis). Of small intrarenal artery (×160)

Obliterative fibrosis and hyalinization (sclerosis). Of intrarenal artery of moderate size (×160)

FIGURE 6-18 BENIGN ESSENTIAL HYPERTENSION

Benign essential hypertension is a poorly defined condition of multifaceted origin characterized by persistent, moderate increase of systemic blood pressure. Over time, progressive damage occurs to the resistance vessels, leading to **hyaline arteriosclerosis** in the kidneys and other organs. The small and medium intrarenal arteries become involved, which leads to fibrosis, hyalinization (sclerosis), and narrowing of the lumen. The hyaline material is composed of degenerated vascular cells and plasma proteins that have leaked into the vessel. Fibrosis results from active laying down of collagen by vascular cells. The narrowing of the arterioles and small arteries results in multifocal ischemia and small scars throughout the renal cortex giving rise to a thinned cortex and a finely granular surface. These changes lead to progressive renal insufficiency.

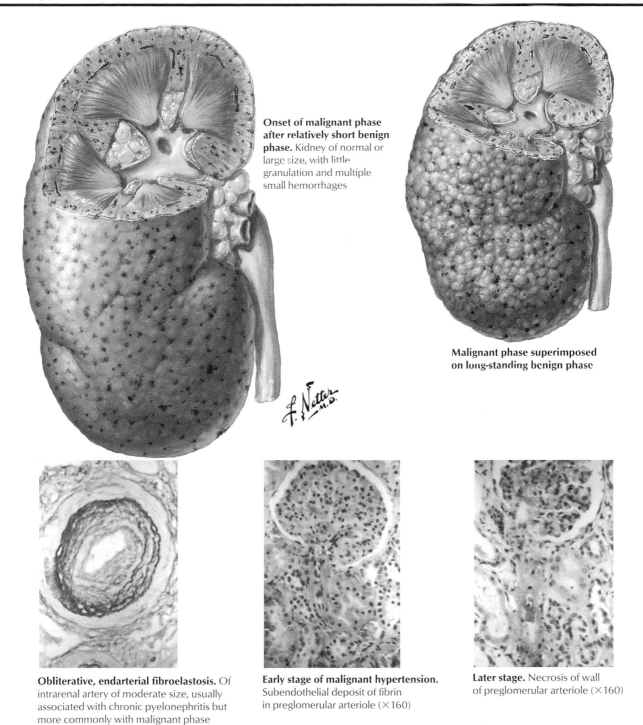

Onset of malignant phase after relatively short benign phase. Kidney of normal or large size, with little granulation and multiple small hemorrhages

Malignant phase superimposed on long-standing benign phase

Obliterative, endarterial fibroelastosis. Of intrarenal artery of moderate size, usually associated with chronic pyelonephritis but more commonly with malignant phase of hypertension (×160). "Onion-skinning"

Early stage of malignant hypertension. Subendothelial deposit of fibrin in preglomerular arteriole (×160)

Later stage. Necrosis of wall of preglomerular arteriole (×160)

FIGURE 6-19 MALIGNANT PHASE OF ESSENTIAL HYPERTENSION: RENAL PATHOLOGY

Malignant hypertension is closely associated with renal ischemia due to parenchymal or renovascular abnormalities or to rapid progression of renal changes in essential hypertension. The kidney may be of normal size with minimal granularity or shrunken and scarred, depending on the extent and duration of preexistent moderate hypertension. The characteristic gross feature of malignant hypertension is the presence of multiple petechial hemorrhages, reflective of multifocal severe ischemia, which produce the "flea-bitten" kidney. **Hyperplastic arteriolosclerosis**, the characteristic microscopic lesion in widespread obliterative fibroelastosis of arterioles and small arteries, is accompanied by glomerular and interstitial hemorrhage and fibrin deposition. Severe malignant hypertension produces fibrinoid necrosis of the afferent glomerular arterioles.

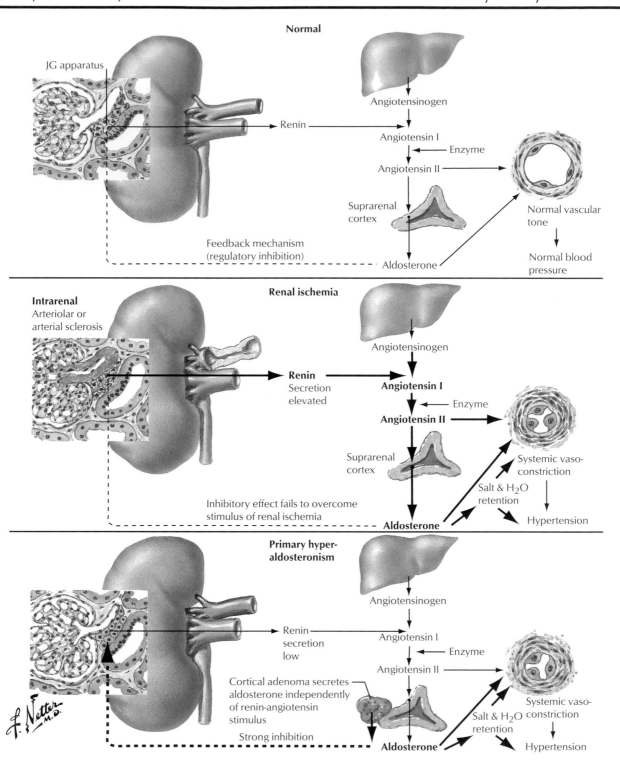

FIGURE 6-20 RENOVASCULAR HYPERTENSION

Various stenosing or obstructing lesions of the extrarenal vasculature, especially stenosis of the main renal artery, often result in **hypertension**. Such lesions include arteriosclerotic plaques, various forms of fibromuscular dysplasia, obstruction, and trauma. An appropriate evaluation is needed to determine whether the lesion is unilateral and whether the hypertension is likely to be relieved by surgery. The renin-angiotensin system has an important role in both extrarenal renovascular hypertension and hypertension due to intrarenal disease. Renal ischemia leads to increased renin excretion, which is followed by production of increased levels of angiotensin I and II and increased release of aldosterone. In primary hyperaldosteronemia, aldosterone is increased, and levels of renin and angiotensin are low.

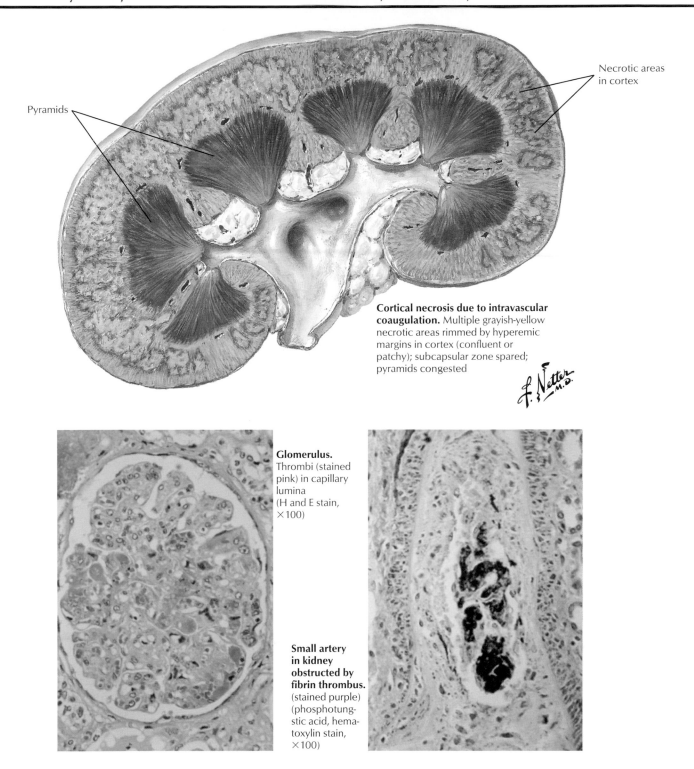

Pyramids

Necrotic areas in cortex

Cortical necrosis due to intravascular coaugulation. Multiple grayish-yellow necrotic areas rimmed by hyperemic margins in cortex (confluent or patchy); subcapsular zone spared; pyramids congested

F. Netter M.D.

Glomerulus. Thrombi (stained pink) in capillary lumina (H and E stain, ×100)

Small artery in kidney obstructed by fibrin thrombus. (stained purple) (phosphotung- stic acid, hema- toxylin stain, ×100)

FIGURE 6-21 HEMOLYTIC-UREMIC SYNDROME

Intravascular coagulation and thrombotic microangiopathy (**hemolytic-uremic syndrome** [HUS]) is characterized by hemoly- sis, thrombocytopenia, intravascular coagulation, hypertension, and renal failure. HUS occurs as an idiopathic disease, usually in infants and young children, or during the course of systemic disease (e.g., malignant hypertension, eclampsia, and dissemi- nated carcinomatosis). The histologic picture is dominated by fibrin-platelet thrombi in many glomerular capillaries and in small arteries, which sometimes exhibit fibrinoid necrosis. The accumulation of pale, finely granular or fibrillar material between the endothelium and the capillary basement membranes of the glomeruli is an important feature of HUS. Immunofluorescence shows that the deposits contain fibrinogen and globulin. The affected capillary walls are thick, and the lumens are narrow. The combination of arteriolar thrombosis and capillary wall thicken- ing constitutes the entity of thrombotic microangiopathy.

Microscopic views

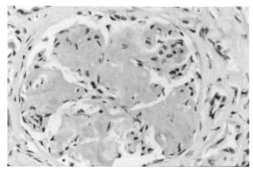

Extensive amyloid deposits in glomerulus of human kidney (Congo red and hematoxylin stain)

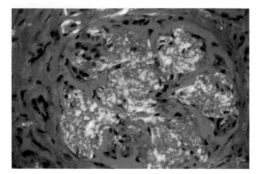

Same section, viewed under polarizing microscope, demonstrating green birefringence

Electron microscopic findings

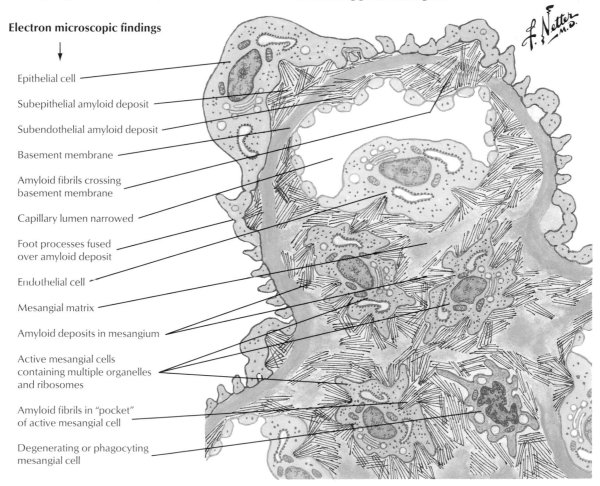

Epithelial cell

Subepithelial amyloid deposit

Subendothelial amyloid deposit

Basement membrane

Amyloid fibrils crossing basement membrane

Capillary lumen narrowed

Foot processes fused over amyloid deposit

Endothelial cell

Mesangial matrix

Amyloid deposits in mesangium

Active mesangial cells containing multiple organelles and ribosomes

Amyloid fibrils in "pocket" of active mesangial cell

Degenerating or phagocyting mesangial cell

FIGURE 6-22 RENAL AMYLOIDOSIS

The kidneys are frequently involved in various forms of amyloidosis. Marked proteinuria is the usual mode of presentation, and overt nephrotic syndrome occurs in most cases. Homogeneous hyaline deposits of amyloid involve the arterioles and the glomeruli. When examined under polarized light, Congo red–stained sections show typical apple-green birefringence as a result of the β-pleated sheet configuration of the amyloid protein. Electron microscopy reveals that amyloid deposits are composed of masses of nonbranching fibrils of 7.5 to 10 nm in diameter, which are much smaller than collagen fibrils found in the foci of ordinary fibrosis.

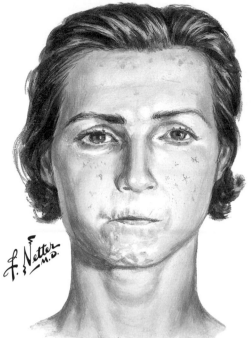

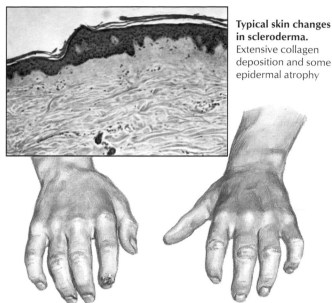

Typical skin changes in scleroderma. Extensive collagen deposition and some epidermal atrophy

Characteristics. Thickening, tightening, and rigidity of facial skin, with small, constricted mouth and narrow lips, in atrophic phase of scleroderma

Sclerodactyly. Fingers partially fixed in semiflexed position; terminal phalanges atrophied; fingertips pointed and ulcerated

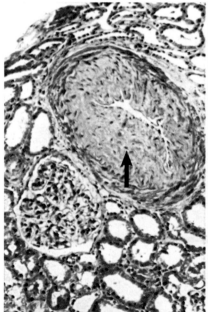

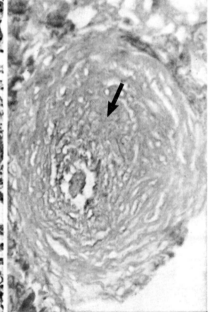

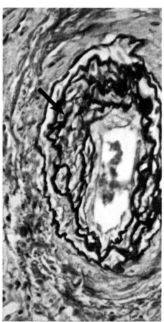

Arcuate artery in acute scleroderma. Mucoid swelling of intima in medium-sized artery of kidney, most ofter seen in acute cases

Arcuate artery in acute scleroderma. Colloidal iron stain, demonstrating that intimal swelling is composed largely of mucopolysaccharides

Arcuate artery in chronic scleroderma. Marked intimal thickening, consisting of dense, laminated matrix, rich in elastic fibers, and small amount of collagen

FIGURE 6-23 PROGRESSIVE SYSTEMIC SCLEROSIS AND RHEUMATOID ARTHRITIS

Progressive systemic sclerosis (scleroderma) is a systemic disease characterized by the accumulation of excess collagen and the presence of vascular lesions with little inflammation. The classic form exhibits widespread involvement of skin and internal organs. Vascular lesions are particularly striking in the kidneys. Medium-sized renal arteries exhibit variable combinations of mucoid swelling of the intima and fibroelastic intimal prolifera-tion, similar to the onion-skinning seen in malignant hypertension. When renal involvement becomes clinically apparent, it progresses rapidly, and malignant hypertension, retinopathy, encephalopathy, and renal failure ensue. Renal involvement in rheumatoid arthritis is less common and usually less severe than in other autoimmune diseases. The basic lesion, a multifocal vasculitis, involves small arteries and veins.

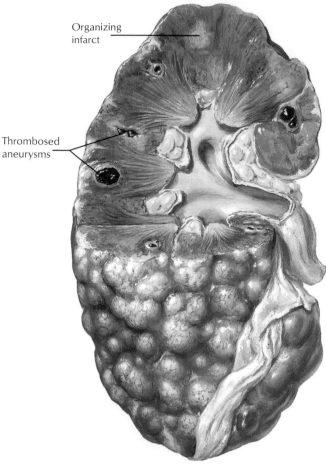

Organizing infarct

Thrombosed aneurysms

Coarsely nodular, irregularly scarred kidney. Cut section reveals organizing infarcts and thrombosed aneurysms in corticomedullary region

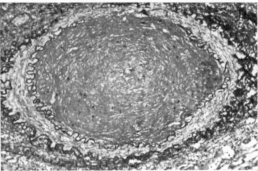

Almost complete obliteration of lumen of arcuate renal artery by intimal fibrosis. Fragmentation of internal elastic membrane and medial fibrosis (elastic van Gieson stain, ×100)

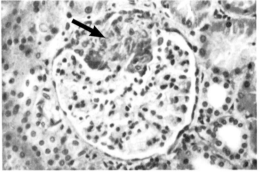

Focal glomerular lesion. Segment of glomerular tuft destroyed by necrotic process with much fibrin and some cellular reaction; patient died from intestinal perforation (H and E stain, ×200)

Renal involvement in hypersensitivity type of polyarteritis nodosa

Necrotizing (fibrinoid) changes in small artery at right of section, with infiltration of all layers by acute and chronic inflammatory cells; the inflammatory process has extended to the interstitium and to the adjacent glomerulus (H and E stain, ×100)

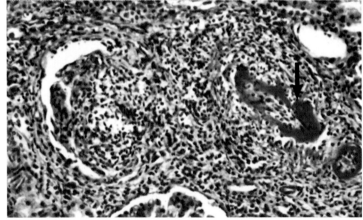

FIGURE 6-24 POLYARTERITIS NODOSA

Polyarteritis nodosa refers to a constellation of inflammatory and necrotizing disease processes that involve medium and small arteries, most commonly in the kidneys, the gastrointestinal tract, and the heart. Classical polyarteritis nodosa produces multifocal involvement of medium or larger arteries. The kidneys may be coarsely nodular and irregularly scarred as a result of regional areas of ischemia and infarction of various ages. Acute lesions are characterized by fibrinoid necrosis of the arterial wall with

inflammatory cellular infiltration by polymorphonuclear leukocytes and plasma cells in the adventitia extending into the media. Healing lesions exhibit medial fibrosis, focal destruction of the internal elastic lamella, and intimal fibrosis. The **hypersensitivity type of polyarteritis nodosa** is dominated by fibrinoid necrosis and inflammation of small arteries. In the kidney, **Wegener granulomatosis** shows segmental and focal necrotizing glomerular lesions and a granulomatous and necrotizing arteriolitis.

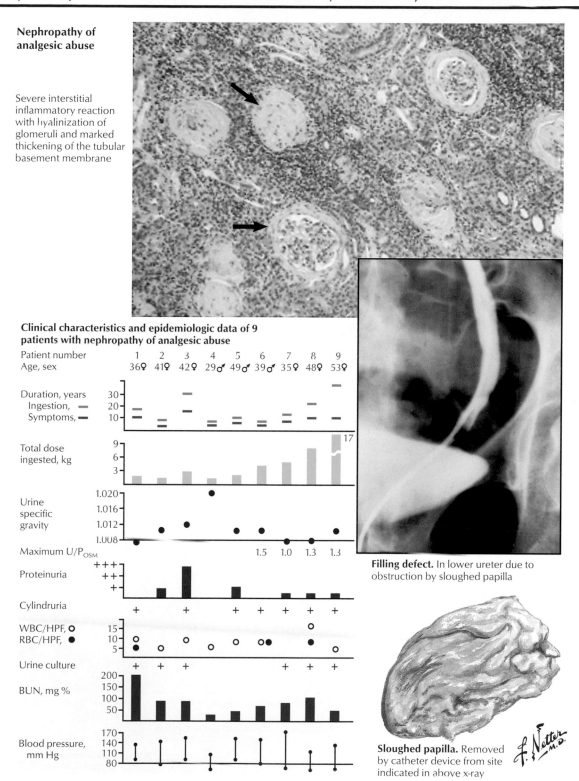

Nephropathy of analgesic abuse

Severe interstitial inflammatory reaction with hyalinization of glomeruli and marked thickening of the tubular basement membrane

Clinical characteristics and epidemiologic data of 9 patients with nephropathy of analgesic abuse

Patient number	1	2	3	4	5	6	7	8	9
Age, sex	36♀	41♀	42♀	29♂	49♂	39♂	35♀	48♀	53♀
Maximum U/P$_{OSM}$						1.5	1.0	1.3	1.3

Filling defect. In lower ureter due to obstruction by sloughed papilla

Sloughed papilla. Removed by catheter device from site indicated in above x-ray

f. Netter M.D.

FIGURE 6-25 TOXIC NEPHROPATHY

Toxic nephropathy encompasses any adverse functional or structural change in the kidney produced by a chemical or biological product. The renal tubules are a frequent target of injury. **Nephrotoxins** include heavy metals (mercury, lead), organic chemicals (carbon tetrachloride, ethylene glycol), drugs (many antibiotics, analgesics), pesticides (e.g., chlorinated hydrocarbons), physical agents (radiation), and products of metabolic disturbances, including hyperuricemia, hypercalcemia, and hypokalemia. Nephrotoxins may act directly on the nephrons or may produce hypersensitivity reactions, which result in vasculitis, nephritis, or nephrotic syndrome. With the toxic nephropathy resulting from excessive intake of mixed analgesic tablets, especially those containing phenacetin, the pathologic process is one of chronic interstitial nephritis with inflammatory cellular infiltration and fibrosis and a tendency for papillary necrosis.

Renal Vein Thrombosis

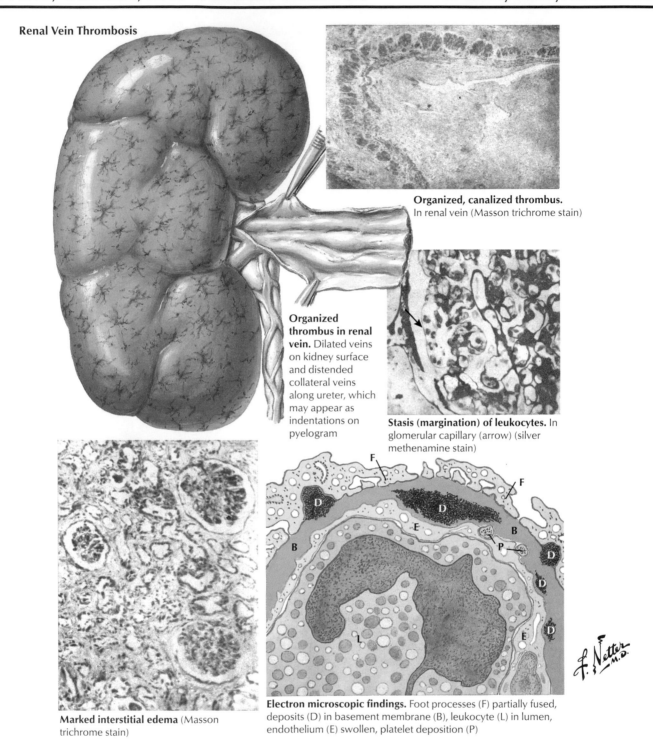

Organized, canalized thrombus. In renal vein (Masson trichrome stain)

Organized thrombus in renal vein. Dilated veins on kidney surface and distended collateral veins along ureter, which may appear as indentations on pyelogram

Stasis (margination) of leukocytes. In glomerular capillary (arrow) (silver methenamine stain)

Marked interstitial edema (Masson trichrome stain)

Electron microscopic findings. Foot processes (F) partially fused, deposits (D) in basement membrane (B), leukocyte (L) in lumen, endothelium (E) swollen, platelet deposition (P)

FIGURE 6-26 RENAL VEIN THROMBOSIS

Renal vein thrombosis is an uncommon cause of nephrotic syndrome. It may occur as a complication of previously existing renal disease or as a primary disease after trauma, particularly in individuals predisposed to venous thrombosis, or as a result of compression of the renal vein by tumors or adhesions. In infants and children, severe dehydration may lead to acute renal vein thrombosis producing renal cortical necrosis and severe renal insufficiency. In adults, the typical presentation is nephrotic syndrome with severe proteinuria. The kidneys become extremely enlarged as a result of interstitial edema, and their surfaces may exhibit small, dilated veins. By electron microscopy, the glomeruli show fusion of epithelial foot processes and the presence of dense osmiophilic deposits on both sides of and sometimes within the basement membrane. These deposits have been shown to consist of IgG, IgM, complement, and fibrin-fibrinogen.

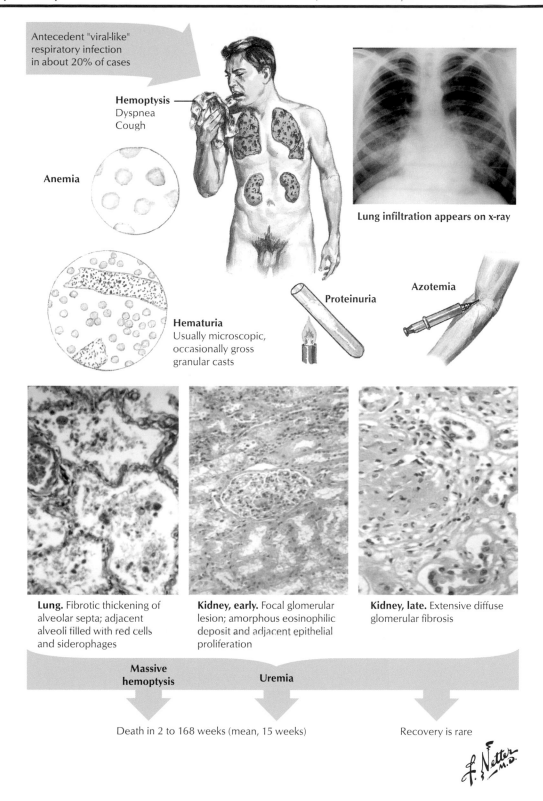

Antecedent "viral-like" respiratory infection in about 20% of cases

Hemoptysis
Dyspnea
Cough

Anemia

Lung infiltration appears on x-ray

Proteinuria

Azotemia

Hematuria
Usually microscopic, occasionally gross granular casts

Lung. Fibrotic thickening of alveolar septa; adjacent alveoli filled with red cells and siderophages

Kidney, early. Focal glomerular lesion; amorphous eosinophilic deposit and adjacent epithelial proliferation

Kidney, late. Extensive diffuse glomerular fibrosis

Massive hemoptysis

Uremia

Death in 2 to 168 weeks (mean, 15 weeks)

Recovery is rare

FIGURE 6-27 LUNG PURPURA WITH NEPHRITIS

Lung purpura with nephritis (**Goodpasture syndrome**) is an acute condition involving the lungs and the kidneys. The characteristic feature is profound hemoptysis, which may lead to severe anemia and very low serum iron levels. Chest radiography typically shows cardiomegaly and striking pulmonary opacities. The pathologic counterpart is a **hemorrhagic alveolitis**. Kidney involvement, which may develop simultaneously with or subsequent to the pulmonary lesion, manifests clinically by gross or microscopic albuminuria and pathologically by necrotic and proliferative lesions. Hypertension generally does not develop.

Hypokalemic (Potassium-Depletion) Nephropathy

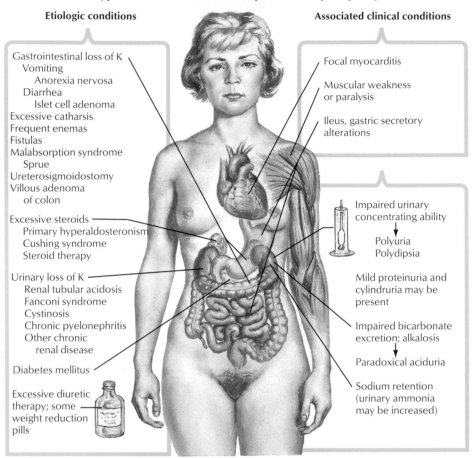

Etiologic conditions

Gastrointestinal loss of K
   Vomiting
      Anorexia nervosa
   Diarrhea
      Islet cell adenoma
Excessive catharsis
Frequent enemas
Fistulas
Malabsorption syndrome
   Sprue
Ureterosigmoidostomy
Villous adenoma
   of colon

Excessive steroids
   Primary hyperaldosteronism
   Cushing syndrome
   Steroid therapy

Urinary loss of K
   Renal tubular acidosis
   Fanconi syndrome
   Cystinosis
   Chronic pyelonephritis
   Other chronic
      renal disease

Diabetes mellitus

Excessive diuretic
therapy; some
weight reduction
pills

Associated clinical conditions

Focal myocarditis

Muscular weakness
or paralysis

Ileus, gastric secretory
alterations

Impaired urinary
concentrating ability
↓
Polyuria
Polydipsia

Mild proteinuria and
cylindruria may be
present

Impaired bicarbonate
excretion; alkalosis
↓
Paradoxical aciduria

Sodium retention
(urinary ammonia
may be increased)

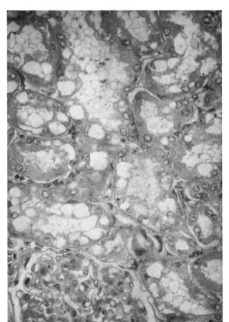

Extensive vacuolization
of renal tubules in
hypokalemic nephropathy
(H and E stain, ×250)

FIGURE 6-28 HYPOKALEMIC NEPHROPATHY

Hypokalemic nephropathy may result from excessive fluid loss through the gastrointestinal tract, excess fluid loss in the urine, excessive sterol levels, or miscellaneous conditions. Renal dysfunction includes impaired urinary concentrating ability, impaired bicarbonate excretion, alkalosis with paradoxical aciduria, and sodium retention. The characteristic histologic finding is marked vacuolization of renal tubular epithelium, which is more marked in the proximal convoluted tubules than in the distal. Clinical manifestations include focal myocarditis, muscle weakness or paralysis, and ileus.

Calcium Nephropathy

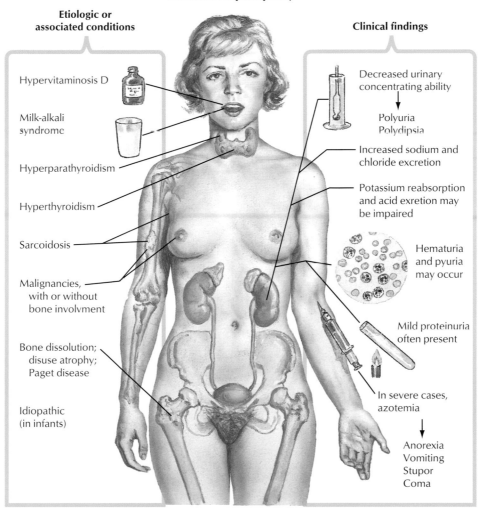

Etiologic or associated conditions

Hypervitaminosis D

Milk-alkali syndrome

Hyperparathyroidism

Hyperthyroidism

Sarcoidosis

Malignancies, with or without bone involvment

Bone dissolution; disuse atrophy; Paget disease

Idiopathic (in infants)

Clinical findings

Decreased urinary concentrating ability
↓
Polyuria
Polydipsia

Increased sodium and chloride excretion

Potassium reabsorption and acid exretion may be impaired

Hematuria and pyuria may occur

Mild proteinuria often present

In severe cases, azotemia
↓
Anorexia
Vomiting
Stupor
Coma

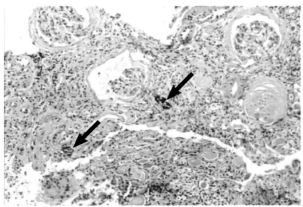

Calcium nephropathy. Periglomerular fibrosis and varying degrees of glomerular hyalinization; multifocal calcium deposits (arrows); intratubular protein material simulating thyroidization of pyelonephritis (H and E stain, ×100)

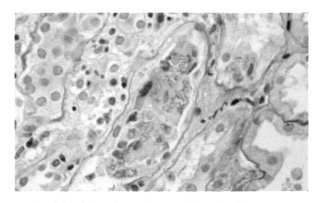

Renal tubule. Intraluminal accumulation of calcium and cellular debris (PAS stain, ×400, enlarged)

FIGURE 6-29 CALCIUM NEPHROPATHY

A variety of metabolic states and systemic diseases may result in an excess calcium load to the kidneys. Clinical findings include decreased urinary concentrating ability; increased sodium and chloride excretion; hematuria; mild proteinuria; and, in severe cases, azotemia, anorexia, stupor, and coma. Pathologically, multifocal calcification of interstitial tissue, distal convoluted tubules, and collecting ducts may be seen. Glomeruli frequently show partial or complete hyalinization, and chronic inflammatory changes are frequently present.

Myelomatosis with Renal Involvement

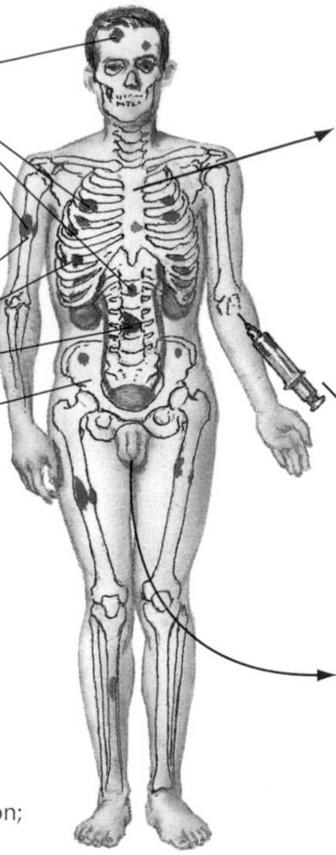

Myelomatous deposits in skull, ribs, spine, pelvis, and/or long bones

Bone pain

Pathologic fractures common

Weight loss

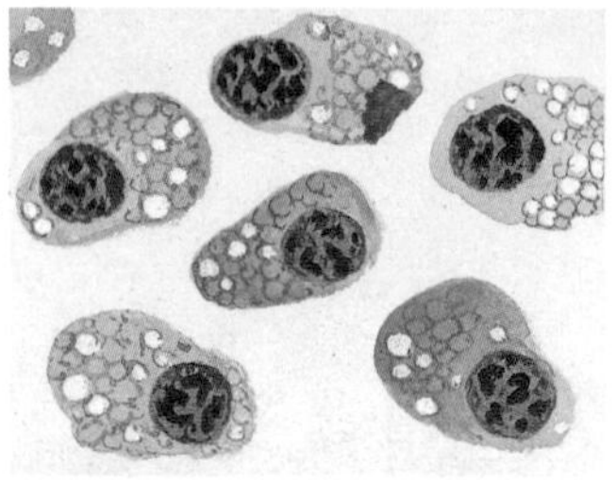

Bone marrow biopsy. Characteristic malignant myeloma cells (may also be found occasionally in circulation)

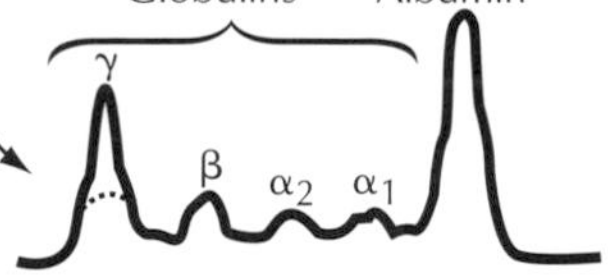

Globulins   Albumin

γ β α_2 α_1

Presence of abnormal proteins in serum (γ spike); also hypercalcemia

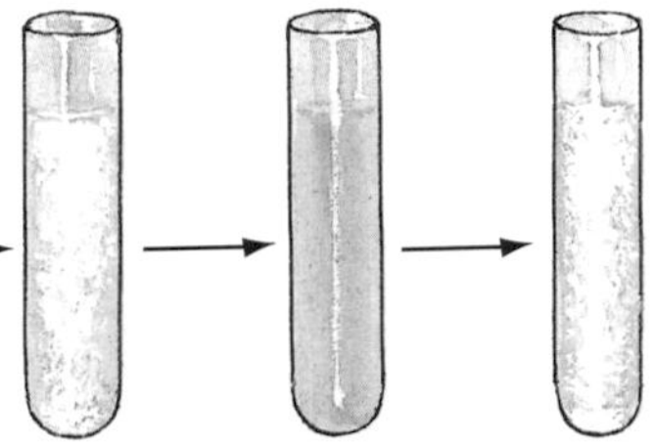

Bence Jones protein in urine in 60% of cases (precipitates at 45 to 60 °C, redissolves at boiling, and reprecipitates on cooling to 60 to 55 °C)

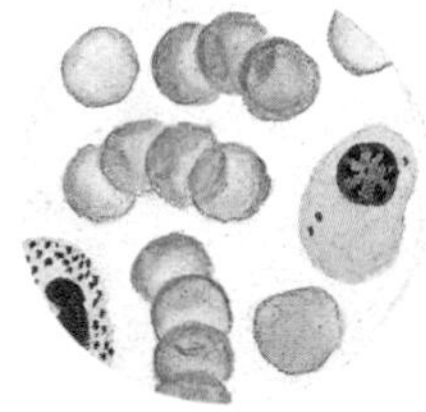

55°C   100°C   55°C

Anemia. Rouleau formation; increased blood viscosity

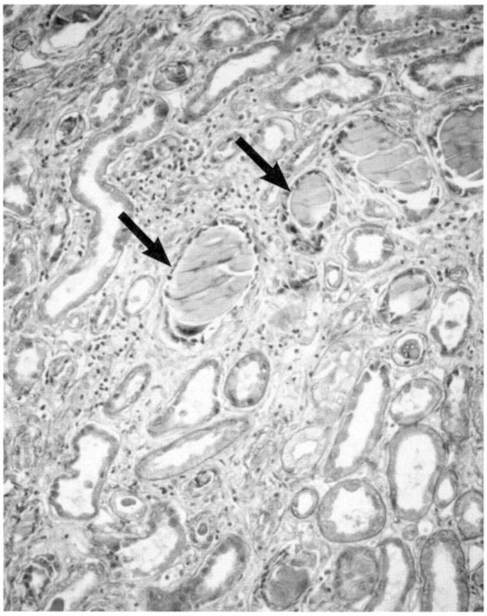

Myeloma kidney. Many dilated tubules containing eosinophilic amorphous casts; atrophy of epithelium; giant cell formation

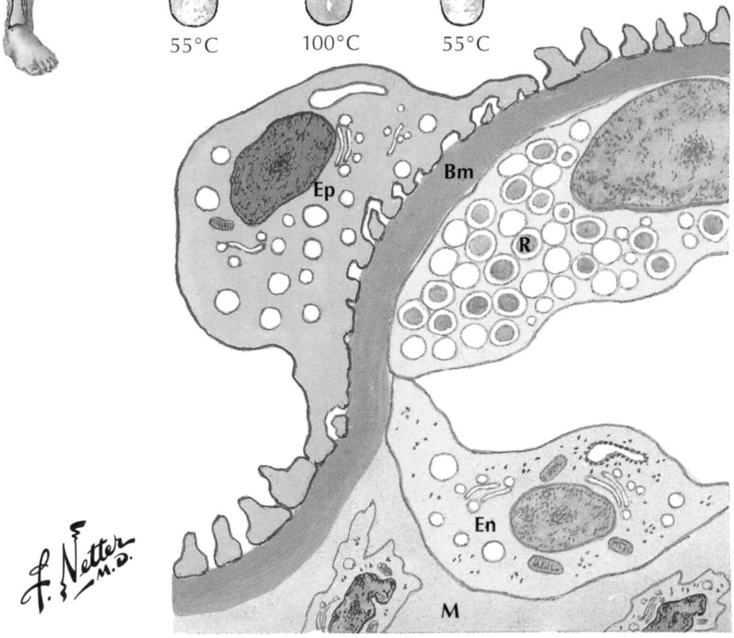

Diagram of electron microscopic findings in glomeruli. Epithelial (Ep) and endothelial (En) cells and mesangium (M) show changes often seen in other proteinuric conditions; focal loss or fusion of foot processes; basement membrane (Bm) thickened but free of deposits; occasional cell on luminal side suggestive of plasma cell transformation with Russell bodies (R)

FIGURE 6-30 MYELOMA

Multiple myeloma is a part of the clinical spectrum of paraproteinemias in which neoplastic plasma cells infiltrate bone, lymph nodes, and various soft tissues and elaborate abnormal serum proteins. These proteins typically produce a monoclonal γ-globulin spike on serum electrophoresis. Approximately 15% of individuals with multiple myeloma also have amyloidosis. In at least 60% of cases, with or without amyloidosis, the kidneys excrete immunoglobulin fragments known as Bence Jones proteins into the urine. The kidneys exhibit glomerular lesions associated with proteinuria as well as markedly dilated tubules containing proteinaceous casts.

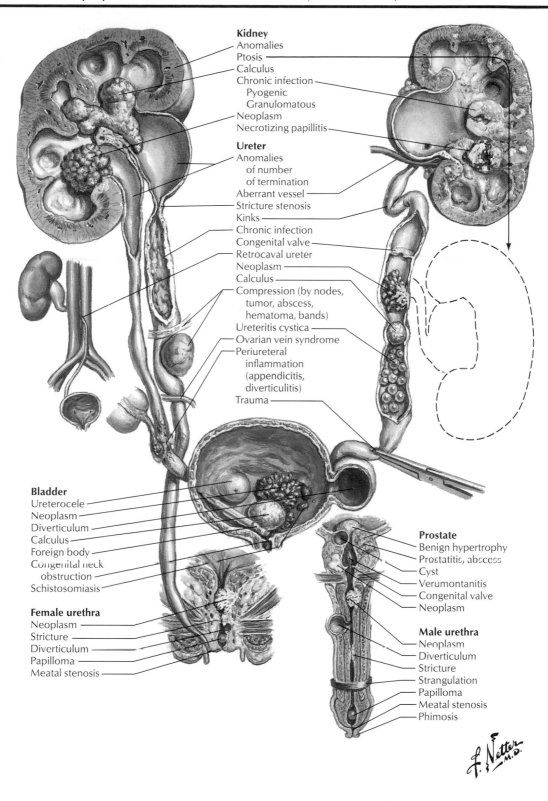

Kidney
Anomalies
Ptosis
Calculus
Chronic infection
    Pyogenic
    Granulomatous
Neoplasm
Necrotizing papillitis

Ureter
Anomalies
    of number
    of termination
Aberrant vessel
Stricture stenosis
Kinks
Chronic infection
Congenital valve
Retrocaval ureter
Neoplasm
Calculus
Compression (by nodes,
    tumor, abscess,
    hematoma, bands)
Ureteritis cystica
Ovarian vein syndrome
Periureteral
    inflammation
    (appendicitis,
    diverticulitis)
Trauma

Bladder
Ureterocele
Neoplasm
Diverticulum
Calculus
Foreign body
Congenital neck
    obstruction
Schistosomiasis

Female urethra
Neoplasm
Stricture
Diverticulum
Papilloma
Meatal stenosis

Prostate
Benign hypertrophy
Prostatitis, abscess
Cyst
Verumontanitis
Congenital valve
Neoplasm

Male urethra
Neoplasm
Diverticulum
Stricture
Strangulation
Papilloma
Meatal stenosis
Phimosis

FIGURE 6-31 OBSTRUCTIVE UROPATHY

Obstructive uropathy, a common cause of severe or fatal renal failure, is caused by pathologic changes in the urinary tract produced by obstruction to the flow of urine. It may be unilateral or bilateral, depending on the site of obstruction. The likelihood of complications is greatly increased by urinary tract infection, a common finding of obstruction. Acute urinary tract obstruction is often associated with obvious clinical symptoms, whereas chronic obstruction may be insidious or clinically silent. **Hydro-**

nephrosis, a dilatation of the renal collecting system resulting from severe obstruction to the flow of urine, may be bilateral depending on the site of obstruction. Severe hydronephrosis with renal parenchymal atrophy is unusual except in persons with congenital hydronephrosis. Asymptomatic or silent hydronephrosis, which occurs in adults, may become clinically significant because it increases susceptibility to trauma and infection.

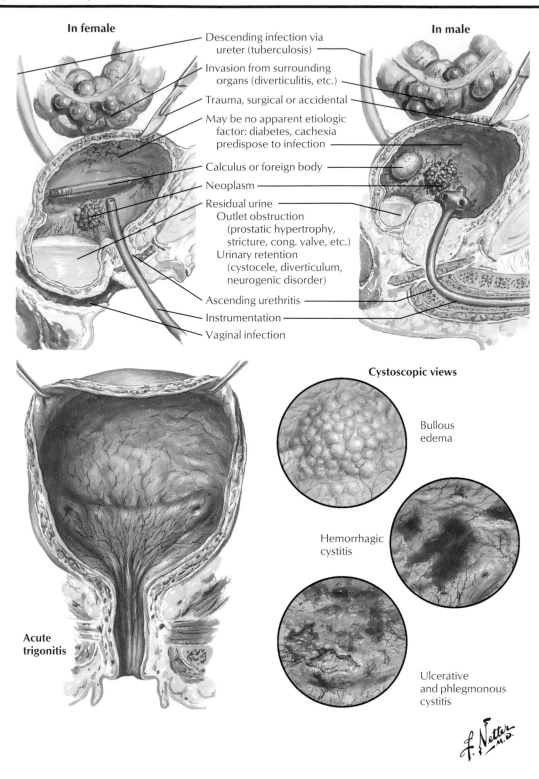

In female

In male

- Descending infection via ureter (tuberculosis)
- Invasion from surrounding organs (diverticulitis, etc.)
- Trauma, surgical or accidental
- May be no apparent etiologic factor: diabetes, cachexia predispose to infection
- Calculus or foreign body
- Neoplasm
- Residual urine
  Outlet obstruction (prostatic hypertrophy, stricture, cong. valve, etc.)
  Urinary retention (cystocele, diverticulum, neurogenic disorder)
- Ascending urethritis
- Instrumentation
- Vaginal infection

Acute trigonitis

Cystoscopic views

Bullous edema

Hemorrhagic cystitis

Ulcerative and phlegmonous cystitis

FIGURE 6-32 CYSTITIS

Cystitis results from an inflammation of the urinary bladder. Cystitis usually is a self-limited condition or one easily treated with antibiotics. In some circumstances, such as poorly controlled DM or chronic urinary tract obstruction, cystitis is a severe condition that progresses to involve the upper urinary tract and kidneys and leads to renal failure. In adult women, cystitis is usually limited to the trigone and rarely develops into a severe ulcerative or hemorrhagic disease. In adult men and in children of both sexes, cystitis usually signifies the presence of an underlying anatomical or physiologic abnormality. On cystoscopy, various patterns of involvement may be seen, including cystitis cystica, which is manifest as multiple epithelial-lined cysts. The chief complication of cystitis is spread of infection to the kidneys.

Possible routes of kidney infection

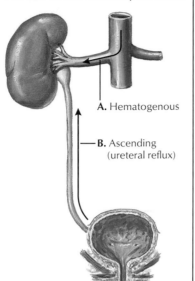

A. Hematogenous

B. Ascending (ureteral reflux)

Predisposing factors in acute pyelonephritis

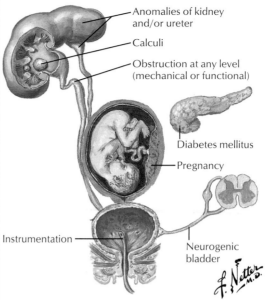

Anomalies of kidney and/or ureter

Calculi

Obstruction at any level (mechanical or functional)

Diabetes mellitus

Pregnancy

Instrumentation

Neurogenic bladder

Acute pyelonephritis. Radiating yellowish-gray streaks in pyramids and abscesses in cortex; moderate hydronephrosis with infection; blunting of calyces (ascending infection)

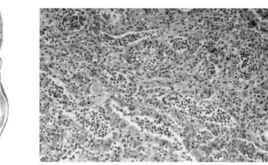

Acute pyelonephritis. With exudate chiefly of polymorphonuclear leukocytes in interstitium and collecting tubules

Chronic pyelonephritis. Thinning of renal parenchyma. With wedge-shaped subcapsular scars; blurring of corticomedullary junction; dilated, fibrosed pelvis and calyces seen in many but not all cases of chronic pyelonephritis

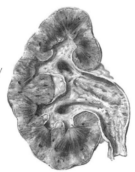

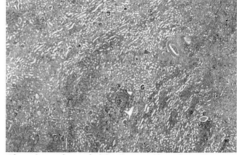

Chronic pyelonephritis. Areas of lymphocytic infiltration alternating with areas of relatively normal parenchyma

FIGURE 6-33 PYELONEPHRITIS

Pyelonephritis, an infectious disease of the kidney, is usually induced by pyogenic microorganisms, particularly *Escherichia coli* and other gram-negative bacteria. The primary process is inflammation of the renal interstitium and the tubules. In **acute pyelonephritis**, the swollen kidney exhibits multiple small abscesses seen as linear, yellowish areas radiating continuously from the corticomedullary junction to the surface and sometimes extending through the medulla into the papillae. Microscopically, the yellow lesions correspond to a heavy interstitial infiltrate of

polymorphonuclear leukocytes, with pus formation and liquefaction necrosis. The lesions are generally patchy with preserved glomeruli and vessels. The characteristic gross feature of **chronic pyelonephritis** is a coarsely granular contracted kidney with significant loss of renal parenchyma in the cortex and the medulla. Chronic interstitial inflammation (lymphocytes, macrophages) is widespread; many tubules are destroyed, and those remaining are dilated, lined by flattened epithelium, and filled with proteinaceous casts.

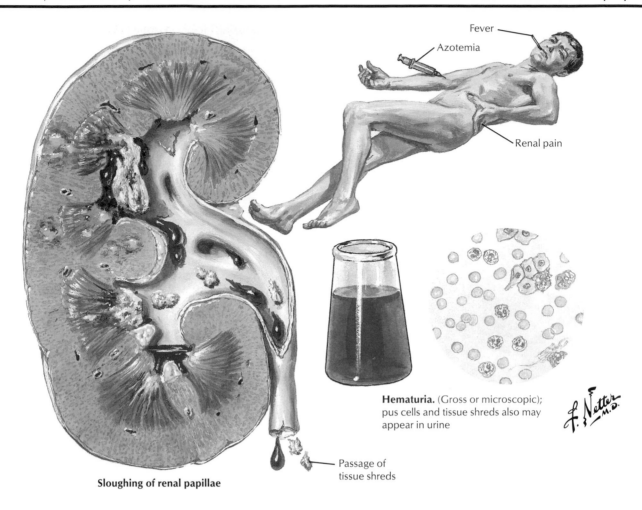

Sloughing of renal papillae

Hematuria. (Gross or microscopic); pus cells and tissue shreds also may appear in urine

Passage of tissue shreds

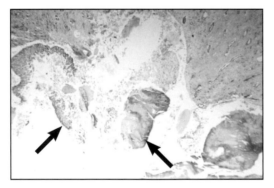

Papillary necrosis with sloughing. Leaving a concave inner border of the medulla. Detached dead fragments can be found in the urine

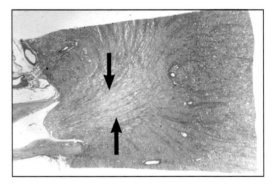

Papillary necrosis without inflammatory reaction. Believed by some to be characteristic of analgesic papillary necrosis

FIGURE 6-34 PAPILLARY NECROSIS

When coagulation necrosis of the renal papillae and portions of the medulla occurs, the necrotic tissue may be sloughed into the renal pelvis and passed into the ureter. The patient typically becomes ill with fever, renal colic, hematuria, oliguria, and azotemia, which may progress to fatal uremia. In some patients, particularly those with long-standing azotemia, sloughing of the papillae may occur over a prolonged period without overt ARF.

Papillary necrosis occurs most often in older people and in those with DM or pyelonephritis, particularly if there is lower urinary tract obstruction. In such individuals, a zone of neutrophilic infiltration at the periphery of the necrotic papilla is usually present. In patients who ingest excessive amounts of analgesic drugs, the papillary necrosis seems to result from a chemical toxicity without significant inflammation.

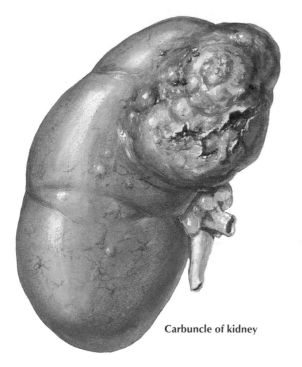

Carbuncle of kidney

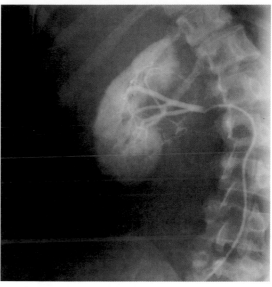

Arteriogram. Numerous vessels around mass surrounded by homogeneous blush in upper pole of kidney, suggestive or inflammatory process (carbuncle); also marked scoliosis

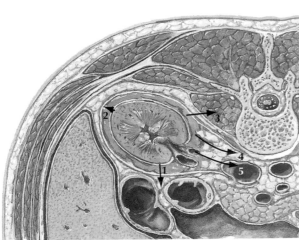

Perirenal abscess

Routes of spread

1 = through renal fascia (of Gerota) to retroperitoneal tissues; 2 = to flank; 3 = to psoas muscle; 4 = to midline (prevertebral); 5 = to inferior vena cava; 6 = to retrohepatic and subphrenic areas; 7 = through diaphragm to pleural cavity; 8 = to pelvic retroperitoneal tissues

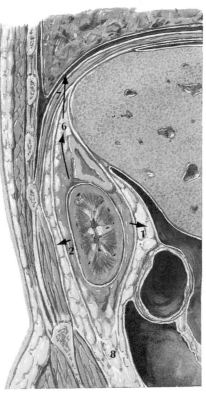

FIGURE 6-35 RENAL CARBUNCLE AND PERIRENAL ABSCESS

Renal carbuncle and **perirenal abscess** are septic conditions caused by infections with *Staphylococcus* species. These conditions, which may begin as an innocuous skin furuncle, reach the renal or perirenal tissue by hematogenous or lymphogenous spread. A renal carbuncle is an abscess in the renal cortex that typically results from the confluence of several smaller abscesses. This lesion occasionally produces a perirenal abscess

through rupture into the collecting system or through the capsule. The perirenal abscess usually develops as a primary abscess in the perirenal fat inside the Gerota fascia. Both renal carbuncle and perirenal abscess produce a marked leukocytosis of the blood, with variable findings on urinalysis. An intrarenal or perirenal mass lesion is detected by imaging studies.

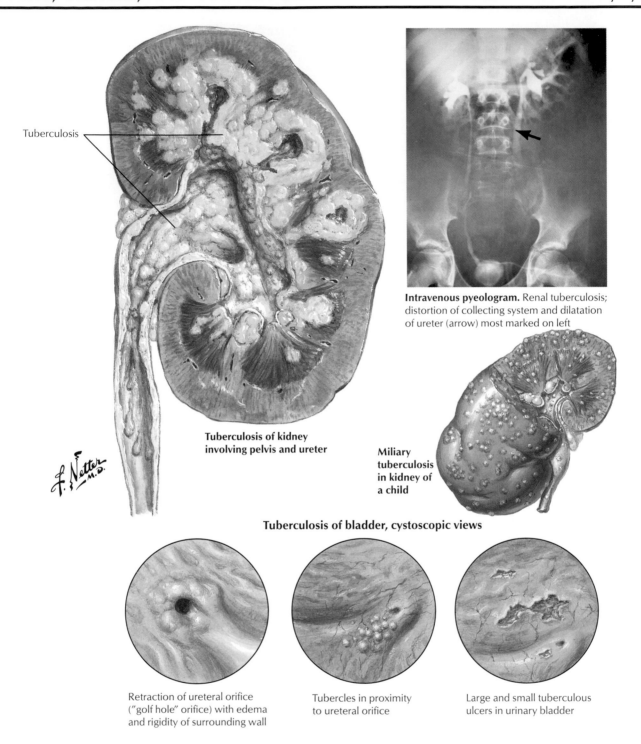

Intravenous pyeologram. Renal tuberculosis; distortion of collecting system and dilatation of ureter (arrow) most marked on left

Tuberculosis

Tuberculosis of kidney involving pelvis and ureter

Miliary tuberculosis in kidney of a child

Tuberculosis of bladder, cystoscopic views

Retraction of ureteral orifice ("golf hole" orifice) with edema and rigidity of surrounding wall

Tubercles in proximity to ureteral orifice

Large and small tuberculous ulcers in urinary bladder

FIGURE 6-36 TUBERCULOSIS OF THE URINARY TRACT

Tuberculosis of the urinary tract develops as a consequence of hematogenous dissemination of the tubercle bacilli (usually *Mycobacterium tuberculosis*). Urinary tract involvement has a peak incidence between the ages of 30 and 50 years and occurs more frequently in males. Bilateral involvement, particularly of the upper poles of the kidneys, is common. After the initial involvement of the kidneys, spread may occur to other compo-nents of the urinary tract. In countries where the dairy industry is closely regulated, the infecting organism is usually the human strain, but infection by the bovine strain is prevalent in other parts of the world. The lesions are those of a caseating granulomatous process with predisposition to cavitation and calcification. The kidneys are a common site of involvement in miliary tuberculosis in children.

Life cycle of *Schistosoma haematobium*

Schistosomula develop into male and female adult worms in portal and mesenteric veins

Schistosomula migrate via heart to portal vein

Worms copulate and migrate to vesical veins; eggs are deposited here in great numbers and are extruded through bladder mucosa

Miracidia enter snails and undergo cycle

Eggs hatch, releasing miracidia in water

Eggs passed in urine

Cercariae penetrate unbroken skin or mucous membranes by means of enzymatic secretions of cephalic glands

Cercariae emerge from snails

Schistosomiasis of the urinary bladder

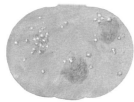

Schistosomal tubercles and nonspecific patches of edema and congestion

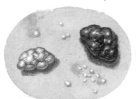

Schistosomal papillomas and tubercles

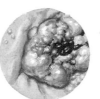

Nodular carcinoma in a schistosomal bladder

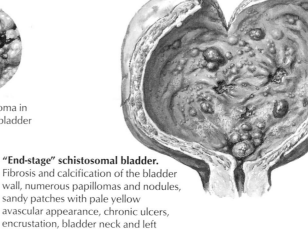

"End-stage" schistosomal bladder.
Fibrosis and calcification of the bladder wall, numerous papillomas and nodules, sandy patches with pale yellow avascular appearance, chronic ulcers, encrustation, bladder neck and left ureteral orifice obstructed

FIGURE 6-37 URINARY SCHISTOSOMIASIS

Blood fluke parasites have a worldwide distribution. Infection with *Schistosoma haematobium* leads to **urinary schistosomiasis**. In the acute phase of the infection, cercarial penetration produces local skin erythema and itching, which is usually followed in 4 to 6 weeks by a febrile and toxic illness with eosinophilia. Spontaneous clinical resolution occurs, although the adult worm continues to lay eggs. Chronic illness resulting from lesions caused by the eggs occurs months or years later. Initially, a granulomatous reaction occurs around schistosome eggs, producing pseudotubercles. Dystrophic calcification of the eggs and adjacent tissue is common. The progression of the lesions is toward a fibrotic stage, which is frequently associated with anatomical distortion of the genitourinary tract. The chronic infection predisposes to the development of carcinoma of the urinary bladder. The disease may progress to bilateral obstructive uropathy with renal dysfunction.

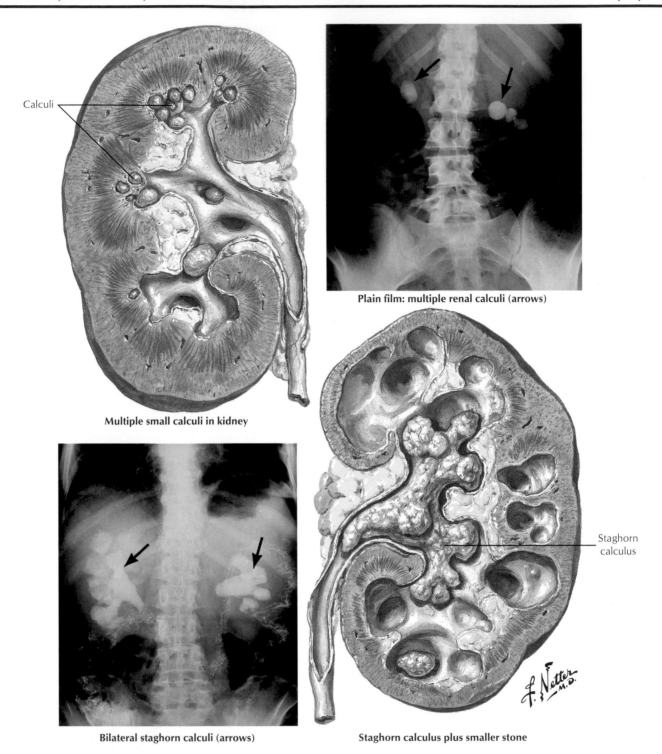

Calculi

Plain film: multiple renal calculi (arrows)

Multiple small calculi in kidney

Staghorn calculus

Bilateral staghorn calculi (arrows)

Staghorn calculus plus smaller stone

FIGURE 6-38 URINARY TRACT CALCULI

Clinically significant complications of **urinary calculi** involve up to 10% of the population. The calculi affect men more than women, with peak occurrence between 20 and 50 years of age. The etiology is poorly defined, although factors leading to highly concentrated urine predispose to stone formation. Most stones originate in the kidney and are composed of calcium oxalate and other calcium salts embedded in an organic matrix. Certain metabolic diseases (hyperoxaluria and disorders of amino acid metabolism) predispose to stone formation. Renal calculi may remain in the pelvis of the kidney (staghorn calculus) or pass down the ureter, which produces the severe pain of renal colic. Destruction of renal parenchyma may result from progressive growth of the calculus, obstruction, or infections. Occasionally, calculi form in the ureter or urinary bladder as a result of urinary stasis secondary to various congenital or acquired anomalies.

Solitary cysts of the kidney

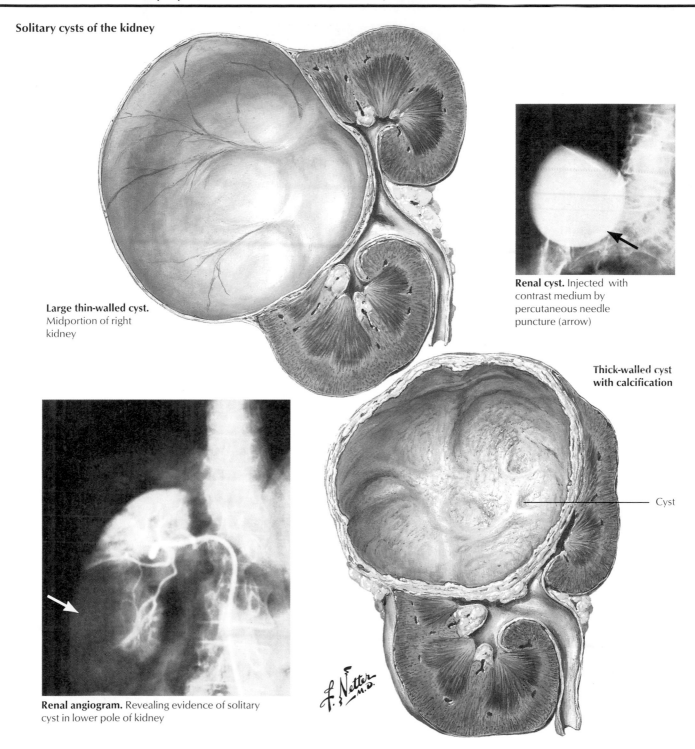

Large thin-walled cyst.
Midportion of right
kidney

Renal cyst. Injected with
contrast medium by
percutaneous needle
puncture (arrow)

**Thick-walled cyst
with calcification**

Cyst

Renal angiogram. Revealing evidence of solitary
cyst in lower pole of kidney

FIGURE 6-39 RENAL CYSTIC DISEASES: SIMPLE CYSTS

A general classification of **renal cystic diseases** is as follows: (1) autosomal dominant (adult) polycystic disease of the kidney; (2) autosomal recessive (childhood) polycystic disease of the kidney; (3) unilateral multicystic disease of the kidney (unilateral renal dysplasia); (4) simple cysts (single, multiple, and multilocular); and (5) cysts of miscellaneous origin, such as retention or inflammatory cysts, and cysts secondary to hematoma, *Echinococcus* infections, pyelonephritis, and other specific diseases. Simple cysts may be solitary or multiple, thin walled or thick walled, trabeculated or multilocular. The cystic fluid may be clear or hemorrhagic, and the wall may occasionally have foci of dystrophic calcification. Rarely, adenocarcinoma of the wall may occur. Simple cysts are usually located in the cortex and bulge through the renal capsule. Sometimes, the cysts may be more deeply located and produce obstruction to urine outflow. Cysts must be kept in mind in the differential diagnosis of mass lesions in the kidney.

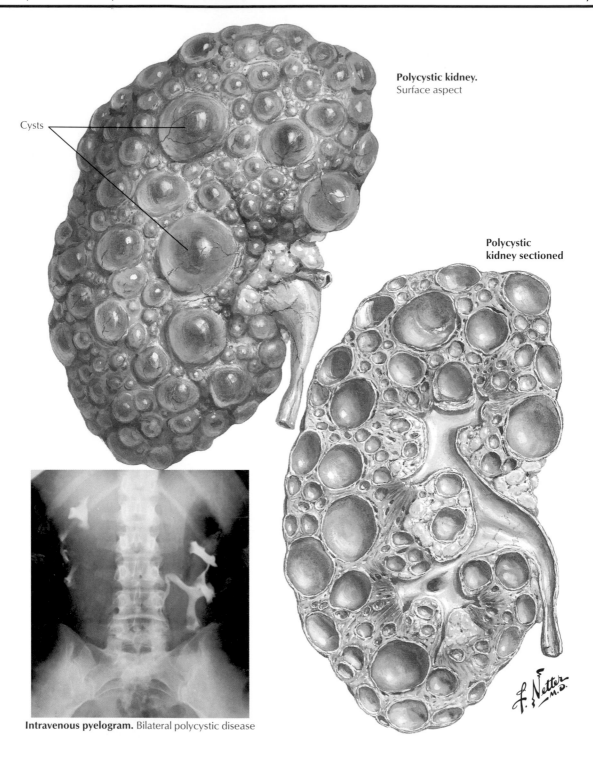

Cysts

Polycystic kidney.
Surface aspect

**Polycystic
kidney sectioned**

Intravenous pyelogram. Bilateral polycystic disease

FIGURE 6-40 RENAL CYSTIC DISEASES: ADULT POLYCYSTIC KIDNEY

Adult polycystic kidney disease has an autosomal dominant inheritance pattern, with individual cases resulting from a mutation of the *PKD1* gene on chromosome 16, the *PKD2* gene on chromosome 4, or a yet-to-be-localized *PKD3* gene. In contrast, infantile or childhood polycystic disease has an autosomal recessive inheritance pattern and represents a severe form of renal dysplasia. Adult polycystic kidney disease is relatively common, occurring in 1 of 400 to 1000 live births and accounting for approximately 10% of chronic renal failure in

adults. Kidney damage is a slowly developing but progressive process that eventually reaches clinical significance in all affected individuals surviving into the ninth decade of life. In the more advanced stages, destruction of renal tissue results in azotemia and physical discomfort from the sheer size of the large cystic masses. Hypertension occurs frequently, as do urinary tract infections. Associated conditions include intracranial berry aneurysms. The patients inevitably become dependent on hemodialysis and are candidates for kidney transplantation.

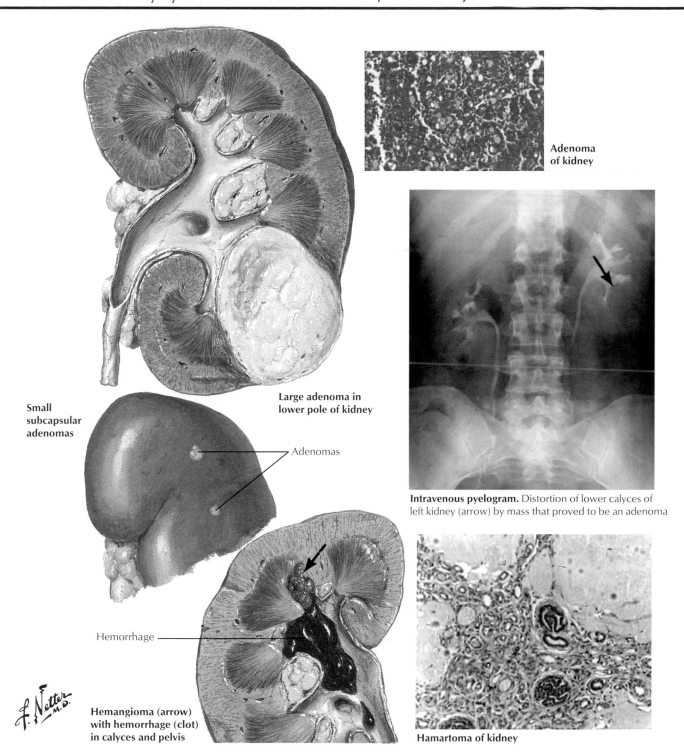

Adenoma
of kidney

Small
subcapsular
adenomas

Large adenoma in
lower pole of kidney

Adenomas

Intravenous pyelogram. Distortion of lower calyces of
left kidney (arrow) by mass that proved to be an adenoma

Hemorrhage

Hemangioma (arrow)
with hemorrhage (clot)
in calyces and pelvis

Hamartoma of kidney

FIGURE 6-41 BENIGN RENAL TUMORS

Benign tumors of the kidney may mimic malignant tumors and
should be considered in the differential diagnosis of a renal cyst.
Renal adenomas are typically small cortical nodules, which often
grow within small cysts. They are usually papillomatous structures but may have a tubular or alveolar growth pattern. Occasionally, a large, single adenoma is found. The cells of adenomas
are usually cuboidal and show well-differentiated cytology and

growth pattern. The adenoma should be considered premalignant
and prone to give rise to clones of malignant cells. Tumors larger
than 3 cm in diameter are likely to metastasize. Connective tissue
tumors that arise in the kidney include fibroma, lipoma, myoma,
hemangioma, and angiomyolipoma (hamartoma), the latter
occurring as part of the tuberous sclerosis complex.

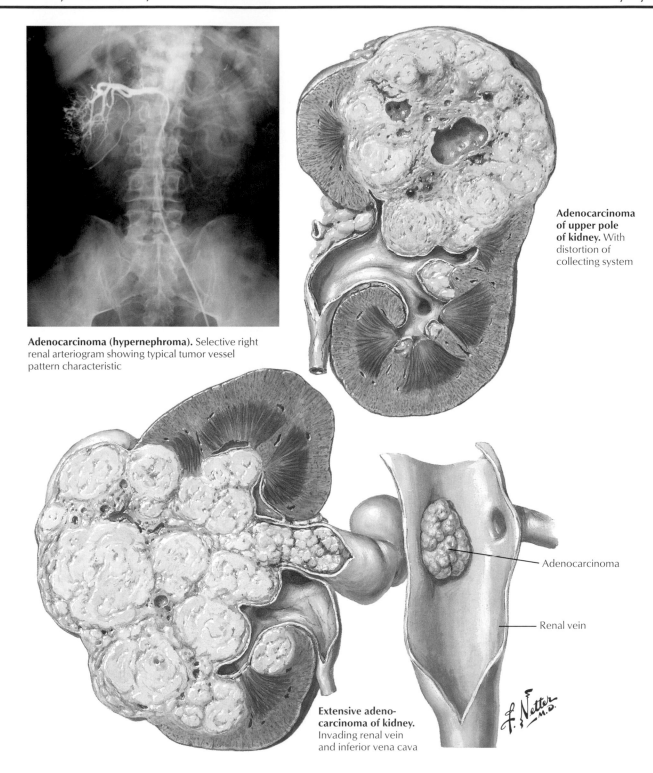

Adenocarcinoma (hypernephroma). Selective right renal arteriogram showing typical tumor vessel pattern characteristic

Adenocarcinoma of upper pole of kidney. With distortion of collecting system

Adenocarcinoma

Renal vein

Extensive adenocarcinoma of kidney. Invading renal vein and inferior vena cava

FIGURE 6-42 MALIGNANT TUMORS OF THE KIDNEY

Malignant tumors of the kidney may be primary tumors originating in the parenchyma, pelvis, or capsule or they may be metastatic, usually with bilateral involvement. Fibrosarcoma, myosarcoma, liposarcoma, and angioendothelioma are rare primary tumors. **Renal adenocarcinoma**, which encompasses all malignant epithelial renal tumors, accounts for approximately three fourths of all renal malignancies, usually occurs in middle age, and affects males twice as often as females. Typically, the unilateral and solitary tumor, which is usually encapsulated, firm, and solid, arises from either pole or the central region of the kidney. Renal vein invasion is common. Growth of the primary lesion may lead to a mass in the flank, microscopic or gross hematuria, and renal colic.

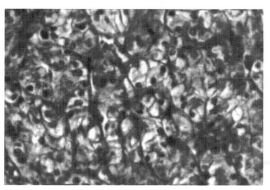

Clear cell adenocarcinoma of kidney (H and E). This type occasionally referred to as *hypernephroma*

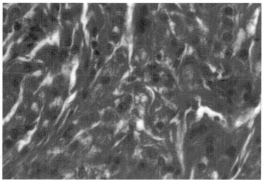

Adenocarcinoma of kidney. Composed of granular cells resembling cells of distal tubule (H and E)

Site of extension and metastasis of renal adenocarcinoma

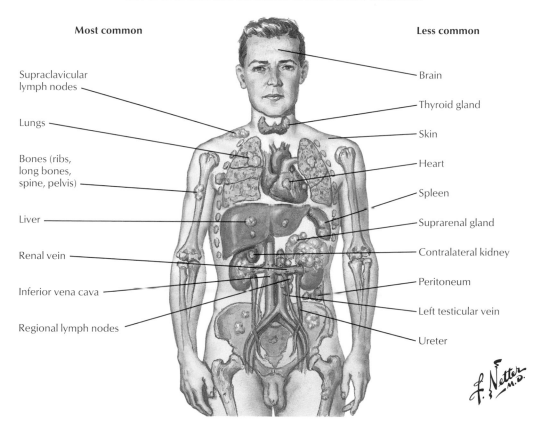

FIGURE 6-42 MALIGNANT TUMORS OF THE KIDNEY (CONTINUED)

Subtypes of renal cell adenocarcinoma (in order of frequency) are clear cell carcinoma (70 to 80%), papillary carcinoma (10 to 15%), chromophobe renal carcinoma (5%), and collecting duct carcinoma (1%). Histologically, adenocarcinoma shows a variety of patterns, including vacuolated clear cells, granular cells, and anaplastic cells. The extent of local spread and the presence of metastases are more important than the histological pattern. Renal cell carcinoma often metastasizes via the blood, but lymphatic spread also occurs.

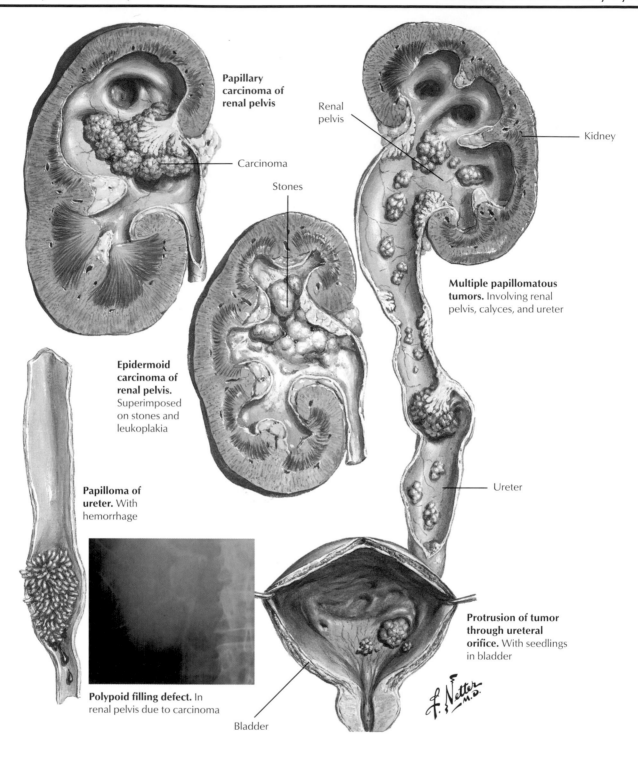

Papillary carcinoma of renal pelvis

Carcinoma

Renal pelvis

Kidney

Stones

Multiple papillomatous tumors. Involving renal pelvis, calyces, and ureter

Epidermoid carcinoma of renal pelvis. Superimposed on stones and leukoplakia

Papilloma of ureter. With hemorrhage

Ureter

Protrusion of tumor through ureteral orifice. With seedlings in bladder

Polypoid filling defect. In renal pelvis due to carcinoma

Bladder

FIGURE 6-43 TUMORS OF THE PELVIS AND THE URETER

Tumors of the renal collecting system, which usually arise from the epithelium as urothelial cell (transitional cell) papillomas or urothelial cell carcinomas, comprise approximately 10% of renal tumors. Squamous cell carcinoma, adenocarcinoma, and metastases are less common. **Urothelial cell papilloma** is cytologically bland but must be considered premalignant, whereas urothelial cell carcinomas exhibit overt cytologic atypia. Urothelial cell tumors of the renal pelvis, ureter, and bladder occur predominately in older men. They may be single or multiple and are usually papillomatous and unilateral. **Squamous cell (epidermoid) carcinoma** is frequently associated with renal calculi and infection. The lesions, which are usually flat and firm and often ulcerated, are likely to invade the renal parenchyma and metastasize early. These tumors usually present with microscopic or gross hematuria.

Bladder tumor prognosis based on degree of infiltration (Jewett classification)

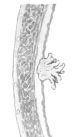 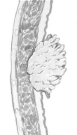 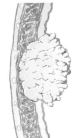 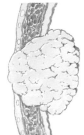

Stage A: growth involving only mucosa and tunica propria

Stage B-1: less than 1/2 of muscle thickness involved

Stage B-2: more than 1/2 of muscle thickness involved

Stage C: complete penetration of bladder wall

Prognosis good　　　　**Prognosis poor**

Bladder tumors (cystoscopic views)

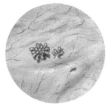 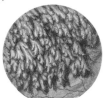

Small villous papillomas

Papilloma at ureteral orifice

Very large villous tumor

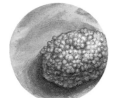 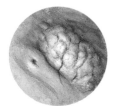 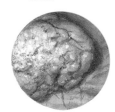

Large infiltrating papilloma with short adherent fronds

Sessile infiltrating carcinoma

Large malignant tumor with necrosis

Bladder tumors (histology)

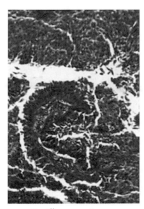 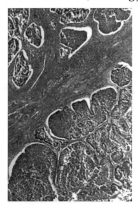 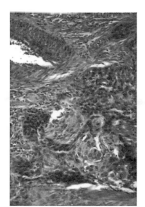

Papillary carcinoma

Infiltrating carcinoma

Squamous cell carcinoma

FIGURE 6-44 TUMORS OF THE BLADDER

Urinary bladder tumors typically arise from the mucosa and are composed of urothelial cells. The full spectrum of lesions includes papillomas, papillary lesions of low malignant potential, flat urothelial carcinoma, and papillary carcinomas. Other forms of bladder cancer include undifferentiated carcinomas, squamous (epidermoid) carcinomas (in areas of leukoplakia), adenocarcinoma (which may be mucin producing), and the rare epithelial mesenchymal tumors. The lesions occur principally in older adults, mostly males, and in 25% of cases are multiple. Exposure to and ingestion of environmental toxins are important in the pathogenesis of these lesions. The prognosis for patients with bladder tumors is strongly influenced by the degree of tumor infiltration of the bladder wall, or tumor stage (Jewett classification), but histologic grading of the degree of differentiation and cytologic atypia also provides useful information (Broder classification).

Wilms tumor

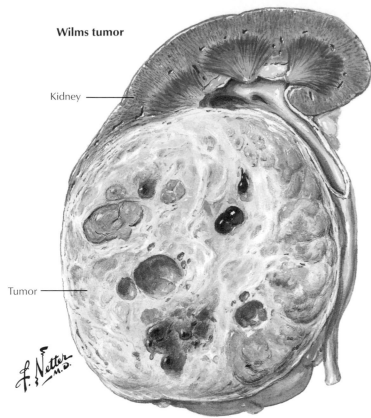

Kidney

Tumor

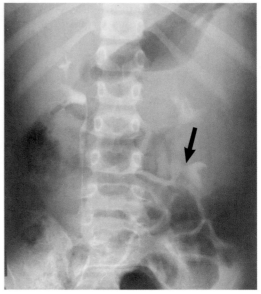

Intravenous pyelogram. Distortion of collecting system of left kidney by Wilms tumor in an infant (arrow)

Wilms tumor. With pseudocapsule and characteristic variegated structure

Clinical features of Wilms tumor

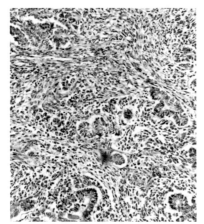

Stroma of sarcomalike spindle cells. With islands of malignant columnar cells in irregular tubular arrangements typical of Wilms tumor

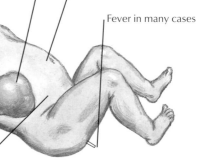

Occurs in infants and young children

Mass in loin or abdomen often first manifestation (differentiate from solitary cyst or multicystic kidney, large hydronephrosis, neuroblastoma)

Pressure phenomena may occur; gastrointestinal, venous (edema), respiratory

Fever in many cases

Metastasizes chiefly to local nodes, lungs, and liver; rarely to bone, in contrast to neuroblastoma, where bone is principal site

Loss of weight, anemia, cachexia may appear late; hematuria often absent; hypertension may appear

FIGURE 6-45 NEPHROBLASTOMA

The differential diagnosis of an upper abdominal mass in an infant or child includes the more common benign conditions such as ureteropelvic junction obstruction, with or without associated pyelonephritis, multicystic kidney disease, and malignant tumors, particularly neuroblastoma and nephroblastoma (Wilms tumor, WT). **Nephroblastoma** is a usually unilateral, intrinsic renal neoplasm containing both epithelial and connec-

tive tissue elements with various degrees of cellular differentiation. It is thought to arise from the metanephrogenic blastoma. Definitive differential diagnosis and rapid treatment are important because the tumor has a propensity for metastasis, primarily to lungs, the liver, the lymph nodes, and, less frequently, the bones. The prognosis has improved with the combined use of chemotherapy, radiation therapy, and surgery.

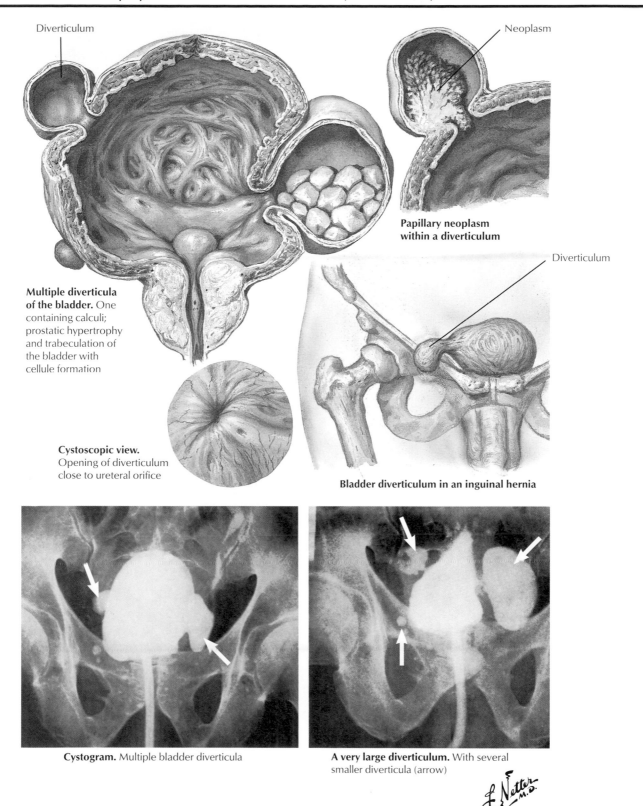

Multiple diverticula of the bladder. One containing calculi; prostatic hypertrophy and trabeculation of the bladder with cellule formation

Papillary neoplasm within a diverticulum

Cystoscopic view. Opening of diverticulum close to ureteral orifice

Bladder diverticulum in an inguinal hernia

Cystogram. Multiple bladder diverticula

A very large diverticulum. With several smaller diverticula (arrow)

FIGURE 6-46 DIVERTICULA OF THE BLADDER

Diverticula of the bladder begin as small outpouchings or evaginations of the bladder wall between hypertrophied muscle bundles in the setting of bladder outlet obstruction. As obstruction progresses, weakening of the detrusor muscle, the external muscle layer of the bladder, gradually allows the formation of one or more true diverticula. The opening of the diverticulum is usually narrow, the lumen is covered with urothelium, and the wall is constructed primarily of connective tissue with focal strands of muscle fibers. The incidence of bladder diverticula is much greater in men and is usually a consequence of bladder outlet obstruction resulting from prostatic enlargement. Congenital diverticula are likely secondary to obstruction.

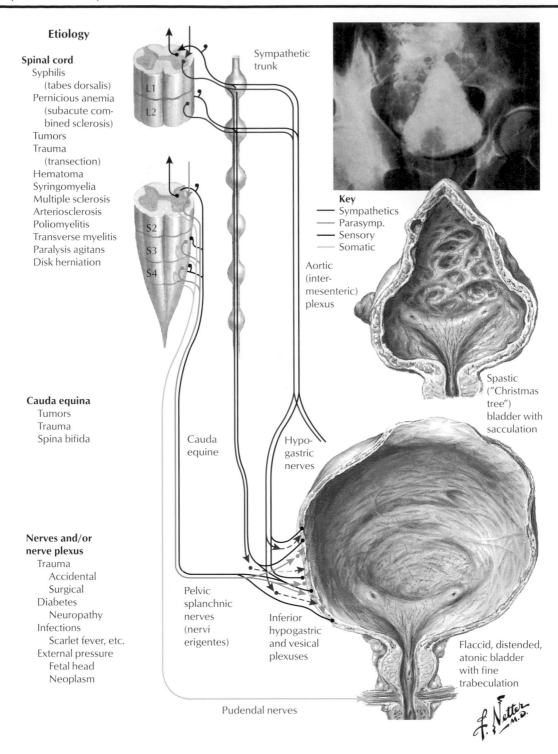

Etiology

Spinal cord
Syphilis
(tabes dorsalis)
Pernicious anemia
(subacute com-
bined sclerosis)
Tumors
Trauma
(transection)
Hematoma
Syringomyelia
Multiple sclerosis
Arteriosclerosis
Poliomyelitis
Transverse myelitis
Paralysis agitans
Disk herniation

Cauda equina
Tumors
Trauma
Spina bifida

Nerves and/or nerve plexus
Trauma
Accidental
Surgical
Diabetes
Neuropathy
Infections
Scarlet fever, etc.
External pressure
Fetal head
Neoplasm

L1
L2

S2
S3
S4

Sympathetic trunk

Key
Sympathetics
Parasymp.
Sensory
Somatic

Aortic (inter-mesenteric) plexus

Cauda equine

Hypo-gastric nerves

Pelvic splanchnic nerves (nervi erigentes)

Inferior hypogastric and vesical plexuses

Pudendal nerves

Spastic ("Christmas tree") bladder with sacculation

Flaccid, distended, atonic bladder with fine trabeculation

FIGURE 6-47 NEUROGENIC BLADDER

Neurologic impairment of bladder function may result from a variety of conditions. The site of the injury or disease determines the nature of the abnormality because the innervation of different parts of the bladder arises from different portions of the nervous system. Treatment of neurogenic bladder is aimed at prevention of eventual damage to the upper urinary tract from infection, urolithiasis, and obstruction. When effective control is absent, chronic neurogenic bladder may cause chronic urinary infection with secondary stone formation, leading to deterioration of kidney function and eventual uremia. Prevention includes use of indwelling urinary catheters, good hydration to maintain high urine volume, bladder irrigation to dissolve calcium salts, and treatment with antibiotics.

CHAPTER 7

DISEASES OF THE MALE REPRODUCTIVE SYSTEM

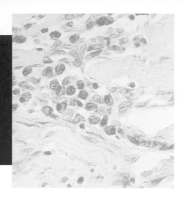

The male reproductive system develops in close relation with the urinary tract, and the two are usually thought of as the **urogenital system**. After formation of the metanephric duct and the induction of nephrons, a distal part of the meso-nephric (**Wolffian**) duct becomes integrated into the lateral walls of the urogenital sinus with separation into ureters and male ejaculatory channels. The testes develop from the gonadal ridge, and their seminiferous tubules combine with the secretory channels formed by the Wolffian duct. The prostate develops from epithelial invaginations in the distal urethra. Therefore, congenital diseases of the genital system may also be associated with disorders of the urinary tract. A summary of the many infectious and inflammatory diseases of the male reproductive system is shown in Table 7-1.

DISEASES OF THE PENIS AND THE URETHRA

A variety of disorders may result in urinary or sexual dysfunction: **structural and functional anomalies**, including malformations; urethral stenosis and phimosis; fibromatosis (**Peyronie disease**); and priapism. In addition, the penis is a frequent site of **inflammatory diseases**, including sexually transmitted diseases (STDs) and some benign and malignant tumors. STDs and related infections, such as papilloma virus and candidiasis, have recently received considerable attention because of their rising incidence, association with HIV infection, and copathogenetic effects in the development of certain cancers. **Squamous cell carcinoma** (SCC) of the penis represents only 0.5% of all cancers in men in the United States but is significantly more frequent in some parts of Africa and Asia. Most penile SCCs are confined to the penis and can be cured by amputation. Delayed diagnosis or the presence of occult metastases at initial presentation, however, worsens the prognosis.

DISEASES OF THE PROSTATE GLAND AND THE SEMINAL TRACTS

Prostatitis occurs fairly frequently in men older than 50 years and is usually nonbacterial. In all ages, bacterial prostatitis usually follows urinary tract infection, but hematogenous forms may occur. Among the more common causative organisms are *Escherichia coli*, *Chlamydia* species, *Mycoplasma*, and *Trichomonas vaginalis*.

Benign prostatic hyperplasia (BPH) is common in older men, affecting more than 50% at the age of 60 years and more than 75% at the age of 80 years. The etiology of BPH is unknown, but recent studies suggest a relation with disturbed 5-dihydrotestosterone synthesis. Clinical features result from compression of the prostatic urethra with resultant obstruction of urine outflow, muscular hypertrophy of the bladder, and retrograde back pressure, ultimately causing hydroureter and hydronephrosis.

Cancer of the prostate (adenocarcinoma, ACP) is among the most frequent malignant tumors in men, causing approximately 30,000 deaths per year in the United States. One of 10 American men has clinically apparent prostate cancer during his life. The etiology of ACP is unknown. Hormonal imbalances (estrone to testosterone ratio) and exogenous carcinogens may play important roles in the pathogenesis. ACP constitutes 98% of prostatic neoplasias. Because the clinical features of ACP are similar to those of BPH, with which it often coexists, only 10% of patients with ACP present at an early stage. Demonstration of prostate-specific antigen (PSA) in serum and/or biopsy specimens may be helpful in the primary diagnosis and follow-up. The treatment and prognosis of ACP are stage dependent.

MALE INFERTILITY

Three mechanisms account for most reproductive problems in males. The most common is testicular damage from radiation, alcohol, varicocele, cryptorchism, or orchitis. Genetic disorders with gonadal dysgenesis include **Klinefelter syndrome** and **Turner syndrome**. Blockage of excretory ducts may result from infections or occlusion.

TESTICULAR DISORDERS

Testicular tumors are divided into 2 major classes: germ cell tumors and gonadal stromal tumors (sex cord tumors). More than 90% of testicular tumors are germ cell tumors, most frequently seminoma, embryonal carcinoma, and teratoma. Seminoma accounts for approximately one half of all germ cell tumors. The so-called classic type, occurring at the ages of 25–55 years, is radiosensitive and, after treatment of solitary tumors, is associated with 5-year survival greater than 90%. Embryonal carcinoma, which occurs at younger ages (20–35 years), is the second most common germ cell tumor. It is histologically more pleomorphic and may include human chorionic gonadotropin- (β-HCG) or α-fetoprotein–producing cells (transition to choriocarcinoma or teratoma). These tumors tend to respond well to chemotherapy; in localized cases, 5-year survival may exceed 95%. Sex cord tumors include **Sertoli cell tumor** and **Leydig cell tumor**.

TABLE 7-1 INFECTIOUS AND INFLAMMATORY DISEASES OF THE MALE REPRODUCTIVE SYSTEM

Diseases of the Glans Penis and Prepuce (Balanitis, Balanoposthitis)

Simple balanitis (infants, older men)	Congenital or acquired phimosis, secondary bacterial infection
Balanoposthitis (adults)	Adhesions, phimosis secondary to obstruction (edema, cancer, elephantiasis), trauma, chemical irritation, sexually transmitted infections
Erosive balanitis	Phimosis, anaerobic organisms (spirochetes, vibrios)
Gangrenous balanitis	Phimosis, anaerobic organisms (spirochetes, vibrios)
Vesicular or ulcerative balanitis	Herpes progenitalis due to herpes simplex virus (HSV) type 2, histoplasmosis, keratosis blenorrhagia, pemphigus, scabies
Atrophic (leukoplakic) balanoposthitis	Dysplasia of epithelium
Venereal warts (Condylomata accuminata)	Human papilloma viruses (HPV), especially types 6, 11, 42, and 44

Diseases of the Uretha

Acute and subacute urethritis	*Neisseria gonorrhoeae* (gonorrheal urethritis), *Trichomonas vaginalis*, *Chlamydia trachonatis* serotypes D-K, other infections

Diseases of the Penis, Scrotum, and Inginual Lymph Nodes

Chancre of glans, penile body, scrotum	Syphillis due to *Treponema pallidum*
Ulcerative lesions with lymphadenopathy	Chancroid (*Haemophilis ducreyi*), lymphogranuloma venereum (*Chlamydia trachomatis* serotypes L1, L2, L3), Granuloma inguinale (*Calymmatobacterium granulomatis*)
Elephantiasis	*Wuchereria bancrofti* (filaria), nonfilarial elephantitis (lymphedema)

Diseases of the Prostate

Acute prostatitis	*Neisseria gonorrhoeae*, staphylococci (instrumentation), nonspecific
Prostatic abscesses	Complication of urethritis and prostatitis, systemic infections
Chronic prostatitis	Insidious onset or extension of actue prostatitis, various pyogenic bacteria, tuberculosis (*Mycobacterium tuberculosis*)

Diseases of the Scrotum

Tinea cruris (jock itch)	Superficial fungal infection (Epidermophyton and Trichophyton groups)
Erythrasma	*Nocardia minutissima*
Dermatitis venenata and other contact dermatoses	Chemical irritants, drug eruption (*Dermatitis medicamentosa*)
Eczema (chronic)	Allergic reactions, atopic dermatitis
Intertrigo	Erythema due to chemical irritation with secondary infection with cocci and fungi
Scabies	Mite infestation (*Sarcoptes scabiei*)
Pediculosis pubis (phthiriasis)	Crab louse infestation (*Phthirius pubis*)
Furuncle (abscess) of the scrotum	Pyogenic bacteria, esp. *Staphylococcus aureus*
Erysipelas of the scrotum	Pyogenic bacteria, esp. *Streptococcus pyogenes*
Gangrene of the scrotum	Mechanical, chemical or thermal injuries with secondary infection, idiopathic gangrene (Fournier's gangrene)

Diseases of the Testis

Orchitis, epididymitis, epididymoorchitis	Multiple organisms, spread from local or systemic infections
Acute pyogenic orchitis, abscess of the testis	Pyrogenic bacteria
Mumps orchitis	Mumps virus
Epididymitis	Specific (gonorrheal, syphilitic, etc.), nonspecific, traumatic
Granulomatous orchitis	Syphlitic orchitis, syphilitic gumma, tuberculosis (*M. tuberculosis*)

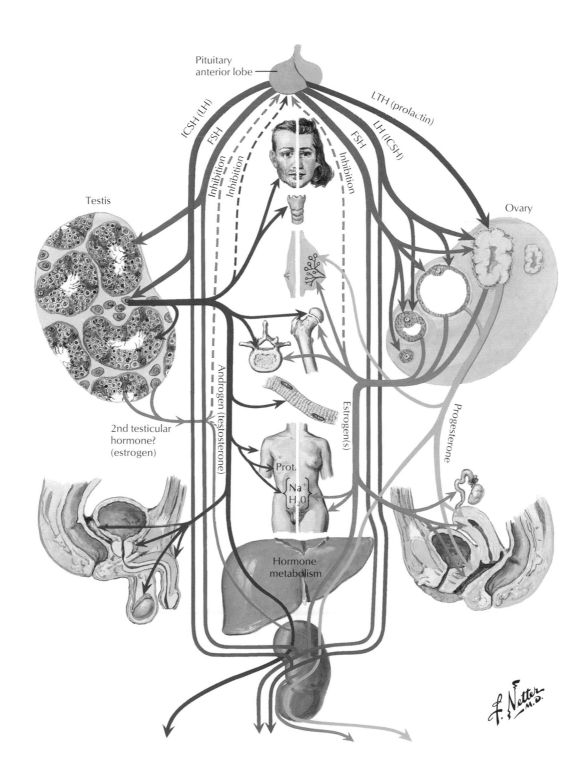

FIGURE 7-1   FUNCTIONAL GONADAL RELATIONS

The 3 gonadotrophic hormones of the pituitary adenohypophysis are (1) follicle-stimulating hormone (FSH); (2) luteinizing hormone (LH) of the female, known as interstitial cell–stimulating hormone (ICSH) in the male; and (3) luteotropin (prolactin, LTH). These pituitary hormones determine the development of the male and female gonads. The germinal epithelia of the testes and ovaries are responsible for the production of sperm and ova,

respectively. Various stromal cells of the gonads are responsible for the production of the androgen and estrogen hormones, which act on the organs of the reproductive tract, the secondary sex organs, and other parts of the body. There is a feedback loop for interdependent regulation of the production of the gonadal and pituitary hormones.

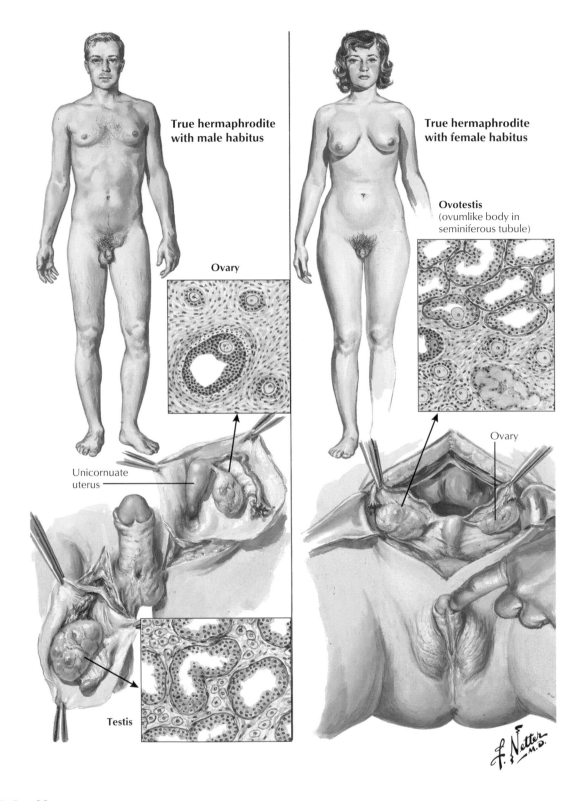

True hermaphrodite with male habitus

Ovary

Unicornuate uterus

Testis

True hermaphrodite with female habitus

Ovotestis
(ovumlike body in seminiferous tubule)

Ovary

FIGURE 7-2   HERMAPHRODITISM

True hermaphroditism, defined as the presence of both testicular and ovarian tissue in the same patient, is rare. The chromosomal karyotype usually is euploid, with either a 46, XX or a 46, XY pattern, but may be aneuploid (45X/XY). Complex alterations in sex chromosomal gene expression lead to abnormal development of the gonads, including the formation of 1 or 2 ovotestes, an ovary on one side and a testis on the other, or a combination of these arrangements. The internal and external genitalia and secondary sexual characteristics correlate with the composition of the gonadal structures. Male pseudohermaphrodites have gonads with the histologic features of testes and varying degrees of feminine characteristics. Female pseudohermaphrodites have ovaries, but their external genitalia appear male. Male and female **pseudohermaphroditism** both generally result from a spectrum of neoplastic and nonneoplastic endocrine disorders.

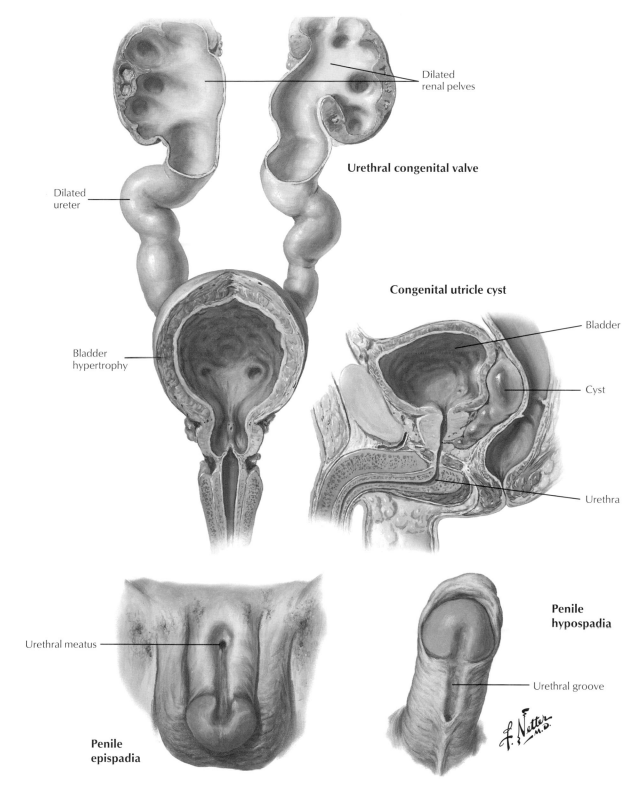

Dilated renal pelves

Urethral congenital valve

Dilated ureter

Congenital utricle cyst

Bladder hypertrophy

Bladder

Cyst

Urethra

Urethral meatus

Penile hypospadia

Urethral groove

Penile epispadia

FIGURE 7-3   CONGENITAL ANOMALIES: CONGENITAL VALVES, EPISPADIA, AND HYPOSPADIA

Certain congenital anomalies of the urinary bladder and urethra are clinically important. **Congenital valves** of the posterior urethra are thin folds of mucosa that develop in the prostatic urethra and extend from the verumontanum to the sides of the urethra. Obstruction to urine flow leads to bladder hypertrophy and dilatation, bilateral hydronephrosis, and, ultimately, fatal renal failure. **Epispadia** is a rare anomaly of the male urethra that involves the dorsum of the penis and can range from minimal

deformity (glanular epispadia) to moderate deformity (penile epispadia) to complete epispadia. **Hypospadia**, which are more common, develop on the ventral aspect of the penis because of the failure of the genital folds to close fully and can be a component of pseudohermaphroditism. Epispadia and hypospadia are often associated with developmental anomalies of the urinary tract (extrophy of the urinary bladder, undescended testicles), infections, and sterility.

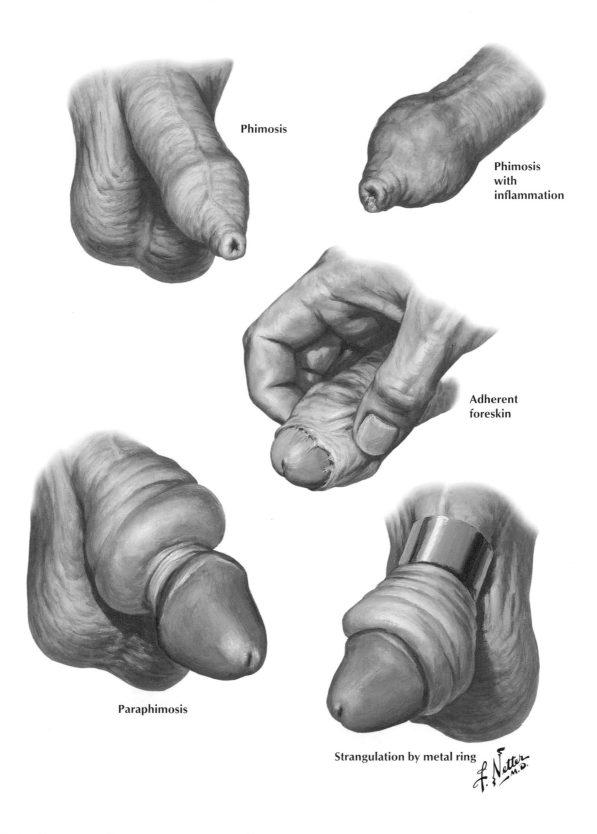

Phimosis

Phimosis with inflammation

Adherent foreskin

Paraphimosis

Strangulation by metal ring

FIGURE 7-4   PHIMOSIS, PARAPHIMOSIS, AND STRANGULATION

Phimosis is the presence of a redundant prepuce that cannot be retracted over the glans penis. If the condition is not relieved, fibrous adhesions may develop between the prepuce and the glans. Infection can significantly complicate the condition by producing an inflammatory exudate and edema. **Paraphimosis** is a retained retraction of a tight foreskin behind the coronary sulcus. Compression of the constricted veins and lymphatics leads to marked edematous swelling of the distal prepuce and glans. **Strangulation** may result from constriction of the penis by external devices, such as metal rings.

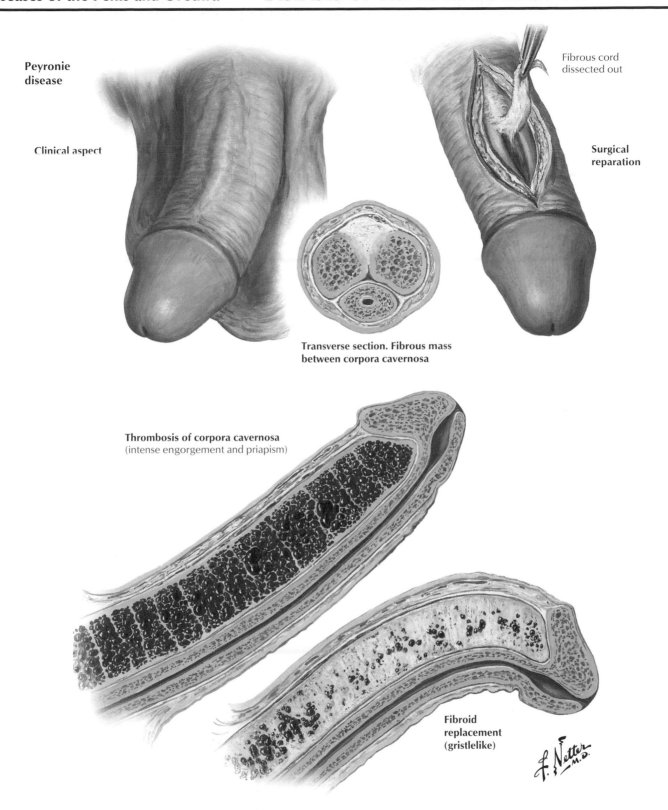

Peyronie disease

Clinical aspect

Fibrous cord dissected out

Surgical reparation

Transverse section. Fibrous mass between corpora cavernosa

Thrombosis of corpora cavernosa (intense engorgement and priapism)

Fibroid replacement (gristlelike)

FIGURE 7-5   PEYRONIE DISEASE, PRIAPISM, AND THROMBOSIS

Peyronie disease (fibrous cavernitis, or plastic induration of the penis), a chronic, self-limiting disease of middle or older age, can be mistaken for malignancy. The position of the erect penis is distorted, and penile erection is painful because of the deposition of inelastic fibrous tissue (plaques) in the tunicae or intracavernous septum of the corpora cavernosa of the penis. **Priapism**, a painful and persistent erection of sudden onset, may be idiopathic or may occur in association with a systemic disorder, such as leukemia, gout, or sickle cell anemia, or with neoplastic or inflammatory lesions of the nervous system. *True priapism* is erection of the corpora cavernosa without erection of the glans penis or corpora spongiosum. A major complication of persistent erection is **thrombosis** of the corpora cavernosa. The organization of the thrombus into fibrous tissue leads to permanent impairment of penile erection.

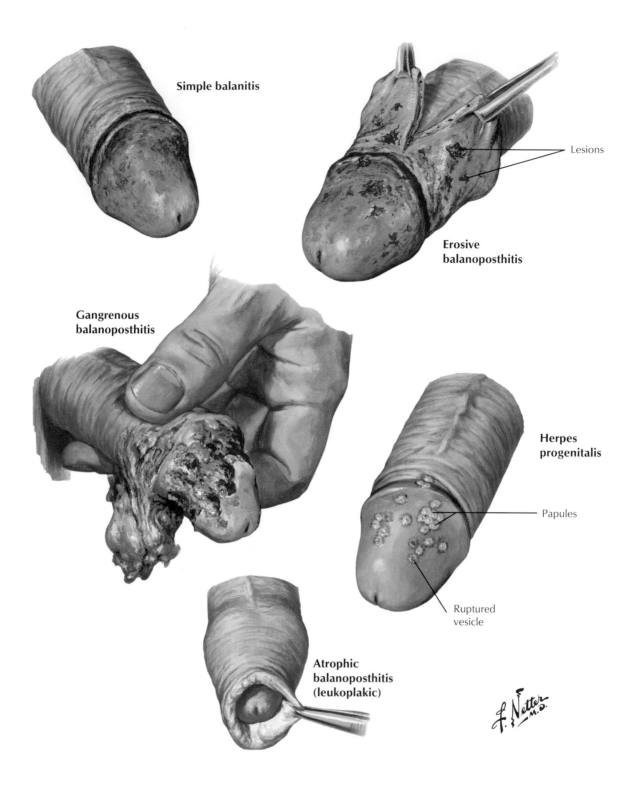

Simple balanitis

Lesions

Erosive balanoposthitis

Gangrenous balanoposthitis

Herpes progenitalis

Papules

Ruptured vesicle

Atrophic balanoposthitis (leukoplakic)

FIGURE 7-6 BALANITIS

Balanitis is inflammation of the glans penis. Balanoposthitis is a similar process involving the glans and the prepuce, usually associated with congenital or acquired phimosis, which predispose to growth of anaerobic microorganisms. **Simple balanitis** is a superficial infection presenting as a swollen, hyperemic, tender, and itchy lesion, whereas **erosive balanoposthitis** is characterized by the formation of painful necrotic erosive lesions. **Gangrenous**

balanoposthitis is a rapidly progressive form of erosive balanoposthitis. In **herpes progenitalis**, which is caused by herpesvirus type 2, red papules on the glans penis develop into vesicles that rupture, leaving superficial ulcers. The lesions heal but tend to recur. Recurring episodes of any form of balanitis may lead to formation of thickened white epithelium, so-called atrophic (leukoplakic) balanoposthitis.

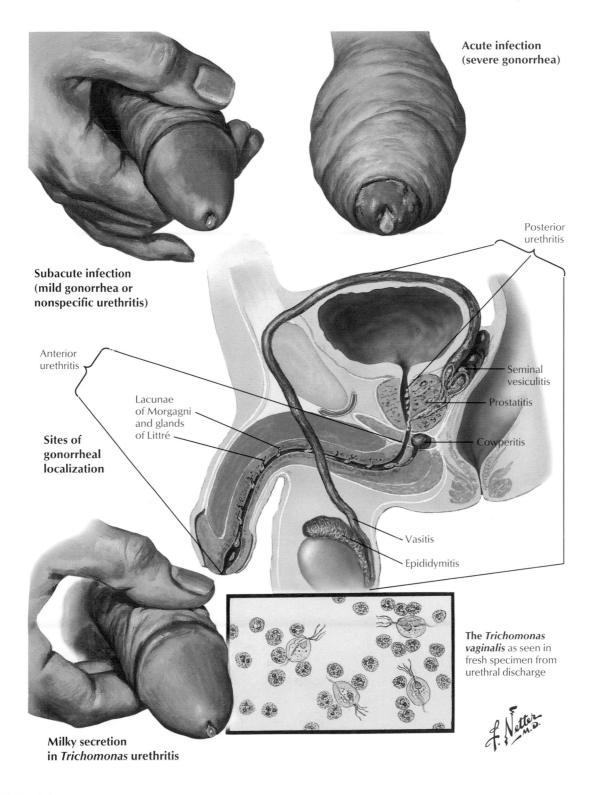

Acute infection
(severe gonorrhea)

Subacute infection
(mild gonorrhea or
nonspecific urethritis)

Posterior
urethritis

Anterior
urethritis

Sites of
gonorrheal
localization

Lacunae
of Morgagni
and glands
of Littré

Seminal
vesiculitis

Prostatitis

Cowperitis

Vasitis

Epididymitis

The *Trichomonas
vaginalis* as seen in
fresh specimen from
urethral discharge

Milky secretion
in *Trichomonas* urethritis

FIGURE 7-7   URETHRITIS

Urethritis results from infections with *Neisseria gonorrhea,
Trichomonas vaginalis, Chlamydia trachomatis,* or, less commonly, other microbes. In gonorrheal urethritis, a superficial infection of the urethral mucosa is followed by extension into the crypts and glands of the penile urethra, leading to involvement of the entire urethra, with an inflammatory exudate and purulent discharge in response to toxins released by the organisms. Complications include infections of the corpus spongiosum and posterior urethra, resulting respectively in painful erections and frequent, painful urination. Infection can extend from the prostate and posterior urethra down the spermatic cord to involve the epididymis. A rare complication is bacterial endocarditis due to gonococcal sepsis. Other forms of urethritis are usually more contained infections. Nonspecific urethritis can occur in isolation or with acute conjunctivitis and arthritis as Reiter syndrome.

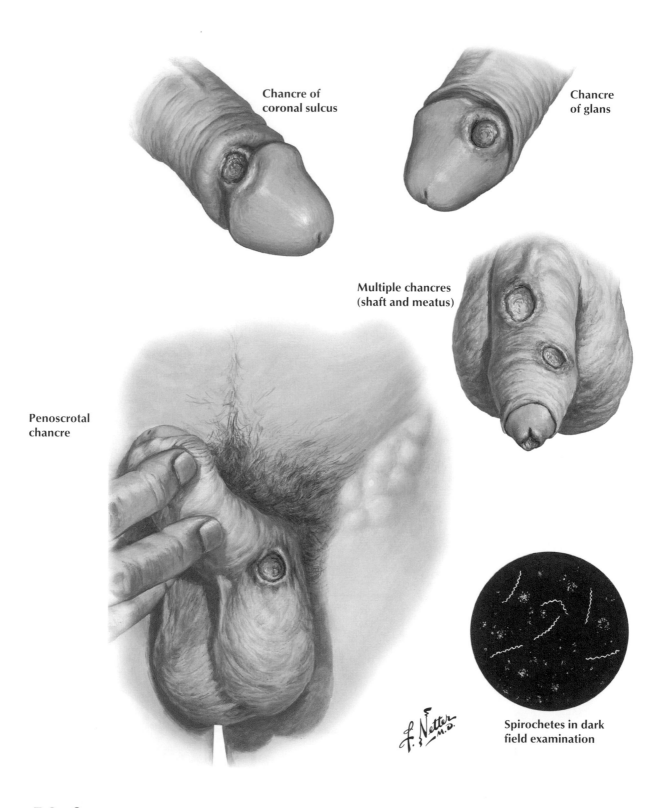

Chancre of coronal sulcus

Chancre of glans

Multiple chancres (shaft and meatus)

Penoscrotal chancre

Spirochetes in dark field examination

FIGURE 7-8   SYPHILIS

The initial stage of **syphilis** is characterized by the development of a painless chancre, the hallmark primary lesion. The chancre, which usually develops slowly as an eroded papule, often accompanied by enlargement of the inguinal lymph nodes, heals gradually over several weeks. Definitive diagnosis is made by detection of the *Treponema pallidum* organism by darkfield examination of fluid from the primary lesion or a lymph node because the serologic test results for syphilis are often negative during the initial phase of infection. In untreated cases, secondary syphilis quickly follows, with systemic dissemination of organisms and skin rash. After a latent period, tertiary syphilis develops, involving the cardiovascular system, the nervous system, or both.

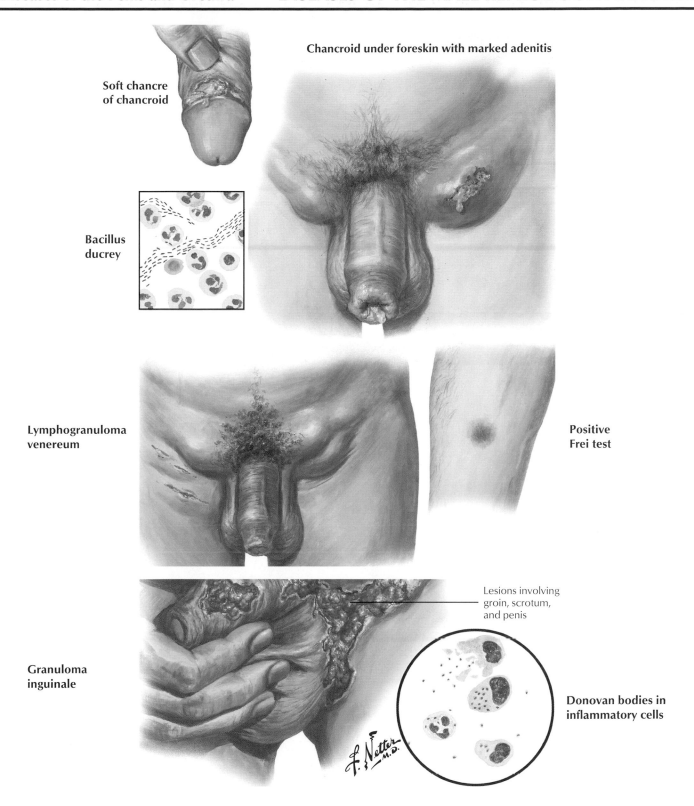

Soft chancre of chancroid

Chancroid under foreskin with marked adenitis

Bacillus ducrey

Lymphogranuloma venereum

Positive Frei test

Lesions involving groin, scrotum, and penis

Granuloma inguinale

Donovan bodies in inflammatory cells

FIGURE 7-9   CHANCROID, LYMPHOGRANULOMA VENEREUM, AND GRANULOMA INGUINALE

Chancroid (soft chancre) usually develops on the penis as a result of venereal infection with *Haemophilus ducreyi*. The infection spreads to the inguinal lymph nodes, producing secondary infection, extensive necrosis, pain, and tenderness. **Lymphogranuloma venereum** is caused by *Chlamydia trachomatis* serotypes L1, L2, and L3, usually transferred during sexual intercourse. The small, inconspicuous vesicle or papule that typically develops on the glans penis is followed by inguinal lymphadenitis and perilymphadenitis, which often progress to a chronic, persistent infection, with suppuration of the inguinal lymph nodes, fistulae, and multiple skin abscesses. Syphilis, chancroid, and lymphogranuloma venereum can coexist. **Granuloma inguinale** is a chronic disease of the genitalia characterized by ulcer formation. Prevalent in the tropics, this disease is not necessarily of venereal origin. The lesion, caused by *Calymmatobacterium granulomatis*, is recognizable as Donovan bodies in inflammatory cells.

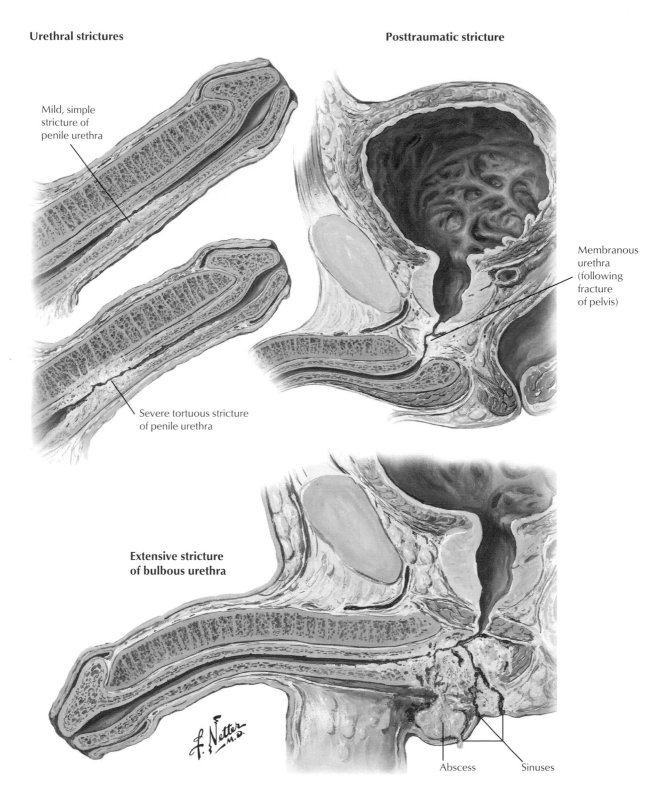

Urethral strictures

Mild, simple stricture of penile urethra

Severe tortuous stricture of penile urethra

Extensive stricture of bulbous urethra

Posttraumatic stricture

Membranous urethra (following fracture of pelvis)

Abscess   Sinuses

f. Netter M.D.

FIGURE 7-10 STRICTURES

Strictures may involve any portion of the urethra, including the meatus and the penile, bulbous, membranous, and prostatic urethra. Narrowing in the urethral lumen may be long or short, single or multiple, and slight or severe. Strictures may develop after urethritis as a result of venereal and other infections or secondary to indwelling urinary catheters. Posttraumatic strictures develop after severe blows, straddle injuries, and various punctures and tears related to instrumentation. Urethral strictures may be accompanied by infection elsewhere in the genitourinary tract, including prostatitis, epididymitis, cystitis, and pyelonephritis. Urethral abscess and urinary sinuses or fistulae are particularly serious complications. Symptoms include difficulty in urination, hematuria, and pyuria.

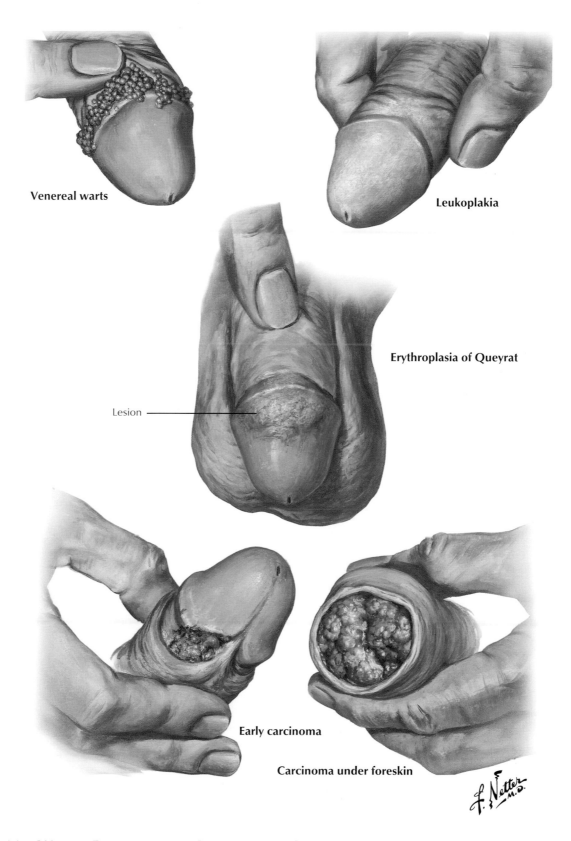

Venereal warts

Leukoplakia

Erythroplasia of Queyrat

Lesion

Early carcinoma

Carcinoma under foreskin

FIGURE 7-11   WARTS, PRECANCEROUS LESIONS, AND CANCER

Venereal warts (condyloma acuminatum, verrucae) caused by human papillomaviruses (HPVs) usually occur around the base of the glans with a phimotic prepuce. **Erythroplasia of Queyrat,** a premalignant lesion of the glans penis, consists of slightly raised, red, velvety plaques composed of hypertrophied epidermis.

Leukoplakia, a premalignant complication associated with chronic inflammation and glycosuria, can involve the entire prepuce or the glans. It develops as patches of indurated, leathery, blue-white skin. **Early carcinoma of the penis** starts as a

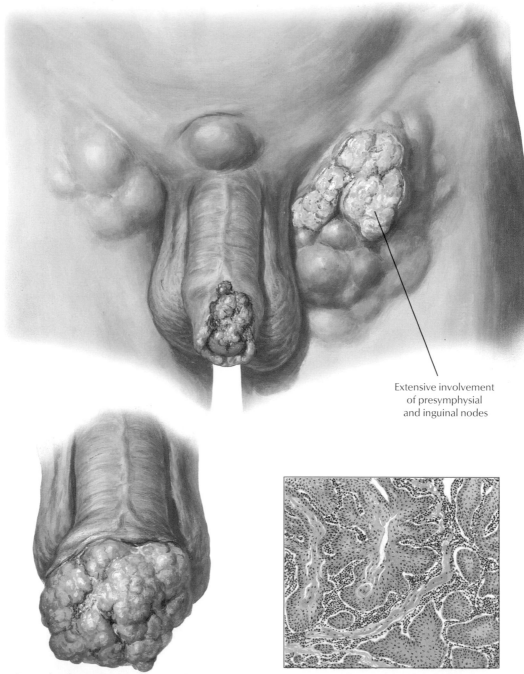

Advanced carcinoma of penis

Extensive involvement of presymphysial and inguinal nodes

Extensive fungating carcinoma of penis

Squamous cell carcinoma of penis, histology

FIGURE 7-11 WARTS, PRECANCEROUS LESIONS, AND CANCER *(CONTINUED)*

small growth around the corona of the glans penis. The lesion often becomes ulcerated; untreated, it develops into a large fungating mass. Almost all penile cancers are **squamous cell carcinomas** (SCCs). At least half of patients have nodal metastases at the time of presentation because the initial lesion is painless and may be obscured by a phimotic prepuce.

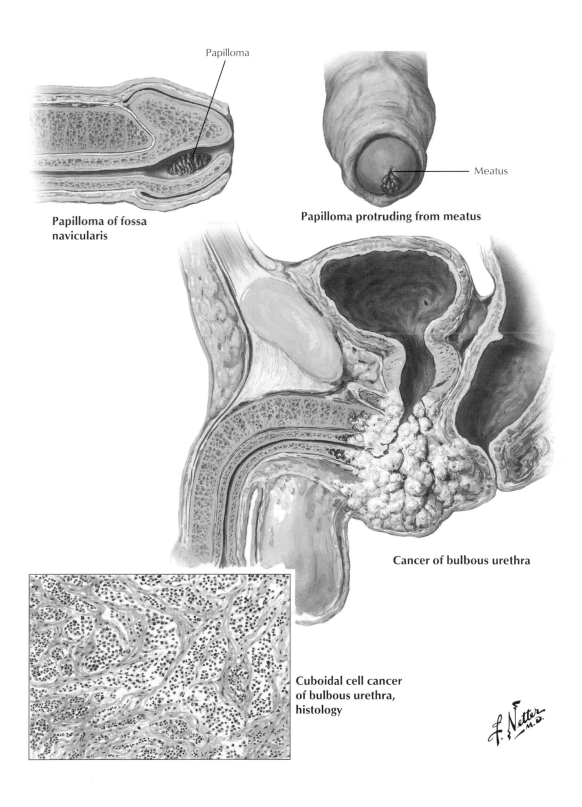

Papilloma

Papilloma of fossa
navicularis

Meatus

Papilloma protruding from meatus

Cancer of bulbous urethra

**Cuboidal cell cancer
of bulbous urethra,
histology**

FIGURE 7-12 PAPILLOMA AND CANCER OF THE URETHRA

Papillomas (polyps) and **verrucae** (condylomas) are benign tumors of the urethra that usually develop just within the urethral meatus in the fossa navicularis as a result of inflammation in the urethral glands. They can cause urinary urgency, frequency and pain, hematuria, and disturbances in sexual function. **Primary carcinoma of the urethra**, a rare malignancy with an indolent course and an unfavorable prognosis, usually occurs in older men. The lesions develop equally often in the penile urethra and in more proximal portions of the urethra. Patients often present with a perineal abscess or a urethral stricture that is suspiciously increasing in size. Undetected tumors most commonly metastasize to regional inguinal lymph nodes.

Acute prostatitis

Chronic prostatitis

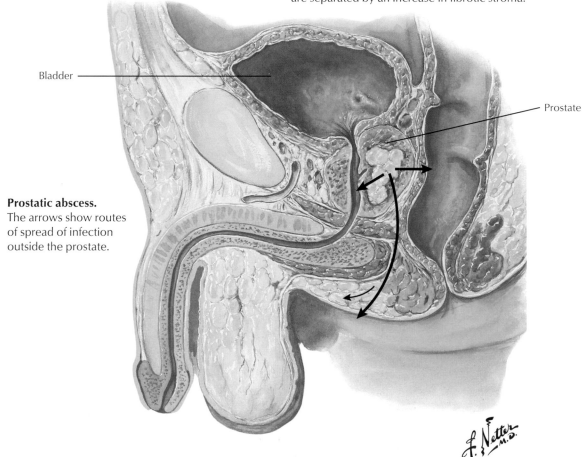

Histology. Polymorphonucleur leukocytes infiltrate the prostatic acini and the stroma.

Histology. A mixed infiltrate of neutrophils and lymphocytes is present and the acini are separated by an increase in fibrotic stroma.

Bladder

Prostate

Prostatic abscess.
The arrows show routes of spread of infection outside the prostate.

f. Netter M.D.

FIGURE 7-13   PROSTATITIS

Acute prostatitis develops as an occasional complication of urinary tract instrumentation. The offending organisms are staphylococci or gram-negative bacilli; acute gonococcal prostatitis is uncommon in the antibiotic era. Polymorphonuclear leukocytes infiltrate the prostatic acini and the stroma. Prostatic abscess is a rare complication. **Chronic prostatitis**, with or without chronic seminal vesiculitis, usually develops without a history of an acute phase and presents as urinary or sexual dysfunction, sometimes with a thin, mucopurulent urethral

discharge. Predisposing conditions include indwelling catheters, urinary tract instrumentation, urinary tract infection, spread of infection from distant foci, and prolonged sexual activity. There is a mixed neutrophilic and lymphocytic infiltrate, and foci of fibrosis may develop. Although a mixed population of bacteria may be identified, lack of demonstrable bacteria is more common. Granulomatous lesions representing tuberculous prostatitis occur rarely.

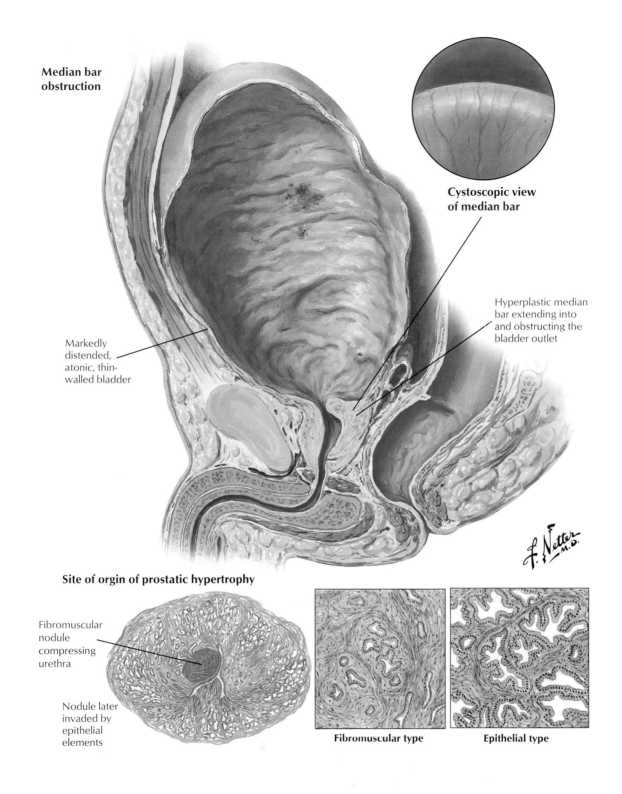

Median bar obstruction

Cystoscopic view of median bar

Hyperplastic median bar extending into and obstructing the bladder outlet

Markedly distended, atonic, thin-walled bladder

Site of orgin of prostatic hypertrophy

Fibromuscular nodule compressing urethra

Nodule later invaded by epithelial elements

Fibromuscular type

Epithelial type

FIGURE 7-14   NODULAR HYPERPLASIA: BENIGN PROSTATIC HYPERTROPHY

Nodular hyperplasia of the prostate is a disease associated with aging. Benign prostatic hypertrophy or hyperplasia (BPH) describes the benign proliferation (hyperplasia) of prostatic acinar epithelium and stroma with variable fibromuscular and epithelial predominance. Hyperplastic lesions typically arise in short glands adjacent to the proximal urethra in the middle lobe of the prostate (transitional zone). As the nodules increase in size, they compress the normal tissue of the more peripherally situated lateral and posterior lobes into a thin rim adjacent to the capsule. Formation of a **median bar** is one mechanism by which hyperplastic tissue obstructs the outlet of the urinary bladder. Significant BPH is confirmed by the detection of an enlarged, firm,

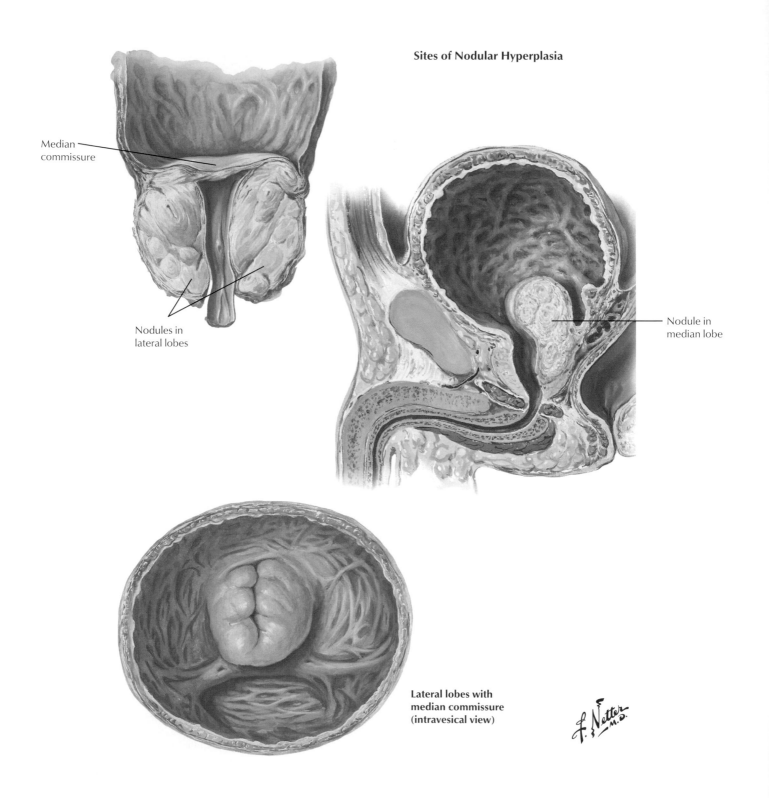

Sites of Nodular Hyperplasia

Median commissure

Nodules in lateral lobes

Nodule in median lobe

Lateral lobes with median commissure (intravesical view)

FIGURE 7-14   NODULAR HYPERPLASIA: BENIGN PROSTATIC HYPERTROPHY (*CONTINUED*)

rubbery prostate gland on rectal examination. BPH can adopt a number of gross configurations that obstruct the bladder outlet, including the median bar, the bilobular pattern (2 lateral lobes), and the trilobular pattern (2 lateral lobes plus median lobe). The pathogenesis of BPH involves hormonally driven proliferation and growth of prostatic tissue in the setting of androgen and estrogen imbalance. BPH leads to progressive urinary dysfunction, recurrent urinary tract infections, and obstructive uropathy. Surgical intervention is usually palliative if not curative.

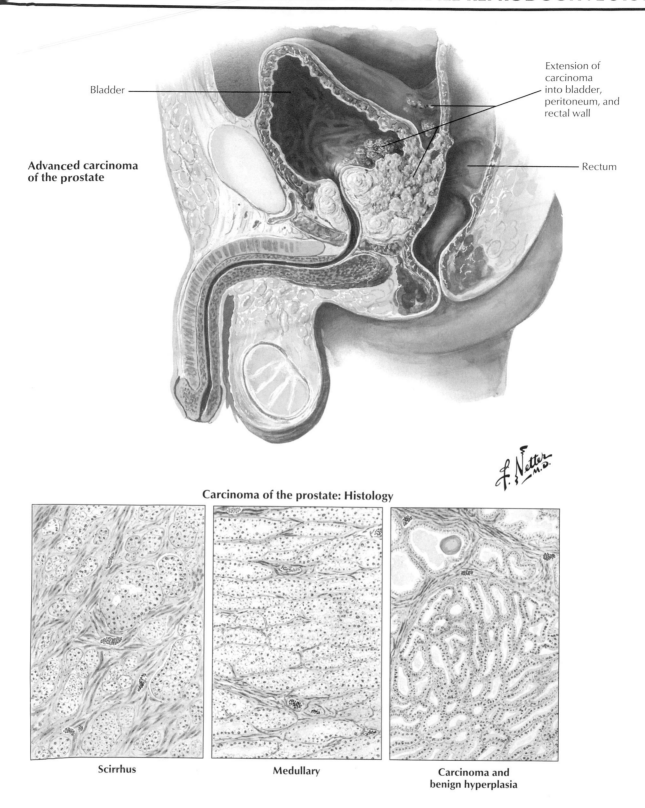

Advanced carcinoma of the prostate

Bladder

Extension of carcinoma into bladder, peritoneum, and rectal wall

Rectum

Carcinoma of the prostate: Histology

Scirrhus

Medullary

Carcinoma and benign hyperplasia

FIGURE 7-15   CARCINOMA OF THE PROSTATE: TYPES, EXTENSION, AND METASTASES

American men older than 50 years have a lifetime risk of clinical carcinoma of the prostate of approximately 10%. It occurs twice as frequently in African-Americans as in whites. This malignant tumor typically originates in the posterior lobe of the gland, with or without coexistent benign hyperplasia. **Prostate cancer** is frequently an adenocarcinoma composed of atypical epithelium (single cell layer without basal cells), which form small acini that grow in a crowded and disorganized pattern intermixed with

abundant fibrous stroma (**scirrhous form**). Prostate cancer is scored on architecture by the Gleason scoring system. The unusual soft medullary type may elude early detection. Occult carcinomas are small lesions found incidentally at autopsy, in tissue resected for BPH, or in biopsy tissue for elevated prostate-specific antigen (PSA). Other prostatic cancers grow progressively to infiltrate much of the parenchyma of the gland, including eventually the posterior capsule. Perineural invasion is probably

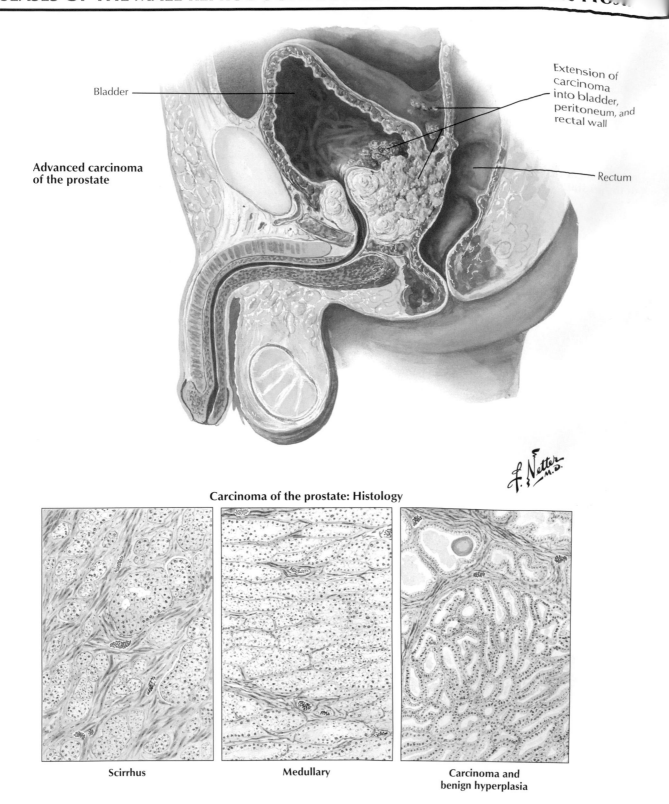

Advanced carcinoma of the prostate

Bladder

Extension of carcinoma into bladder, peritoneum, and rectal wall

Rectum

Carcinoma of the prostate: Histology

Scirrhus

Medullary

Carcinoma and benign hyperplasia

FIGURE 7-15   CARCINOMA OF THE PROSTATE: TYPES, EXTENSION, AND METASTASES (CONTINUED)

important in local extension and development of metastases. Prostatic cancer extends initially by contiguous spread to the bladder and surrounding tissues. It spreads eventually to distant sites by invasion of the bloodstream and lymphatics. Approximately two thirds of patients with advanced disease have bony metastases. Typically, the metastatic foci stimulate bone growth, producing osteoblastic metastases that manifest as radiodense ~ions, although radiolucent, osteoclastic metastases occur

rarely. Lymph node and visceral metastases can be localized or widespread. Because androgens stimulate the growth of normal and neoplastic prostatic epithelium, carcinogenesis likely relates to an imbalance in production of androgens and estrogens. However, of utmost importance for cure of prostatic cancer is early detection and treatment before the malignancy has extended beyond the prostatic capsule to involve adjacent pelvic structures or spread to distant sites.

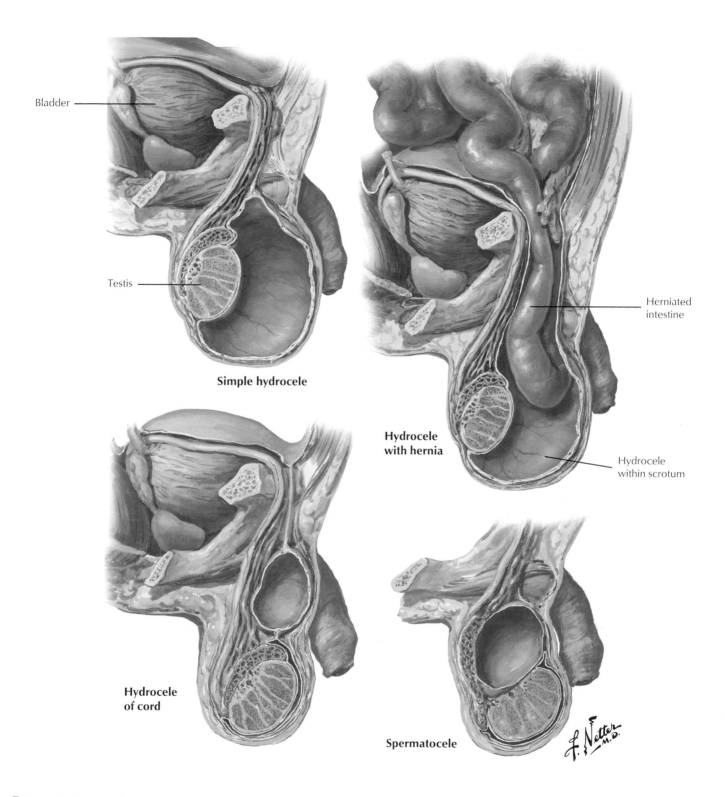

FIGURE 7-16   HYDROCELE AND SPERMATOCELE

Hydrocele, an accumulation of serous fluid in the 2 peritoneal layers of the tunica vaginalis, results from abnormalities in the descent of the testicles from the retroperitoneal position in the abdominal cavity to the scrotum. The common **simple hydrocele** is a distended, fluid-filled segment of a normally formed tunica vaginalis. **Congenital hydrocele**, with or without hernia, involves a communication with the abdominal cavity. **Hydrocele of the cord** develops as a circumscribed sac of peritoneum localized in

the cord. **Acute hydrocele** typically occurs secondary to trauma, tumors, or infection of the testicle and epididymis, particularly gonorrhea and tuberculosis. **Chronic hydrocele** may or may not have an apparent underlying cause. A **spermatocele** is a cyst within the scrotum that develops due to obstruction of the sperm transporting system. Rarely, enlargement of the spermatic cord is due to a malignant tumor, typically some type of sarcoma.

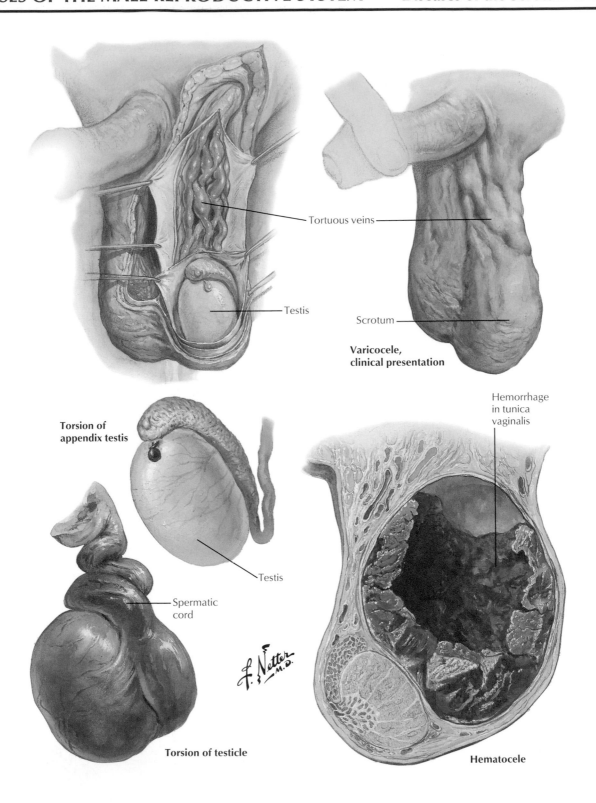

Tortuous veins

Testis

Scrotum

Varicocele, clinical presentation

Torsion of appendix testis

Testis

Spermatic cord

Torsion of testicle

Hemorrhage in tunica vaginalis

Hematocele

FIGURE 7-17   VARICOCELE, HEMATOCELE, AND TORSION

Varicocele, a collection of dilated, tortuous veins of the pampiniform plexus in the scrotum, is nearly always left sided and asymptomatic. Most varicoceles occur in young males and are without demonstrable etiology. The sudden onset of varicocele after the age of 30 years is secondary to retroperitoneal disease, such as tumors, hydronephrosis, or vascular anomalies. **Hematocele** is due to hemorrhage into the tunica vaginalis caused by an injury to the spermatic vessels, particularly trauma or operation, or it may occur spontaneously related to underlying vascular disease, infection, or neoplasm. **Torsion** (twisting) of the spermatic cord results in compression of the vasculature followed by infarction or complete gangrene of the testicle. Excessive mobility of the testis due to various developmental anomalies is the common predisposing factor. Torsion of the tiny vestigial appendix testis may cause acute pain in the scrotum, which can simulate acute epididymitis or can even mimic acute appendicitis from a referred pain pattern.

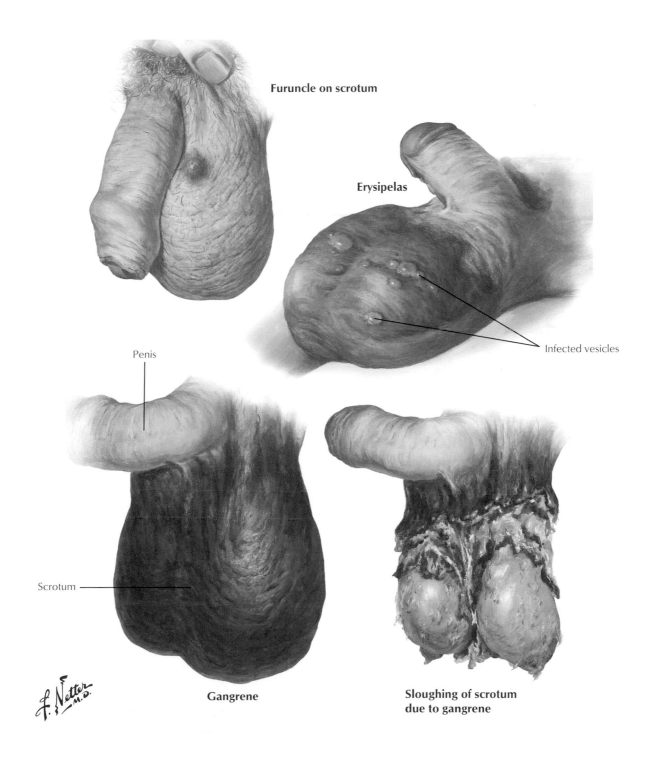

Furuncle on scrotum

Erysipelas

Infected vesicles

Penis

Scrotum

Gangrene

Sloughing of scrotum
due to gangrene

FIGURE 7-18   INFECTION AND GANGRENE

Reduced air circulation and evaporation of sweat in a tight space, irritation of scrotal skin by rubbing against adjacent structures, and ready access to bacteria are common causes of infection in the scrotum. Furuncles develop from hair follicles or sweat glands infected with *Staphylococcus aureus*. **Scrotal erysipelas**, a widespread superficial infection of scrotal skin, is usually caused by *Streptococcus pyogenes*. **Gangrene of the scrotum** with extensive necrosis and sloughing of skin can develop as a result of extravasation of infected urine into the subcutaneous tissues or mechanical, chemical, or thermal injuries to the scrotum, particularly in individuals with diabetes mellitus, alcoholism, or other chronic diseases. Abrupt onset and rapid progression of gangrene in apparently healthy individuals are initiated by an occult infection (idiopathic or Fournier gangrene). Prompt debridement and antibiotic therapy are mandatory.

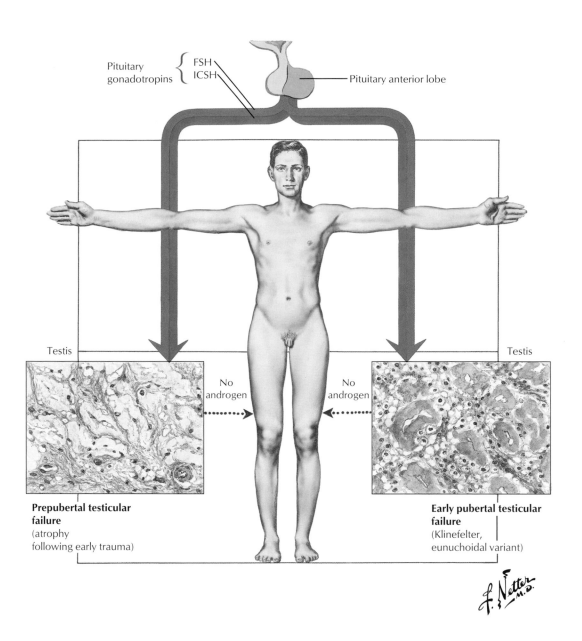

FIGURE 7-19 TESTICULAR FAILURE: PRIMARY HYPERGONADOTROPIC HYPOGONADISM AND PREPUBERTAL FAILURE

Hypogonadism connotes testicular deficiency in androgen production by the interstitial (Leydig) cells, although failure of the sperm-producing germinal cells is also involved. Eunuchism and eunuchoidism are, respectively, the absence of the testis and severe reduction of androgen production. Primary testicular failure, which typically begins in the prepubertal or very early pubertal period, is the result of various intrinsic developmental defects in the testis with intact pituitary function. This picture is

characterized as *primary* or **hypergonadotropic eunuchoidism** or **hypergonadotropic hypogonadism**. Testicular atrophy also can occur from acquired causes, such as infections (e.g., mumps) and trauma. Klinefelter syndrome, a genetic disease with a sex chromosomal abnormality, usually XXY, presents at puberty with small testes with hyalinized seminiferous tubules and features of eunuchoidism.

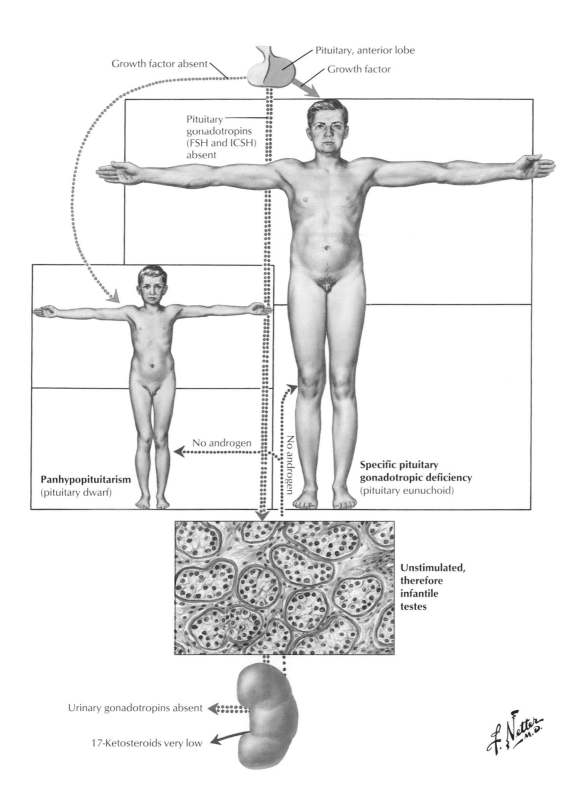

Growth factor absent

Pituitary, anterior lobe

Growth factor

Pituitary gonadotropins (FSH and ICSH) absent

No androgen

No androgen

No androgen

Panhypopituitarism (pituitary dwarf)

Specific pituitary gonadotropic deficiency (pituitary eunuchoid)

Unstimulated, therefore infantile testes

Urinary gonadotropins absent

17-Ketosteroids very low

FIGURE 7-20   TESTICULAR FAILURE: SECONDARY HYPOGONADOTROPIC HYPOGONADISM

Testicular deficiency is secondary to failure of the pituitary to produce gonadotrophic hormones (secondary hypogonadotropic hypogonadism) in approximately 80% of hypogonadal male patients. Although the exact cause of the hypofunction is often unknown, it is important to rule out a pituitary tumor (chromophobe adenoma) or a hypothalamic tumor or other intracranial lesion. Histologically, the testis is immature, with small tubules containing undifferentiated spermatogonia and Sertoli cells and few interstitial Leydig cells. The phenotype may be eunuchoid with a specific pituitary gonadotrophic deficiency or that of a pituitary dwarf with panhypopituitarism. Many patients present with hybrid features of both primary and secondary hypogonadism.

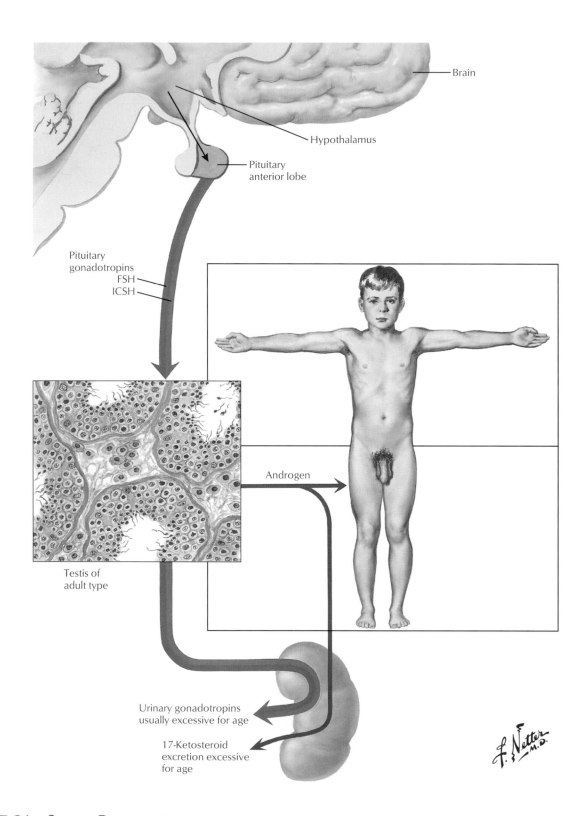

FIGURE 7-21   SEXUAL PRECOCITY

Sexual precocity involves not only premature enlargement of the penis, pubic hair, and testes (macrogenitosomia), but also growth of the skeleton, muscles, body hair, and other structures. Sexual precocity may result from premature development or abnormalities of the hypothalamus and pituitary. Histology of the testis shows a mature pattern with significant development of both tubules and interstitial cells. Urinary gonadotropins and

17-ketosteroids are usually excessive for age. The endocrine type (pseudosexual precocity) results from an adenoma, carcinoma, or hyperplasia of the adrenal cortex or an interstitial cell (Leydig cell) tumor of the testis. These patients can combine the macrogenitosomia and premature musculoskeletal development with Cushing syndrome, hypertension, or both. The testes remain infantile in both germinal and interstitial development.

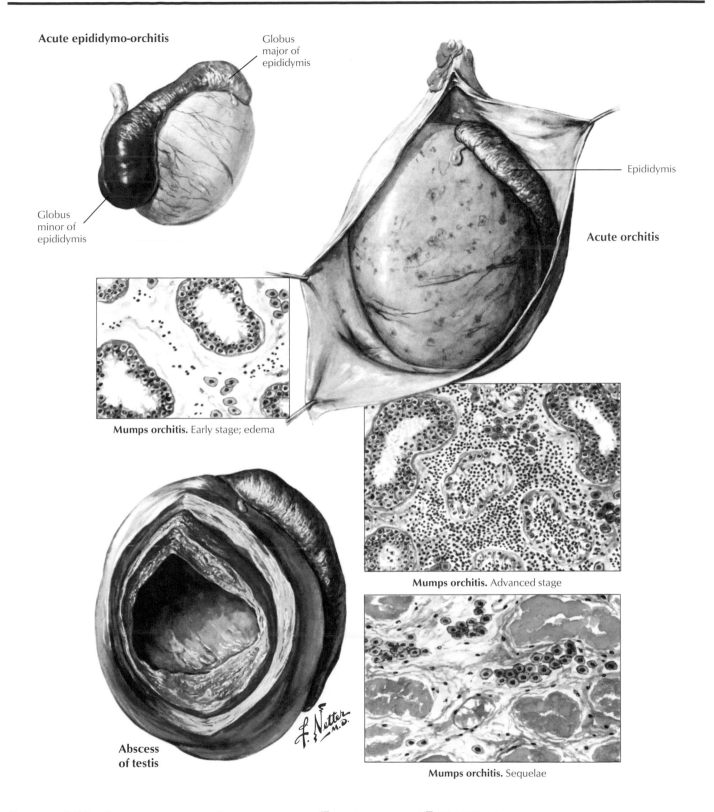

Acute epididymo-orchitis

Globus major of epididymis

Globus minor of epididymis

Epididymis

Acute orchitis

Mumps orchitis. Early stage; edema

Mumps orchitis. Advanced stage

Abscess of testis

Mumps orchitis. Sequelae

FIGURE 7-22   INFECTION AND ABSCESS OF THE TESTIS AND THE EPIDIDYMIS

Orchitis may develop alone but more commonly occurs secondary to epididymitis. It may also result from systemic infections or be caused by bacterial toxins from distant localized infections, such as tonsillitis, sinusitis, or cellulitis. **Acute pyogenic orchitis** (epididymoorchitis) may progress to involve the testis, resulting in a large abscess. Mumps orchitis, which complicates approximately 20% of postpubertal mumps cases, progresses from transitory edema to marked interstitial inflammation (lympho-cytes, macrophages, and plasma cells). If severe, it can result in tubular sclerosis and testicular atrophy. Most cases are unilateral, and sterility is rare. **Epididymitis** without orchitis is common in adults. It may result from a specific infection (e.g., gonorrhea, syphilis, or tuberculosis), a nonspecific inflammation, or trauma. The source of organisms can be infected urine, prostate, or seminal vesicles, with spread via the vas deferens to the epididymis.

251

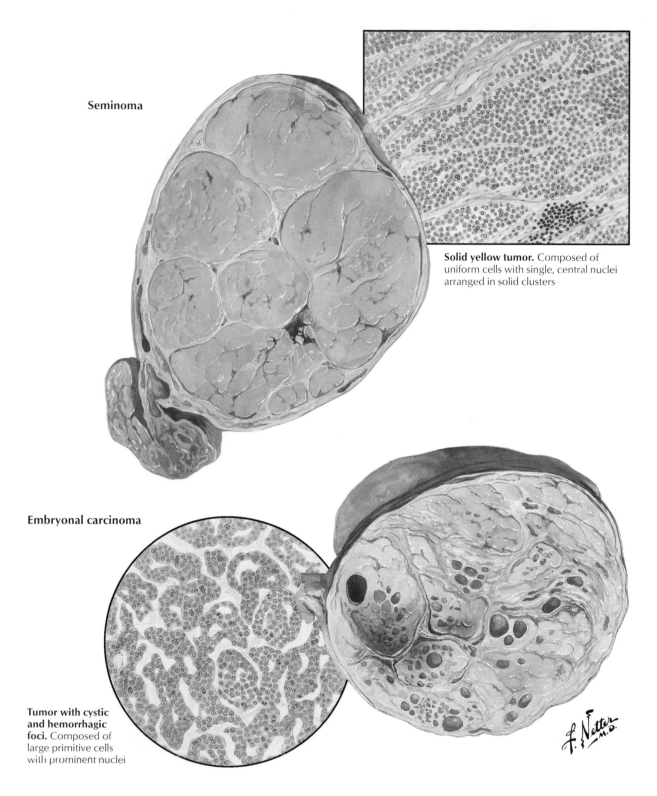

Seminoma

Solid yellow tumor. Composed of uniform cells with single, central nuclei arranged in solid clusters

Embryonal carcinoma

Tumor with cystic and hemorrhagic foci. Composed of large primitive cells with prominent nuclei

f. Netter M.D.

FIGURE 7-23   TESTICULAR TUMORS: SEMINOMA AND EMBRYONAL CARCINOMA

Malignant neoplasms of the testis, which usually occur in men aged 15-40 years, are more frequent in undescended testicles. **Seminomas** are nonencapsulated but well circumscribed tumors with a lobulated architecture and a yellow, orange, or pink color. Histologically, they are composed of uniform cells with single, prominent, central nuclei arranged in compact lobules separated by thin fibrous septa. The stroma typically contains lymphocytes and plasma cells. These tumors are highly radiosensitive and

curable if they do not contain a malignant trophoblastic component. **Embryonal carcinomas** have foci of hemorrhage and necrosis in a yellow lobulated mass. Histologically, they are composed of primitive cells with prominent nuclei that grow in glandular, lobular, or tubular patterns and, occasionally, exhibit chorioepitheliomatous tissue. Embryonal carcinoma usually has relative radioresistant elements, may have spread beyond the testis at diagnosis, and carries a guarded prognosis.

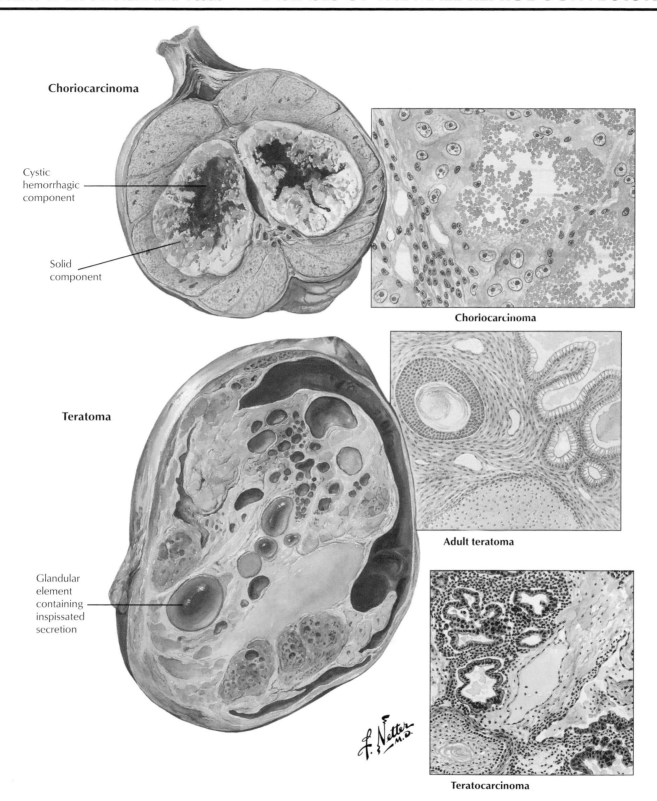

Choriocarcinoma

Cystic hemorrhagic component

Solid component

Choriocarcinoma

Teratoma

Adult teratoma

Glandular element containing inspissated secretion

Teratocarcinoma

FIGURE 7-24   TESTICULAR TUMORS: CHORIOCARCINOMA, TERATOMA, AND TERATOCARCINOMA

Choriocarcinomas are highly malignant neoplasms that occur most often as focal components of embryonal carcinomas and **teratocarcinomas**. They rarely occur as pure primary tumors. Histologically, choriocarcinomas consist of atypical syncytial and cytotrophoblastic cells surrounding blood spaces, which form structures resembling chorionic villi. Teratomas have a variable gross appearance with solid and cystic areas and a variable histologic appearance reproducing various mature glandular and solid tissues derived from the 3 germ layers. However, mature (adult) teratomas in males should be considered to have malignant potential because of the frequent occurrence of cryptic foci of poorly differentiated elements. Teratocarcinoma represents a group of tumors in which malignant elements of embryonal carcinoma, chorioepithelioma, and seminoma are present in conjunction with differentiated teratoid structures.

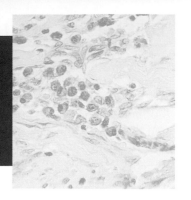

CHAPTER 8

DISEASES OF THE FEMALE REPRODUCTIVE SYSTEM

Female sex organs develop from the same primitive structures as male sex organs. The ovary evolves from the embryonic urogenital ridge, and the Wolffian (mesonephric) duct remains vestigial without male stimulation. Paramesonephric ducts (**müllerian ducts**) form the anlage of the fallopian tubes, uterus, and vagina. External genitalia are essentially female in design and develop male features only when stimulated by dihydrotestosterone.

Common diseases of the female reproductive system are discussed in the following chapter according to their anatomical sites. They comprise congenital alterations, inflammation, and infections (Table 8-1); benign and malignant tumors; and pregnancy-related disorders.

DISEASES OF THE VULVA

The vulva includes such structures as the mons pubis, the labia majora and minora, the clitoris, and the introitus (vestibule). Diseases of the vulva affect the skin (e.g., vulvitis, tumors) and the adnexal glands (cysts, **bartholinitis,** tumors).

DISEASES OF THE VAGINA

The vagina connects the uterus with the vestibule and is lined by a hormone-sensitive squamous epithelium. Consequently, loss of estrogen stimulation favors infections and causes atrophic vaginitis. Diseases of the vagina involve the epidermis (e.g., inflammation, polyps, squamous cell carcinoma [SCC]), the adnexal glands (adenosis, adenocarcinoma), or ductal remnants (**Gartner duct cysts**).

DISEASES OF THE UTERUS

The uterus is subdivided for diagnostic and therapeutic reasons into the uterine cervix, the endometrium, and the myometrium. Common diseases include functional disturbances, inflammation, and neoplasia. Cervicitis, which often results from sexually transmitted disease (STD), is common, whereas endometritis is rather rare. STDs include infections by papilloma virus, herpes simplex virus type II, syphilis, and gonorrhea (also see chapter 7). Chlamydia species cause infections of the female reproductive system with increasing frequency.

Cervical intraepithelial neoplasia (CIN) is a common atypical proliferation of squamous epithelium, frequently related to infection with certain papilloma viruses (human papillomaviruses [HPVs] 16 and 18), which carries the risk of progressing to SCC. Early diagnosis of CIN by exfoliative cytology (PAP smear) followed by appropriate treatment has helped to decrease the annual incidence of SCC by 50% to 85%.

Squamous cell carcinoma of the cervix is the second or sixth most common tumor of females (depending on the efficiency of cervical cytologic screening). There are 15 new cases annually per 100,000 women in the United States. The chief clinical feature of SCC is vaginal bleeding after intercourse or douching; it may be silent in sexually inactive women. The 5-year survival after treatment is stage-dependent and ranges from 90% in patients diagnosed in International Federation of Gynecology and Obstetrics (FIGO) stage I to 10% in those diagnosed in stage IV.

Endometrial hyperplasia and **endometrial adenocarcinoma** (EAC) represent a continuum of proliferative diseases (hyperplasias) that start as a benign disturbance and proceed stepwise to malignancy. Atypical hyperplasia with complex glandular crowding and cytologic atypia signals the transition to carcinoma. Afflicting approximately 34,000 women per year in the United States, EAC is the fourth most frequent cancer in women. The incidence decreased recently when the administration of menopausal estrogens was reduced, suggesting that prolonged estrogenic stimulation may support its pathogenesis. The essential clinical feature of EAC is perimenopausal or postmenopausal bleeding. The prognosis for patients with EAC depends on the tumor stage and additional risk factors; the 10-year survival rate is approximately 65%.

DISEASES OF THE FALLOPIAN TUBES

Inflammation (salpingitis) and ectopic pregnancy (EP) are the most common diseases in this region. Salpingitis caused by *Escherichia coli,* chlamydia, or gonorrhea, frequently as STDs, may cause abscesses, adhesions, obstructions, and sterility. EPs may be related to preceding salpingitis and occur in the United States at a rate of approximately 1.5 per 100 live births. More than 95% of EPs are located in the fallopian tubes. They constitute life-threatening diseases because of their risk of tubal rupture and massive hemorrhage. Adenocarcinoma of the salpinx is a rare disease.

DISEASES OF THE OVARY

Besides various endocrinopathies, **ovarian tumors** are the most important diseases in this region. There are more than 25 types of ovarian tumors and many subtypes. They are classified into major groups: tumors of the germinal epithelium (e.g., serous and mucinous cystadenoma/carcinoma), tumors of the germ cell (dysgerminoma, teratoma, choriocarcinoma), tumors of the gonadal stroma (granulosa cell tumor, Sertoli-Leydig cell tumor, thecoma), and benign hilus cell tumors (composed of Leydig cells). The most common, **serous cyst-adenocarcinoma** (SAC), occurs in approximately 1% of women, favoring older women. SAC does not secrete hormones and usually causes symptoms of pain and abdominal distention only as it increases in size. It spreads readily by lymphatic channels and peritoneal dissemination. The prognosis is poor, with an overall 5-year survival of 35%.

PREGNANCY AND ITS DISEASES

Diseases discussed in this section comprise a large variety of disorders: structural and functional alterations (placenta previa, EP, abortion), various infections and tumors, diseases of the fetus (**erythroblastosis fetalis**), and toxemia of pregnancy and eclampsia.

TABLE 8-1   INFECTIOUS AND INFLAMMATORY DISEASES OF THE FEMALE REPRODUCTIVE SYSTEM

Conditions	Causes
Dermatoses of the vulva	
Folliculitis and furunculosis	*Staphylococcus aureus,* mixed organisms
Herpes genitalis (progenitalis)	Herpes simplex virus type 2
Intertrigo	Chafing plus dermatophytosis (fungal infection)
Tinea cruris	Ringworm of the groin, usually *Epidermophyton floccosum*
Molluscum contagiosum	Poxvirus
Psoriasis	Systemic noninfectious inflammatory disorder
Infections and other lesions of the vulva, vagina, and cervix	
Diabetic vulvitis	Mycotic (fungal) infection
Gonorrhea	*Neisseria gonorrhoeae*
Syphilis	*Treponema pallidum*
Chancroid	*Haemophilus ducreyi*
Lymphogranuloma venereum	*Chlamydia trachomatis* types L1, L2, L3
Granuloma inguinale	*Calymmatobacterium granulomatis* (originally *Donovania* species)
Bartholin gland cyst and abscess	*Neisseria gonorrhoeae,* other pathogenic bacteria
Common vulvovaginitis, urethritis, and cervicovaginitis	*Candida albicans* (moniliasis), *Chlamydia trachomatis* (serotypes D-K), *Trichomonas vaginalis*, other organisms, including gram-positive and -negative bacteria (nonspecific vaginitis)
Genital (venereal) warts (condylomata acuminata)	Human papillomaviruses, especially types 6, 11, 42, and 44 (low risk for cervical cancer)
Tuberculosis	*Mycobacterium tuberculosis*
Chemical vaginitis	Douches (high-concentration chemicals)
Traumatic vaginitis	Foreign bodies, pessaries
Pelvic inflammatory disease	
Vulvitis, cervicitis, endometritis, salpingitis, oophoritis	*Neisseria gonorrhoeae, Chlamydia trachomatis,* polymicrobial puerperal infections—staphylococci, streptococci, coliform bacteria, *Clostridium perfringens*
Puerperal infections	
Endometritis, vaginitis, sepsis	*Streptococcus* species, *Staphylococcus* species, gram-negative bacteria

PATHOLOGY OF THE MAMMARY GLAND

The female breast, like the endometrium and the cervical-vaginal epithelium, responds sensitively and with varying histology to alterations in female sex hormones during adolescence, the menstrual cycle, pregnancy, and menopause. Knowledge of the normal histologic reaction patterns in the breast gland is essential for the interpretation of pathologic changes. The most frequent disorders today are various forms of hyperplasia (**fibrocystic disease**) and **mammary carcinoma** (MCa). MCa is the most frequent tumor in females of the Western world, with a lifetime incidence of approximately 1 woman in 9. Approximately one third of patients die of the disease.

Genetic factors play a significant role in breast cancer, and its risk is significantly increased among first-degree relatives of affected individuals. Several genes, including BRCA1 and 2, have been implicated. In addition, there are obvious hormonal and environmental influences on the pathogenesis of MCa. Because the initial growth of the tumor usually remains clinically inapparent or is camouflaged by preexistent fibrocystic disease, regular breast examination is essential for early diagnosis and survival.

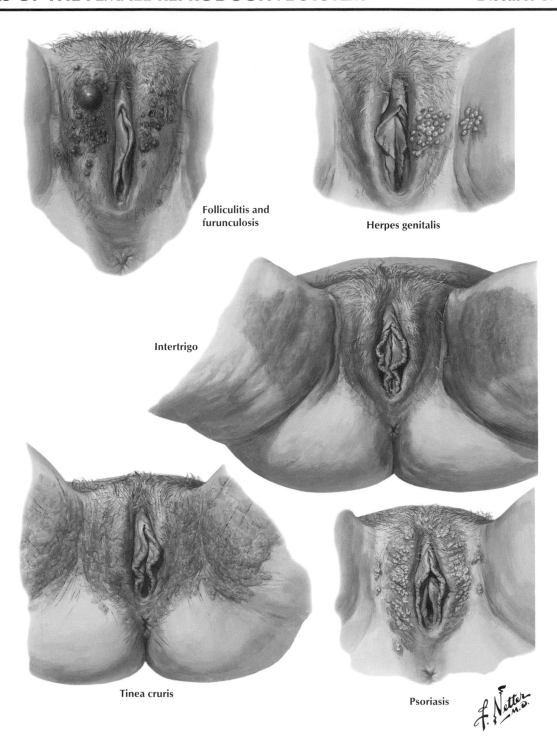

Folliculitis and furunculosis

Herpes genitalis

Intertrigo

Tinea cruris

Psoriasis

FIGURE 8-1 DERMATOSES

The skin of the vulva can be involved by the same spectrum of dermatoses that affect the skin of the rest of the body. Some common dermatoses are shown here, and the causes are listed in Table 8-1. **Folliculitis** is a papular or pustular inflammation involving the apertures of the hair follicles, and **furuncles** are larger and more deeply seated lesions with a central core of purulent exudate. **Herpes genitalis** or **progenitalis** is a recurring, localized condition, beginning as groups of vesicles on an edematous, erythematous base and subsequently forming small ulcers that dry, crust, and heal. **Intertrigo** and **tinea cruris** are superficial dermatoses associated with fungal infection. Vulvar lesions of psoriasis, a systemic noninfectious inflammatory disorder, are typically pruritic, red, and covered with silvery-white scales. The presence of similar lesions on the scalp and extensor surfaces of the extremities and nail changes help to establish the diagnosis.

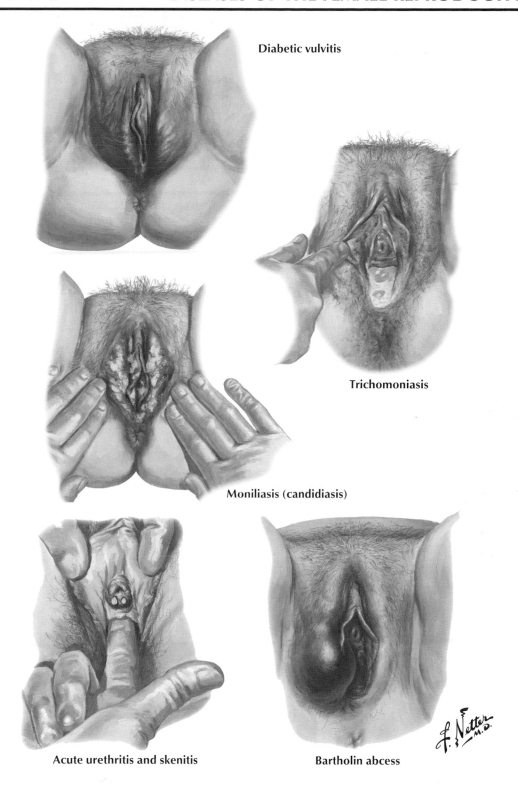

Diabetic vulvitis

Trichomoniasis

Moniliasis (candidiasis)

Acute urethritis and skenitis

Bartholin abcess

FIGURE 8-2   DIABETIC VULVITIS, TRICHOMONIASIS, MONILIASIS, AND GONORRHEA

Presenting features of **vulvitis** or **vulvovaginitis** include pruritus vulvae, vaginal discharge, burning on urination, and dyspareunia. Diabetic vulvitis is characterized by an inflamed, dark-red or beefy appearance with a superimposed superficial fungal infection. The vulvovaginitis produced by *Trichomonas vaginalis* has a thick, odoriferous, bubbly discharge in the vestibule. Vulvovaginitis caused by *Candida albicans* and related yeast fungi (moniliasis) is characterized by white, cheesy, irregular plaques, partially adherent to the congested mucosa of the vagina and cervix (vaginal thrush). Acute **gonorrhea** often presents with vaginitis beginning 1 to several days after contact; occasionally, the disease may not manifest until after the following menses, when ascending infection has resulted in acute salpingitis. Examination of the external genitalia may reveal a congested vestibule with a purulent discharge and inflammation of the urethra, Skene ducts, and Bartholin ducts.

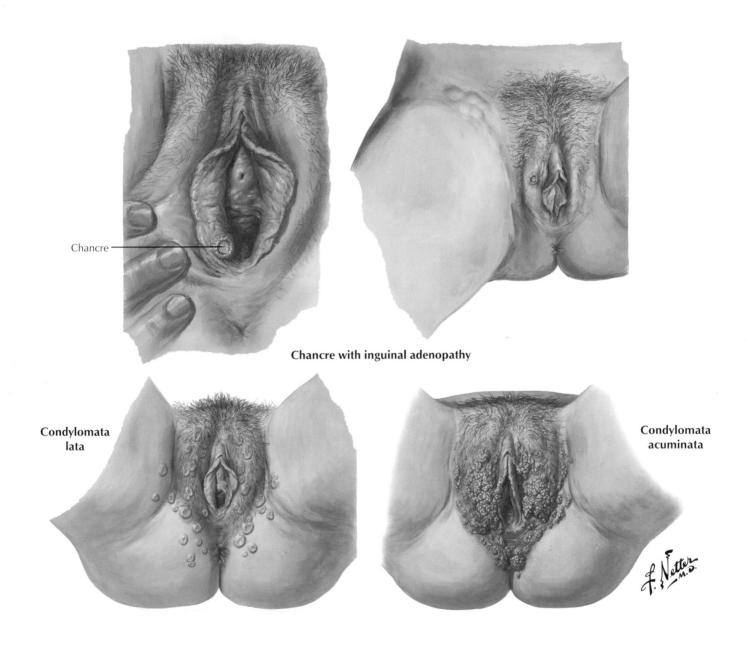

Chancre

Chancre with inguinal adenopathy

Condylomata
lata

Condylomata
acuminata

FIGURE 8-3   SYPHILIS AND GENITAL (VENEREAL) WARTS

The painless ulcerated **chancre**, the primary lesion of **syphilis**, typically develops on the labia majora or vaginal mucosa approximately 3 to 4 weeks after infection and is easily overlooked. Inguinal lymphadenopathy develops slowly and is usually well demarcated 6 weeks after infection. Histologically, the chancre shows edema, congestion, and infiltration with lymphocytes, plasma cells, epithelioid macrophages, and multinuclear giant cells. The diagnosis is made by the demonstra-

tion of the spirochetes of *Treponema pallidum* by dark field examination of wet preparations of the lesions. **Condylomata lata**, the lesions of secondary syphilis, are slightly elevated, disk-shaped papules with depressed centers. **Condyloma acuminata** (genital or venereal warts) are caused by an infection with HPVs, often not the precancerous 16 and 18. The confluent, cauliflowerlike growths of squamous epithelium form multiple soft, pointed, watery excrescences about the labia and perineum.

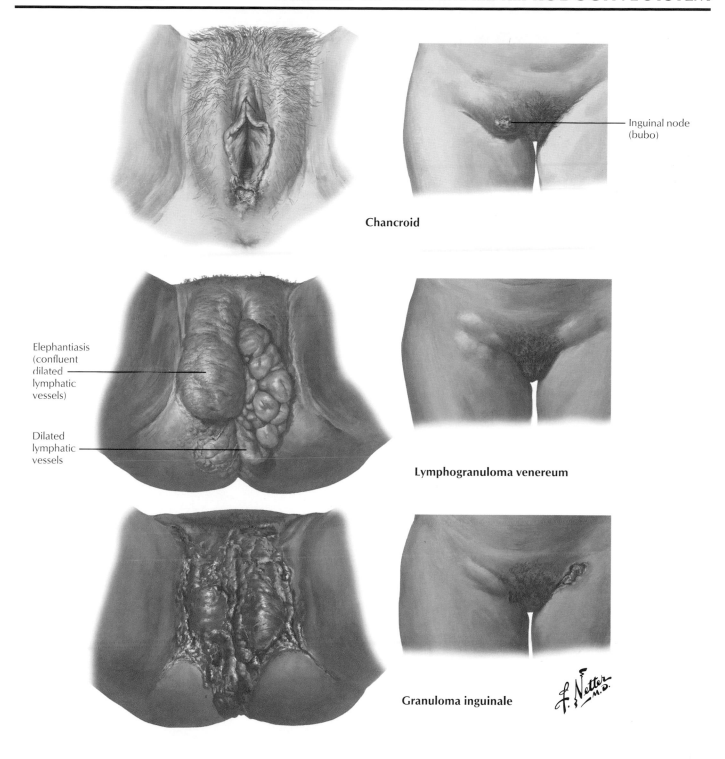

Inguinal node
(bubo)

Chancroid

Elephantiasis
(confluent
dilated
lymphatic
vessels)

Dilated
lymphatic
vessels

Lymphogranuloma venereum

Granuloma inguinale

f. Netter M.D.

FIGURE 8-4   CHANCROID, LYMPHOGRANULOMA VENEREUM, AND GRANULOMA INGUINALE

Chancroid, a venereal infection caused by the Ducrey bacillus (*Haemophilus ducreyi*), is a painful ulcerated, inflamed lesion that develops 3 to 10 days after infection. It is associated with suppurative inguinal nodes or buboes. **Lymphogranuloma venereum,** which is caused by strains of *Chlamydia trachomatis,* begins as a papule, a pustule, or an erosion on the vulva or within the vagina. Lymphatic spread leads to the development of inguinal adenitis, a painful matted mass of glands with periadeni-

tis and occasional suppuration and draining sinuses. Complications include rectal stricture. **Granuloma inguinale** is a chronic infectious disease that is widespread in the tropics and common in the southern United States. After a variable incubation period, the primary lesion develops as a vivid, circumscribed, granulomatous nodule involving the vulva, the vaginal mucosa, or the cervix. Healing occurs slowly, with the lesion persisting for many months or years.

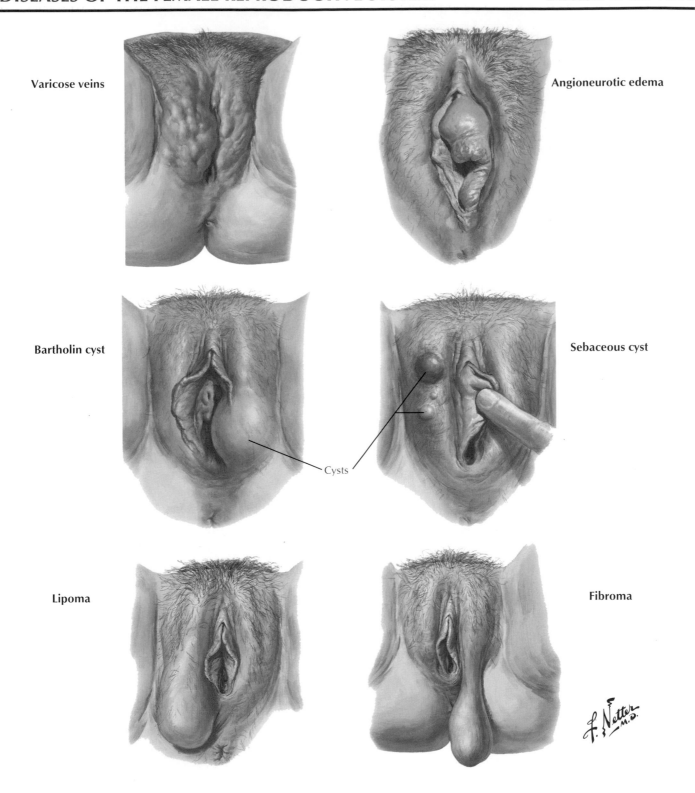

Varicose veins

Angioneurotic edema

Bartholin cyst

Cysts

Sebaceous cyst

Lipoma

Fibroma

FIGURE 8-5   CIRCULATORY DISTURBANCES, CYSTS, AND BENIGN TUMORS

Varicose veins of the vulva are associated with varicose veins of the lower extremities that develop as a result of retarded venous flow caused by increased intrapelvic pressure during pregnancy. **Angioneurotic edema** is a transient recurrent allergic reaction that manifests as painless swelling of the vulva and other areas of the body. **Bartholin cysts** result from obstruction of the excretory duct or one of its subdivisions due to specific or nonspecific infections and accidental or operative trauma. **Sebaceous cysts** result from occlusion of a sebaceous duct, which causes sebum and epithelial debris to be retained in the gland. **Benign tumors of the vulva** include the fibroma, fibromyoma, **lipoma**, papilloma, urethral caruncle, hydradenoma, angioma, myxoma, neuroma, and endometrial growths. **Fibromas**, which arise from vulvar connective tissue, become pedunculated as they increase in size and weight. Lipomas of the vulva are soft proliferations of benign adipose tissue.

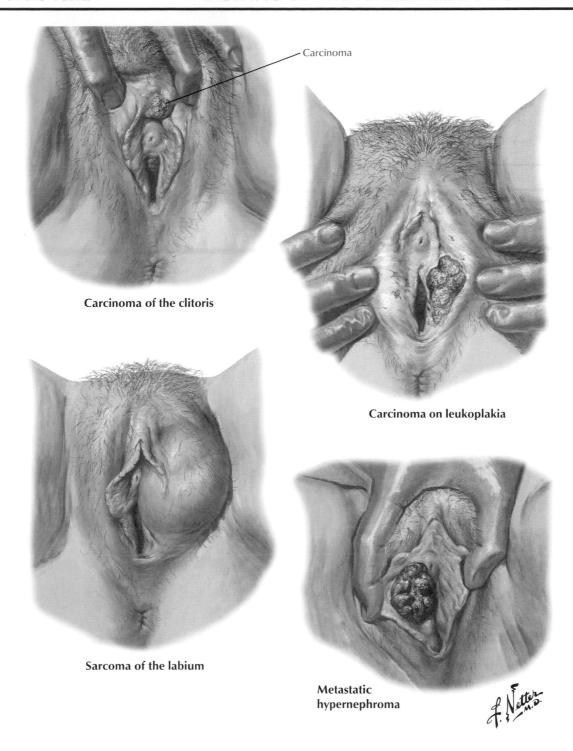

Carcinoma

Carcinoma of the clitoris

Carcinoma on leukoplakia

Sarcoma of the labium

Metastatic hypernephroma

FIGURE 8-6 MALIGNANT TUMORS

Primary vulvar lesions account for approximately 5% of the malignant tumors of the female genital tract. **Primary carcinoma of the vulva or clitoris** almost always develops in elderly women. Most are SCCs, and approximately 50% are preceded by **leukoplakia**. The typical course is the development of a small, firm nodule that progressively enlarges and ulcerates. Lymphatic extension to the regional inguinal nodes occurs early, but distant metastases are rare. Basal cell carcinoma or adenocarcinoma of a Bartholin gland or other glandular tissue are less common. **Secondary carcinoma** of the vulva is uncommon, but it may occur particularly with renal cell carcinoma (**hypernephroma**), choriocarcinoma of the uterus, and carcinoma of the uterine body or cervix. **Sarcoma** of the vulva, which includes fibrosarcoma, spindle cell carcinoma, lymphosarcoma, myxosarcoma, and liposarcoma is also uncommon, but it is usually very malignant.

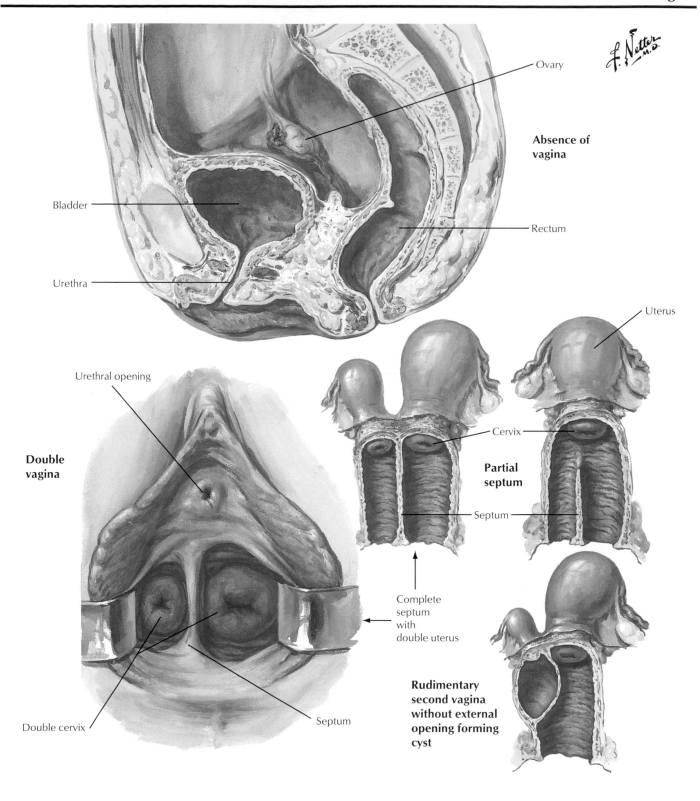

FIGURE 8-7   CONGENITAL ANOMALIES OF THE VAGINA

Most congenital anomalies of the uterus and vagina are caused by a failure of the müllerian ducts to fuse completely or to develop after fusion. Absence of the vagina (**gynatresia**) results from complete lack of union of the müllerian ducts. Each ovary, because it is derived from a different embryonic structure, is normal; the fallopian tubes may be rudimentary. A less extreme failure in müllerian development leads to a double vagina. The partial septate vagina is a milder degree of congenital malformation caused by a failure of the core of solid müllerian epithelium to slough completely at its lowermost portion. Another variation is a rudimentary second vagina. Failure of proper interaction and development of the lower müllerian ducts and the urogenital sinus can lead to an imperforate hymen (external gynatresia).

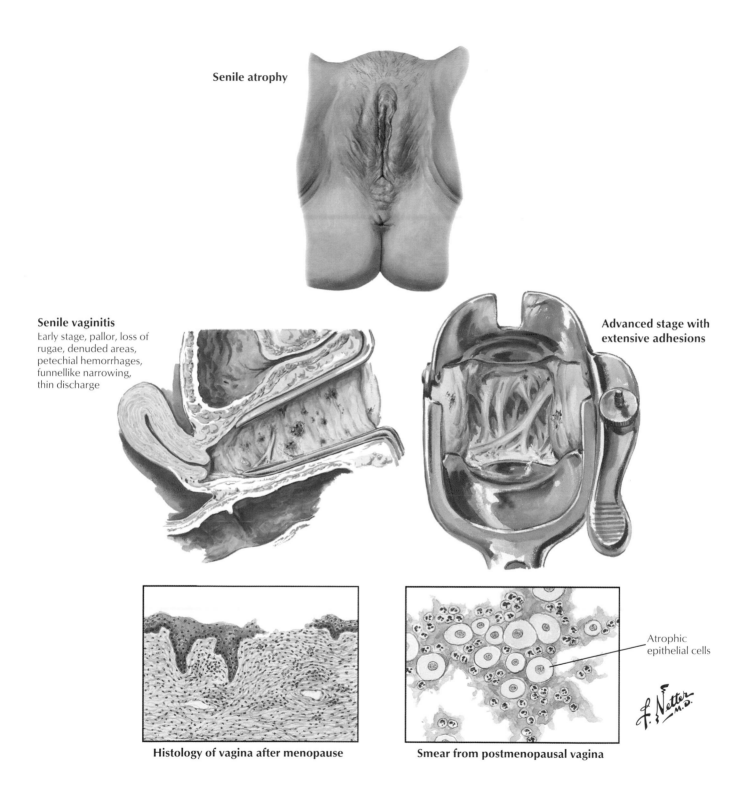

Senile atrophy

Senile vaginitis
Early stage, pallor, loss of rugae, denuded areas, petechial hemorrhages, funnellike narrowing, thin discharge

Advanced stage with extensive adhesions

Atrophic epithelial cells

Histology of vagina after menopause

Smear from postmenopausal vagina

FIGURE 8-8   VAGINAL ATROPHY

The decline in estrogen levels after the onset of menopause leads to vulvar and **vaginal atrophy**. The vagina is narrowed, especially near the apex, making visualization of the cervix difficult. The thin mucosa exhibits pallor and petechial hemorrhages, and some ulcerations may be present. *Trichomonas* or mixed bacterial infections may be present. As the condition advances, attempts at regeneration and repair lead to the formation of adhesions. Histologically, the epithelium is thin and focally interrupted, and the stroma is edematous and contains focal infiltrates of lymphocytes and polymorphonuclear leukocytes. Cytology of a cervical smear shows atrophic epithelial cells and neutrophils. Senile vaginitis is a common cause of postmenopausal bleeding.

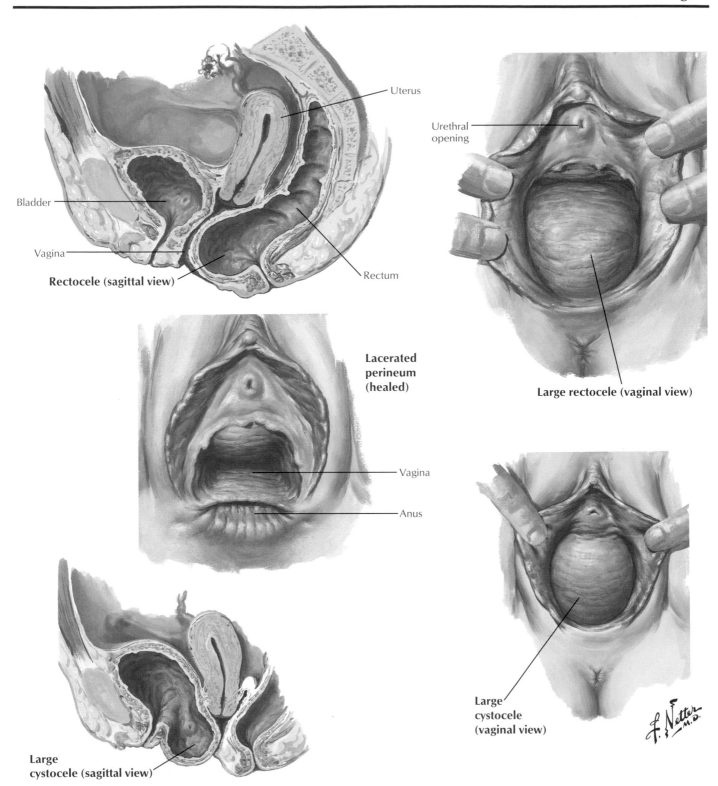

Uterus

Urethral opening

Bladder

Vagina

Rectocele (sagittal view)

Rectum

Large rectocele (vaginal view)

Lacerated perineum (healed)

Vagina

Anus

Large cystocele (vaginal view)

Large cystocele (sagittal view)

FIGURE 8-9 CYSTOCELE AND RECTOCELE

A **cystocele**, a hernialike structure, occurs when the spreading and tearing of the principal muscular supports of the vagina and rupture of pelvic fascia during childbirth cause the bladder to push forward and downward through the anterior vaginal wall. **Fistulae** may develop between the vagina and urinary bladder and rectum, diverting the urinary or fecal streams and causing incontinence. The extent of the defect depends on the number and difficulty of previous deliveries and the quality of prepartum and postpartum care. A severe cystocele may produce urinary retention leading to recurrent attacks of **cystitis** with dysuria, frequency, nocturia, and stress incontinence and may necessitate surgical repair. The consequences of unrepaired posterior obstetric lacerations of the vagina depend on the direction and extent of the tear. **Rectocele** and varying degrees of prolapse of the pelvic floor may occur in subsequent months. Rectoceles are graded according to size; third degree is a hernia to or beyond the introitus.

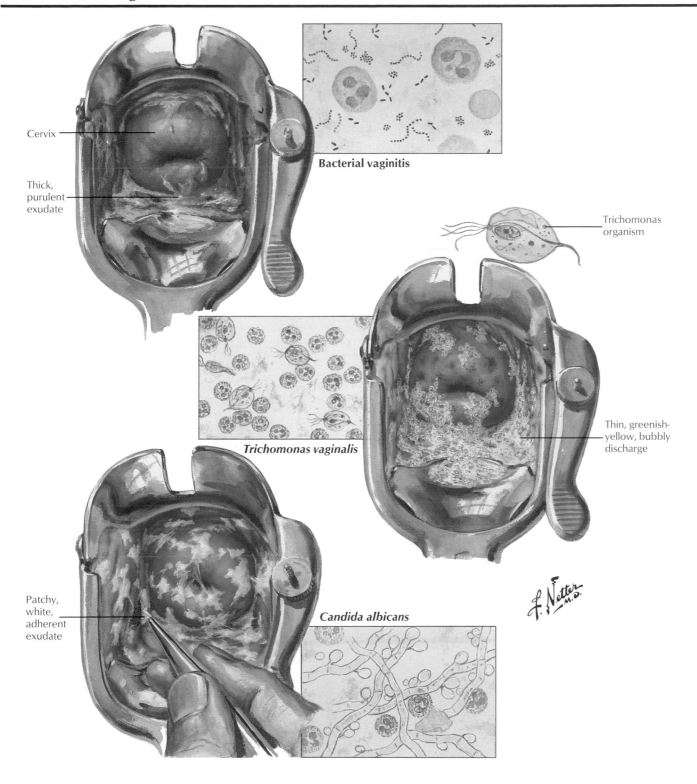

Cervix

Thick, purulent exudate

Bacterial vaginitis

Trichomonas organism

Thin, greenish-yellow, bubbly discharge

Trichomonas vaginalis

Candida albicans

Patchy, white, adherent exudate

FIGURE 8-10   TRICHOMONIASIS, MONILIASIS, NONSPECIFIC VAGINITIS, AND CHEMICAL AND TRAUMATIC VAGINITIS

Nonspecific or simple **vaginitis** occurs when the normal vaginal flora of microorganisms proliferate, stimulated by conditions such as age, debility, systemic disease, ovulation, menstruation, or pregnancy. Characteristic features of the infection caused by the protozoan parasite *Trichomonas vaginalis* are a vaginal and cervical epithelium with small petechial hemorrhages producing a "strawberry" appearance and a thin, greenish-yellow discharge containing many small bubbles, producing a foamy appearance.

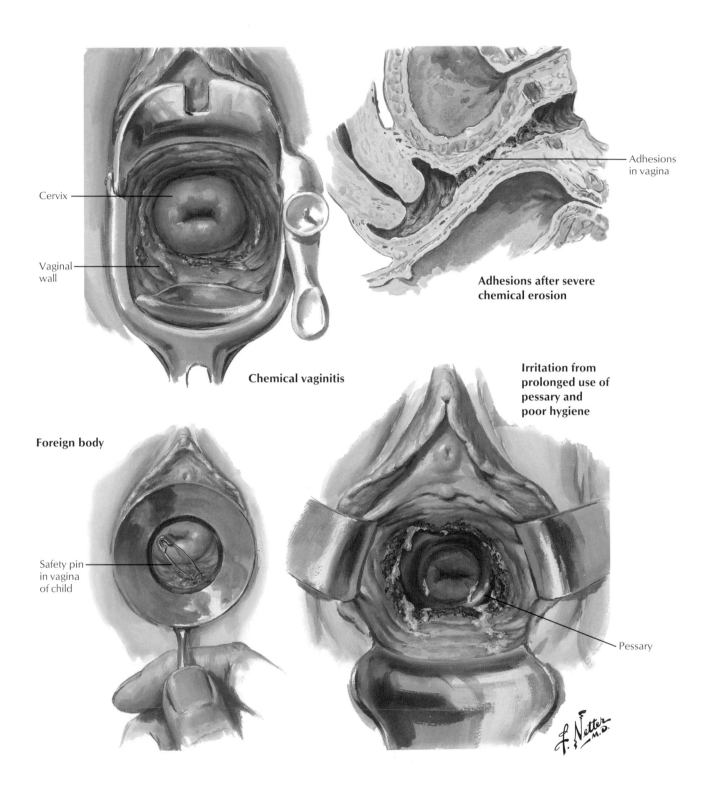

Cervix

Vaginal wall

Adhesions in vagina

Adhesions after severe chemical erosion

Chemical vaginitis

Foreign body

Irritation from prolonged use of pessary and poor hygiene

Safety pin in vagina of child

Pessary

FIGURE 8-10   TRICHOMONIASIS, MONILIASIS, NONSPECIFIC VAGINITIS, AND CHEMICAL AND TRAUMATIC VAGINITIS (CONTINUED)

Vaginal infection due to the fungus *C albicans* (moniliasis) causes an aphthous ulcerative infection with patchy, white exudate that leaves a raw, bleeding surface when it is removed. Predisposing factors are diabetes and previous use of antibiotics. Vaginitis can be produced by chemical irritation from substances in douches and from foreign bodies in the vagina.

Syphilis

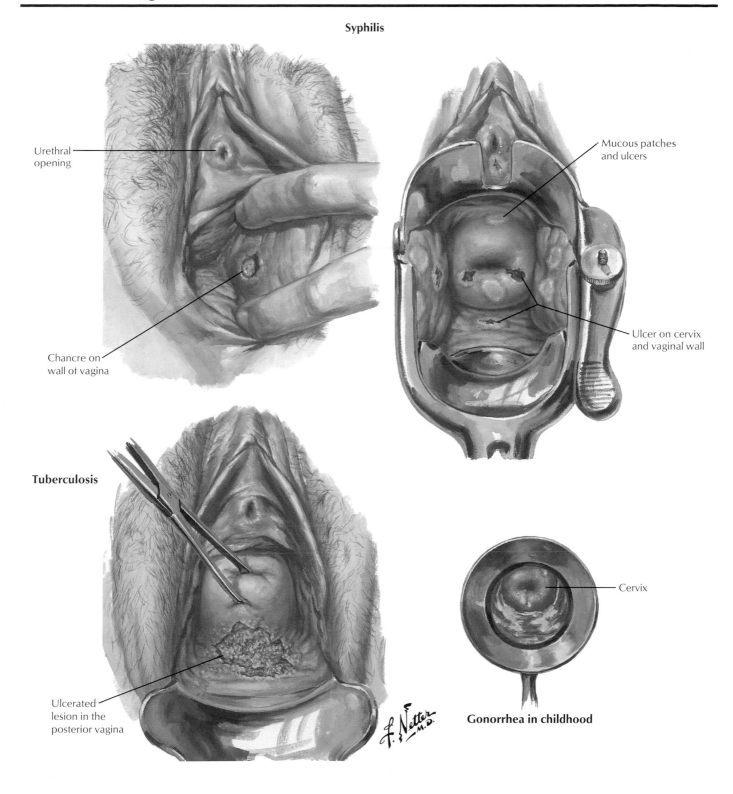

Urethral opening

Chancre on wall of vagina

Mucous patches and ulcers

Ulcer on cervix and vaginal wall

Tuberculosis

Ulcerated lesion in the posterior vagina

Cervix

Gonorrhea in childhood

FIGURE 8-11   SYPHILIS, GONORRHEA, AND TUBERCULOSIS

In the vagina, the syphilis **chancre**, with its raised indurated border surrounded by a shallow ulceration, is most likely to be near the vestibule, and inguinal lymphadenopathy may be present. In the primary stage, serologic test results are often negative, and dark field examination results of a smear from the lesion are positive for treponemes. In late **syphilis**, white mucosal patches that coalesce and ulcerate focally may be present in the vagina and the external genitalia. **Gonorrhea** involves the cervix, but spares the vagina during reproductive life because the vaginal epithelium is resistant to infection by *Neisseria gonorrhoeae*. Gonorrheal vaginitis is a recognized but rare clinical entity in the postmenopausal period and in childhood. **Tuberculosis**, which rarely affects the vagina, is secondary to tuberculosis of the fallopian tubes, the uterus, and the cervix. Typical ulcerated lesions usually involve the posterior vagina.

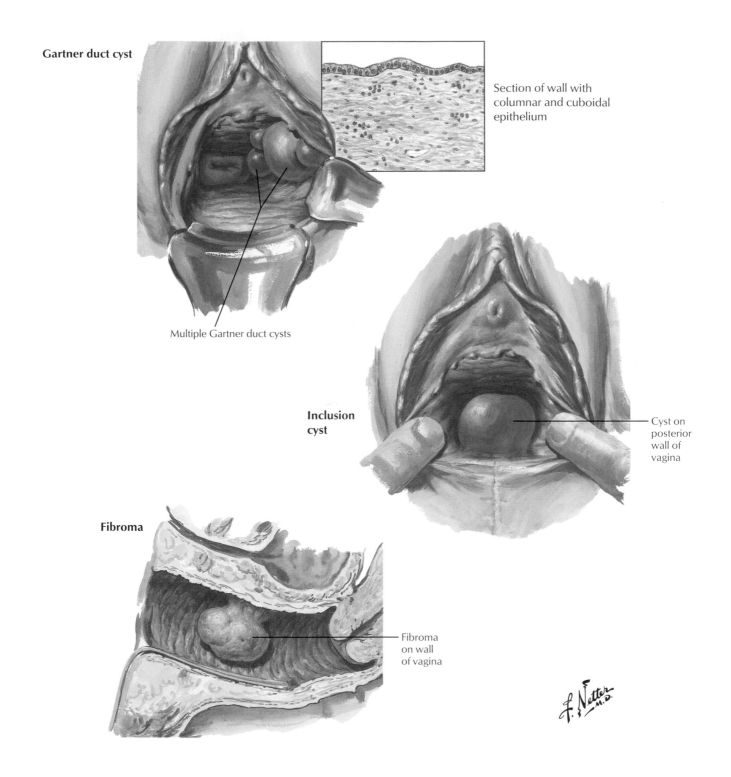

Gartner duct cyst

Section of wall with columnar and cuboidal epithelium

Multiple Gartner duct cysts

Inclusion cyst

Cyst on posterior wall of vagina

Fibroma

Fibroma on wall of vagina

FIGURE 8-12   CYSTS AND PRIMARY BENIGN AND MALIGNANT TUMORS

Most vaginal tumors are **benign cysts**. **Gartner duct cysts** are formed from embryonic epithelial remnants of Wolffian ducts, are located on the anterolateral vaginal walls, may be simple or multiple, and occasionally attain large enough size to produce pain and other symptoms. Congenital cysts of müllerian origin (**inclusion cysts**) may occur in the fornices or lower in the vagina. Malignant tumors include **primary carcinoma of the vagina,** which is usually an SCC that begins as a small growth of the

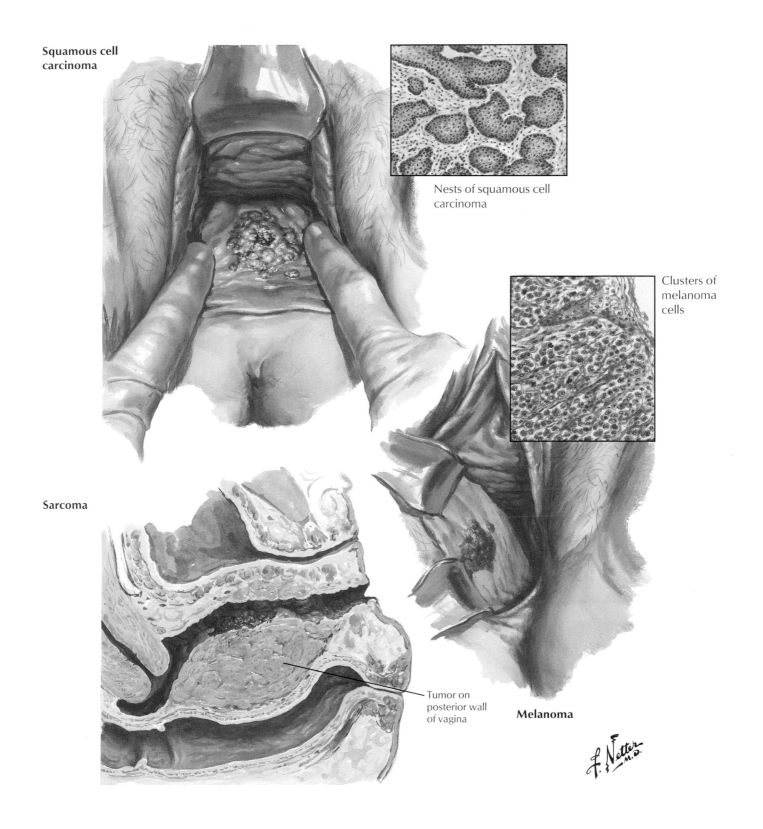

Squamous cell carcinoma

Nests of squamous cell carcinoma

Clusters of melanoma cells

Sarcoma

Tumor on posterior wall of vagina

Melanoma

FIGURE 8-12   CYSTS AND PRIMARY BENIGN AND MALIGNANT TUMORS *(CONTINUED)*

posterior vaginal wall and progresses to infiltrate the vagina and eventually the adjacent pelvic viscera and regional lymphatics, and the rare vaginal sarcomas, fibrosarcoma, and variants in adults and sarcoma botryoides in children. Melanoma of the vagina is unusual, but can occur as an apparently primary lesion or, more commonly, as part of metastatic disease.

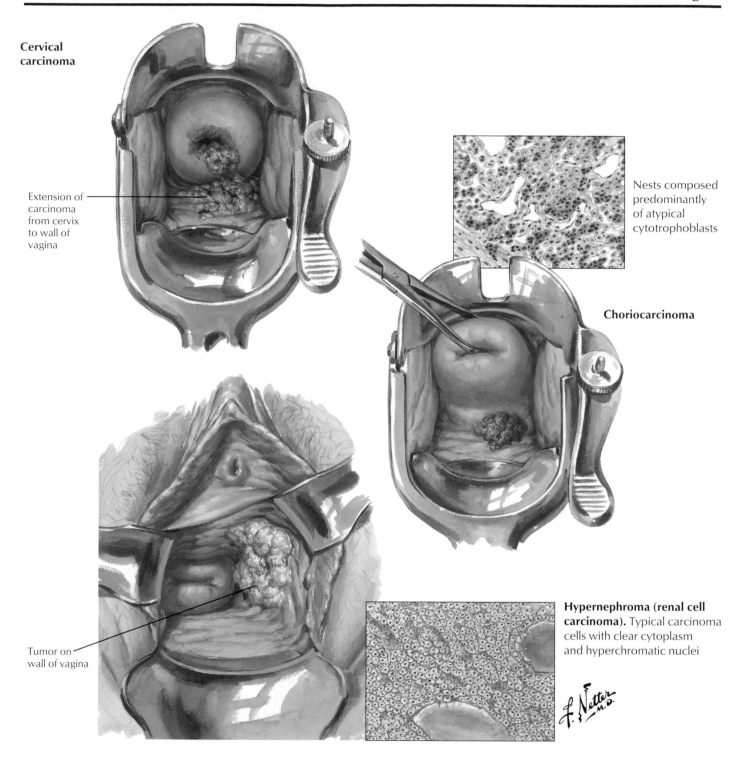

Cervical carcinoma

Extension of carcinoma from cervix to wall of vagina

Nests composed predominantly of atypical cytotrophoblasts

Choriocarcinoma

Tumor on wall of vagina

Hypernephroma (renal cell carcinoma). Typical carcinoma cells with clear cytoplasm and hyperchromatic nuclei

FIGURE 8-13 MALIGNANT TUMORS: METASTASES AND EXTENSION

Approximately 60% of vaginal malignant tumors are secondary to other tumors, most often carcinomas of the cervix or endometrium. After hysterectomy for endometrial carcinoma, the vaginal vault is a common site of recurrence. Vulvar carcinomas may involve some or most of the vagina. The vagina is the most frequent site of **metastases** from uterine choriocarcinoma and may be the earliest clinical manifestation. A history of recent pregnancy may be elicited. The dark-purple hemorrhagic gross appearance and the histologic picture are characteristic. The

lesion is made up of clusters of syncytiotrophoblasts and cytotrophoblasts, with the trophoblastic cells exhibiting large, hyperchromatic nuclei and frequent mitoses. Renal cell carcinoma, or **hypernephroma**, may metastasize to the vagina, forming a nodular, yellow tumor mass, usually composed of clear cells with hyperchromatic nuclei. Metastases or extensions may involve the vagina before or after treatment of carcinomas of the ovary, the bladder, or the rectum.

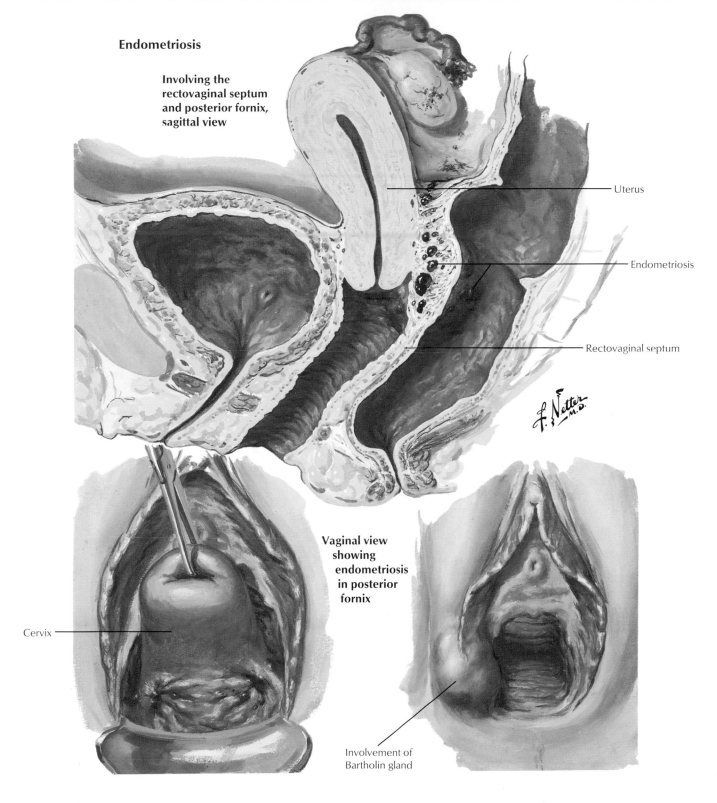

Endometriosis

Involving the rectovaginal septum and posterior fornix, sagittal view

Uterus

Endometriosis

Rectovaginal septum

Cervix

Vaginal view showing endometriosis in posterior fornix

Involvement of Bartholin gland

FIGURE 8-14　ENDOMETRIOSIS OF THE VULVA, THE VAGINA, AND THE CERVIX

Endometriosis is characterized by the presence of hormonally responsive endometrial glands or stroma in abnormal locations outside the uterus. Endometrial tissue can result from retrograde menstruation through the fallopian tubes, metaplasia of coelomic epithelial implants, or vascular or lymphatic dissemination of tissue from the endometrium. Vaginal endometriosis is associated with similar lesions in the ovary and rectovaginal septum. The sagittal section shows a distribution of endometriosis on the surface of the ovary and other implants on the adjacent peritoneum of the posterior cul-de-sac and the lateral pelvic wall. Blue-domed endometrial cysts extend down the rectovaginal septum, which causes the anterior rectal wall to adhere to the posterior surface of the uterus. Occasionally, there may be involvement of the vulva or perineum and, rarely, a Bartholin gland.

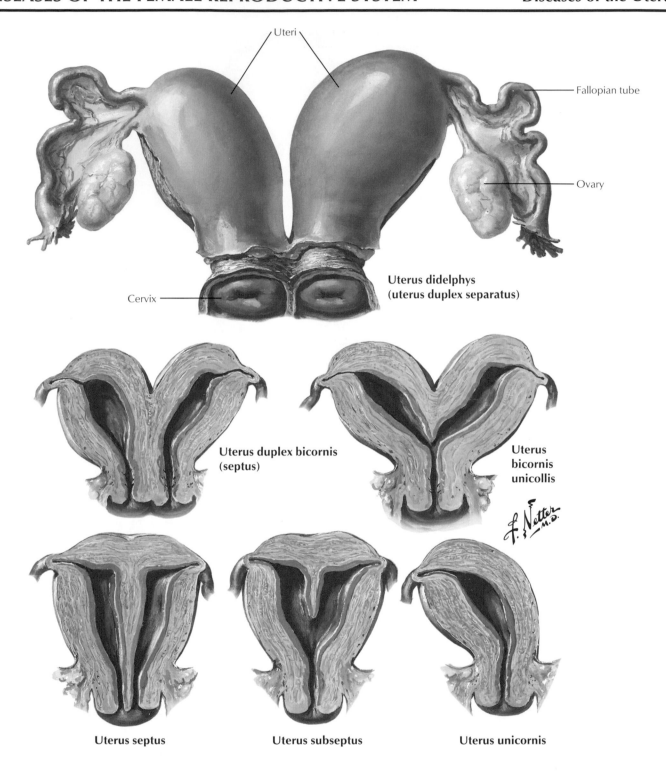

Uterus didelphys (uterus duplex separatus)

Uterus duplex bicornis (septus)

Uterus bicornis unicollis

Uterus septus

Uterus subseptus

Uterus unicornis

FIGURE 8-15 CONGENITAL ANOMALIES OF THE UTERUS

A variety of congenital anomalies are related to the embryologic derivation of the female genital tract from the müllerian ducts. Complete failure of fusion of the müllerian ducts results in the formation of 2 separate genital tracts with completely independent uteri and a fallopian tube attached to the lateral angle of each uterus (**uterus didelphys**). Each uterus can function separately and sustain a normal pregnancy. More frequently, partial fusion of the müllerian ducts takes place, as is the case in the **uterus duplex bicornis**. If failure of fusion occurs only at a higher level, the result is 2 uterine bodies with a single cervix, the **uterus bicornis unicollis**. In some cases, the uterine cavities are completely or partially separated by a thin septum, giving rise to uterus septus or uterus subseptus, respectively. **Uterus unicornis** is a half uterus arising from only 1 formed müllerian duct. **Uterine aplasia** with blind fallopian tubes also is known to occur.

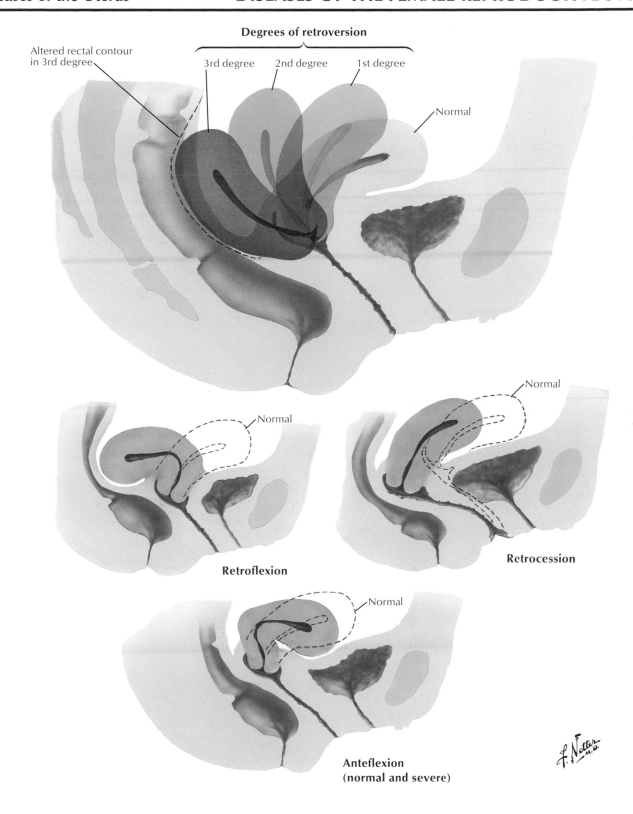

Degrees of retroversion

Altered rectal contour in 3rd degree

3rd degree   2nd degree   1st degree

Normal

Normal

Normal

Retroflexion

Retrocession

Normal

Anteflexion (normal and severe)

FIGURE 8-16   DISPLACEMENTS AND PROLAPSE

Displacement of the uterus occurs when it becomes fixed or rests chronically in an abnormal position. The anatomical configurations are **retroversion**, **retroflexion**, **retrocession**, and **anteflexion**. **Prolapse** refers to descent of the uterus down the vaginal canal so that it lies below its normal position. Some degree of retroversion is present. Usually, this occurs after parturition when the stretched uterine ligamentous supports cannot counteract the usual intraabdominal pressure and the involuting uterus lacks normal myometrial tone. In first-degree prolapse, the cervix does not protrude at the introitus. In second-degree prolapse (procidentia), the cervix protrudes. In complete procidentia, the entire uterus

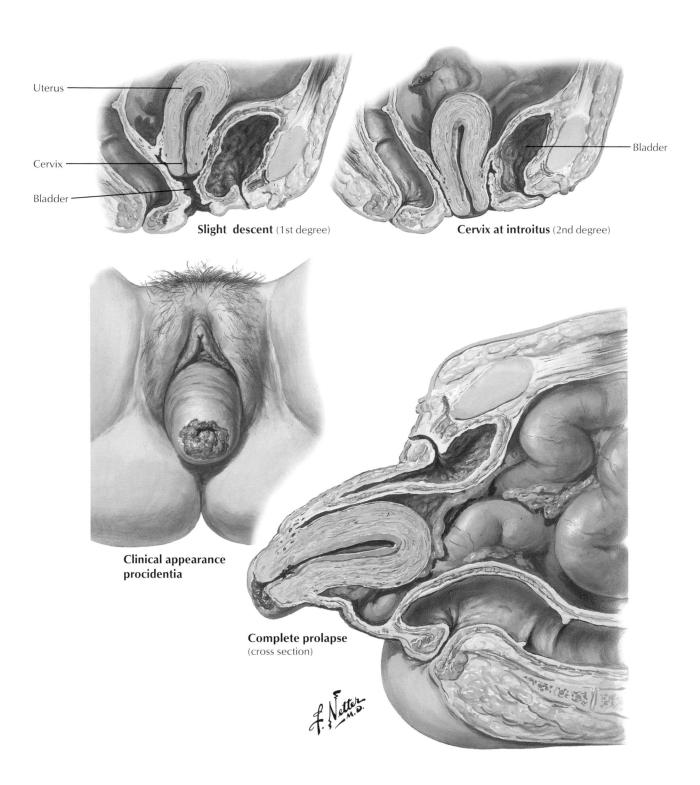

Uterus

Cervix

Bladder

Bladder

Slight descent (1st degree)

Cervix at introitus (2nd degree)

Clinical appearance procidentia

Complete prolapse (cross section)

FIGURE 8-16   DISPLACEMENTS AND PROLAPSE *(CONTINUED)*

protrudes. **Cystocele** and **rectocele** are frequent complications. Spontaneous rupture of the uterus is a rare complication of parturition or may occur during procedures such as dilatation and curettage, especially when there is preexisting displacement with anatomical malposition of the uterus.

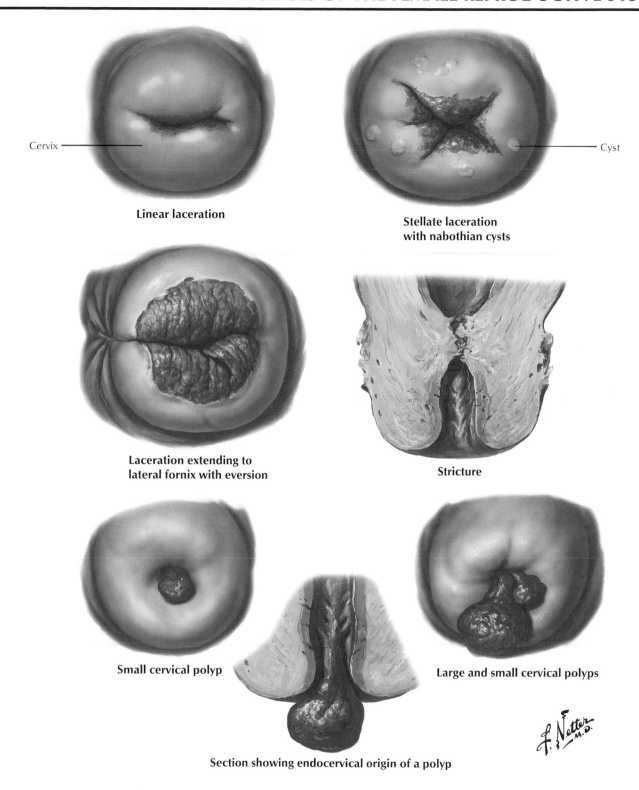

Cervix

Cyst

Linear laceration

**Stellate laceration
with nabothian cysts**

**Laceration extending to
lateral fornix with eversion**

Stricture

Small cervical polyp

Large and small cervical polyps

Section showing endocervical origin of a polyp

FIGURE 8-17   LACERATIONS, STRICTURES, AND POLYPS

Lacerations of the external cervical os are common after parturition, and, barring infection, most heal spontaneously. More complex lacerations penetrate deeply into the endocervical stroma or extend into the lateral fornix, which permits eversion of the lining of the endocervical canal, predisposing to infection. **Stricture** of the internal cervical os, which can result in hematometra (retained menstrual flow and endometrial debris), occurs after posttraumatic or postinfectious scarring, after radiation

therapy, and in rare cases of partial or complete congenital atresia. The uterine mucosa can form **polyps**, which differ from endometrial polyps etiologically and clinically. Endocervical polyps, which are usually benign, typically contain all the elements of the endocervical mucosa (columnar epithelium, fibrous stroma, and glands). As the polyps grow to produce protruding soft, red, granular lesions, they can produce mild vaginal bleeding. The etiology of cervical polyps is unknown.

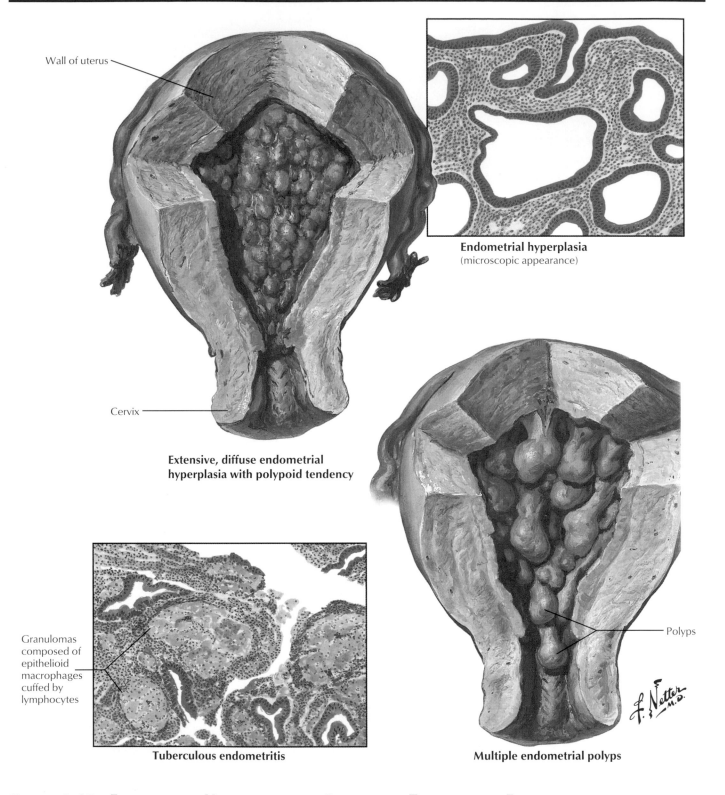

Wall of uterus

Endometrial hyperplasia
(microscopic appearance)

Cervix

**Extensive, diffuse endometrial
hyperplasia with polypoid tendency**

Granulomas
composed of
epithelioid
macrophages
cuffed by
lymphocytes

Polyps

Tuberculous endometritis

Multiple endometrial polyps

FIGURE 8-18 ENDOMETRIAL HYPERPLASIA AND POLYPS AND TUBERCULOUS ENDOMETRITIS

Endometrial hyperplasia occurs under conditions that produce a constant stimulus of estrogen, which prevents the progestational or secretory phase of the menstrual cycle to take place. The gross appearance of endometrial hyperplasia is a thickened and edematous mucosa. Estrogenic stimulation produces an overgrowth of glands, stroma, and microvessels. In long-standing cases, the glands show irregular cystic dilatation with a lining of low cuboidal epithelium, which leads to the "Swiss cheese" pattern. The exuberant growth may be difficult to distinguish from well-differentiated adenocarcinoma. Atypical hyperplasia is defined as complex glandular crowding and cytologic atypia. Endometrial hyperplasia may give rise to single or multiple endometrial polyps. The diagnosis of endometrial hyperplasia usually is made from pathologic examination of endometrial curettings from a woman with abnormal uterine bleeding. Occasionally, examination reveals an infectious process, including tuberculosis. **Tuberculous endometritis** is characterized by caseating granulomas in the endometrial stroma.

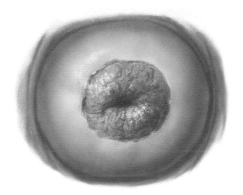

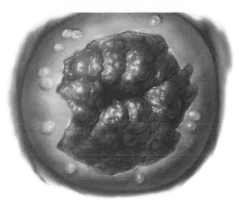

Congenital erosion.
In nulliparous cervix

Extensive erosion with proliferation.
Papillary erosion; also nabothian cysts

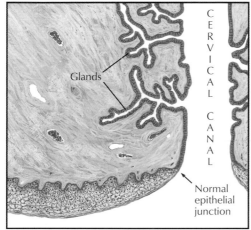

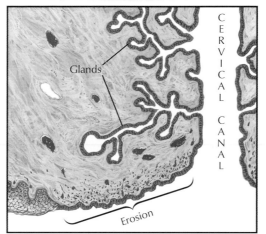

Normal portio vaginalis.
(schematic section)

Portio vaginalis.
(schematic section
showing erosion)

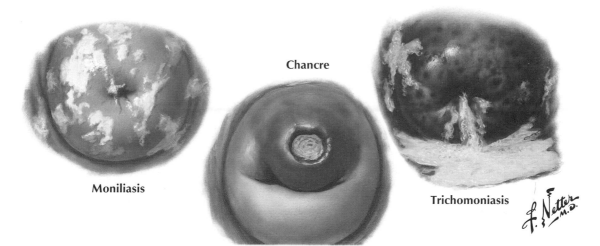

Moniliasis

Chancre

Trichomoniasis

FIGURE 8-19   CERVICITIS: EROSIONS, MONILIASIS, TRICHOMONIASIS, AND SYPHILIS

Exposure of the mucous glands in the endocervical canal, which is often due to erosions from congenital defects or childbirth injuries, is a key factor in initiating cervical infections. The even, concentric appearance of congenital erosions contrasts sharply with the jagged papillary granulomas that usually result from inadequately treated lacerations of childbirth. Spontaneous healing does not occur because the inward growth of squamous epithelium does not cover the infected areas. In areas where healing has occurred, the covering epithelium blocks the exit of previously exposed glands, which produces retention cysts of various sizes (**nabothian cysts**).

Gonorrhea in Women

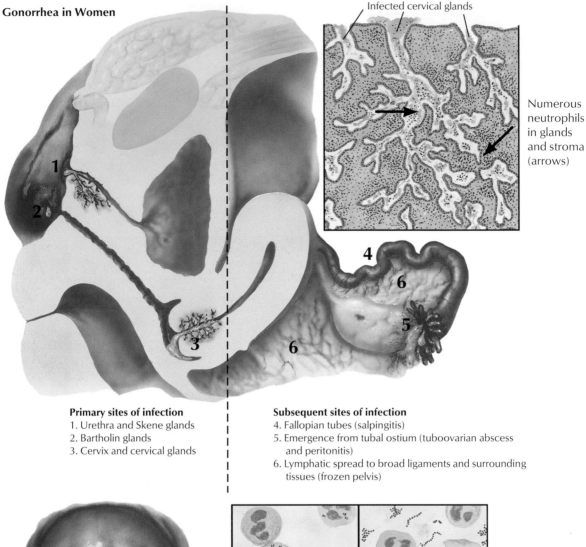

Infected cervical glands

Numerous neutrophils in glands and stroma (arrows)

Primary sites of infection
1. Urethra and Skene glands
2. Bartholin glands
3. Cervix and cervical glands

Subsequent sites of infection
4. Fallopian tubes (salpingitis)
5. Emergence from tubal ostium (tuboovarian abscess and peritonitis)
6. Lymphatic spread to broad ligaments and surrounding tissues (frozen pelvis)

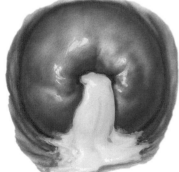

Appearance of cervix in acute infection

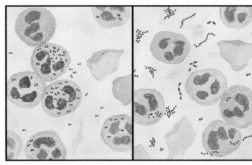

Gonorrheal infection (Gram stain)

Nonspecific infection (Gram stain)

FIGURE 8-20   CERVICITIS: GONORRHEA AND PYOGENIC INFECTIONS

Gonorrheal infection caused by the gram-negative diplococcus *Neisseria gonorrhoeae* is the most common cause of **acute cervicitis**. The infection begins in the lower genital tract and does not ascend to the adnexa until the next menstruation. Initially, acute infection involves the deeply branching cervical and endocervical glands, the urethra and the Skene glands, and the Bartholin glands in the vulva. At the time of menses, the gonorrheal infection ascends through the uterus to the fallopian tubes, which become swollen, inflamed, and tortuous. Inflammation of the endosalpinx leads to extrusion of pus from the edematous fimbriae into the posterior cul-de-sac, causing pelvic peritonitis. Lymphatic involvement of the mesosalpinx can predispose to bacteremia and septicemia. A minority of cases of acute cervicitis is caused by pyogenic infections of cervical glands exposed by unhealed lacerations of childbirth. Gram staining of smears may reveal a mixed bacterial population and neutrophils.

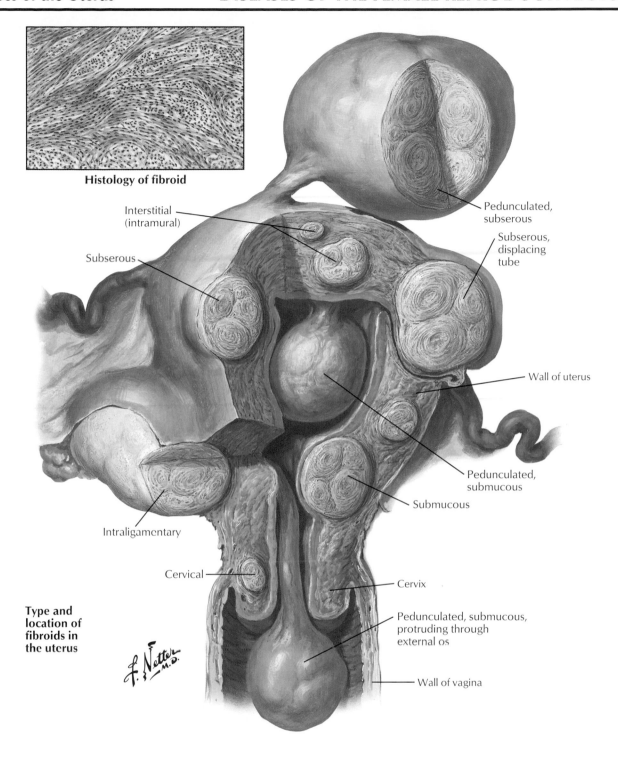

Histology of fibroid

Interstitial (intramural)

Subserous

Pedunculated, subserous

Subserous, displacing tube

Wall of uterus

Pedunculated, submucous

Submucous

Intraligamentary

Cervical

Cervix

Pedunculated, submucous, protruding through external os

Wall of vagina

Type and location of fibroids in the uterus

F. Netter, M.D.

FIGURE 8-21 LEIOMYOMA (FIBROID)

Uterine myomata, the most common tumors in the female pelvis, have an incidence of approximately 4% to 11% in adult women. Commonly called **fibroids**, these tumors are composed of benign proliferations of uterine smooth muscle cells with a typical whorled pattern on histologic examination and are, therefore, **leiomyomata**. The tumors, which vary in size, location, and position (intramural, subserous, or submucosal), occur most frequently in the fifth decade of life and are more common in black women. **Leiomyomata** also are found in the cervix and broad ligament (intraligamentary myoma). The most common symptom, profuse or prolonged uterine bleeding, occurs in approximately 50% of cases. The uterine bleeding and the growth of the leiomyomata may have a common cause in excess estrogen stimulation, so that excision of the leiomyoma may or may not cure the uterine bleeding.

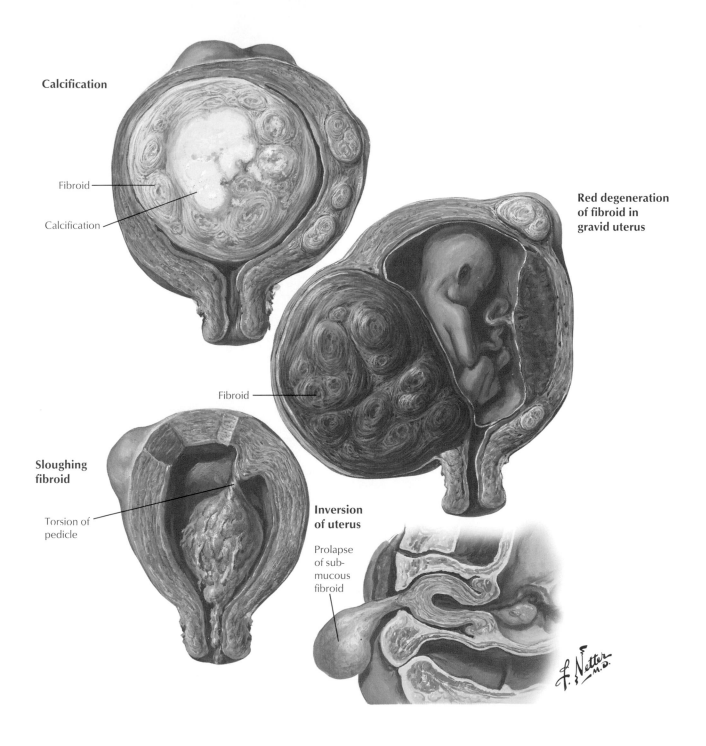

Calcification

Fibroid

Calcification

Red degeneration
of fibroid in
gravid uterus

Fibroid

Sloughing
fibroid

Torsion of
pedicle

Inversion
of uterus

Prolapse
of sub-
mucous
fibroid

FIGURE 8-22 LEIOMYOMA: SECONDARY CHANGES

The evaluation of infertility should take uterine leiomyomata into account, particularly if there are submucous myomas. Indications for surgery, either removal of the leiomyoma (leiomyectomy) or hysterectomy, include recurrent uterine bleeding, pelvic pressure, pelvic pain, and rapid growth suggesting sarcomatous transformation. Pedunculated submucous leiomyomas are prone to torsion of the pedicle, cutting off the blood supply and causing sloughing and necrosis. Occasionally, a myoma on a long pedicle can prolapse through the cervix and cause complete inversion of the uterus. Large leiomyomas sometimes exceed their blood supply, leading to cystic degeneration and calcification. Leiomyomas may not affect a successful pregnancy but, if located in the cervix, may obstruct the passage of the fetal head through the birth canal. During pregnancy, the vascular supply to an interstitial leiomyoma may become compromised, leading to necrosis and hemorrhage, so-called red degeneration, which may become a serious complication.

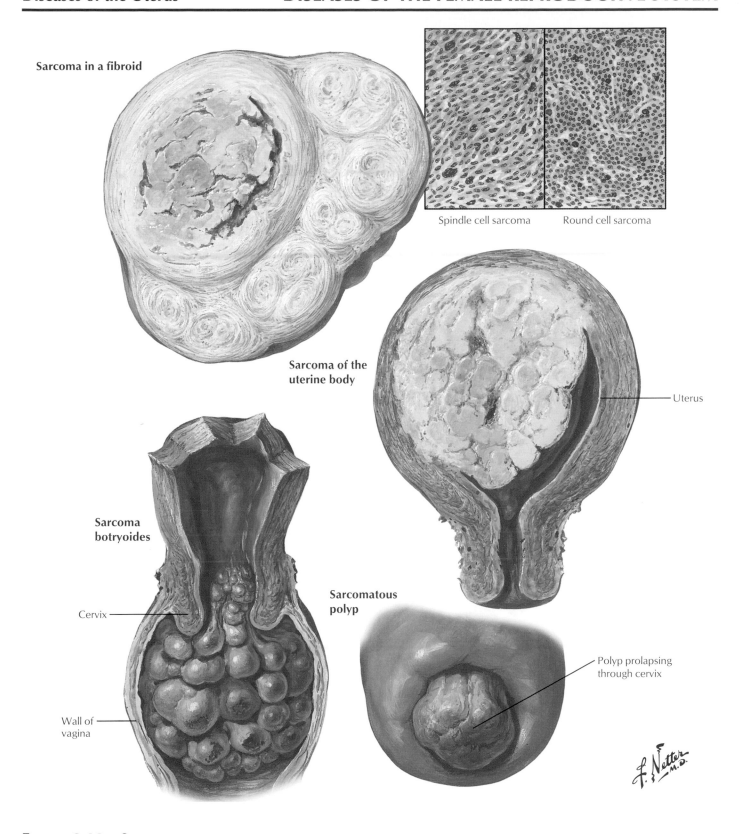

Sarcoma in a fibroid

Spindle cell sarcoma   Round cell sarcoma

Sarcoma of the
uterine body

Uterus

Sarcoma
botryoides

Cervix

Wall of
vagina

Sarcomatous
polyp

Polyp prolapsing
through cervix

FIGURE 8-23 SARCOMA

Sarcoma of the uterus accounts for approximately 3% to 4% of malignancies of the female genital tract. Uterine sarcomas, whether primary or secondary to a preexisting fibroid (rate of sarcomatous degeneration is approximately 1%), grow rapidly and have a grave prognosis. Sarcomas arising in a fibroid appear grossly as soft, meaty areas, often with foci of central necrosis or hemorrhage due to an inadequate blood supply. The size and extent of tumor are more important for prognosis than is location or histologic characteristics. Histologically, the sarcoma cells may be spindle-shaped or round and show nuclear pleomorphism and mitoses. Occasionally, uterine polyps show sarcomatous degeneration. **Sarcoma botryoides** ("grape" sarcoma) is a rare and almost invariably fatal condition that occurs only in young children.

Cervical Cell Pathology in Squamous Tissue

Grades and cell types

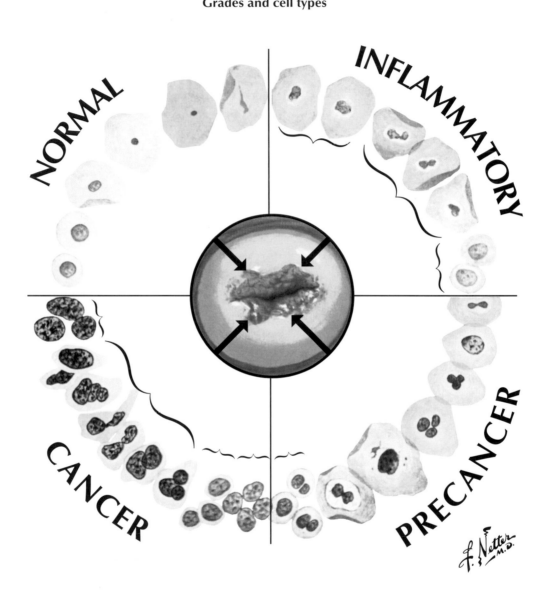

FIGURE 8-24   CERVICAL CANCER: CYTOLOGY

Cervical carcinoma, a slow-growing neoplasm confined for several years to the surface epithelium as a noninvasive growth, is caused by infection by strains of HPV, including HPV-16, 18, 31, and 33. The in situ lesions in the early stage of the disease can be detected by screening with exfoliative cytology of cervical scrapings and vaginal smears (Pap smear) and confirmed by cervical biopsy. In cytologic preparations, cells of the squamous epithelium are classified as basal, parabasal, intermediate,

precornified, cornified (keratinizing), and hypercornified. These epithelial cells show a variety of changes during inflammatory processes. The squamous cells show changes generally classified as CIN, ranging from mild dysplasia (CIN grade I) to **carcinoma in situ** (CIN III), and invasive cancer. These changes are characterized by progressive nuclear enlargement, hyperchromasia, atypia, loss of maturation, and anaplasia. Viral changes may be especially prominent in CIN I.

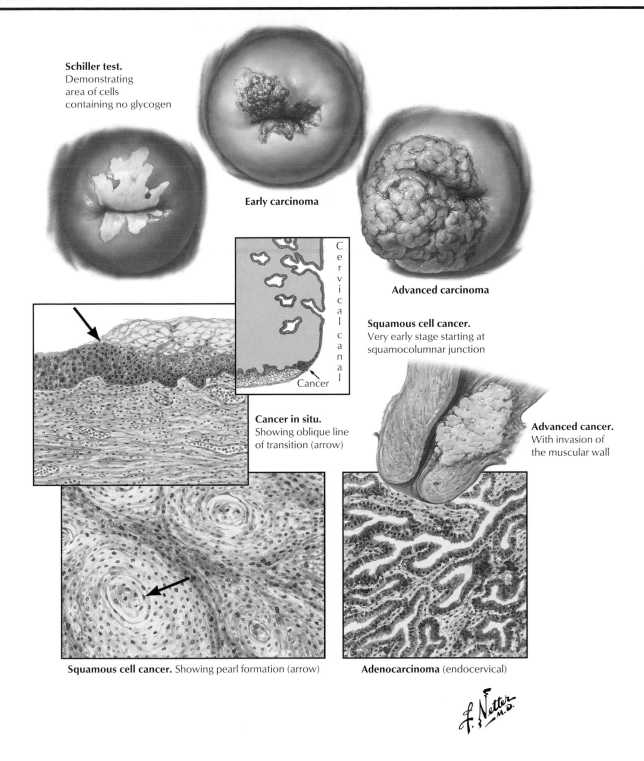

Schiller test. Demonstrating area of cells containing no glycogen

Early carcinoma

Advanced carcinoma

Cervical canal

Cancer

Cancer in situ. Showing oblique line of transition (arrow)

Squamous cell cancer. Very early stage starting at squamocolumnar junction

Advanced cancer. With invasion of the muscular wall

Squamous cell cancer. Showing pearl formation (arrow)

Adenocarcinoma (endocervical)

FIGURE 8-25　CERVICAL CANCER: STAGES AND TYPES

Surface carcinoma, CIN grade III, typically originates at the squamocolumnar junction of the cervix and appears histologically as a complete lack of normal basal to surface maturation of the epithelium, coupled with marked nuclear atypia of the cervical epithelial cells. Invasive **SCC** is characterized by the extension of sheets of atypical squamous cells forming foci of keratinization (epithelial pearls) into the cervical stroma. **Adenocarcinoma** arises from the endocervical glands and invades the stroma by atypical glandular epithelium. **Cervical cancer** follows a standard pattern of extension involving the lymphatic channels and direct invasion of adjacent organs. It is characterized histologically according to degree of differentiation (anaplasia) from grade I to grade IV and clinically according to spread of disease from stage 0 to stage IV. Death is more common from uremia secondary to obstructions from local disease than from late metastases to the liver, the lungs, or the bones.

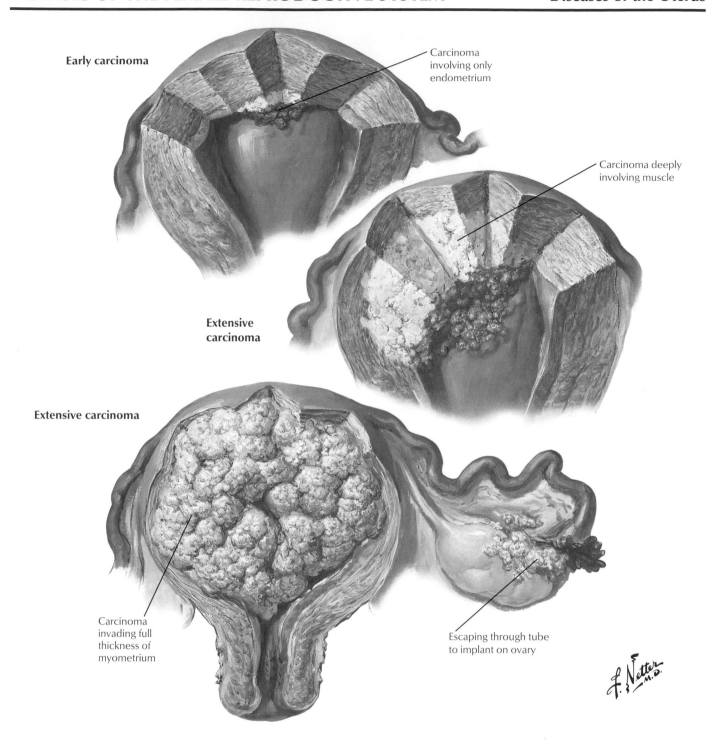

Early carcinoma

Carcinoma involving only endometrium

Carcinoma deeply involving muscle

Extensive carcinoma

Extensive carcinoma

Carcinoma invading full thickness of myometrium

Escaping through tube to implant on ovary

FIGURE 8-26   CANCER OF THE UTERINE CORPUS: STAGES AND TYPES

The differential diagnosis of abnormal vaginal bleeding or discharge, particularly in postmenopausal women, should include **adenocarcinoma of the uterus**. Detection of **endometrial carcinoma** in a curettage specimen is diagnostic. Stage 0 designates lesions limited to focal areas of the mucosa. Stage I refers to tumor involving the full thickness of the mucosa, with invasion of the myometrium but limited to the uterus. Stage II indicates tumor that has involved the corpus uteri and the cervix. Stage III and IV designate a cancer that has extended beyond the

uterus, including direct extension through the uterine wall or transmigration of cancer cells through the fallopian tubes with implantation on the ovaries. Fractional curettage defines the site of origin of the carcinoma: (1) those that involve only the corpus, (2) those arising only from the endocervix, and (3) those involving both the corpus and endocervix. The importance of the site of origin for staging and therapy reflects different routes of lymphatic spread and invasion.

Extensive carcinoma

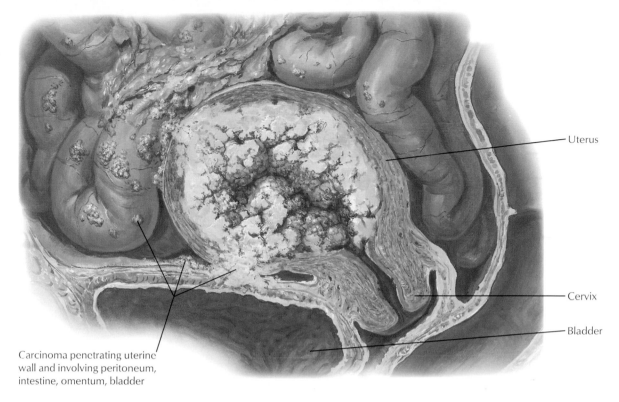

Uterus

Cervix

Bladder

Carcinoma penetrating uterine wall and involving peritoneum, intestine, omentum, bladder

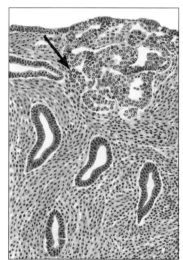

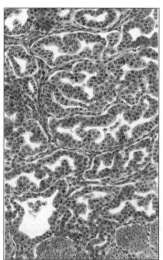

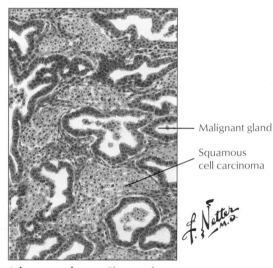

Malignant gland

Squamous cell carcinoma

Carcinoma in situ (stage 0). Focus of crowded glands with atypical cells (arrow)

Adenocarcinoma. Large cluster of abnormal glands with atypical cells

Adenoacanthoma. Sheets of squamous cell carcinoma mixed with malignant glands

FIGURE 8-27 CANCER OF THE UTERINE CORPUS: HISTOLOGY AND EXTENSION

The histopathologic diagnosis of **adenocarcinoma** can be difficult, particularly differentiation from an atypical adenomatous hyperplasia of the endometrium. Foci of adenocarcinoma are characterized by crowded, back-to-back glands lined by thickened layers of epithelial cells exhibiting nuclear hyperchromasia and atypia. Most lesions are pure adenocarcinomas, but some lesions, termed **adenoacanthomas**, have islands or sheets of squamous carcinoma intermingled with the malignant glands.

Location and stage of disease are of paramount importance prognostically, but the more anaplastic tumors may be expected to grow more rapidly and to metastasize earlier than the more mature adenocarcinomas. Successful therapy depends on surgical removal of the disease while it is confined to the uterus. Radiation treatment is used as adjunct therapy. Death from distant metastases to vital organs occurs more often in endometrial carcinoma than in cervical neoplasms.

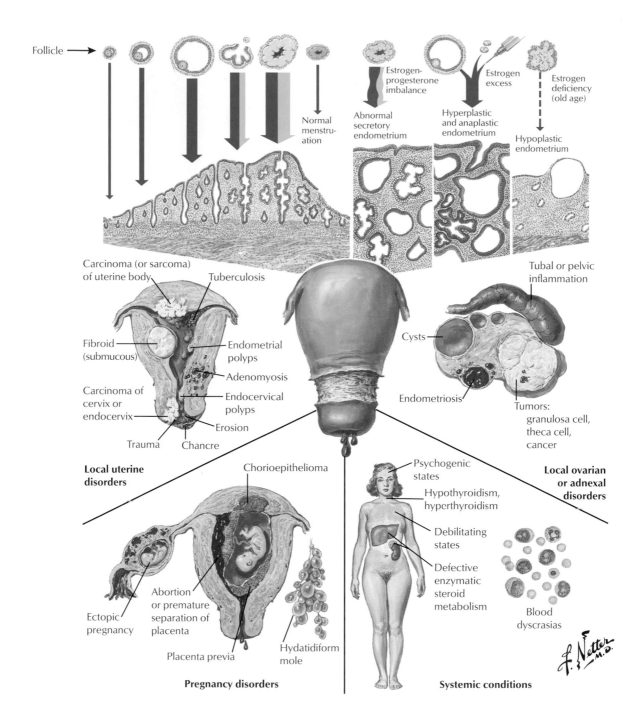

FIGURE 8-28   FUNCTIONAL AND PATHOLOGIC CAUSES OF UTERINE BLEEDING

Normal desquamation of the uterine mucosa with menstrual bleeding is controlled through a delicate balance of pituitary and ovarian hormones and the response of the target tissue, the endometrium. Steroid withdrawal bleeding is often associated with persistent estrogen phases and anovulatory cycles. It may follow a state of estrogen-progesterone imbalance, which produces an abnormal secretory endometrium. Excess estrogen produces hyperplastic and anaplastic endometrium, while an estrogen deficiency produces a hypoplastic endometrium. The major categories of pathologic states that can cause or be accompanied by **menorrhagia** (heavy or prolonged menstrual flow) or **metrorrhagia** (spotting or bleeding between menstrual flows) are illustrated.

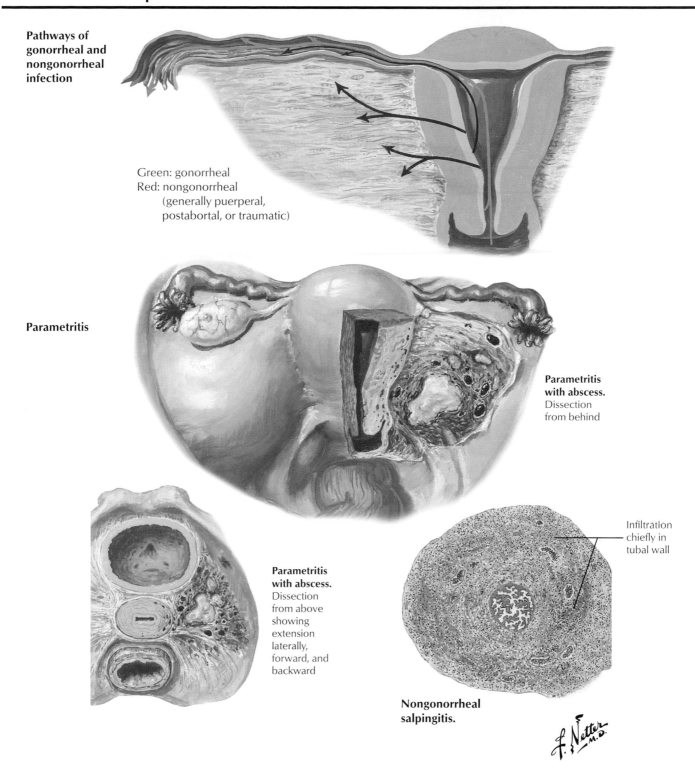

Pathways of gonorrheal and nongonorrheal infection

Green: gonorrheal
Red: nongonorrheal
(generally puerperal, postabortal, or traumatic)

Parametritis

Parametritis with abscess. Dissection from behind

Parametritis with abscess. Dissection from above showing extension laterally, forward, and backward

Infiltration chiefly in tubal wall

Nongonorrheal salpingitis.

FIGURE 8-29   ACUTE SALPINGITIS: PATHWAYS OF INFECTION AND PARAMETRITIS

Because the fallopian tubes traverse between the uterus and the ovaries, infection can spread from either the uterus or the ovaries to involve the fallopian tubes producing an **acute salpingitis**. The opening of the tubes into the peritoneal cavity predisposes the tubes to peritoneal infections, especially appendicitis. Infection by the hematogenous route also may occur as in tuberculosis. Gonococci and most other bacteria reach the tubes by way of the mucous membranes of the vagina and the uterus. Gonococci produce a relatively superficial infection of the mucosa, whereas streptococci and staphylococci typically spread from the mucosa into the uterine wall and invade the adjacent lymphatics, blood vessels, and adjacent pelvic connective tissue, where the most prominent changes with these infections occur. These changes constitute a **purulent parametritis**, lymphangitis, and thrombophlebitis. Occasionally, a parametrial abscess forms.

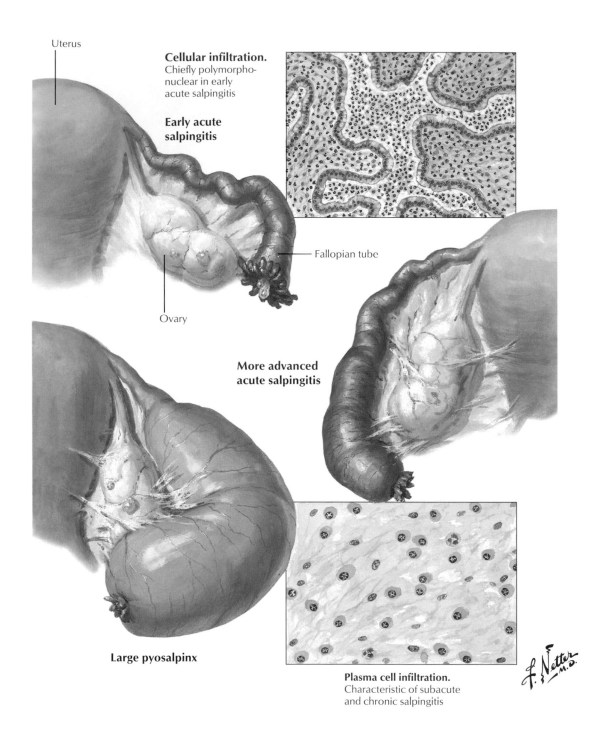

Uterus

Cellular infiltration. Chiefly polymorpho-nuclear in early acute salpingitis

Early acute salpingitis

Fallopian tube

Ovary

More advanced acute salpingitis

Large pyosalpinx

Plasma cell infiltration. Characteristic of subacute and chronic salpingitis

FIGURE 8-30   ACUTE SALPINGITIS: PYOSALPINX

Acute salpingitis is characterized by an edematous, hyperemic, and tortuous fallopian tube with thickened mucosal folds, pus-filled lumen, and a fibrinous or fibrinopurulent exudate on the serosa (**perisalpingitis**). In gonorrheal salpingitis, the infiltrate is located chiefly in the mucosa. In nongonorrheal salpingitis, the entire wall is inflamed. The loss of epithelium and inflammatory exudate often leads to adhesions of the edematous folds of mucosa. The acute stage is followed by a subacute and eventu-ally by a chronic inflammatory stage. Complications include unilateral or bilateral partial or complete closure of the ampullary ostium, the uterine end, or both the uterine and ampullary sections of the tubes. The closure leads to progressive distention of the tube, forming a sausage-shaped structure called a **pyosal-pinx**. The thick contents of the tube liquefy gradually to become serous or serosanguinous fluid, thus transforming the pyosalpinx into a **hydrosalpinx**.

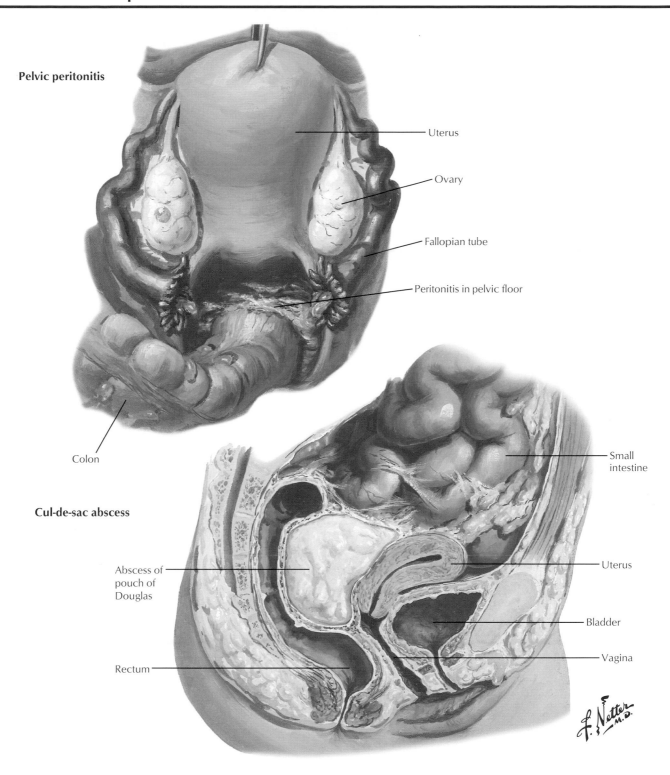

Pelvic peritonitis

Uterus

Ovary

Fallopian tube

Peritonitis in pelvic floor

Colon

Cul-de-sac abscess

Abscess of pouch of Douglas

Small intestine

Uterus

Bladder

Vagina

Rectum

FIGURE 8-31   PELVIC PERITONITIS: ABSCESS

Pelvic peritonitis can result from spillage of the purulent contents of an infected fallopian tube with a patent ampullary ostium or, with obstructed tubes, from spread of tubal lymphangitis and perisalpingitis or rupture of a tube. The severity and extent of the peritonitis depend on the type and virulence of the pathogenic bacteria, the resistance of the patient, and the efficacy of treatment. A pelvoperitoneal abscess, or **abscess of pouch of Douglas**, results when the pus that has accumulated in the cul-de-sac between the uterus and the rectum becomes sealed off from the rest of the peritoneal cavity by fibrous adhesions between the pelvic organs and the overlying intestinal loops. Pelvic peritonitis usually results in formation of multiple adhesions, which can lead to uterine retroflexion and accompanying pelvic symptomatology. Kinking and fibrosis of the fallopian tubes can lead to infertility.

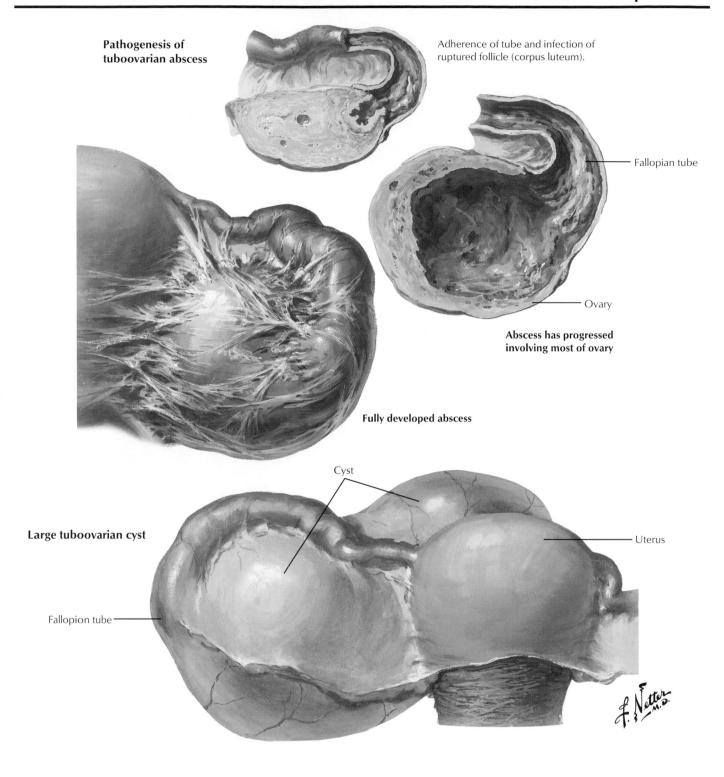

Pathogenesis of tuboovarian abscess

Adherence of tube and infection of ruptured follicle (corpus luteum).

Fallopian tube

Ovary

Abscess has progressed involving most of ovary

Fully developed abscess

Cyst

Large tuboovarian cyst

Uterus

Fallopion tube

FIGURE 8-32   TUBOOVARIAN ABSCESS

Salpingo-oophoritis is an inflammatory disease involving the ovaries and the fallopian tubes. A **tuboovarian abscess** forms when a pyosalpinx communicates with a ruptured ovarian follicle or corpus luteum. The ovary may be the site of a bacterial infection or may be involved secondarily from inflammation of the adjacent tube. Generally, follicular or luteal abscesses develop as complications of pelvic peritonitis, whereas ovarian

stromal abscesses are usually due to hematogenous dissemination of bacteria. In rare cases, a tuboovarian abscess may gradually become a **tuboovarian cyst**, which consists of the dilated tube in communication with a large ovarian cyst. The pelvis also may contain **mesonephric cysts** (congenital cysts) and **multiple loculated cysts** from *Echinococcus* infestations (the tapeworm, *Echinococcus granulosus*).

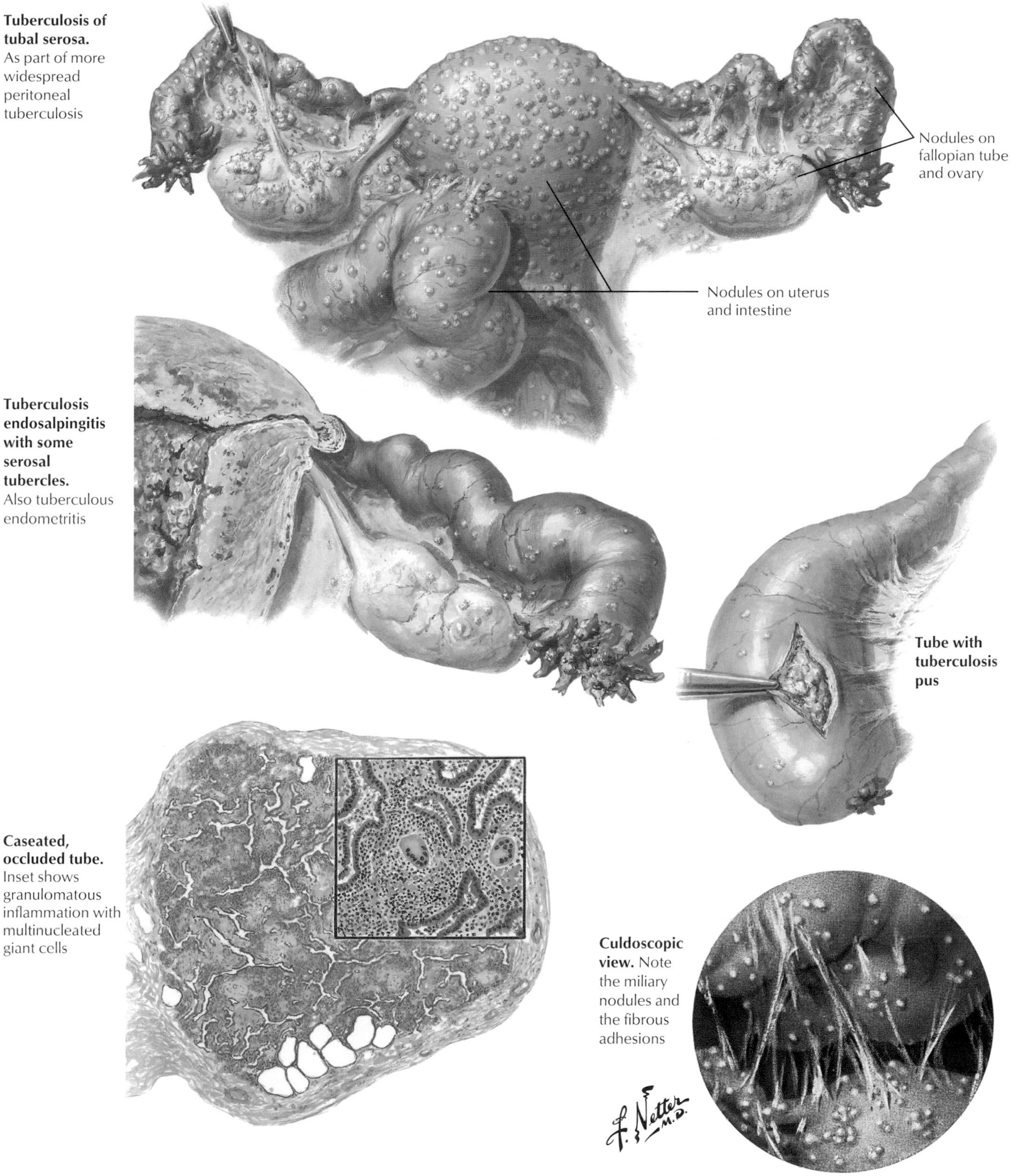

Tuberculosis of tubal serosa. As part of more widespread peritoneal tuberculosis

Nodules on fallopian tube and ovary

Nodules on uterus and intestine

Tuberculosis endosalpingitis with some serosal tubercles. Also tuberculous endometritis

Tube with tuberculosis pus

Caseated, occluded tube. Inset shows granulomatous inflammation with multinucleated giant cells

Culdoscopic view. Note the miliary nodules and the fibrous adhesions

FIGURE 8-33   TUBERCULOSIS

Hematogenous dissemination of *Mycobacterium tuberculosis*, usually from a primary focus in the lungs or hilar lymph nodes, can result in tuberculous infection of the uterus, tubes, and pelvic peritoneum. Usually, both tubes are involved in association with **tuberculous peritonitis**, and the uterus is involved in approximately half of the cases. Grossly, multiple small nodules consis-tent with the miliary pattern of tuberculosis are observed. The tubes exhibit caseous necrosis and granulomatous inflammation. The pelvic infectious process can be insidious, and the diagnosis can be difficult to make. The disease process can be exacerbated if diffuse peritonitis develops or if a secondary pyogenic bacterial infection occurs.

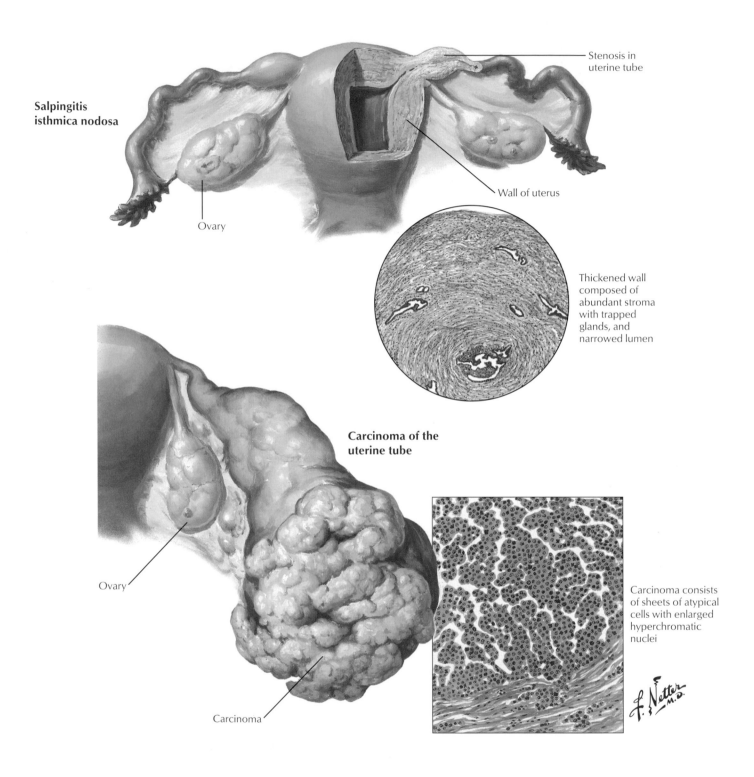

Salpingitis isthmica nodosa

Stenosis in uterine tube

Ovary

Wall of uterus

Thickened wall composed of abundant stroma with trapped glands, and narrowed lumen

Carcinoma of the uterine tube

Ovary

Carcinoma

Carcinoma consists of sheets of atypical cells with enlarged hyperchromatic nuclei

FIGURE 8-34   SALPINGITIS ISTHMICA NODOSA AND CARCINOMA

Salpingitis isthmica nodosa, a benign proliferation of stroma and glands similar to uterine adenomyosis, results in an enlargement with stenosis of the inner, isthmic portion of the tubes. Primary neoplasms of the uterine tubes are uncommon and may arise from epithelium (papillomas, adenomas, carcinomas, choriocarcinomas) or the mesenchymal tissue (fibromas, angiomas, leiomyomas, myomas). The carcinomas may be primary in the tubal mucosa or may occur as a metastasis from a primary carcinoma of the ovary, the uterus, or the gastrointestinal tract. The primary carcinomas have the appearance of a distended tube filled with a protuberant growth of neoplastic tissue with multiple papillary projections. The lesions spread by peritoneal implantation as well as by lymphatic and hematogenous metastases. Diagnosis is usually late, and the prognosis is poor.

Turner Syndrome

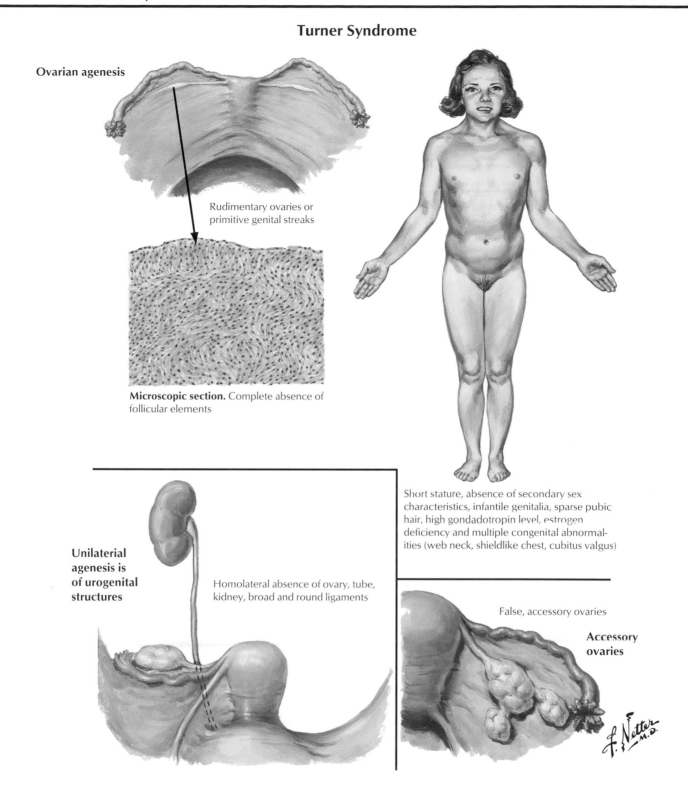

Ovarian agenesis

Rudimentary ovaries or primitive genital streaks

Microscopic section. Complete absence of follicular elements

Short stature, absence of secondary sex characteristics, infantile genitalia, sparse pubic hair, high gondadotropin level, estrogen deficiency and multiple congenital abnormalities (web neck, shieldlike chest, cubitus valgus)

Unilateral agenesis is of urogenital structures

Homolateral absence of ovary, tube, kidney, broad and round ligaments

False, accessory ovaries

Accessory ovaries

Figure 8-35   Developmental Abnormalities

Turner syndrome (ovarian agenesis, ovarian dwarfism) is due to a major defect in ovarian development. This syndrome results from complete or partial monosomy of the X chromosome with a 45, XO karyotype in most subjects and various deletions in 1 of the 2 X chromosomes in the remaining subjects. Turner syndrome is characterized by short stature, infantile genitalia, primary amenorrhea, failure of development of secondary sex features, and multiple congenital abnormalities (web neck, shieldlike chest, cubitus valgus, coarctation of the aorta). The ovaries are rudimentary and consist of stroma without germ cells or follicles. **Less common developmental anomalies** include absence of one ovary and tube, ectopic ovary, and accessory ovaries.

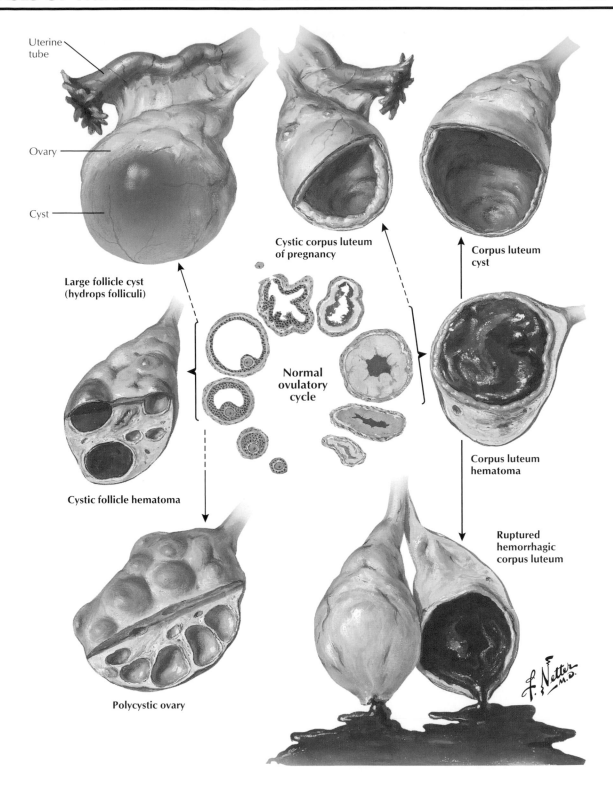

FIGURE 8-36 PHYSIOLOGIC VARIATIONS AND NONNEOPLASTIC CYSTS

Most small and simple cysts in the ovary represent variations of the normal ovulatory cycle. These cysts are derived from ovarian follicles and corpora lutea and are nonneoplastic but may be mimicked by a small neoplastic ovarian cyst. A **corpus luteum of pregnancy** can become large and cystic and can be suspected of being an EP. **Follicle cysts** are distended atretic follicles up to 1 cm in diameter. A polycystic ovary contains multiple cystic follicles. **Hydrops folliculi** refers to an unusually large follicle cyst

that is several centimeters in diameter. A **follicle cyst hematoma** may result from bleeding into the cyst from the vascularized perifollicular thecal zone. A similar mechanism can produce a corpus luteum hematoma. Resorption of the hematoma produces a **corpus luteal cyst,** which can convert to a corpus albicans cyst lined by dense collagen. A ruptured Graafian follicle or hemorrhagic corpus luteum gives rise to intraabdominal bleeding.

Pelvis—Sites of Implantation

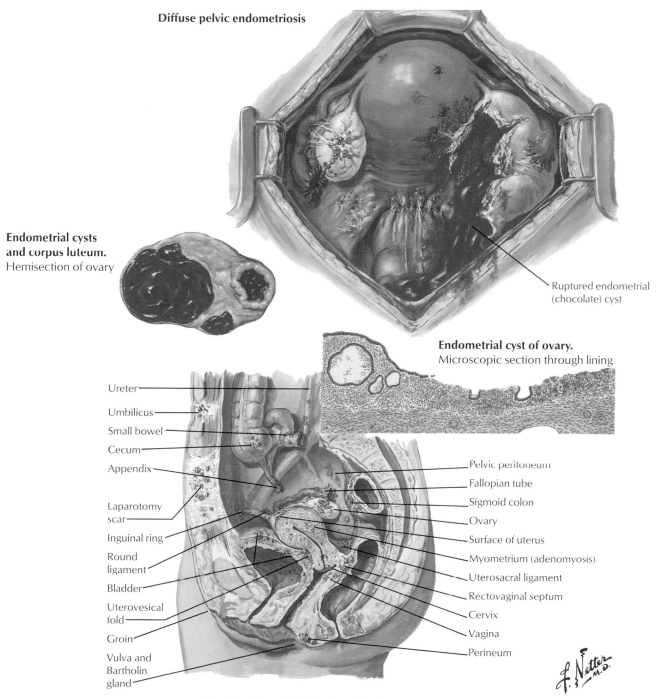

Diffuse pelvic endometriosis

Endometrial cysts and corpus luteum.
Hemisection of ovary

Ruptured endometrial (chocolate) cyst

Endometrial cyst of ovary.
Microscopic section through lining

Ureter
Umbilicus
Small bowel
Cecum
Appendix
Laparotomy scar
Inguinal ring
Round ligament
Bladder
Uterovesical fold
Groin
Vulva and Bartholin gland

Pelvic peritoneum
Fallopian tube
Sigmoid colon
Ovary
Surface of uterus
Myometrium (adenomyosis)
Uterosacral ligament
Rectovaginal septum
Cervix
Vagina
Perineum

Possible sites of distribution of endometriosis

FIGURE 8-37 ENDOMETRIOSIS OF THE PELVIS

Pelvic endometriosis results from the nonneoplastic growth of aberrant or ectopic endometrium in response to stimulation by estrogen and progesterone. Pelvic lesions result from periodic proliferation of the aberrant tissue, infiltration of local structures, recurrent bleeding, and fibrosis. Symptoms include sterility, dysmenorrhea, sacral and pelvic pain, and abnormal uterine bleeding. Endometriosis of the ovary occurs as small surface implants, small hemorrhagic cysts within the cortex, or large dark-brown cysts filled with old blood with the appearance of thick chocolate (**chocolate cysts**). The distribution of the cysts and associated fibrous adhesions render them prone to rupture on manipulation with escape of large quantities of thick, chocolate-colored fluid. The cyst wall may exhibit a lining of typical endometrial stroma and glands, but older lesions may show little evidence of endometrial tissue.

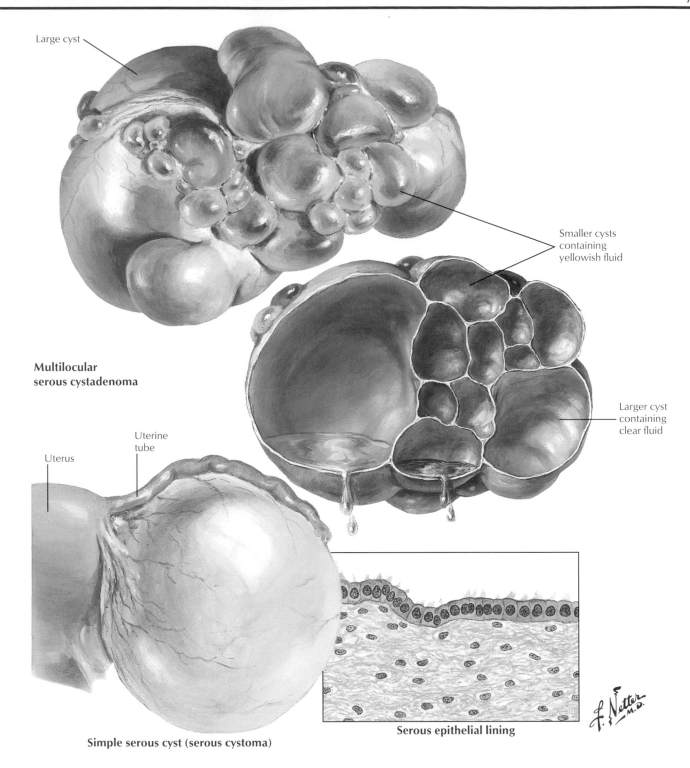

Large cyst

Smaller cysts containing yellowish fluid

Multilocular serous cystadenoma

Larger cyst containing clear fluid

Uterus

Uterine tube

Serous epithelial lining

Simple serous cyst (serous cystoma)

FIGURE 8-38   SEROUS CYSTOMA AND SEROUS CYSTADENOMA

Cystadenomas comprise a group of common benign ovarian neoplasms. Serous cysts include a connective tissue and an epithelial component, with variable predominance of these components. The simple **serous cyst** (serous cystoma) is a unilocular cyst lined by a simple cuboidal layer of serous epithelium. It is usually unilateral, smooth surfaced, and grayish-white and contains clear, serous, watery fluid. The

serous cystadenoma is a unilocular or multilocular serous cyst of the ovary that contains glandlike, epithelial foci in its wall. These lesions are frequently bilateral and are composed of multiple interconnecting cysts of various sizes. Histologically, the cyst walls are lined by a single layer of cuboidal or low columnar ciliated epithelium.

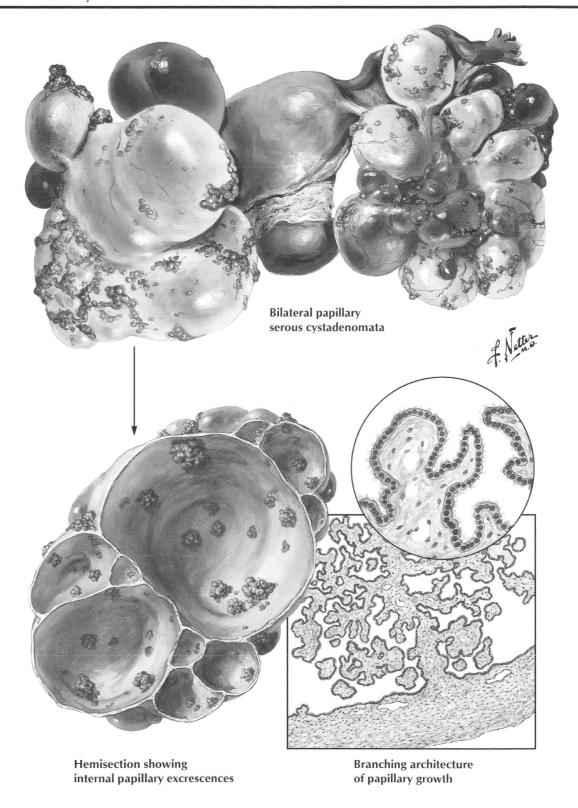

**Bilateral papillary
serous cystadenomata**

**Hemisection showing
internal papillary excrescences**

**Branching architecture
of papillary growth**

FIGURE 8-39   PAPILLARY SEROUS CYSTADENOMA

Papillary serous cystadenomas are serous cysts that are typically bilateral and multilocular and exhibit intracystic or extracystic papillary and adenomatous growths, which indicates an increased proliferative tendency. The lesions have the potential to spread slowly in the peritoneal cavity and recur after surgery, thus fitting into the borderline malignant category. The papillary excrescences are the most striking feature of these tumors.

Histologically, the cyst wall is composed of fibrous tissue with an inner lining of a single cell layer of serous epithelium. Focal calcifications or psammoma bodies may be present. The cysts and papillae may show focal areas of piling of epithelium or cytologic atypia. They usually occur during the reproductive years (age 20-50 years).

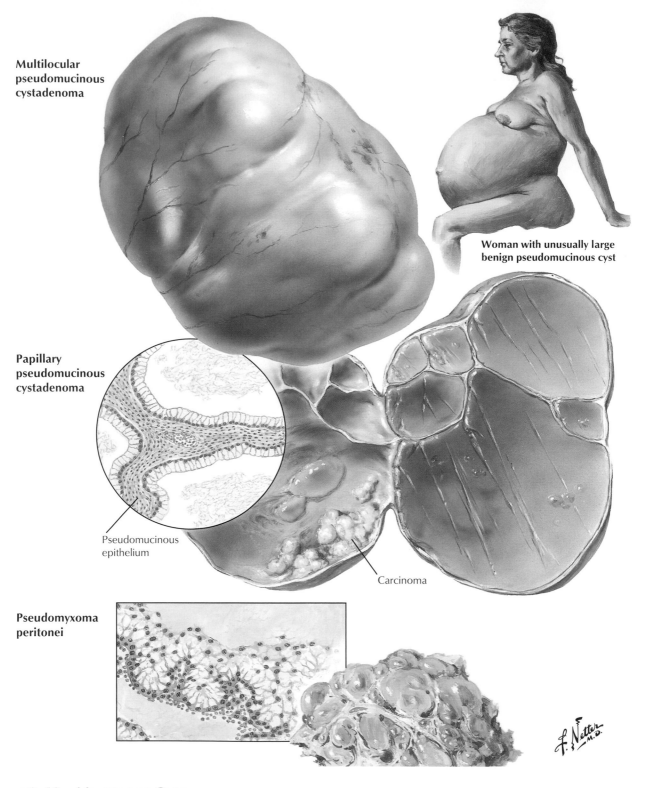

Multilocular pseudomucinous cystadenoma

Woman with unusually large benign pseudomucinous cyst

Papillary pseudomucinous cystadenoma

Pseudomucinous epithelium

Carcinoma

Pseudomyxoma peritonei

FIGURE 8-40   MUCINOUS CYSTADENOMA

Mucinous cystadenomas are cystic ovarian neoplasms lined with mucous-producing epithelium. Typically, they are unilateral and smooth surfaced, are composed of multiple distended lobules, and occur during the reproductive years. They vary in size, some becoming so large as to distend the abdomen. Microscopically, benign, variants of mucinous cystadenomas show the connective tissue capsule and dividing septa lined by a single layer of tall columnar cells with clear cytoplasm and uniform basal nuclei. More aggressive borderline malignant and malignant lesions

exhibit localized, firm infiltrations of the cyst wall with papillary projections on the interior of the cyst. **Pseudomyxoma peritonei** arises from a mucinous ovarian lesion or, more commonly, from a primary mucinous tumor of the appendix, with subsequent implantation and growth of pseudomucinous epithelium in the peritoneal cavity and progressive enlargement of the abdomen leading to increased abdominal pressure and impairment of bladder and bowel function.

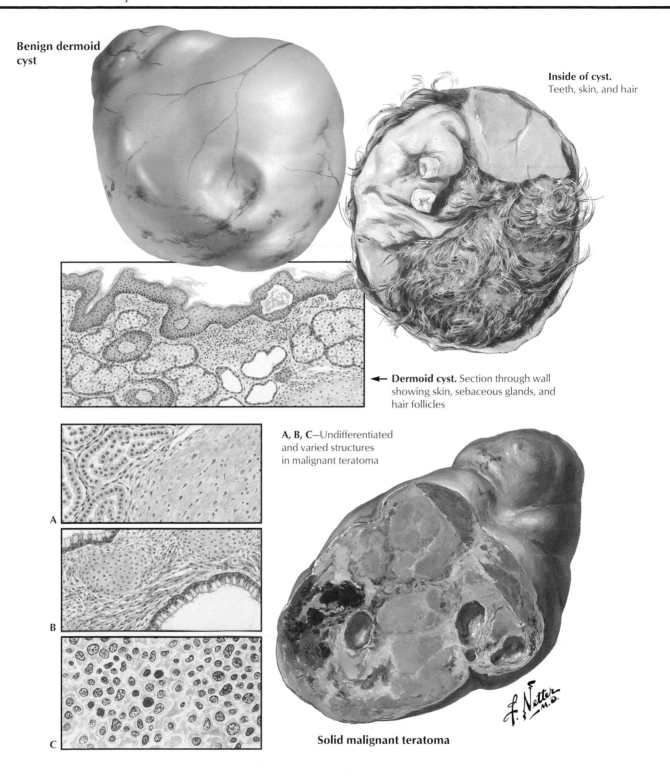

Benign dermoid cyst

Inside of cyst. Teeth, skin, and hair

← **Dermoid cyst.** Section through wall showing skin, sebaceous glands, and hair follicles

A, B, C—Undifferentiated and varied structures in malignant teratoma

Solid malignant teratoma

FIGURE 8-41   TERATOMA: DERMOID CYST AND SOLID TERATOMA

The **dermoid cyst** (benign teratoma of the ovary) is a common benign cystic neoplasm of germ cell origin with well-differentiated components of the 3 germ layers. The tumors, which are sometimes bilateral and can vary in size, are round or oval, are heavy, have a smooth, gray-white or yellow surface, and contain variable combinations of fatty sebaceous material and strands of hair. Histologically, the wall is lined by squamous epithelium; contents include well-differentiated tissues of ectodermal, mesodermal, and endodermal origin. Malignant

transformation, most often as SCC, occurs in approximately 2% of cases. **Solid (embryonal) teratomas** are rare malignant neoplasms occurring typically in younger women. On cut section, malignant teratomas have a variegated appearance with foci of necrosis, hemorrhage, and cystic degeneration. Microscopically, well-differentiated areas coexist with poorly differentiated elements showing embryonal, undifferentiated, sarcomatous, or carcinomatous features.

301

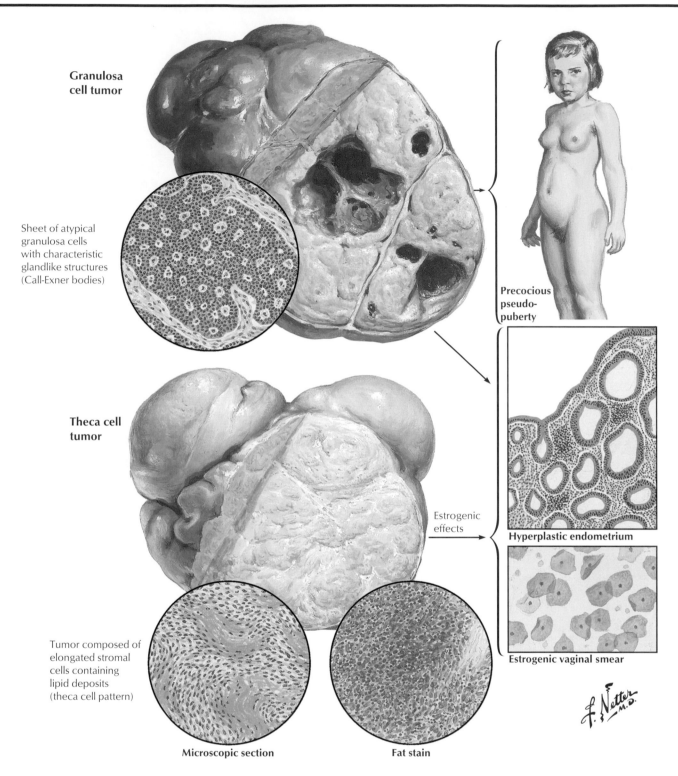

Granulosa cell tumor

Sheet of atypical granulosa cells with characteristic glandlike structures (**Call-Exner bodies**)

Theca cell tumor

Tumor composed of elongated stromal cells containing lipid deposits (**theca cell pattern**)

Precocious pseudo-puberty

Estrogenic effects

Hyperplastic endometrium

Estrogenic vaginal smear

Microscopic section

Fat stain

FIGURE 8-42   FEMINIZING NEOPLASMS: GRANULOSA CELL TUMOR AND THECA CELL TUMOR

The **granulosa cell tumor** is a usually benign, but occasionally malignant feminizing neoplasm composed of cells with features and organizational pattern of granulosa cells of the **Graafian follicle**, including small glandlike structures mimicking immature follicles (**Call-Exner bodies**). Grossly, the tumors are usually unilateral, soft, and yellow, with focal cystic areas. These hormone-producing tumors occur with approximately equal frequency in young adult and postmenopausal women and may occasionally occur in prepubertal girls, leading to precocious pseudopuberty. **Theca cell tumors** are benign, unilateral, solid, estrogen-producing neoplasms composed of cells resembling the theca interna. They occur in menopausal and postmenopausal women and rarely in young adults. Histologically, the tumor is composed of interlacing bands of elongated, stromal cells with oval nuclei and vacuolated fat-containing cytoplasm (theca cell features) separated by collagenous bands.

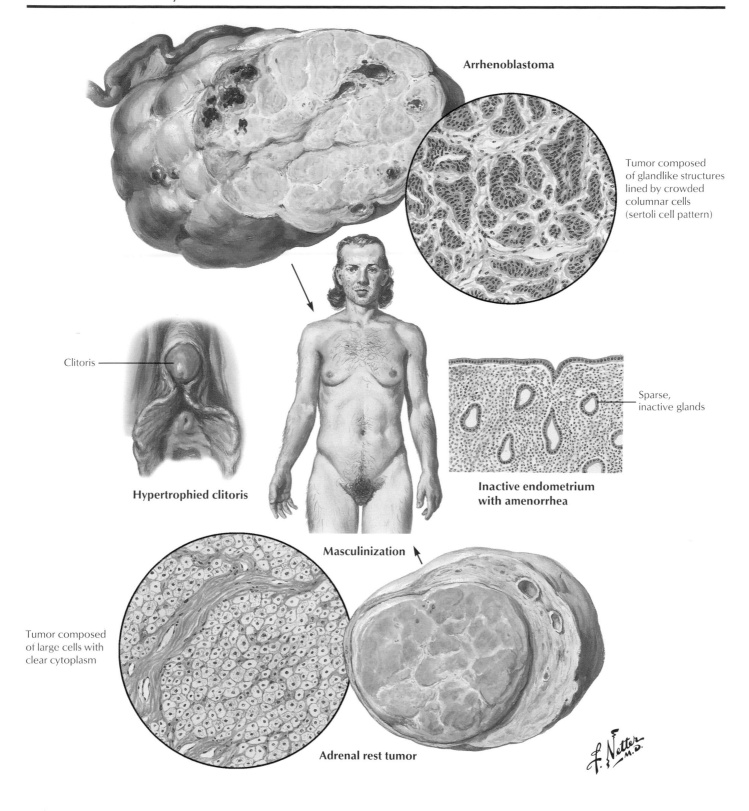

Arrhenoblastoma

Tumor composed of glandlike structures lined by crowded columnar cells (sertoli cell pattern)

Clitoris

Hypertrophied clitoris

Sparse, inactive glands

Inactive endometrium with amenorrhea

Masculinization

Tumor composed of large cells with clear cytoplasm

Adrenal rest tumor

FIGURE 8-43   MASCULINIZING NEOPLASMS: ARRHENOBLASTOMA AND ADRENAL REST TUMOR

The **arrhenoblastoma** (sertoli–Leydig cell tumors) is composed of cells that show features of testicular differentiation in the maturing gonad. Most of these tumors occur in young to middle-aged women; 25% are malignant. The tumors are unilateral, solid, smooth, lobulated, encapsulated, gray-yellow neoplasms with numerous foci of necrosis, hemorrhage, and cystic change in cut section. Several patterns occur, including cuboidal or columnar cells forming tubules or glands (**sertoli cells**), large polygonal

interstitial or **Leydig cells**, and, in some, more primitive areas with poorly organized spindle-shaped or epithelioid cells. **Adrenal rest tumors** may arise from aberrant adrenal rests in the ovary. These rare tumors are composed of large polygonal cells with central nuclei and clean cytoplasm. Leydig cell tumors are rare neoplasms derived from the hilus cells of the ovary. Virilism associated with these neoplasms includes hypertrophied clitoris, hirsutism, acne, and increased muscularization.

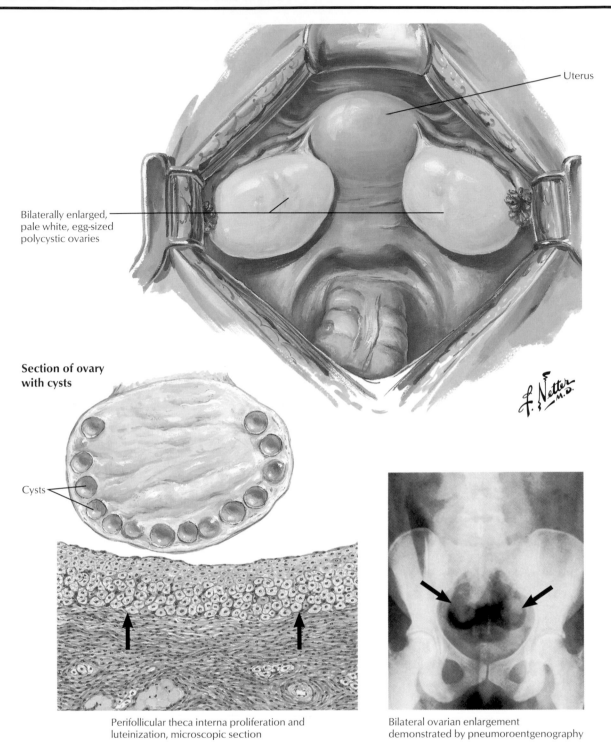

Uterus

Bilaterally enlarged, pale white, egg-sized polycystic ovaries

Section of ovary with cysts

Cysts

Perifollicular theca interna proliferation and luteinization, microscopic section

Bilateral ovarian enlargement demonstrated by pneumoroentgenography

FIGURE 8-44   STEIN-LEVENTHAL SYNDROME

Stein-Leventhal syndrome, characterized by amenorrhea, sterility, hirsutism, and obesity, is often associated with polycystic ovaries. Grossly, the ovaries are enlarged symmetrically and contain many cystic follicles, 2 to 15 mm in diameter, just below the outer, thickened tunica albuginea. Microscopically, there is evidence of hyperthecosis. The theca interna layer surrounding many of the atretic follicles shows prominent proliferation and luteinization, whereas the ovarian parenchyma is hyperplastic with increased cellularity. Stein-Leventhal syndrome is an endocrinologic disturbance involving increased production of luteinizing hormone of the anterior pituitary and ovary (increased luteinizing hormone stimulating the theca cells to produce androgens). Bilateral wedge resection of one half to two thirds of each ovary can lead to renewed menses and fertility in some cases.

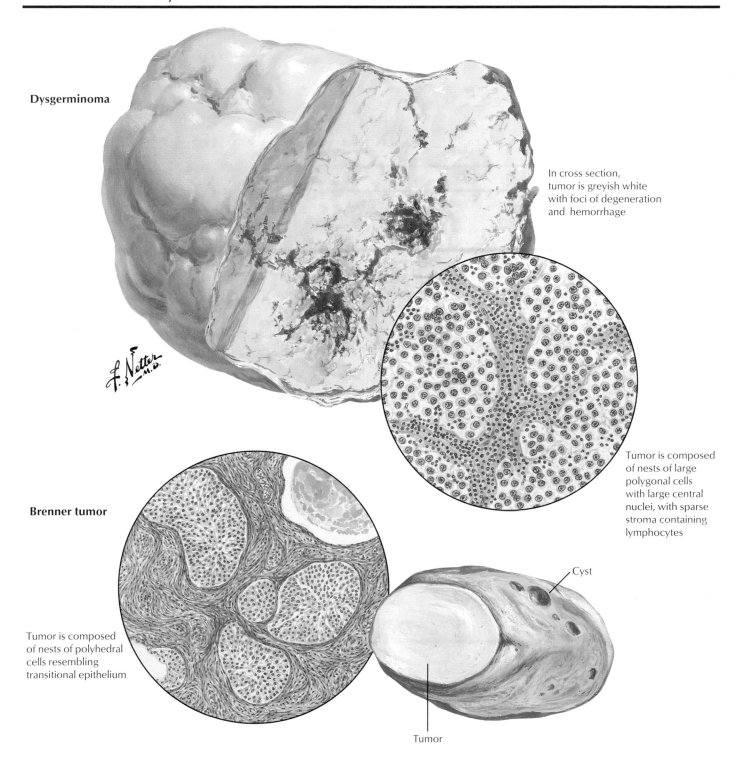

Dysgerminoma

In cross section, tumor is greyish white with foci of degeneration and hemorrhage

Tumor is composed of nests of large polygonal cells with large central nuclei, with sparse stroma containing lymphocytes

Brenner tumor

Tumor is composed of nests of polyhedral cells resembling transitional epithelium

Cyst

Tumor

FIGURE 8-45   DYSGERMINOMA AND BRENNER TUMOR

The **dysgerminoma** is a unilateral, malignant epithelial tumor analogous to the seminoma of the testis. It may be associated with gonadal maldevelopment or pseudohermaphroditism. Most occur in young adults. The dysgerminoma is a solid oval tumor of variable size composed of cords or nests of large, round or polygonal cells with centrally placed, round, uniform nuclei with prominent nucleoli, mitoses, and often an interspersed infiltrate of lymphocytes. Dysgerminomas are malignant but exhibit variability in aggressive growth and spread beyond the capsule.

These tumors are radio-sensitive. The **Brenner tumor** is an uncommon, benign, unilateral, fibroepithelial neoplasm composed of masses of polyhedral cells surrounded by connective tissue that resemble transitional cells of the urinary bladder. Microscopically, the masses of epithelial cells resemble a pavement epithelium. Multiple or solitary small cysts may be present. Most Brenner tumors occur after the age of 40 years or postmenopausally.

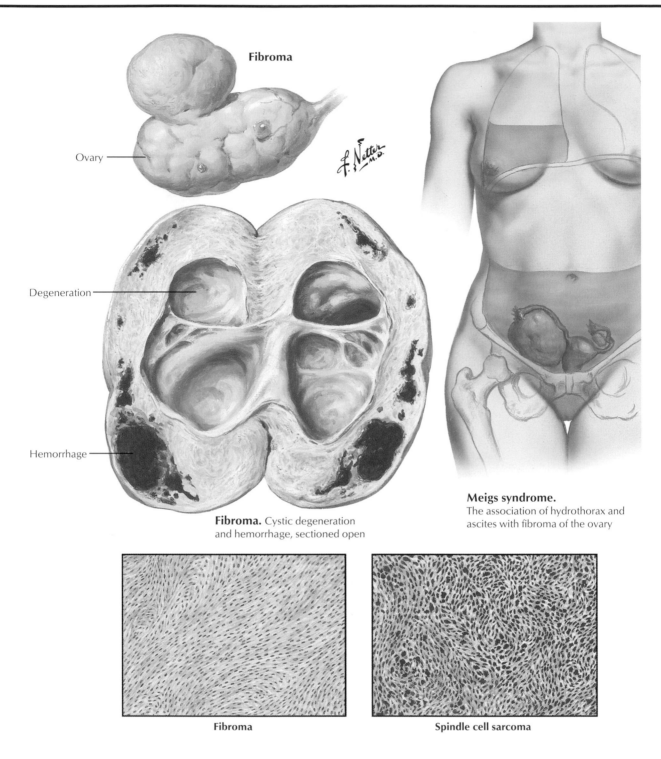

Fibroma

Ovary

Degeneration

Hemorrhage

Fibroma. Cystic degeneration and hemorrhage, sectioned open

Meigs syndrome.
The association of hydrothorax and ascites with fibroma of the ovary

Fibroma

Spindle cell sarcoma

FIGURE 8-46 STROMATOGENOUS NEOPLASMS: FIBROMA, MEIGS SYNDROME, AND SARCOMA

Ovarian fibromas, benign tumors of ovarian stroma, may be small surface pedunculated lesions or large pelvic masses. They are usually unilateral, although a single ovary may show multiple tumors. Most fibromas are found in postmenopausal women, but they can occur at any age. The ovarian fibroma is the most common tumor associated with **Meigs syndrome** of hydroperitoneum (ascites) and hydrothorax. **Fibromas** are well-encapsulated, solid, oval, grayish-white tumors composed of dense, white, interweaving bundles of connective tissue and, in the larger

neoplasms, focal areas of cystic degeneration and hemorrhage. Microscopically, the tumor is composed of interlacing whorls of spindle-shaped cells with uniform, small nuclei. Removal of the pelvic tumor typically results in resorption of the hydrothorax and hydroperitoneum. **Fibrosarcoma** of the ovary is a rare neoplasm composed predominantly of spindle cells with irregular hyperchromatic nuclei. Extension may be by direct invasion or via the vasculature.

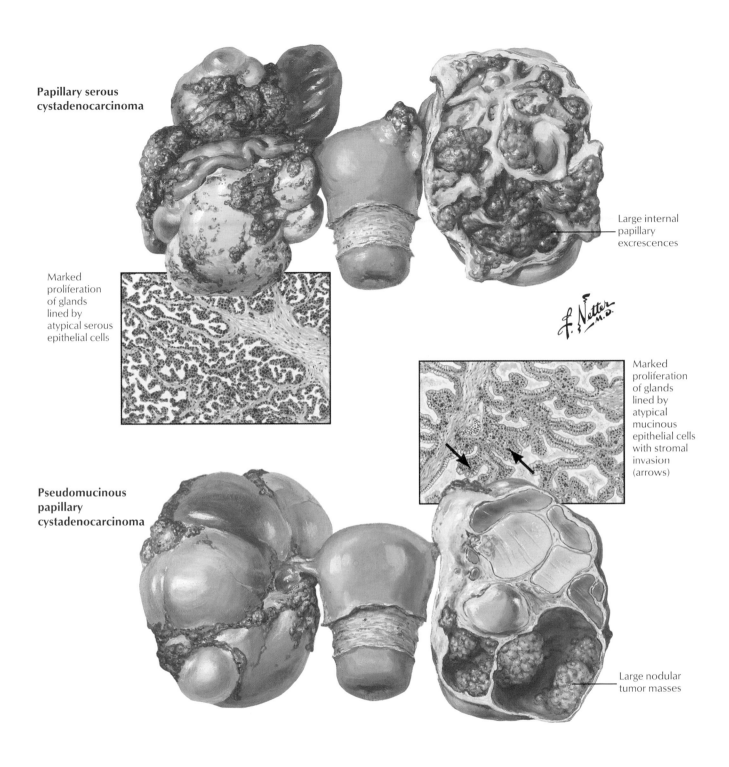

Papillary serous cystadenocarcinoma

Marked proliferation of glands lined by atypical serous epithelial cells

Large internal papillary excrescences

Marked proliferation of glands lined by atypical mucinous epithelial cells with stromal invasion (arrows)

Pseudomucinous papillary cystadenocarcinoma

Large nodular tumor masses

FIGURE 8-47   PRIMARY CYSTIC CARCINOMA

Ovarian carcinomas are either primary or secondary (metastatic) carcinomas. The primary carcinomas may be solid or cystic. **Ovarian carcinoma** is a major category of malignancy of the female genital tract, ranking next to carcinoma of the cervix and uterine fundus. Most ovarian carcinoma occurs between 40 and 60 years of age. Most ovarian carcinomas are papillary SACs. **Mucinous cystadenocarcinoma** is less common, and mucinous cysts are less likely to be malignant than are papillary lesions.

Most ovarian carcinomas are relatively large at the time of diagnosis. Histologic features of malignancy include crowding and piling up of cells with marked nuclear atypia. Bilateral ovarian involvement occurs in one third to one half of cases, depending on the type of malignancy. SACs are more likely to be bilateral than are **pseudomucinous cystadenocarcinomas**. SCCs may develop in a dermoid cyst.

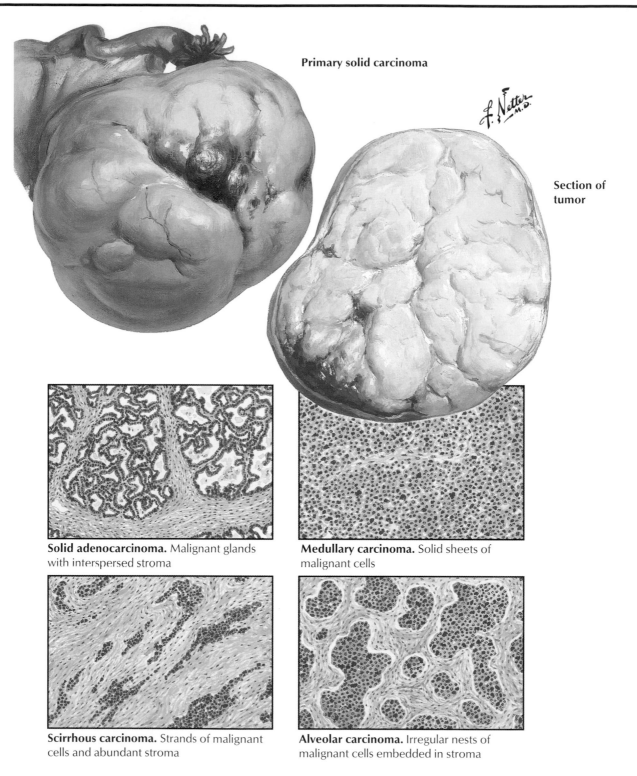

Primary solid carcinoma

Section of tumor

Solid adenocarcinoma. Malignant glands with interspersed stroma

Medullary carcinoma. Solid sheets of malignant cells

Scirrhous carcinoma. Strands of malignant cells and abundant stroma

Alveolar carcinoma. Irregular nests of malignant cells embedded in stroma

FIGURE 8-48   PRIMARY SOLID CARCINOMA

Primary solid ovarian carcinomas, also designated as the **undifferentiated** or **unclassified group**, are classified as solid **adenocarcinoma**, **medullary carcinoma**, **scirrhous carcinoma**, **alveolar carcinoma**, plexiform carcinoma, and adenocarcinoma with squamous cell metaplasia (adenoacanthoma) on the basis of the pattern and arrangement of the epithelial and connective tissue elements. Carcinoma of the ovary spreads by various routes, including local infiltration, to involve adnexal structures, metastatic spread via retroperitoneal channels to the opposite ovary, lymphatic extension to other pelvic organs and lymph nodes, implantation on the peritoneal lining of the abdominal cavity, and spread to distant organs by either lymphatic or hematogenous routes. Prognosis is strongly influenced by the type of tumor and the extent of involvement at the time of diagnosis.

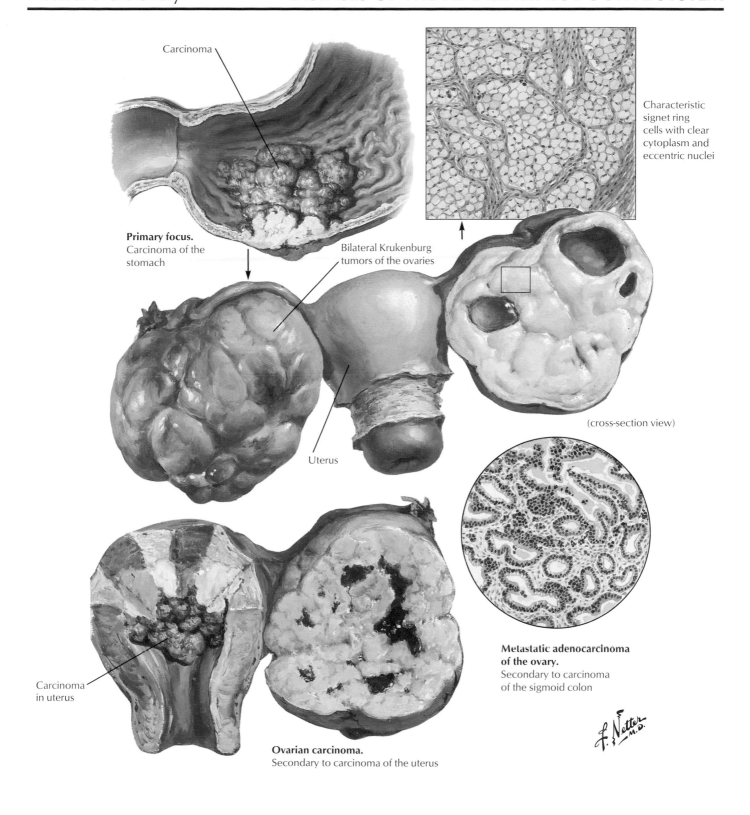

Carcinoma

Characteristic signet ring cells with clear cytoplasm and eccentric nuclei

Primary focus. Carcinoma of the stomach

Bilateral Krukenburg tumors of the ovaries

(cross-section view)

Uterus

Carcinoma in uterus

Metastatic adenocarcinoma of the ovary. Secondary to carcinoma of the sigmoid colon

Ovarian carcinoma. Secondary to carcinoma of the uterus

FIGURE 8-49   SECONDARY OVARIAN CARCINOMA

The ovary is a common site of metastatic invasion by carcinoma. The primary sites include the breast, lungs, stomach, colon, pancreas, liver, uterus, tubes, opposite ovary, and urinary bladder. Metastatic ovarian carcinoma occurs most frequently from the fourth to the sixth decades of life. Ascites is a common finding. There is bilateral involvement in up to 75% of cases, and lesions can vary in size from minute to large. The cut surface may be solid and uniform or cystic and mottled, depending on the extent of hemorrhage and necrosis. Other abdominal foci of tumor may be present. The histologic features generally mirror the primary lesion. **Krukenberg tumor** is a secondary ovarian carcinoma containing characteristic signet ring cells in which the nucleus is flattened to one side by secretion, distending the cell and creating clean cytoplasm. Primary carcinoma of the stomach metastatic to the ovary is a classic cause of Krukenberg tumor. The prognosis in secondary ovarian carcinoma is generally grave.

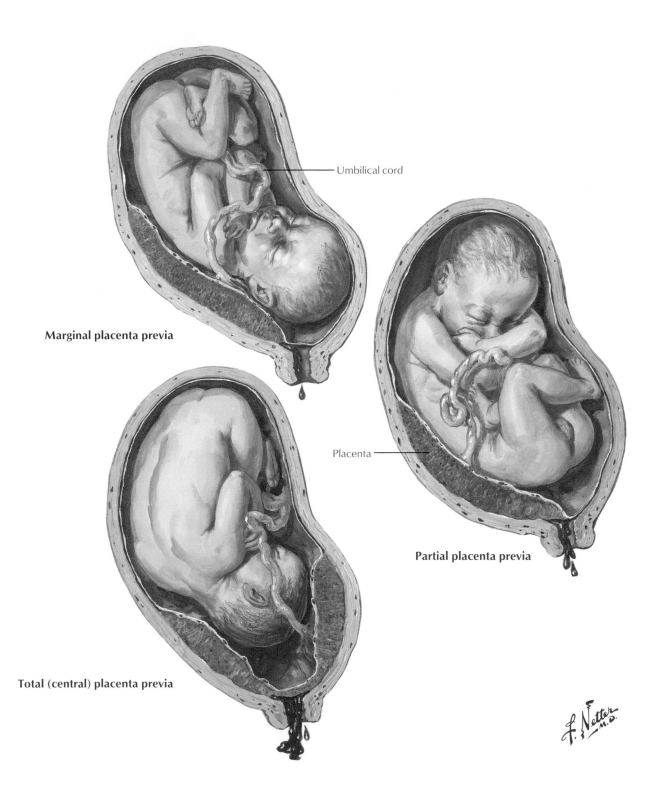

Umbilical cord

Marginal placenta previa

Placenta

Partial placenta previa

Total (central) placenta previa

FIGURE 8-50   PLACENTA PREVIA AND ABRUPTIO PLACENTAE

In **placenta previa**, the placenta is implanted in the lower uterine segment so that it partially or totally obstructs the cervical canal. In **abruptio placenta**, the normally implanted placenta separates prematurely from its uterine attachment in the late second or third

trimester of pregnancy. Placenta previa and abruptio placenta are major causes of uterine bleeding during the last trimester of pregnancy. The bleeding from placental detachment may be internal or external, depending on whether the blood remains

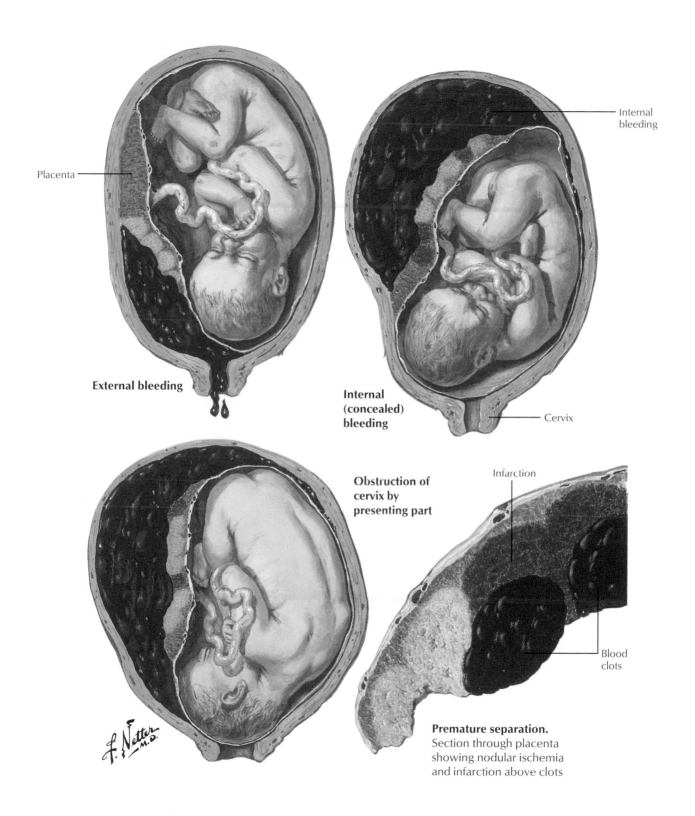

Placenta

External bleeding

Internal
bleeding

**Internal
(concealed)
bleeding**

Cervix

**Obstruction of
cervix by
presenting part**

Infarction

Blood
clots

Premature separation.
Section through placenta
showing nodular ischemia
and infarction above clots

FIGURE 8-50   PLACENTA PREVIA AND ABRUPTIO PLACENTAE *(CONTINUED)*

concealed between the placenta and the uterine wall because of incomplete detachment of the placenta or obstruction of the cervical canal by the fetus. Most cases of abruptio placenta are associated with toxemia of pregnancy or with chronic hyperten-sion complicating the pregnancy, with associated placental ischemia as often is manifest by a large number of placental infarcts. Abruptio placenta is treated by rapid emptying of the uterus and blood transfusions.

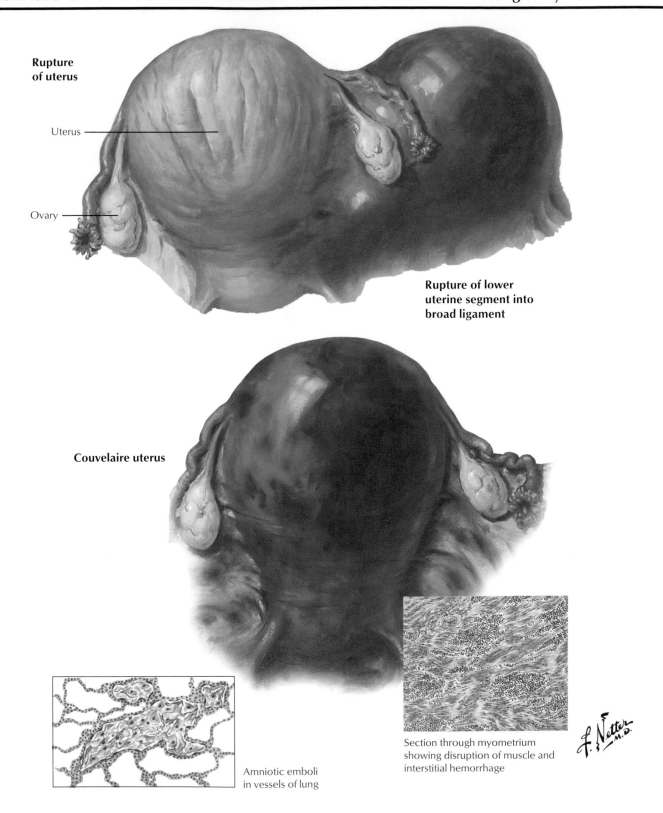

Rupture of uterus

Uterus

Ovary

Rupture of lower uterine segment into broad ligament

Couvelaire uterus

Amniotic emboli in vessels of lung

Section through myometrium showing disruption of muscle and interstitial hemorrhage

FIGURE 8-51   COUVELAIRE UTERUS, RUPTURE OF THE UTERUS, AND MATERNAL PULMONARY EMBOLISM ___

Uteroplacental apoplexy (Couvelaire uterus) is usually associated with severe forms of abruptio placentae. The process is characterized by extensive hemorrhage into the myometrium, the tubes, and the ovaries compounded by defibrination and impaired clotting of the blood. Lifesaving hysterectomy is often necessary to stop the continuous bleeding because the uterus remains atonic after being emptied of the fetus. **Rupture of the uterus**, which may be traumatic or spontaneous, occurs before (rare) or during labor and often results in death of both the mother and the fetus. **Maternal pulmonary embolism** by cellular debris containing amniotic fluid is the apparent cause of some cases of sudden obstetric death, with the typical setting being in multiparas with excessive uterine contractions. The clinical course is one of dyspnea, cyanosis, shock, and death within a few hours.

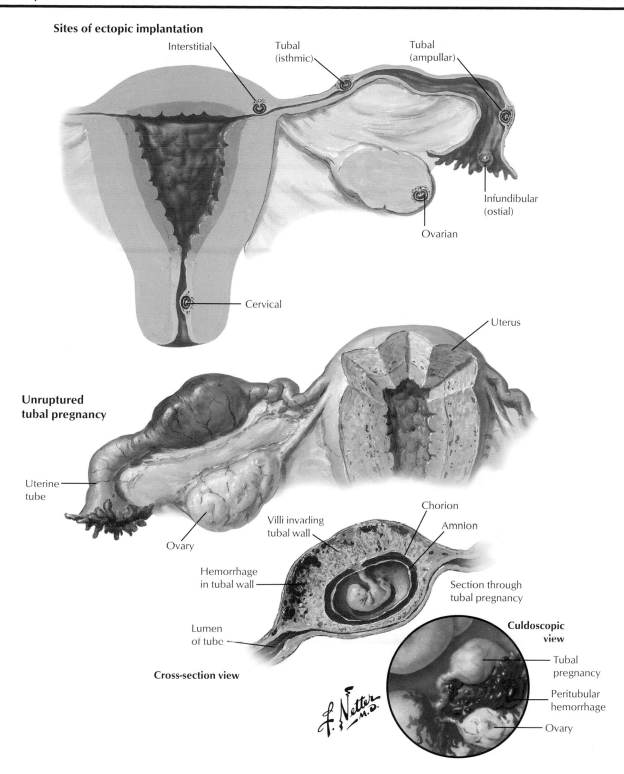

Sites of ectopic implantation

Interstitial

Tubal (isthmic)

Tubal (ampullar)

Infundibular (ostial)

Ovarian

Cervical

Uterus

Unruptured tubal pregnancy

Uterine tube

Ovary

Villi invading tubal wall

Chorion

Amnion

Hemorrhage in tubal wall

Section through tubal pregnancy

Lumen of tube

Cross-section view

Culdoscopic view

Tubal pregnancy

Peritubular hemorrhage

Ovary

FIGURE 8-52   ECTOPIC PREGNANCY: TUBAL PREGNANCY

Ectopic pregnancy is the implantation of a fertilized ovum outside the uterine cavity, which occurs in approximately 1 of 150 to 200 pregnancies. Previous pelvic inflammatory disease with chronic salpingitis is a significant predisposing factor. The site of implantation determines the type: tubal (by far the most common), ovarian, abdominal or peritoneal, and cervical. The subtypes of tubal ectopics—interstitial, isthmic, ampullar, and infundibular—refer to the portion of the tube in which implanta-

tion takes place. **Ampullar implantation** is most common, although the interstitial form has more serious clinical consequences. Early development of an EP is the same as that of a uterine pregnancy, but tubal pregnancy usually ends in abortion through the tube into the peritoneal cavity, or the trophoblast erodes the tubal wall, leading to tubal rupture. A typical presentation is amenorrhea of several weeks followed by bleeding and abdominal pain. It necessitates immediate surgical attention.

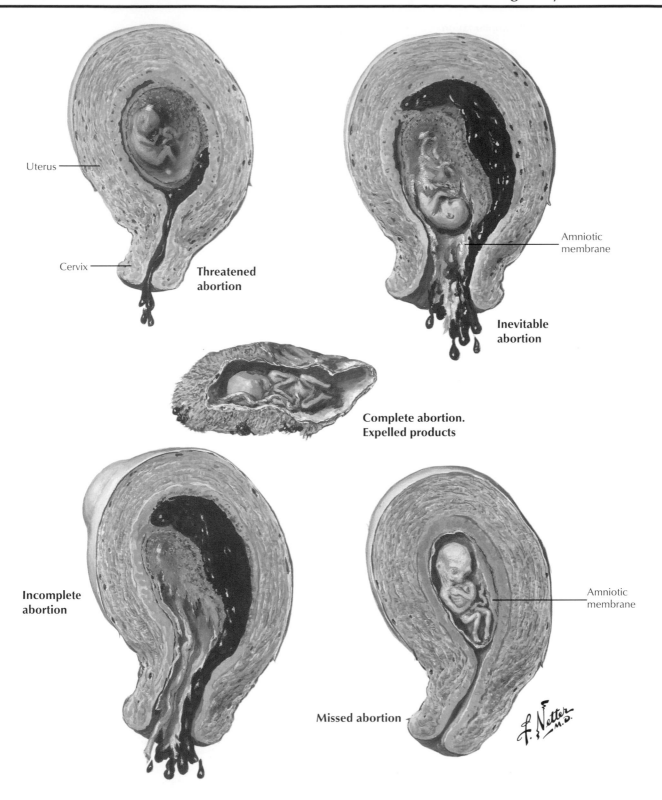

Uterus

Cervix

Threatened abortion

Amniotic membrane

Inevitable abortion

Complete abortion. Expelled products

Incomplete abortion

Amniotic membrane

Missed abortion

FIGURE 8-53   ABORTION

Abortion is the interruption of pregnancy in the first trimester before fetal viability. After viability, early end of pregnancy is called **premature labor**. Maternal or fetal factors, or both, may contribute to an abortion. Maternal factors include systemic infections and toxic agents in the maternal organism. Fetal factors include fetal malformations and congenital abnormalities. Rh incompatibility is an example of combined maternal and fetal factors. Signs and symptoms of abortion are vaginal bleeding followed by expulsive uterine contractions and cervical dilation. Abortion is complete when the entire fetus, placenta, and membranes are expelled and incomplete when the fetus is expelled but all or part of the placenta is retained in the uterus. In missed abortion, the fetus dies, but the placenta is not detached, and the fetus undergoes mummification. In the various types of inevitable abortion, the uterus must be completely evacuated to prevent recurrent hemorrhage and infection.

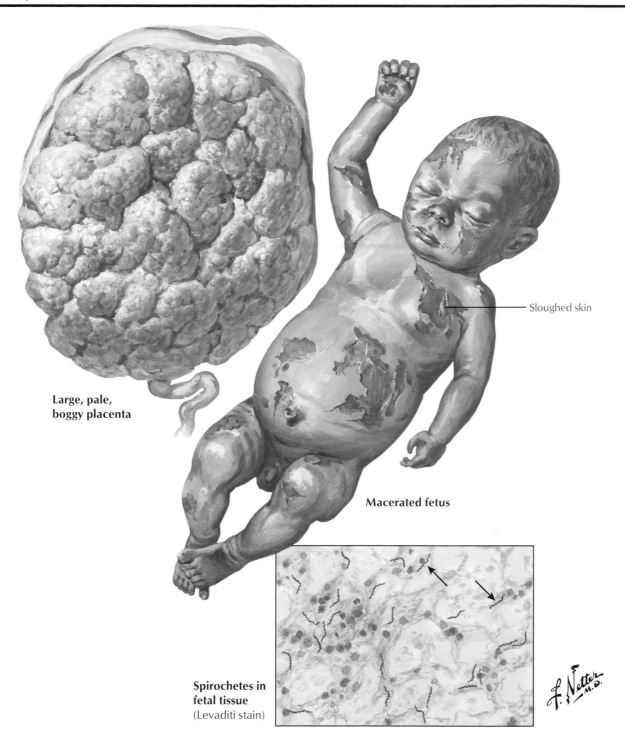

Large, pale, boggy placenta

Sloughed skin

Macerated fetus

Spirochetes in fetal tissue (Levaditi stain)

FIGURE 8-54   SYPHILIS

In various high-risk populations, **syphilis** remains a common cause of late fetal death. The fetus becomes infected through the placenta from the mother. At delivery, the placenta is enlarged, excessively lobulated, pale, and edematous. The cord and membranes are discolored and pale. Most syphilitic fetuses are born dead, but if the fetus is born alive, congenital syphilis soon becomes manifest. A syphilitic fetus is usually shorter than

expected and has maceration of the skin. At autopsy, inflammatory and degenerative changes are usually present in the lungs, liver, spleen, kidneys, and other organs. There is a characteristic osteochondritis with signs of disordered cartilage formation and endochondral ossification. Silver stains can reveal spirochetes of *T. pallidum* in fetal tissues and the placenta.

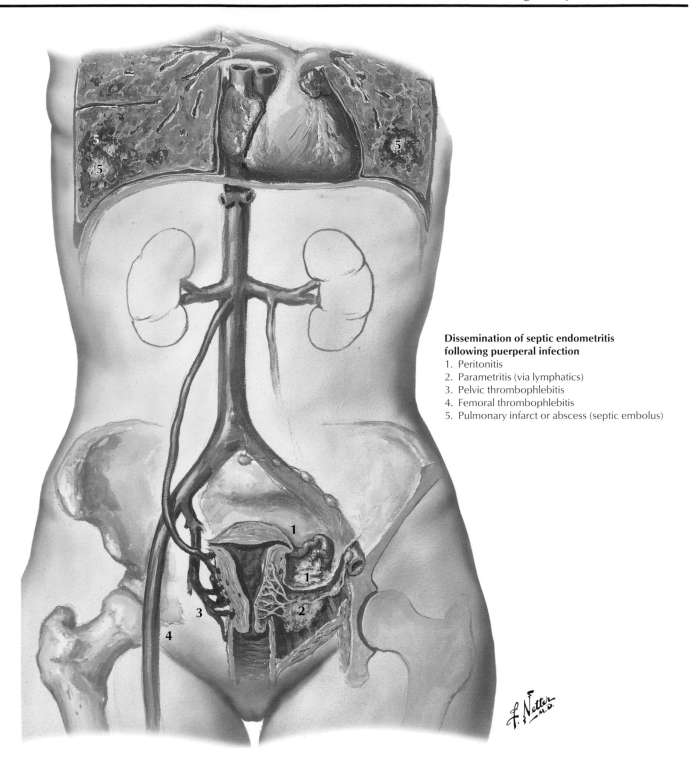

**Dissemination of septic endometritis
following puerperal infection**
1. Peritonitis
2. Parametritis (via lymphatics)
3. Pelvic thrombophlebitis
4. Femoral thrombophlebitis
5. Pulmonary infarct or abscess (septic embolus)

FIGURE 8-55   PUERPERAL INFECTION

Puerperal infection is infection with various microorganisms of the birth canal in the postpartum period. Most cases of puerperal infection are caused by anaerobic and aerobic nonhemolytic varieties of streptococci. However, hemolytic streptococcus, introduced from the outside, is the most common cause of the fulminating and severe forms of puerperal infection. A similar pathophysiology is operative in nonpregnant women with toxic shock syndrome. Less common causes of puerperal infection are staphylococci and anaerobic and coliform bacteria. Blood loss and birth trauma are the most important predisposing factors for puerperal infection. Avoidable factors include faulty aseptic technique during labor and delivery. Endometritis may develop and give rise to puerperal sepsis. Pelvic thrombophlebitis as well as thrombophlebitis of the leg veins also may develop. Distant spread of infection from septic emboli may occur. Rapid diagnosis and antibiotic therapy can prevent a fatal outcome.

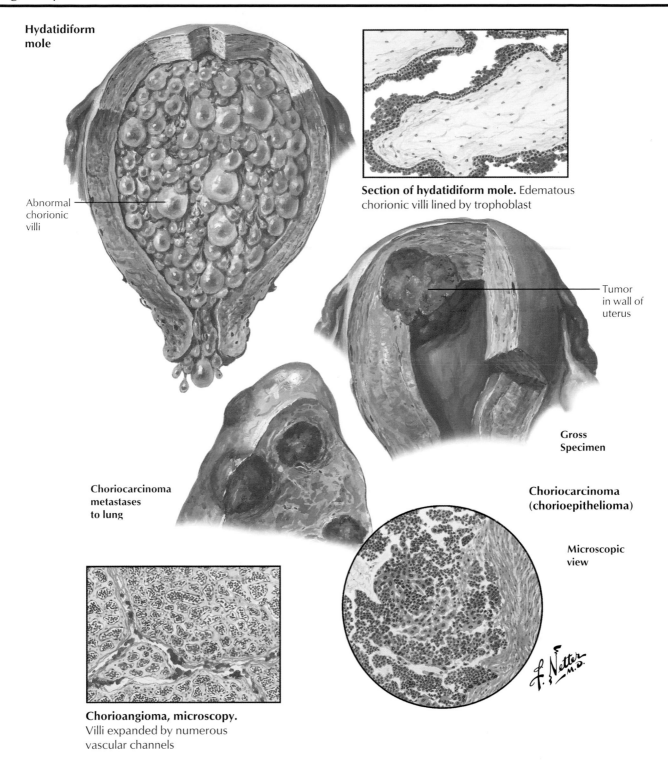

Hydatidiform
mole

Abnormal
chorionic
villi

Section of hydatidiform mole. Edematous
chorionic villi lined by trophoblast

Tumor
in wall of
uterus

Gross
Specimen

Choriocarcinoma
metastases
to lung

**Choriocarcinoma
(chorioepithelioma)**

Microscopic
view

Chorioangioma, microscopy.
Villi expanded by numerous
vascular channels

FIGURE 8-56   INTRAUTERINE NEOPLASMS

Hydatidiform mole and **choriocarcinoma** arise from trophoblastic tissues and cause rapid uterine enlargement, vaginal bleeding, and significantly increased urine and serum levels of human chorionic gonadotropic (HCG) hormone. Beginning as a pregnancy with a defective ovum, a hydatidiform mole is composed of abnormal chorionic villi that appear as grapelike clusters of vesicles and consist of branching structures covered with 2 or more layers of trophoblastic cells but lacking fetal blood vessels. Partial moles have embryo present and contain mixtures of normal and abnormal villi. Complete moles are composed entirely of abnormal villi with no identifiable embryo. A benign or malignant character to the mole is indicated primarily by the degree of cellular atypia of the villi. **Choriocarcinoma** (chorioepithelioma) is a rare but very malignant tumor composed of both syncytial and cytotrophoblastic cells arranged in a disordered pattern without forming chorionic villi. The neoplasm invades the uterine wall aggressively and metastasizes early, particularly to the lungs. Treatment includes evacuation of the contents of the uterus, surgery, and chemotherapy. Chorioangioma is a rare benign lesion.

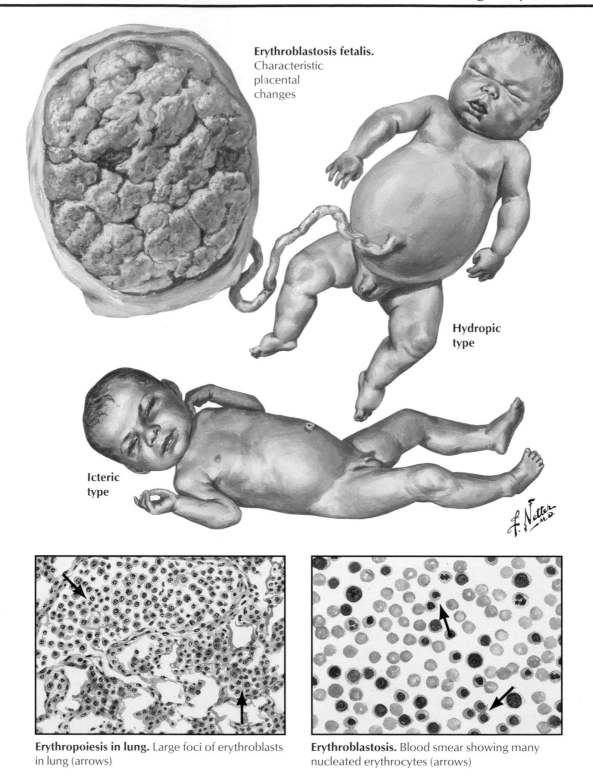

Erythroblastosis fetalis. Characteristic placental changes

Hydropic type

Icteric type

f. Netter M.D.

Erythropoiesis in lung. Large foci of erythroblasts in lung (arrows)

Erythroblastosis. Blood smear showing many nucleated erythrocytes (arrows)

FIGURE 8-57   ERYTHROBLASTOSIS FETALIS

Erythroblastosis fetalis (hemolytic disease of the newborn) results from the progressive destruction of fetal erythrocytes by Rh factor antibodies produced by an Rh-negative mother (approximately 15%) and passed through the placental circulation to the fetus. Predisposing factors include transfusion or intramuscular injection of Rh-positive blood or carrying an Rh-positive fetus in utero. The major features of the disease are hemolytic anemia, icterus, and hydrops. **Hydrops**, the most severe form, results in an enlarged, boggy placenta and a macerated, stillborn infant. This must be distinguished from neonatal syphilis. The **icteric** type occurs in live infants with severe hemolytic anemia. In these infants, fetal blood contains many nucleated red blood cells, and the organs have prominent foci of extramedullary erythropoiesis. In less severe cases, anemia is milder, but the destruction of erythrocytes still leads to icterus and increased indirect bilirubin. Injection of Rh immune globulin to induce immunologic tolerance in the mother may prevent erythroblastosis fetalis.

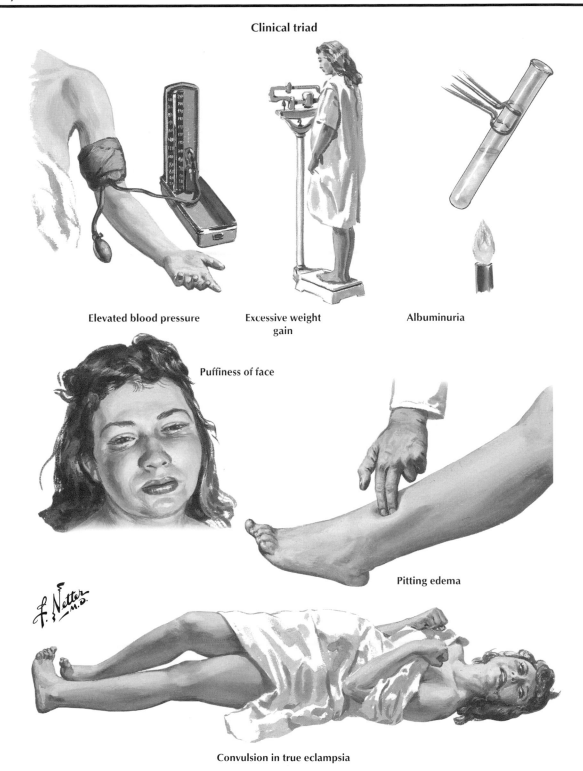

Clinical triad

Elevated blood pressure   Excessive weight gain   Albuminuria

Puffiness of face

Pitting edema

Convulsion in true eclampsia

FIGURE 8-58   ACUTE TOXEMIA OF PREGNANCY: SYMPTOMATOLOGY OF PREECLAMPSIA AND ECLAMPSIA

Toxemia of pregnancy is a generic term for a syndrome of pregnancy characterized by hypertension, proteinuria, and edema with the potential for convulsions or coma. Toxemia includes preeclampsia and eclampsia, and is distinct from essential hypertension associated with pregnancy. Acute toxemia develops during the third trimester of pregnancy—presenting as progressive weight gain, blood pressure higher than 140/90 mm Hg, and proteinuria—and disappears promptly after delivery. Eclampsia is characterized by convulsions and coma, and these manifestations may develop independent of the magnitude of hypertension. Regular, prompt care is the key to prevention.

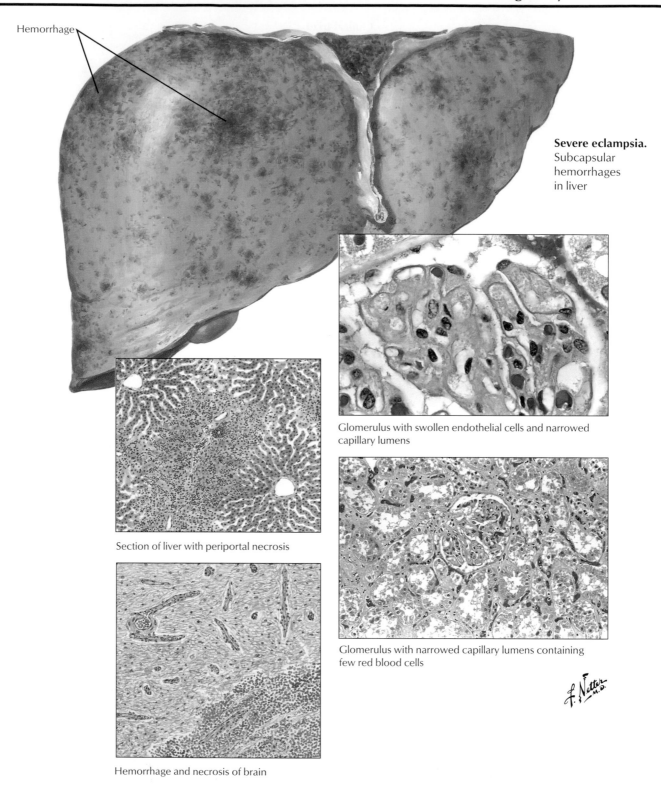

Hemorrhage

Severe eclampsia.
Subcapsular
hemorrhages
in liver

Glomerulus with swollen endothelial cells and narrowed
capillary lumens

Section of liver with periportal necrosis

Glomerulus with narrowed capillary lumens containing
few red blood cells

Hemorrhage and necrosis of brain

FIGURE 8-59   ACUTE TOXEMIA OF PREGNANCY: VISCERAL LESIONS IN PREECLAMPSIA AND ECLAMPSIA

The pathologic effects of **preeclampsia** and **eclampsia** in various organs are qualitatively similar but vary in severity in relation to the clinical course. The liver and other organs can exhibit swollen and multiple foci of hemorrhage and necrosis. The most characteristic renal lesion consists of narrowing of the lumens of glomerular capillaries caused by thickening of the glomerular membranes due to endothelial cell swelling. Obstruction of blood flow through the glomerular tufts can lead to distal tubular

necrosis. Bilateral cortical necrosis, a less common but severe lesion, is caused by severe vasoconstriction and necrosis of the intralobular arteries. The characteristic changes in the brain include edema, petechial hemorrhages, and, in severe cases, larger foci of hemorrhagic necrosis. All of this organ pathology is driven by vasoconstriction often complicated by microthrombosis due to disseminated intravascular coagulation (DIC).

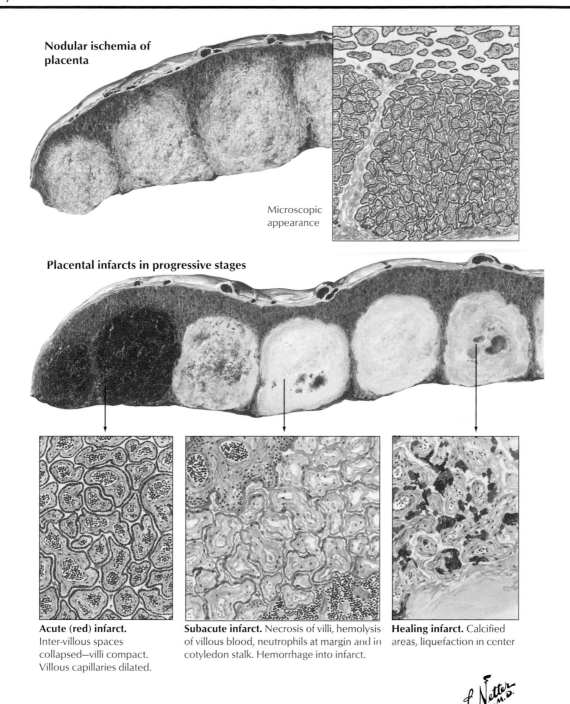

Nodular ischemia of placenta

Microscopic appearance

Placental infarcts in progressive stages

Acute (red) infarct.
Inter-villous spaces collapsed—villi compact. Villous capillaries dilated.

Subacute infarct. Necrosis of villi, hemolysis of villous blood, neutrophils at margin and in cotyledon stalk. Hemorrhage into infarct.

Healing infarct. Calcified areas, liquefaction in center

FIGURE 8-60   ACUTE TOXEMIA OF PREGNANCY: PLACENTAL LESIONS IN PREECLAMPSIA AND ECLAMPSIA AND INFARCTS

There is a close correlation between the occurrence of **acute toxemia** and conditions that predispose to a decrease in the maternal circulation to the placenta, the decidua, or both. Severe reduction of maternal blood flow causes true infarction of one or more of the placental cotyledons. True infarcts are found on the maternal aspect of the placenta, in contrast to other incidental placental lesions. Microscopically, the characteristic feature is necrotic chorionic villi. Acutely, the lesions are **hemorrhagic**

infarcts that become pale as they age and heal without organization (i.e., without formation of granulation tissue and fibrosis). **Placental ischemia** is considered the major event in the pathogenesis of acute toxemia because it leads to increased production of angiotensin and other vasoconstrictors and decreased production of nitric oxide and other vasodilators. In turn, the placental ischemia may be caused by abnormal formation and implantation of the placenta (placentation).

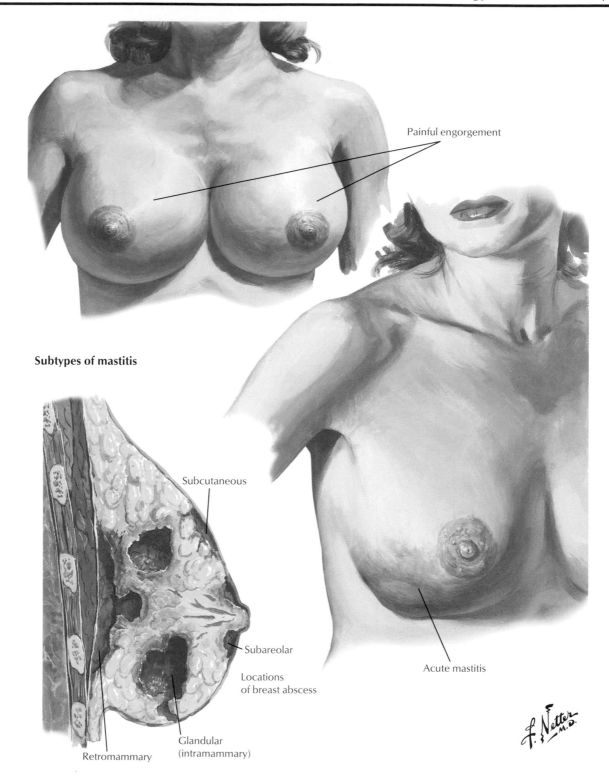

Painful engorgement

Subtypes of mastitis

Subcutaneous

Subareolar

Locations
of breast abscess

Glandular
(intramammary)

Retromammary

Acute mastitis

FIGURE 8-61   PAINFUL ENGORGEMENT AND PUERPERAL MASTITIS

Painful engorgement of the breast usually occurs within the first few days postpartum, before the onset of lactation, or later when active lactation is interrupted. Because of vascular stasis, the breasts become engorged, firm, warm, and painful. **Acute mastitis** occurs during lactation after entry of infectious agents by way of a cracked or traumatized nipple, most commonly in primiparous women. The clinical manifestations are fever, leukocytosis, tenderness, and induration. There are 3 subtypes of mastitis: subareolar, glandular, and interstitial, the latter giving rise to a retromammary abscess. Rare infections of the breast, usually in nonpregnant women, are tuberculosis and syphilis with chancre formation.

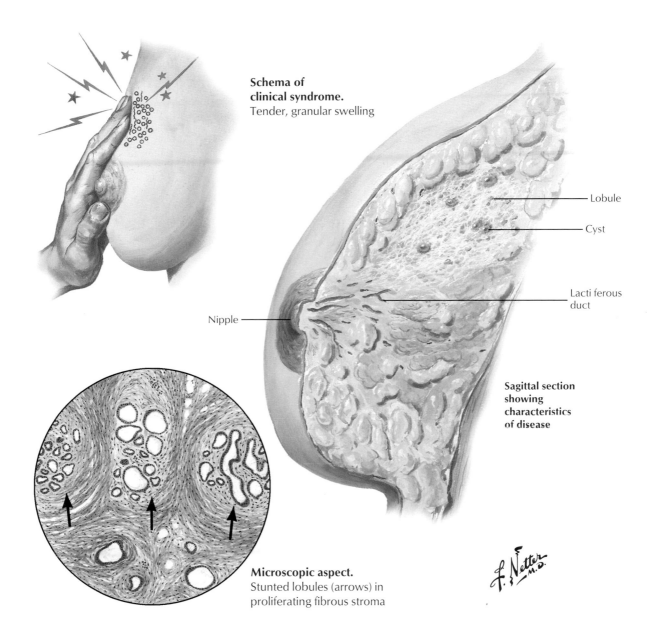

Schema of clinical syndrome.
Tender, granular swelling

Lobule

Cyst

Lacti ferous duct

Nipple

Sagittal section showing characteristics of disease

Microscopic aspect.
Stunted lobules (arrows) in proliferating fibrous stroma

FIGURE 8-62   FIBROCYSTIC DISEASE: EARLY CHANGES

Chronic cystic disease or **fibrocystic disease** of the breast is a mammary disease complex with underlying endocrine disturbance, which comprises 3 principal types of abnormalities: cyst formation, often with apocrine metaplasia, fibrosis, and adenosis. True mastodynia, or intrinsic mammary pain, can be the first manifestation. Palpation typically reveals a swollen granular zone of increased density, which is most frequently located in the upper lateral quadrant, often bilaterally. On biopsy, the painful mammary tissue grossly is more dense and fibrous than normal, and histologically, the lobules are stunted or irregularly shaped, with small cystic dilatations, and they are surrounded by immature, proliferating connective tissue. The defective lobule formation relates to some disturbance of integrated action of the ovarian hormones on the mammary gland, increased estrogen production, inadequate progesterone secretion, or a combination of these.

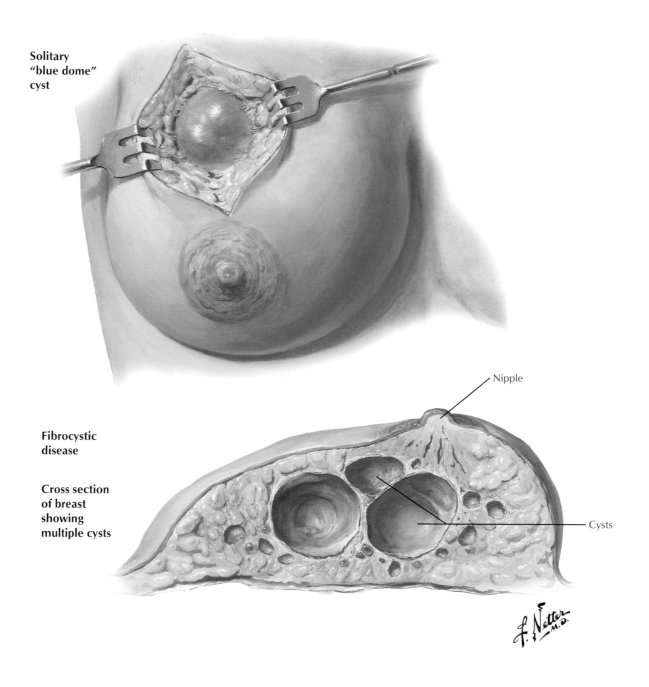

Solitary "blue dome" cyst

Fibrocystic disease

Cross section of breast showing multiple cysts

Nipple

Cysts

FIGURE 8-63   FIBROCYSTIC DISEASE: CYSTIC CHANGES

Some cases of **fibrocystic disease** are dominated by cystic changes. In some subjects, a single cyst of 1 to several centimeters in diameter develops. In other cases, the cysts are multiple, and often but not uniformly, both breasts are affected. The larger cysts have a characteristic blue dome, which bulges into the subcutaneous fat and contains cloudy straw-colored fluid, and a thin, fibrous wall, which may have an epithelial lining of duct cells. The cyst wall is embedded in dense, fibrous stroma. Multiple smaller cysts have similar features.

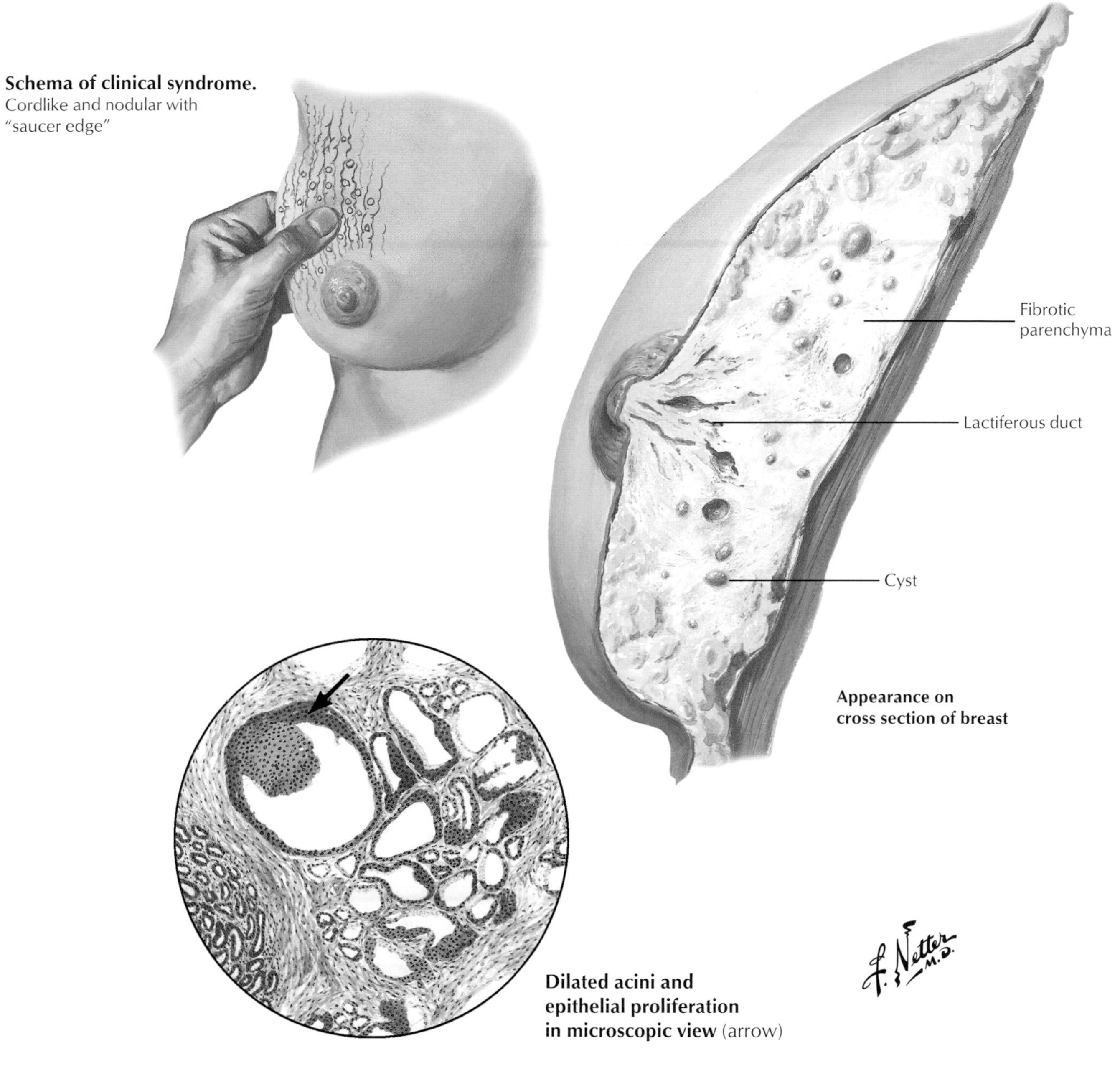

Schema of clinical syndrome.
Cordlike and nodular with "saucer edge"

Fibrotic parenchyma

Lactiferous duct

Cyst

Appearance on cross section of breast

Dilated acini and **epithelial proliferation in microscopic view** (arrow)

FIGURE 8-64   FIBROCYSTIC DISEASE: ADENOSIS

Adenosis is characterized by the development, in one or both breasts, of multiple nodules, varying from 1 mm to 1 cm in size and usually distributed about the periphery of the breast, creating a nodular breast with a saucerlike edge. The affected mammary tissue contains dense fibrous tissue, numerous cysts, and foci of epithelial proliferation. Lobule formation is considerably distorted. Some of the terminal tubules form solid plugs of basal cells, which, on cross section, appear as duct adenomas. Other tubules have greatly enlarged lobular structures, which are penetrated by dense strands of fibrous tissue, giving the appearance of an orderly proliferation of small ductules and acini, known as **sclerosing adenosis**. The incidence of cancer in patients with fibrocystic disease and accompanying ductal proliferative changes is approximately twice as high as is the incidence in the general female population.

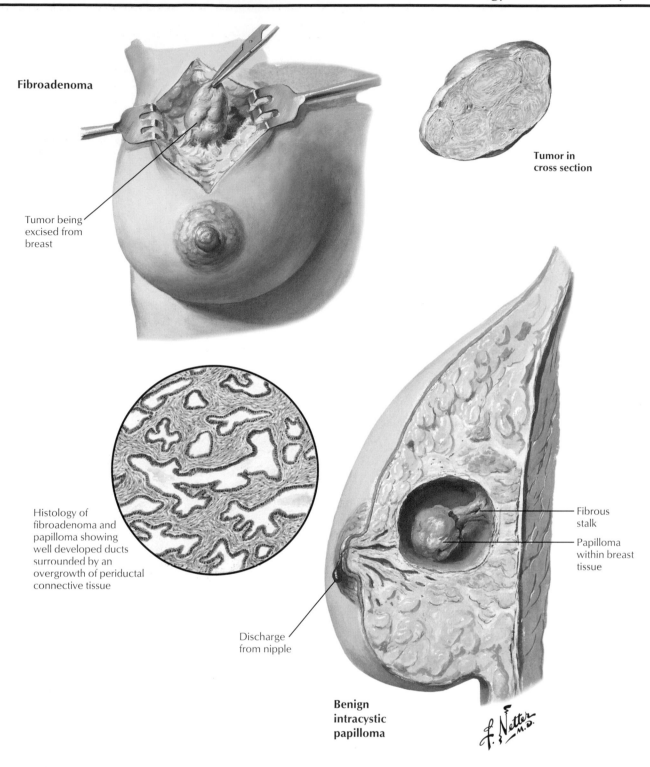

Fibroadenoma

Tumor being excised from breast

Tumor in cross section

Histology of fibroadenoma and papilloma showing well developed ducts surrounded by an overgrowth of periductal connective tissue

Fibrous stalk

Papilloma within breast tissue

Discharge from nipple

Benign intracystic papilloma

FIGURE 8-65   BENIGN FIBROADENOMA AND INTRACYSTIC PAPILLOMA

The **fibroadenoma**, the most common benign mammary tumor of the female breast, usually occurs in young adult women. The typical presentation is a firm, well circumscribed, nodular, freely movable, gradually enlarging mass. On excision, the tumor appears as a lobular mass and consists of well-developed ducts surrounded by marked overgrowth of periductal connective tissue. The growth of fibroadenoma is rapid in early adolescence, in pregnancy, or toward menopause, when estrogenic secretion is increased. Benign intracystic papillomas are fleshy epithelial growths occurring within a mammary duct or a dilated acinus, usually at or near menopause, in the central zone of the breast. They cause either a sanguinous discharge from the nipple or a lump associated with moderate tenderness. **Intracystic papillomas** are encapsulated tumors that contain branching epithelial projections and rest on a fibrous stalk. Multiple papillomas may occur in one or both breasts.

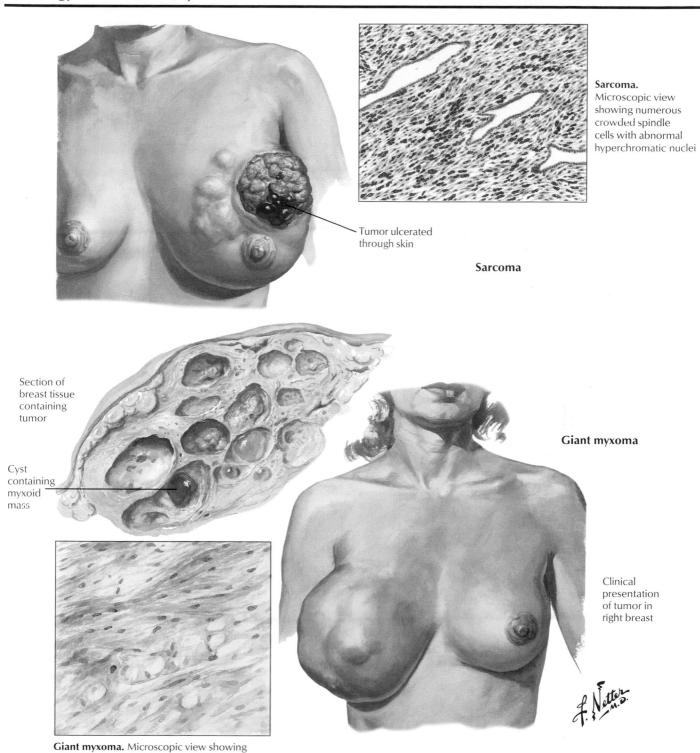

Sarcoma. Microscopic view showing numerous crowded spindle cells with abnormal hyperchromatic nuclei

Tumor ulcerated through skin

Sarcoma

Section of breast tissue containing tumor

Cyst containing myxoid mass

Giant myxoma

Clinical presentation of tumor in right breast

Giant myxoma. Microscopic view showing bland myxoid connective tissue containing uniform spindle cells

FIGURE 8-66   GIANT MYXOMA AND SARCOMA

Giant mammary myxoma, also known as **phyllodes tumor** or **cystosarcoma phyllodes**, is a fibroadenoma that typically occurs near menopause and grows to large size. The tumors are heavy, massive, lobulated, fleshy growths with cystic areas; they remain encapsulated and moveable. Microscopically, the lesions are composed of myxomatous and fibrous connective tissue lined by epithelial cells and containing abundant stromal cells. Most of these tumors behave in a benign fashion. **Mammary sarcoma** is rare among the mammary tumors. Most of these sarcomas are fibrocellular lesions arising in the stroma of the breast or from the stroma of preexisting fibroadenomas. The lesions are characterized by rapid growth, large size, firm consistency, and, commonly, ulceration of the skin, with fungation of the mass.

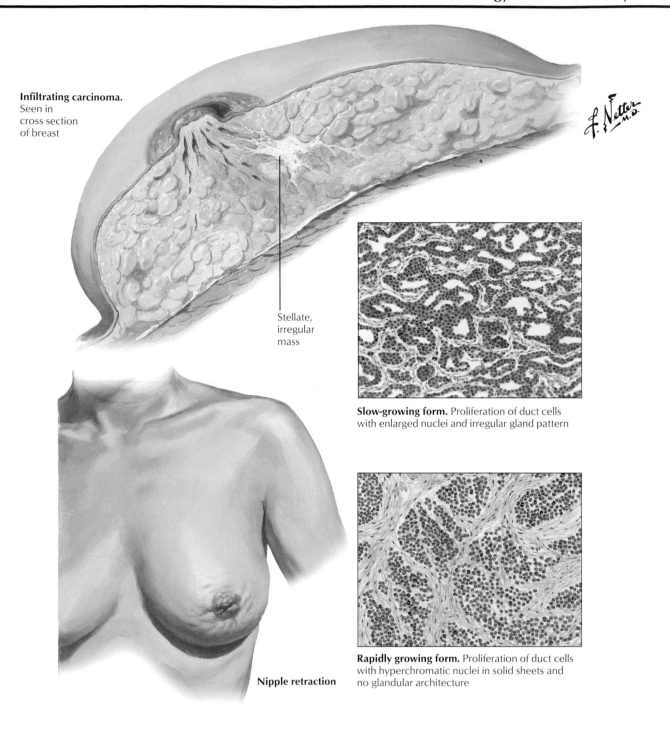

Infiltrating carcinoma. Seen in cross section of breast

Stellate, irregular mass

Slow-growing form. Proliferation of duct cells with enlarged nuclei and irregular gland pattern

Rapidly growing form. Proliferation of duct cells with hyperchromatic nuclei in solid sheets and no glandular architecture

Nipple retraction

FIGURE 8-67   INFILTRATING CARCINOMA

Approximately 15% to 30% of mammary carcinomas are in situ, and 70% to 85% are invasive. Approximately 80% of invasive lesions are **infiltrating ductal carcinoma** (scirrhus carcinoma or carcinoma simplex). They present as a palpable mass and may be associated with nipple retraction. Grossly, these are dense, yellowish-white, stellate, irregular masses with a gritty consistency. Microscopically, the tumor cells have a relatively uniform size; exhibit prominent, hyperchromatic nuclei; grow in small nests or cords; and are accompanied by growth of fibrous tissue

producing the scirrhus feature of the lesions. Invasive lobular carcinoma (5-10% of breast carcinomas) tends to be multicentric in the same breast, to involve both breasts at a high frequency (approximately 20%), and to be hard to detect because of a diffusely invasive pattern. Prognosis is influenced by growth pattern of the tumor; degree of organization and cellular differentiation; expression of various gene products, including estrogen receptors and *BRCA*1 and *BRCA*2; and the presence of regional axillary lymph node and distant metastases.

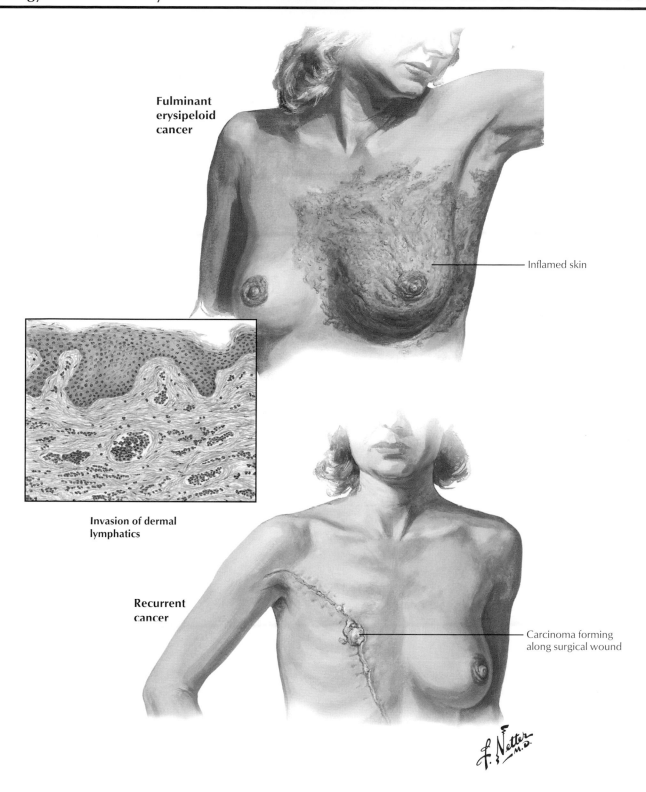

Fulminant
erysipeloid
cancer

Inflamed skin

Invasion of dermal
lymphatics

Recurrent
cancer

Carcinoma forming
along surgical wound

FIGURE 8-68   FULMINANT CARCINOMA

Inflammatory or **acute fulminant carcinoma** usually presents as a rapidly widening area of inflamed skin. The dermal inflammation usually correlates with retrograde spread of the cancer cells through the lymphatics of the skin. The skin is reddened, edematous, and rough, producing the characteristic orange peel effect. The carcinomatous spread is accompanied by a localized and systemic inflammatory process with low-grade fever, increased leukocyte count, and enlarged axillary lymph nodes. The most frequent site of local recurrence of breast cancer is the scar in the chest wall, followed by the axilla and the supraclavicular regions.

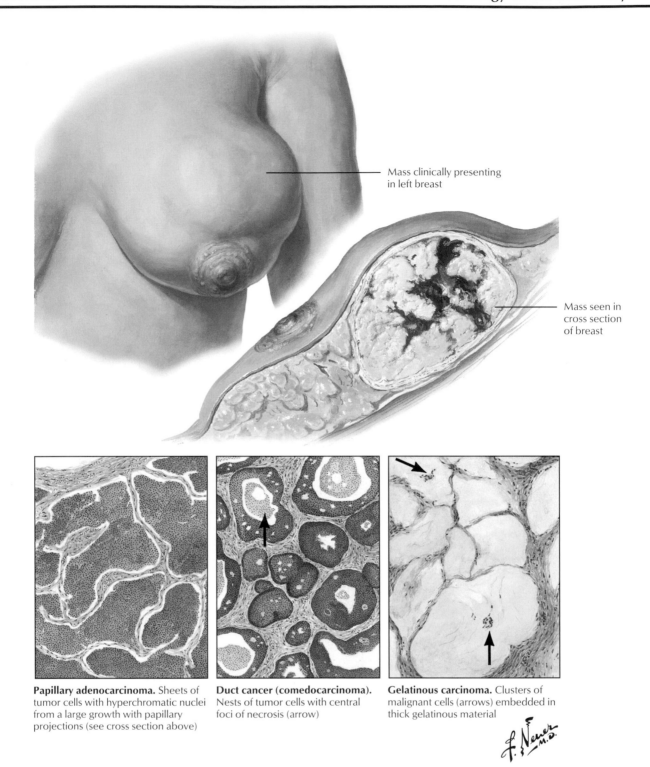

Mass clinically presenting in left breast

Mass seen in cross section of breast

Papillary adenocarcinoma. Sheets of tumor cells with hyperchromatic nuclei from a large growth with papillary projections (see cross section above)

Duct cancer (comedocarcinoma). Nests of tumor cells with central foci of necrosis (arrow)

Gelatinous carcinoma. Clusters of malignant cells (arrows) embedded in thick gelatinous material

FIGURE 8-69   CIRCUMSCRIBED FORMS OF ADENOCARCINOMA

Approximately one fourth of mammary carcinomas have features of well-differentiated **adenocarcinomas**. These lesions include **papillary adenocarcinomas**, carcinomas with gelatinous, mucoid degeneration, and **comedocarcinoma**, a type of intraductal carcinoma that forms plugs and circumscribed rings of carcinoma cells in preexisting ducts. These lesions tend to bulge out from the breast rather than retract inwardly as with the infiltrating carcino-

mas. Skin and axillary node involvement occur much later in the course than with infiltrating scirrhous carcinoma. The tumors typically progress slowly and often reach large size. The majority are detected and removed by mastectomy before metastasis occurs. The lesions may have central foci of necrosis or hemorrhage.

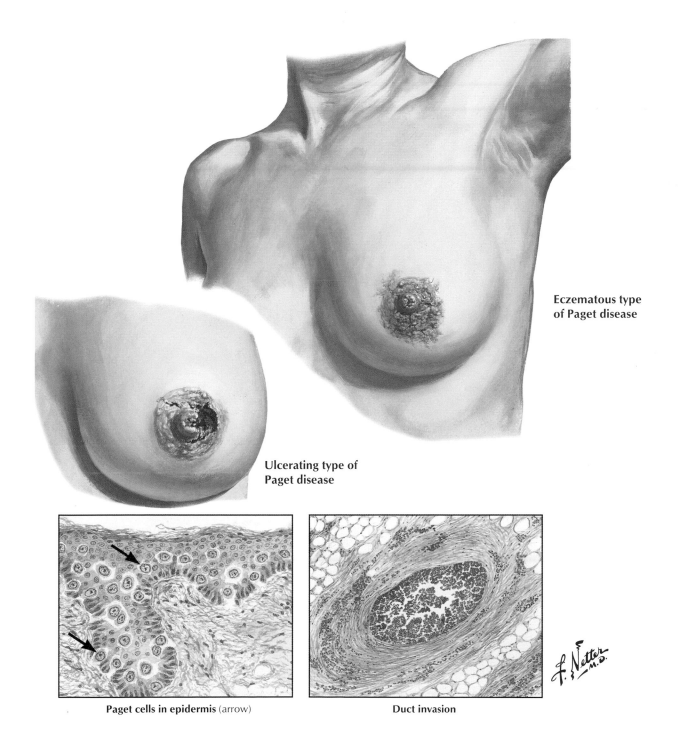

Eczematous type
of Paget disease

Ulcerating type of
Paget disease

Paget cells in epidermis (arrow)

Duct invasion

FIGURE 8-70   PAGET DISEASE OF THE NIPPLE

Paget disease of the nipple is produced by carcinomatous invasion of the nipple or areola and the mouths of the larger ducts by large malignant cells with hyperchromatic or vesicular nuclei and pale staining cytoplasm. Usually, involvement of the nipple precedes the detection of a small primary tumor in the breast. The disease is occasionally bilateral. The involved nipple has a red granular or an exudating crusted appearance and eventually undergoes ulceration. Eventually, a hard mass, which is often associated with enlarged axillary lymph nodes, is palpable.

CHAPTER 9

INTEGUMENTARY SYSTEM (SKIN)

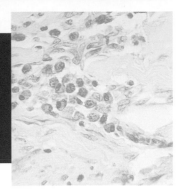

The usual classification of skin diseases differs slightly from the terminology used in general pathology: both the gross appearance of lesions and, at least in part, their pathogenesis determines their class in dermatopathology.

Acute inflammatory diseases of the skin, commonly lasting a few days to several weeks, are numerous and pathogenetically inhomogeneous. Like other dermatologic diseases, they are classified according to the location of changes (i.e., in different strata of epidermis, dermis, and subcutis) and according to their composition and quality (edematous, vesicular, neutrophilic, lymphocytic, mast cell, necrotic, hemorrhagic, vascular, etc). Consequently, there are several classification schemes for dermatologic diseases, and the examples in this chapter do not favor any particular one.

Chronic inflammatory diseases of the skin (chronic inflammatory **dermatoses**), lasting for several months to years, are also pathogenetically inhomogeneous but have in common signs of chronic inflammation with thickening of the skin, keratinic scale formation, and desquamation (shedding). Among them is systemic lupus erythematosus, which because of its complexity cannot be described in detail here but is discussed in texts on clinical immunology and immunopathology.

Vesicular and bullous dermatoses are characterized by epidermal or dermal-epidermal separation (**dyshesive diseases**) with formation of vesicles or bullae (blisters). They are classified according to the site where blisters form: **epidermolytic blisters** comprise superficial intradermal or acantholytic separation and suprabasal epidermal separation, **junctional blisters** are found below the basal cell layer and dermal lamina densa, and **dermolytic blisters** form in the upper subepithelial dermis. Although the etiology of these diseases remains obscure, most if not all bullous dermatoses seem to have an autoimmune pathogenesis. Different types of autoantibodies (e.g., immunoglobulin [Ig] A) to basement membrane antigen or other structures are demonstrable by immunofluorescence studies.

There exists a large variety of **dermatologic infections**, the pathologic changes of which are similar to those in other organs and tissues (taking into account the structural peculiarities of the site of infection): neutrophilic inflammation with or without necrosis and hemorrhage (bacteria, fungi), lymphoplasmacytic infiltration (virus or autoimmune component), and granulomatous (intracellular organisms, fungi, parasites, or autoimmune component). Lesions may be localized (site of entry, lymphatic spread) or systemic (hematogenous spread), occur in superficial or deep parts of the skin, and are usually painful. Infection with certain organisms (*Candida,* zoster and other herpes viruses, papilloma virus, and others) may suggest that the patient has immune deficiency (**opportunistic infections**).

Tumors of the skin may be benign or malignant. Hyperplastic changes of the skin consist primarily of hyperplastic scars (keloids) or hyperplastic glands (**sebaceous hyperplasia**). Benign tumors of the skin are common, and only exceptional cases of conditions such as actinic keratosis (AK) and some forms of nevi progress to malignancy. Benign tumors are usually derived from surface epithelium (**seborrheic keratosis, keratoacanthoma, epithelioma of Malherbe**), ductular cells of skin appendages (**sebaceous adenoma, syringoma**, various cysts), or neuroectodermal cells (nevi). Some benign tumors are associated with viral infections (**verruca vulgaris, molluscum contagiosum**). Benign mesenchymal tumors in the dermis include hemangiomas, lymphangiomas, and fibromas, including **skin tags** (dermatofibroma, fibrous histiocytoma), neurofibromas, and lipomas.

The most frequent **malignant tumors** of the skin are epidermal neoplasms (squamous cell carcinoma [SCC], basal cell carcinoma [BCC]), melanocytic tumors (malignant melanomas [MMs]), and malignant lymphomas. Less frequent are tumors of the skin appendages (sebaceous cell carcinoma, sweat gland carcinoma), other neuroectodermal tumors (malignant neuroectodermal tumor, Merkel cell tumor), and mesenchymal neoplasms (fibrosarcoma, liposarcoma, hemangiosarcoma, lymphangiosarcoma).

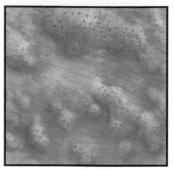

Urticaria: Pink edematous plaques with follicular accentuation caused by the dermal edema

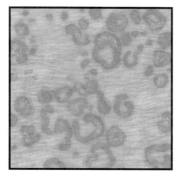

Annular and serpiginous urticaria: This is a less commonly seen variant of urticaria

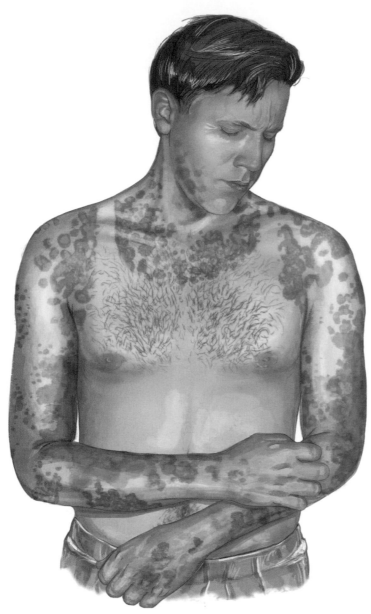

Solar Urticaria: Note the areas affected are those only exposed to the sun in this sleeveless shirt–wearing man

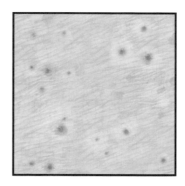

Cholinergic urticaria: This form of urticaria can be induced by increasing the body temperature through exercise or submersion in a warm bath

FIGURE 9-1   URTICARIA AND ACUTE ECZEMATOUS DERMATITIS

Urticaria (hives), an acute pruritic disease of short duration, is caused by a type I immune reaction (allergic, IgE-mediated) that results in local accumulation and degranulation of mast cells with histamine release and edema (pruritic nodule, edematous swelling and plaques, formation of bullae). Urticaria is caused by substances such as drugs, household stuffs, insect bites, and foods that elicit a type I immune reaction. Chronic urticaria lasting more than 6 weeks suggests persistent exposure to food additives, dyes, drugs, dust, or diseases such as thyroiditis or systemic lupus erythematosus. Acute eczematous dermatitis is characterized by erythema, edema, and vesicle formation. In later stages, oozing lesions may become crusted with scaling plaques. The etiopathogenesis is similar to urticaria (IgE-dependent immune reaction), but microscopy shows distinct eosinophilia and epidermal spongiosis. Fungal infection (**dermatophytosis**) must be excluded in the differential diagnosis.

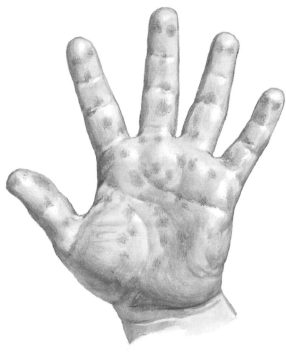

Erythema multiforme frequently
affects the palms.

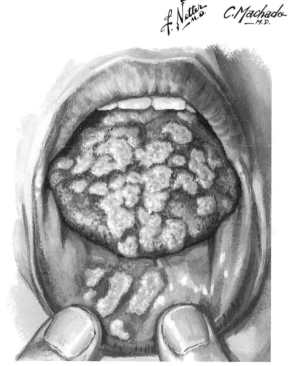

Erythema multiforme exudativum

FIGURE 9-2   ERYTHEMA MULTIFORME

Erythema multiforme (**EMF**), a common hypersensitivity syndrome with associated vasculitis, may coincide with other diseases (e.g., various infections). EMF may occur after the administration of certain drugs (sulfonamides, barbiturates, salicylates) or may accompany malignant diseases (carcinoma, lymphoma) and collagen-vascular disorders (e.g., systemic lupus erythematosus). It represents a hypersensitivity reaction (CD8+ cellular immune reaction), although the immediate causative agent is unknown. Skin eruption is frequently preceded by malaise, fever, and itching or burning sensations. Typical skin changes consist of **target lesions** with centrifugal growth, dusky red plaques, and macules and papules on the feet and the extensor surfaces of the arms and legs. Individual lesions heal within 1 to 2 weeks and show variable hyperpigmentation and hypopigmentation. Urticarial changes may add to the polymorphism (hence the term *multiforme*).

Lichen Planus

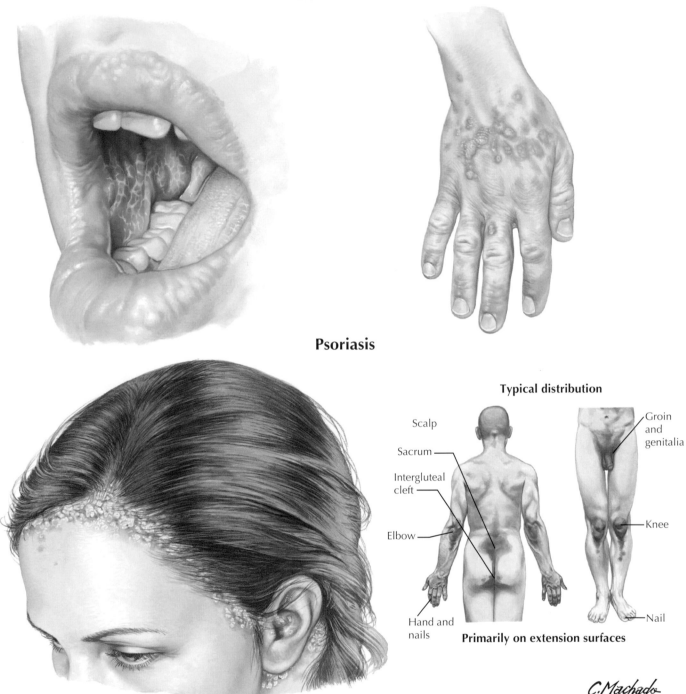

Psoriasis

Typical distribution

Scalp

Sacrum

Intergluteal cleft

Elbow

Hand and nails

Primarily on extension surfaces

Groin and genitalia

Knee

Nail

C. Machado
—M.D.

FIGURE 9-3   LICHEN PLANUS AND PSORIASIS

Lichen planus (LP) is a **papulosquamous dermatosis**. LP affects skin and mucous membranes and consists of small (2-10 mm) polygonal, white to pink, flat pruritic papules with a crisscrossed surface (**Wickham striae**). Externally, the papules are located on the flexor surfaces of the wrists, arms, and legs; internally, they appear on the tongue and buccal mucosa as nonerosive or erosive plaques. Malignant transformation of oral LP to SCC has been reported. Microscopy shows liquefaction degeneration of basal cells with subepithelial lymphocytic infiltration. Rete pegs are elongated with hyperparakeratosis, fissures, and single cell keratinization (**Civatte bodies**). LP is a cellular immune reaction against unidentified epithelial antigens. **Psoriasis** is a chronic inflammatory dermatosis of epidermis and dermis with epidermal hyperplasia and hyperkeratosis and parakeratosis. A deregulated epidermal cell proliferation with disturbed microcirculation has been hypothesized. Skin lesions are large (4-5 cm), demarcated, pink plaques with silver-white keratotic scales showing pinpoint hemorrhages (**Auspitz sign**). Microscopy shows epidermal thickening with elongated rete pegs (**acanthosis**), loss of the stratum granulosum and parakeratosis, thinning of suprapapillary plates with hyperemic vessels in dermal papillae, and a mixed cellular subepidermal-epidermal inflammatory infiltrate.

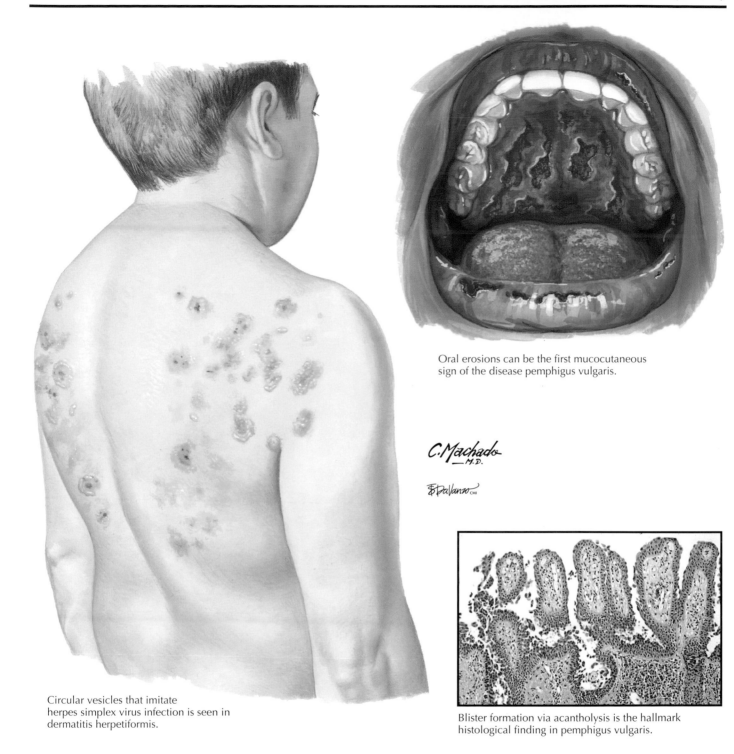

Oral erosions can be the first mucocutaneous sign of the disease pemphigus vulgaris.

Circular vesicles that imitate herpes simplex virus infection is seen in dermatitis herpetiformis.

Blister formation via acantholysis is the hallmark histological finding in pemphigus vulgaris.

FIGURE 9-4   DERMATITIS HERPETIFORMIS AND PEMPHIGUS VULGARIS

Dermatitis herpetiformis is a pruritic vesicular dermatosis often related to gluten-sensitive enteropathy (celiac disease). Burning and itching lesions on the extensor surfaces, the knees and elbows, the back, and the buttocks show a herpeslike (**herpetiform**) pattern. Microscopy shows subepidermal cleft formation with dense neutrophilic infiltration and microabscess formation. Dermoepidermal separation causes blister formation. Immunofluorescence shows granular or fibrillar IgA deposits in dermal papillae, and antiendomysial IgA antibodies can be demonstrated. **Pemphigus vulgaris**, a potentially lethal autoimmune dermatosis, involves skin and mucous membranes, primarily in older patients. It occurs everywhere on the skin except the palms and soles, with blisters that can be laterally dislocated (**Nikolsky sign**). Healing occurs with hyperpigmentation and scarring. Microscopy shows vesicle formation within the **stratum spinosum** with **acantholytic** epithelial cells and few lymphocytes, macrophages, or eosinophils. Serum IgG autoantibodies against **desmoglein III** (intercellular desmosomal component) can be demonstrated. Death occurs in approximately 10% of cases.

Impetigo starts with painless blisters, usually on the face, especially near the nose and mouth. Blisters fill with clear or yellow fluid and crust over.

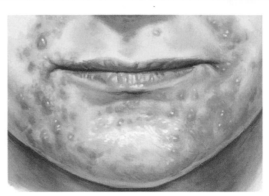

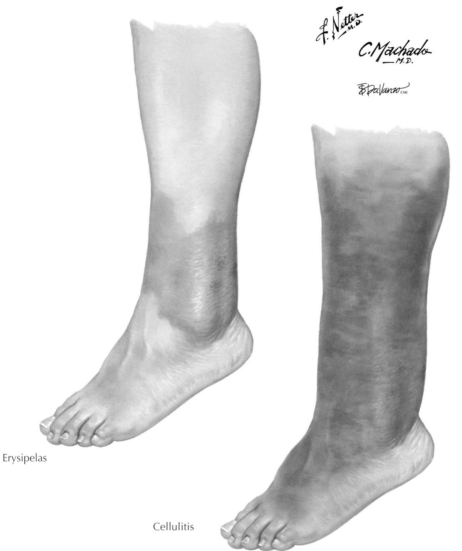

Erysipelas

Cellulitis

FIGURE 9-5 IMPETIGO, CELLULITIS, AND ERYSIPELAS

Impetigo, a superficial staphylococcal infection of the skin, occurs after minor injury. Lesions consist of pustular, vesicular, or bullous eruptions with surrounding erythema and development of honey-yellow adherent crusts. The infection usually heals within a few weeks or months. **Cellulitis** is an acute streptococcal infection of the deeper dermis and subcutaneous tissue that can spread to cover a large area of skin. Lesions consist of poorly demarcated painful erythematous swellings, occasionally complicated by blisters, hemorrhage, or abscess formation.

Cellulitis often occurs in patients with impaired host defense from diabetes mellitus, liver cirrhosis, renal failure, chronic alcoholism, or human immunodeficiency virus (HIV). **Erysipelas** is an acute superficial form of cellulitis with demarcated margins and prominent lymphangitis usually caused by type A streptococci. Patients experience malaise, anorexia, fever, and chills. Blood culture results may be positive in cases with high fever. Lesions clear within 2 to 3 weeks, with frequent recurrences in immunocompromised patients.

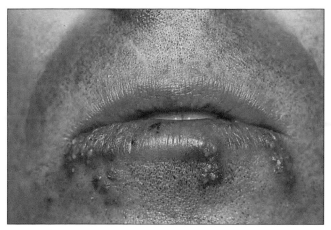

Herpes simplex virus (HSV1) infection. See typical "fever blisters" of lips

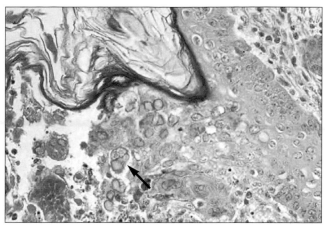

HSV1 infection. Microscopy shows typical nuclear inclusions (arrow) and vesicle formation of epidermis

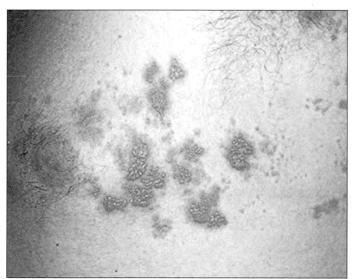

Typical herpes zoster lesions. In reactivated VZV infection

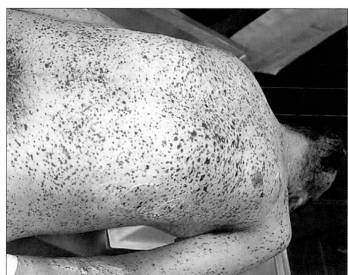

Varicella zoster virus (VZV). Multiple hemorrhagic vesicles, infection in patient with immune deficiency

FIGURE 9-6   HERPES SIMPLEX AND VARICELLA ZOSTER

Along with varicella zoster virus and herpes genitalis, **herpes simplex virus** is among the more common viruses causing acute vesicular dermatitis. Acute primary infection by respiratory droplets or direct contact causes transient stomatitis and pharyngitis associated with mild lymphadenopathy. Grouped vesicles on an erythematous background appear at various sites, including the mucous membranes. Lesions heal spontaneously without scarring within 2 to 6 weeks. Some areas show only erythematous spots or plaques. Reactivated herpes simplex or **varicella zoster** in immunodeficient patients can cause severe systemic herpes with generalized necrotic and hemorrhagic lesions and life-threatening internal disease (hemorrhagic enteritis and encephalitis, necrotizing and hemorrhagic hepatitis).

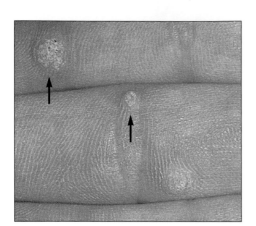

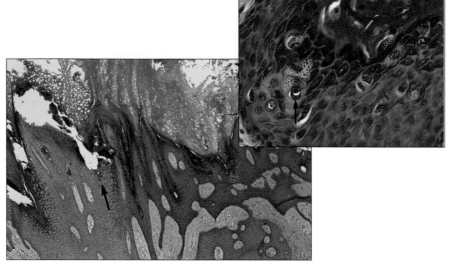

Verruca vulgaris. Multiple lesions on palmar side of fingers (**left**, arrows) showing microscopically severe epidermal hyperplasia, prominent keratohyalin granules (**right**, arrow) and hyperkeratosis. Keratohyalin granules seen in higher magnification (**inset**, arrow)

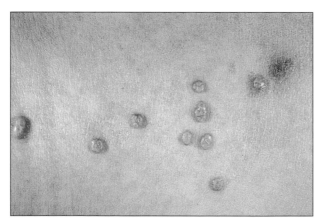

Molluscum contagiosum. (milker nodules) showing typical small centrally depressed nodules

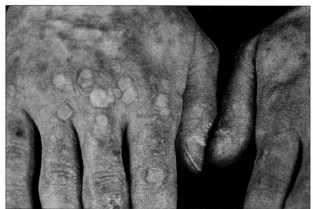

Epidermodysplasia verruciformis. Showing irregular, white nodules and plaques on dorsal surface of hands

FIGURE 9-7   MISCELLANEOUS VIRAL SKIN INFECTIONS

Other viral infections of the skin produce a proliferative epidermal reaction with or without overt inflammatory response. These include **verrucae vulgares** (common warts) and **condylomata acuminata** (genital warts) caused by human papillomavirus (HPV) and **molluscum contagiosum** (Milker nodule) caused by an unclassified poxvirus. There are more than 70 subtypes of HPV, some of which may be oncogenic, including HPV-5, implicated

in **epidermodysplasia verruciformis**; HPV-6, in genital warts; HPV-16, in penile carcinoma; HPV-16 and HPV-18, which in a subset of cases may lead to the development of dysplasia (cervical intraepithelial neoplasia) or carcinoma. The occurrence of proliferative viral infections and their malignant sequelae increase significantly in immunodeficient patients.

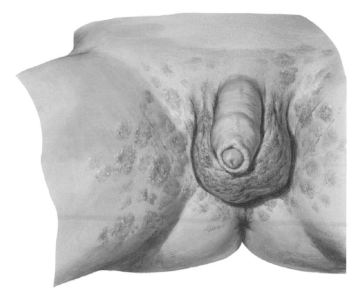

Candida albicans infection, typical "diaper rash"

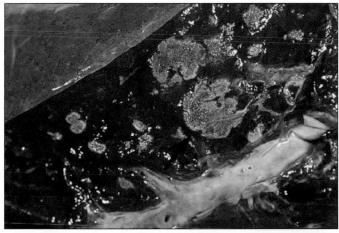

Systemic candida infection. In an immunodeficient patient showing typical dry and granular pulmonary abscesses (arrow)

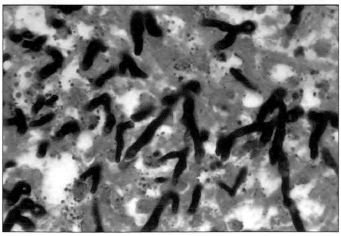

Microscopy of candida organisms. Stained by methenamine silver reaction (black)

FIGURE 9-8   DERMAL CANDIDIASIS

Dermal candidiasis is a fungal infection that occurs frequently in patients with metabolic or immunodeficiency disorders (e.g., diabetes mellitus, long-standing steroid or antibiotic treatment, HIV, inherited immune deficiency). Yeasts, such as *Candida* species, belong to the normal flora of skin and mucous membranes close to the skin (oral cavity, vagina, anus). If the host defense is disturbed, these organisms become pathogenic,

causing mucositis and eventual hematogenous spread. Initially, warm, moist areas, such as the axillae, the groin, and other intertriginous regions, show moist erythematous plaques and papules with red denuded areas and glistening, cigarette paper–like scaling. Fungal organisms can be scraped from lesions and shown with histologic stains or by cultivation.

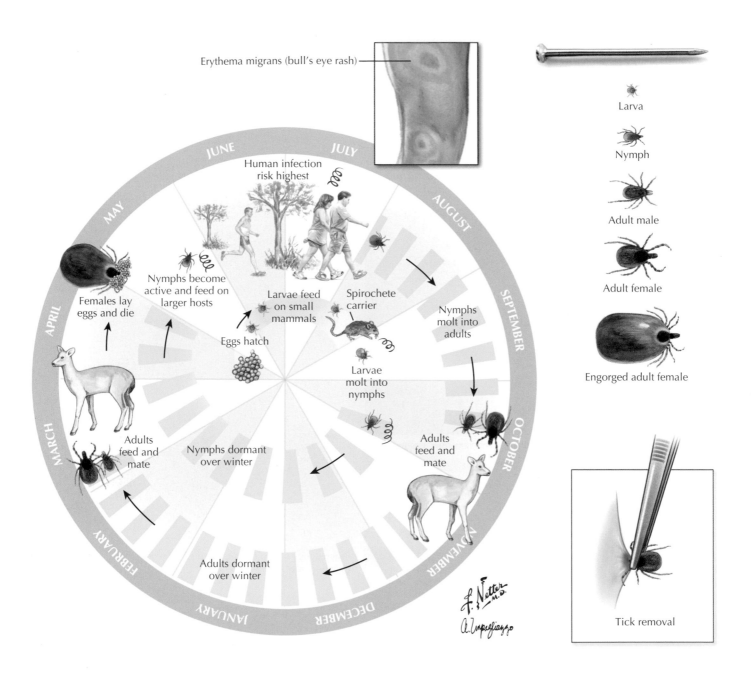

Erythema migrans (bull's eye rash)

Larva

Nymph

Adult male

Adult female

Engorged adult female

JUNE **JULY** **AUGUST** **SEPTEMBER** **OCTOBER** **NOVEMBER** **DECEMBER** **JANUARY** **FEBRUARY** **MARCH** **APRIL** **MAY**

Human infection risk highest

Nymphs become active and feed on larger hosts

Females lay eggs and die

Larvae feed on small mammals

Spirochete carrier

Nymphs molt into adults

Eggs hatch

Larvae molt into nymphs

Adults feed and mate

Adults feed and mate

Nymphs dormant over winter

Adults dormant over winter

Tick removal

FIGURE 9-9 LYME DISEASE

Lyme disease is caused by the spirochete *Borrelia burgdorferi,* which is acquired through tick bites. Ticks invade the skin, causing **erythema migrans**. Starting at the site of the tick bite, erythemalous patches develop and spread in an irregular pattern while the center will return to normal. Lyme disease progresses through several stages, including an acute influenzalike illness, cardiac and neurologic symptoms, and, finally, arthritis and persistent neuropsychiatric disorders.

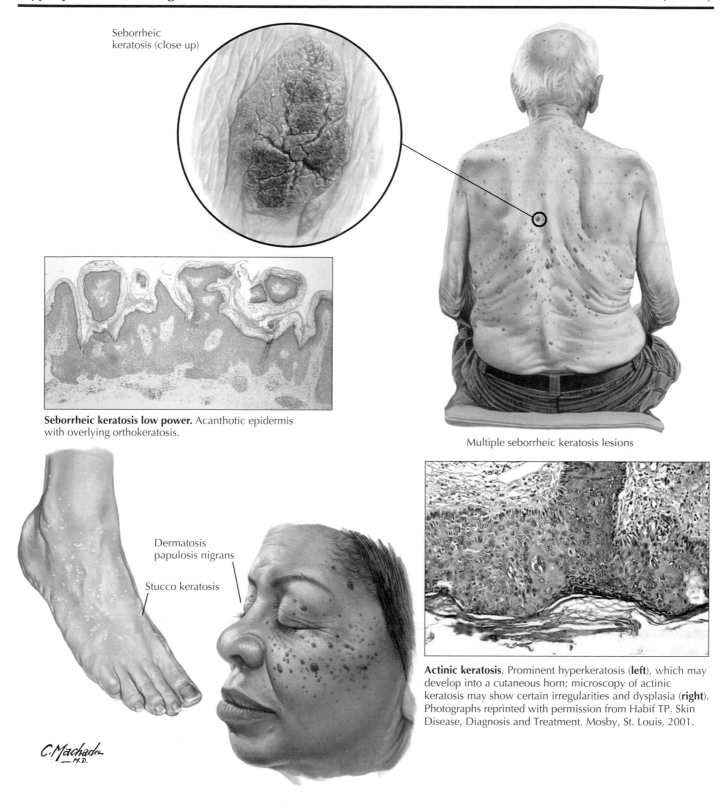

Seborrheic keratosis (close up)

Seborrheic keratosis low power. Acanthotic epidermis with overlying orthokeratosis.

Multiple seborrheic keratosis lesions

Dermatosis papulosis nigrans

Stucco keratosis

Actinic keratosis. Prominent hyperkeratosis (**left**), which may develop into a cutaneous horn; microscopy of actinic keratosis may show certain irregularities and dysplasia (**right**). Photographs reprinted with permission from Habif TP. Skin Disease, Diagnosis and Treatment. Mosby, St. Louis, 2001.

FIGURE 9-10   KERATOSES

Seborrheic keratosis is a common, benign, sharply demarcated, flat or raised, epidermal proliferation with a pink to brownish-black, pigmented, smooth or lobulated surface. A sudden outgrowth of multiple seborrheic keratoses may be associated with malignancies of internal organs (**Leser-Trélat sign**). Microscopy shows epidermal thickening by multiple layers of small basaloid cells and various degrees of melanin pigmentation and

hyperkeratosis. Some pigmented lesions must be distinguished from MM. **AK** is a benign lesion that may eventually progress to SCC. Excessive keratinization frequently produces **cutaneous horns**. AK develops at sites of chronic sun exposure and shows progressive epithelial dysplasia. Some may be pigmented (**spreading pigmented actinic keratosis**) and are difficult to distinguish from lentigo maligna or superficial spreading MM.

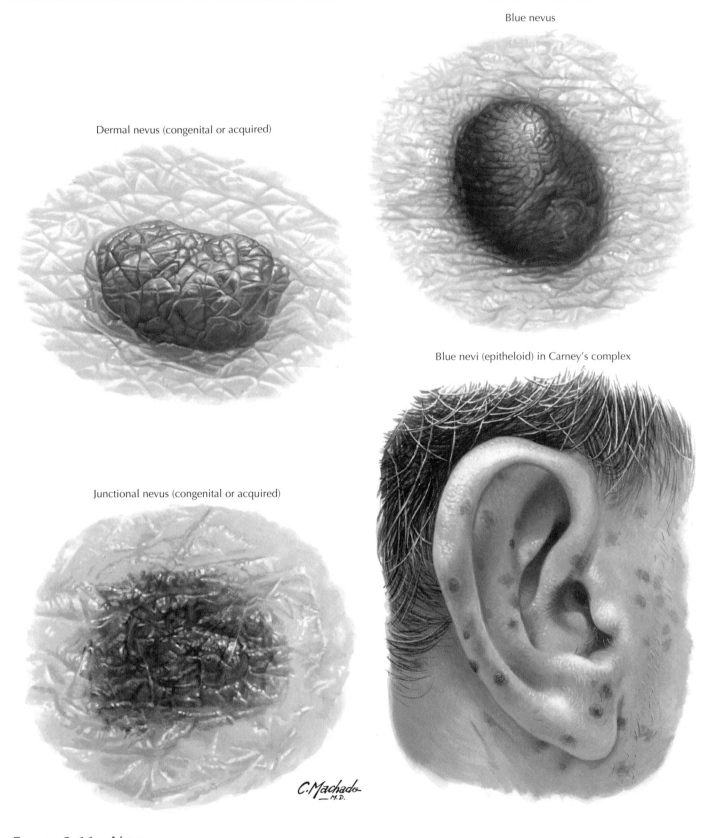

Blue nevus

Dermal nevus (congenital or acquired)

Blue nevi (epitheloid) in Carney's complex

Junctional nevus (congenital or acquired)

C. Machado — M.D.

FIGURE 9-11 NEVI

Nevi (**common moles**) are benign skin tumors of melanocytic origin. **Dysplastic nevi** describe nevi with cellular atypia without invasion. Nevi erupting de novo in areas of the body not exposed to the sun and occurring after the age of 30 years should always be evaluated for malignancy. Microscopy shows bands or nests of melanocytes in the epidermis (**epidermal**) or epidermal junction (**junctional nevus**) or both (**compound nevi**). **Dermal nevi** do not show epidermal involvement. Deep dermal nevi are referred to as **blue nevi**. A gross change to asymmetry and partial poor demarcation with spread and discoloration may indicate malignant transformation.

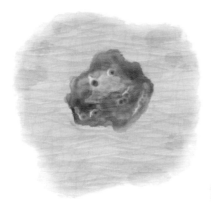

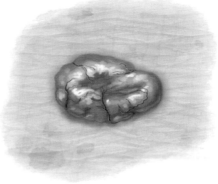

Superficial basal cell carcinoma. Slightly scaly pink to red patch. These tumors are slow growing and occur on chronically sun-exposed skin.

Nodular basal cell carcinoma. Pearly plaque with telangiectatic central ulceration, and rolled border

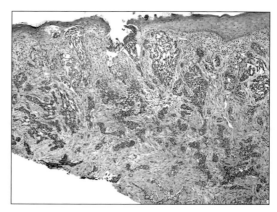

Basophilic tumor lobules and strands extending from the epidermis into the dermis

FIGURE 9-12 BASAL CELL CARCINOMA

Basal cell carcinoma is a primary epidermal malignancy that does not metastasize but shows progressive invasion without sparing even skull bones (**ulcus rodens**). BCC is frequent in the skin of the face, scalp, ears, and neck. In addition, there exists a rare familial basal cell nevus syndrome with multiple tumors on the back and other non–sun-exposed sites. BCC appears as flat, yellowish-pink circumscribed nodules ("pearly" appearance) with prominent telangiectasia and occasional white keratotic scaling. Microscopy shows the replacement of regular squamous epithelium with atypical basal cells with peripheral palisading and signs of invasion. After surgical removal, 92% of patients with primary tumors and 60% with recurrences achieve 5-year survival.

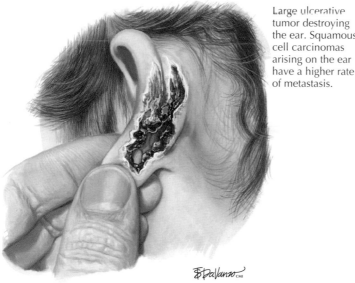

Large ulcerative tumor destroying the ear. Squamous cell carcinomas arising on the ear have a higher rate of metastasis.

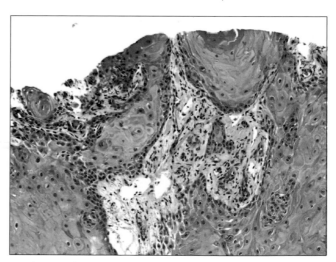

Invasive SCC, high power. Atypical keratinocytes, mitotic figures, and horn pearl formation

FIGURE 9-13 SQUAMOUS CELL CARCINOMA

Squamous cell carcinoma, derived from keratinocytes, is one of the most common malignant tumors in the sun-exposed skin (head, neck, hands) of older people. Chemical carcinogens in tars, oils, arsenicals, and ionizing radiation also may cause SCC. Primary SCC appears as sharply circumscribed, soft or firm red nodules with a "crusted" hyperkeratotic or eroded center spreading within the skin and extending into the dermis along perivascular or perineural spaces (**conduit spread**). Ultimately, tumors metastasize to regional lymph nodes. Microscopy shows variable differentiation and keratinization of squamous cells, with disorganized growth and single cell keratosis, focal or total loss of stratification, and overt invasion. Tumors larger than 2 cm in diameter with deep (0.4 cm) dermal invasion are at risk for metastasis, which occurs in approximately 2% to 6% of tumors in well-vascularized regions and 20% to 30% in other areas (lips, ears, scar tissue). The 5-year mortality in patients with regional metastases is approximately 50%.

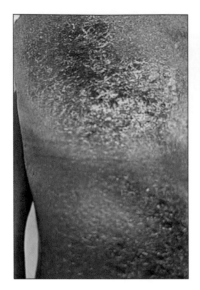
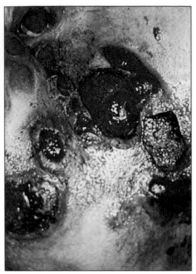
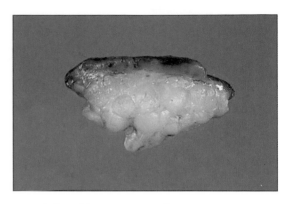

Mycosis fungoides. Eczematous (**left**), tumorous (**middle**), and plaquelike (**right**) infiltrations of skin

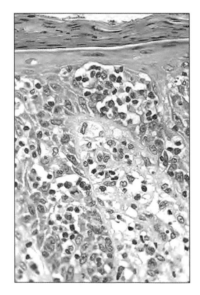
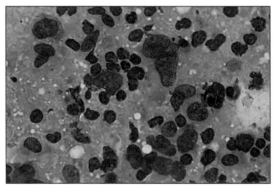

Microscopy. Epidermal invasion (**left**) and atypical giant cells in touch prep (**right**)

FIGURE 9-14   MALIGNANT LYMPHOMAS

Malignant lymphomas of the skin include non-Hodgkin lymphomas and Hodgkin lymphomas. The most frequent non-Hodgkin lymphoma of the skin is the T-cell lymphoma identified as **mycosis fungoides** (MF), preferentially affecting people aged 30 to 50 years. MF is a distinct CD4+ T helper cell lymphoma that may secondarily involve lymph nodes and internal organs. It develops in stages from pre-MF eczematoid or psoriasislike lesions to a patch stage, a plaque stage, and a tumor stage.

Microscopy shows a bandlike polymorphous dermal infiltrate with small to medium lymphoid cells, including approximately 10% to 40% atypical cells with **cerebriform nuclei** (**MF cells**) and pronounced epidermotropism. Atypical cells invade the epidermis to form small aggregates referred to as **Pautrier abscesses.** The median survival time is 5 years, although if lesions are ulcerated and MF invades lymph nodes, the survival time decreases to 1 year.

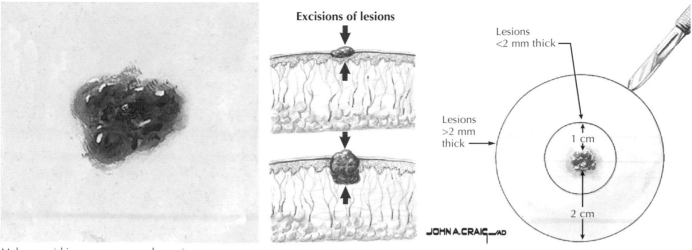

Melanoma (skin or mucous membranes)

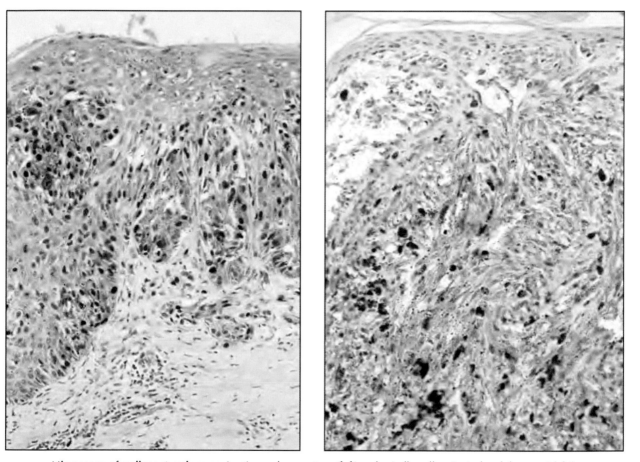

Microscopy of malignant melanoma. Lentigo melanoma type (**left**) and spindle cell variant of nodular type (**right**)

FIGURE 9-15 MALIGNANT MELANOMA

Malignant melanoma, an increasingly common melanocytic neoplasm, comprises approximately 4% of all cancers, with greatest incidence in the sun-exposed skin of red- or fair-haired persons. MM is clinically asymptomatic except for the warning signs: enlargement of a preexisting nevus with irregular border or change in color; itching and pain; or sudden development of pigmented lesions in adults in sites not often exposed to the sun. Late-stage changes are tenderness, bleeding, and ulceration. The types of MM are **lentigo maligna melanoma**, **superficial spreading melanoma**, **nodular melanoma**, and **amelanotic melanoma**. Microscopy shows poorly formed nests of nevus cells with atypia (enlarged nuclei with prominent nucleoli and mitoses), overt signs of invasion, adjacent chronic inflammatory reaction, and lymphatic spread. Size and vertical spread determine clinical staging and prognosis. After lesion removal, the 5-year survival rate is 80% to 95% in patients with early MM and less than 20% in patients with advanced disease.

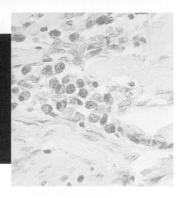

CHAPTER 10

HEMATOPOIETIC AND LYMPHATIC TISSUES

Cells of the hematopoietic and lymphatic tissues serve vital functions of host defense, internal homeostasis, and bodily intactness. They all originate from the same stem cell population and in their functional activities interact in various ways (see chapter 1). Disorders in one cell population may thus cause reactions in the other. For this reason, the hematopoietic and lymphatic systems are discussed together. Just as there are a large number of different cell populations with various differentiation stages and functional activities, so are there a multitude of human diseases of the blood and lymphatic systems. The most common and important are discussed in this chapter. The most common leading symptoms of all these diseases are infection, hemorrhage or thrombosis, and anemia.

RED BLOOD CELL DISORDERS

Red blood cell (RBC) disorders manifest themselves by either a decrease (**anemia**) or an increase (**erythrocytosis**) of RBCs, the latter being reactive or neoplastic in nature. These disorders preferentially affect oxygen transport to tissues; excessive erythrocytosis may be complicated by increased intravascular thrombosis.

WHITE BLOOD CELL DISORDERS (NONLYMPHATIC)

White blood cell (WBC) disorders (nonlymphatic) include reactive and neoplastic changes of hematopoietic tissues. Reactive changes may be either hyperplastic (**leukocytosis**) or hypoplastic/aplastic (**leukopenia**). They arise in response to exogenous or endogenous stimuli and generally are reversible. Neoplastic changes (**myelodysplastic** or **myeloproliferative syndromes, leukemia**) also may occur in response to certain stimuli (e.g., carcinogens, radiation, viral infection) but become autonomous and thus practically irreversible.

NONNEOPLASTIC LYMPHATIC DISORDERS

Lymphatic tissues are the body's main carriers of host defense, both specific and nonspecific. Consequently, nonneoplastic changes in the lymphatic system may result from functional alterations in the immune system as well as from inflammatory, necrotic, or metabolic disorders. Changes in lymph nodes or spleen may be secondary to other disorders, as when the lymph system or bloodstream transports disease products from a primary disease focus (e.g., lymphadenitis in the neck developing secondary to a dental abscess or septic splenitis secondary to bacterial enterocolitis). Investigation of a patient with some form of lymphatic disease therefore must always include a search for a primary cause.

NEOPLASTIC LYMPHATIC DISORDERS

Malignant neoplasias of the lymphatic tissues are collectively identified as **malignant lymphomas** (MLs) or, when malignant cells circulate in the blood, **lymphocytic leukemias**. There are 2 major groups of MLs: **Hodgkin lymphomas (lymphogranulomatosis)** and **non-Hodgkin lymphomas** (NHLs). Hodgkin lymphoma, or Hodgkin disease (HD), is distinguished from NHL by its polymorphic features, including certain inflammatory components such as fibrosis and occasional regression simulating nonneoplastic diseases, which eventually may progress to ML. Although it is a lymphatic malignancy, it is accompanied by a large number of associated nonneoplastic cells, which may influence the course and progression of the disease. NHL, by contrast, begins as malignant clonal proliferations. Transition from HD to NHL and combinations of HD with certain types of NHL have been observed (HD and chronic lymphocytic leukemia [CLL] or follicular center cell lymphoma [FCC]; see Table 10-4).

Along with diagnosing an ML as HD or NHL and determining the subclassification based on histologic, immunologic, and cytogenetic markers, staging of disease extent helps to determine the appropriate treatment and the life expectancy of the patient. Staging of all lymphomas is similar: *stage I* indicates involvement by lymphoma of 1 lymph node site (e.g., axillary, neck); *stage II* indicates involvement of 2 lymph node sites on the same side of the diaphragm (e.g., neck and axillary, or left and right inguinal); *stage III* indicates involvement of lymph nodes on both sides of the diaphragm; and *stage IV* indicates involvement of lymphatic and extralymphatic sites (e.g., liver, spleen, bone marrow). ML may arise from sites other than the lymph nodes. These are grouped together as *extranodal lymphomas* and have different staging.

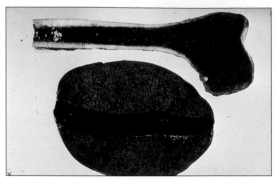

Hematopoietic hyperplasia in hemolytic anemia. Bone marrow (top) and spleen (bottom)

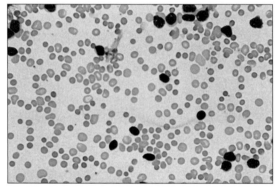

Autoimmune hemolytic anemia

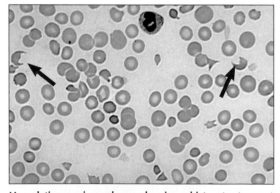

Hemolytic uremic syndrome showing schistocytes (arrows)

TABLE 10-1 CLASSIFICATION OF ANEMIAS*

Category	RBCs	Characteristics
Blood loss, acute	Initially: normochromic, normocytic Later: hypochromic reticulocytosis	Acute volume depletion RBC reduction secondary to fluid influx Rapid RBC regeneration
Blood loss, chronic	Hypochromic	Reduced iron stores
Increased Destruction of Erythrocytes		
Hemolytic anemias		Features of hemolysis and tissue siderosis Bone marrow: significant erythropoietic hyperplasia Splenomegaly
Immunologic	Reticulocytosis	Autoantibodies against RBC (infection or drug induced) Isohemagglutinins (transfusion induced, erythroblastosis fetalis)

Mechanical	Schistocytes	Microangiopathic:
		  Hemolytic uremic syndrome
		  Thrombotic thrombocytopenic purpura
		  Trauma by intracardiac artificial devices
		  Multiple hemangiomas (e.g., hepatic)

Hereditary	Spherocytosis Elliptocytosis Sickle cells Hypochromic, microcytic Heinz bodies	RBC membrane and cytoskeleton deficiencies Hemoglobinopathies: sickle cell anemia, thalassemia Enzyme deficiencies (e.g., of hexose monophosphate shunt)
Deficient Erythropoiesis		
"Stem cell" defect	Normochromic, Normocytic to mildly macrocytic	Aplastic anemia (with pancytopenia), pure red cell aplasia secondary to myelofibrosis (with thrombocytopenia, splenomegaly)
Maturation defect	Megaloblastic Anisocytic Hypochromic Poikilocytic	Pernicious anemia (vitamin B_{12} deficiency), folate deficiency, anemia, iron deficiency (infection, tumor, chronic blood loss)
Hb synthesis defect	Sideroblasts	Sideroblastic anemia

*Hb indicates hemoglobin; RBC, red blood
normochromic: normal color (i.e. normal Hb content); normocytic: normal size and shape of RBC; hemolytic: red cell lysis

FIGURE 10-1 ACQUIRED ANEMIAS

Classification of **anemias** by immediate cause is shown in Table 10-1. Acute blood loss initially causes blood volume depletion; normochromic anemia becomes overt 24 to 48 hours later, after some volume is replaced. Chronic blood loss (e.g., in intestinal ulcers, polyposis, hypermenorrhea) with depletion of the body's iron stores causes hypochromic anemia. Erythrocyte destruction causes several anemias. **Immunohemolytic anemia** arises spontaneously after infection or drug treatment or in **erythroblas-** **tosis fetalis**, the incompatibility of erythrocyte antigens between an Rh-negative mother and her Rh-positive fetus. **Microangiopathic hemolytic anemia** (MAHA) is caused by mechanical shear forces from fibrin strands in small vessels (**hemolytic uremic syndrome**, **disseminated intravascular coagulation**, or multiple hemangiomas) or from artificial devices in the bloodstream (e.g., cardiac valvular prostheses). Peripheral blood smears show fragmented erythrocytes (**schistocytes, fragmentocytes**).

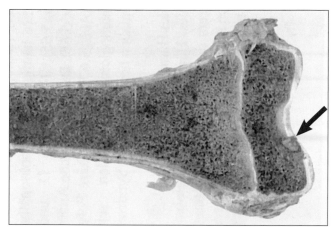
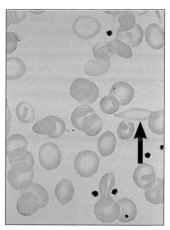

Sickle cell anemia in femur marrow showing diffusely hyperplastic bone marrow and focal necrosis (arrow)

Sickle cell anemia. Blood smear (arrow for sickle cells)

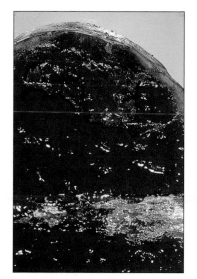
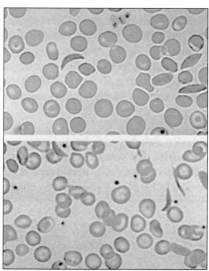

β-Thalassemia. Splenic infarct

β-Thalassemia. Blood smear

FIGURE 10-2   HEREDITARY ANEMIAS

Hereditary anemias with structural abnormalities of RBC membranes, cytoskeleton, or hemoglobin (Hb) show spherocytes (**hereditary spherocytosis**), elliptocytes (**hereditary elliptocytosis**), sickle cells (**sickle cell anemia**), or poikilocytosis, anisocytosis, microcytosis, hypochromasia, and reticulocytosis. Vulnerable RBCs are sequestered in the spleen and undergo hemolysis. Many hereditary anemias thus have clinical features of hemolytic anemia: splenomegaly, bone marrow hyperplasia, and tissue siderosis. **Thalassemias** entail defective synthesis of Hb α or β chains (α, β-thalassemia). A severe form (**Cooley anemia**) shows a reduction or absence of Hb β chains, predominance of fetal hemoglobulin, reactive bone marrow hyperplasia and spleno-megaly, enhanced iron resorption, and iron overload syndrome (hemosiderosis, hemochromatosis). In **sickle cell anemia**, rigid sickle cells undergo hemolysis and cause vasoocclusive disease (capillary stasis and thrombosis) with infarcts in many organs.

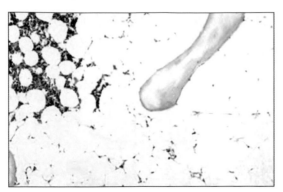
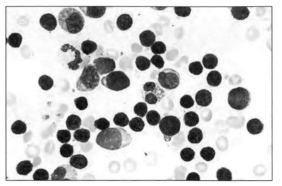

Aplastic anemia. Showing a severely hypoplastic bone marrow (**left**) and a blood smear with immature red cell precursors and a relative increase of lymphocytes (**right**)

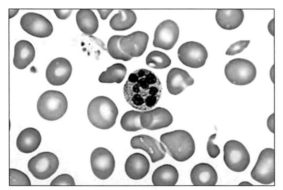
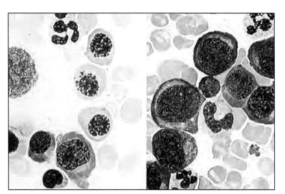

Pernicious anemia. Blood smear showing macrocytes and hypersegmented neutrophils

Pernicious anemia. Marrow smear showing megaloblasts and hypersegmented neutrophils

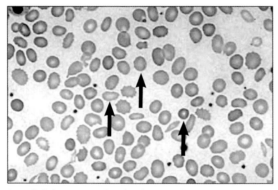
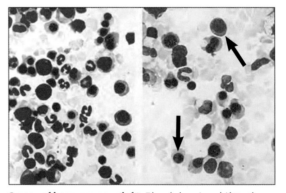

Iron deficiency anemia. Blood smear showing anisocytosis and poikilocytosis (arrows)

Smear of bone marrow (left). Blood showing shift to the left with increased megaloblasts and nucleated erythrocytes (arrows)

FIGURE 10-3 ANEMIAS OF DEFICIENT HEMOPOIESIS

Aplastic anemia is characterized by anemia, neutropenia (reduced number in neutrophils), and thrombocytopenia (reduced number in platelets) and may transform to leukemia. The bone marrow is hypocellular. Patients show pallor, petechial hemorrhages, and increased susceptibility to infection. **Pernicious anemia** (megaloblastic anemia) arises from a deficiency of vitamin B_{12}, folate, or both secondary to reduced resorption in atrophic gastritis or chronic liver diseases. Myelocytes and megakaryocytes in the bone marrow show nuclear abnormalities (e.g., "horseshoe myelocytes," hypersegmented megakaryocytes). **Sideroblastic anemia** is an X chromosome–linked or acquired deficiency of Hb synthesis. It is a hypochromic microcytic anemia with ferric phosphate or hydroxide deposits in mitochondria of erythroblasts (**ring sideroblasts**). Resistant cases necessitate multiple transfusions and thus may be complicated by iron overload syndrome with secondary hemochromatosis, cardiac failure, and diabetes mellitus.

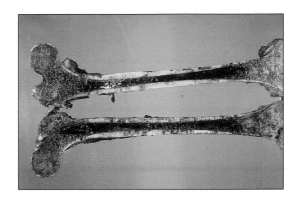

Polycythemia vera. Hematopoietic hyperplasia of bone marrow, femur

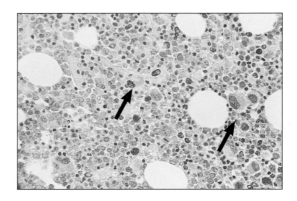

Polycythemia vera. Bone marrow biopsy showing hematopoietic hyperplasia, reduced trilinear maturation, and increased immature megakaryocytes (arrows)

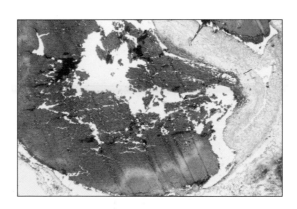

Deep vein thrombosis. Complication of polycythemia vera

FIGURE 10-4   POLYCYTHEMIA VERA

A chronic myeloproliferative disease with autonomous clonal proliferation of myelopoietic stem cells in bone marrow and extramedullary sites (liver, spleen), **polycythemia vera** (PCV; primary erythrocytosis) must be distinguished from other chronic myeloproliferative diseases, such as chronic myelogenous leukemia (CML), primary thrombocythemia (PTH), and osteomyelofibrosis (OMF). The bone marrow in PCV shows panhyperplasia with erythropoietic predominance, depletion of bone marrow iron stores, progressive fibrosis, and clusters of macromegakaryo-cytes. Clinical features include splenomegaly, erythrocytosis of 6 to 10 million cells/µL, Hb level greater than 20 g/dL, and hematocrit greater than 60%. Serum erythropoietin is reduced. Patients show a typical red facies and report headaches and dizziness. Disturbances in blood flow may result in **angina pectoris**, **claudicatio intermittens**, upper intestinal ulcerations, or life-threatening thrombotic complications. Twenty percent to 50% of PCV patients progress to preleukemia and acute leukemia.

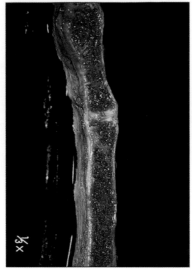

Malaria. Causing bone marrow hyperplasia and dirty gray-red pigmentation

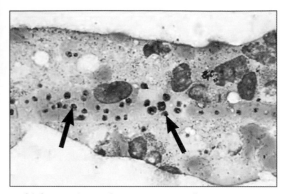

Multiple parasites. In bone marrow capillary (arrows)

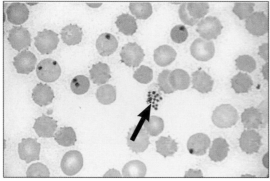

Merazoites. In blood smear

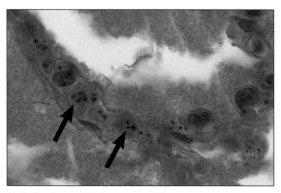

Malaria pigment. Pulmonary capillary

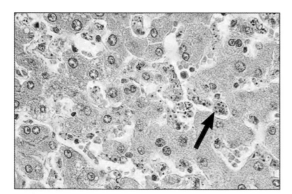

Engorgement of capillaries. Erythrocytes and parasites, liver

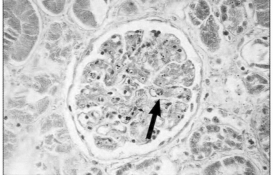

Engorgement of capillaries. Erythrocytes and parasites, kidney

FIGURE 10-5 MALARIA

Plasmodium protozoa (*P vivax, P malariae, P ovale,* and *P falciparum*) are carried by the female *Anopheles* mosquito, whose bite transfers **sporozoites** to the blood. After infecting hepatocytes, they transform to **merozoites** and infect erythrocytes. The 4 species cause diseases of different cycles and severity. *P vivax* and *P ovale* cause **tertian malaria**, *P malariae* causes **quartan malaria**, and *P falciparum* causes **falciparum malaria**, the most lethal form. Initial symptoms are anorexia, headache, bone pain, and chills. Episodic destruction of RBCs by schizogony and release of merozoites causes spiking fevers and shaking chills every third day in tertian and falciparum malaria and every fourth day in quartan malaria. Pathologic changes are hemolytic anemia, reticuloendothelial (RE) cell hyperplasia (liver, lymph nodes, spleen), obstruction of capillaries by infected RBCs (lungs, liver, kidneys, bone marrow, brain), and deposits of **malaria pigment** in RE cells and vascular endothelia.

TABLE 10-2   REACTIVE HEMATOPOIETIC HYPERPLASIA (NONLYMPHATIC)

Involved Cell Compartment	Cause
Erythrophilic, neutrophilic, and megakaryopoiesis	Blood loss or transient myelotoxic agents
Preferentially neutrophilic	Pyogenic bacterial infections, extensive tissue necroses Less extensive: drugs such as SCF, steroids
Neutrophilic and histiocytic (frequently with lymphocytes and eventual granuloma formation)	Chronic infections such as by intracellular organisms (e.g., *Rickettsia, Yersinia, Salmonella,* mycobacteria), mycoses, collagen-vascular diseases (e.g., lupus erythematosus)
Preferentially histiocytic	Protozoal infection (e.g., malaria) Suggestive viral infection (hemophagocytic syndrome) Phagocytosis defects (infantile septic granulomatosis, **Chediak-Higashi syndrome**, and others) Metabolic (various storage diseases: **morbus Gaucher, morbus Niemann-Pick**, and others)
Eosinophilic	Allergic diseases Parasitic infestations Viral infections with immune complex reaction (e.g., Hodgkin disease) Treatment with IL-2
Basophilic	Certain allergic diseases (e.g., food allergies) Certain endocrine disorders (e.g., myxedema) Estrogen treatment

SCF indicates colony stimulating factor; IL, interleukin.

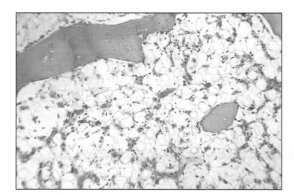

Marrow hypoplasia. Following cancer chemotherapy

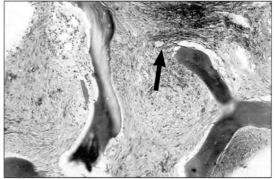

Marrow hypoplasia and focal fibrosis (arrow) in autoimmune agranulocytosis

FIGURE 10-6   HEMATOPOIETIC HYPOPLASIA

Decrease or loss of peripheral blood neutrophilic WBCs (**neutropenia** or **agranulocytosis**) is caused either by enhanced removal or destruction of cells or by their reduced production (i.e., by **bone marrow hypoplasia**). Increased destruction may result from toxins or infections (e.g., drugs, overwhelming infections), autoimmune reactions (e.g., autoimmune neutropenia or agranulocytosis), or increased removal in enlarged spleens (i.e., **hypersplenism** with **neutrophilic sequestration**). In these cases, the bone marrow shows reactive hyperplasia without cytologic abnormalities. In cases of toxic destruction, peripheral blood neutrophils may show **toxic granulations** in their cytoplasm and hypersegmented or fragmented nuclei. The 3 characteristic clinical consequences of hematopoietic hypoplasia are anemia, hemorrhage (in thrombocytopenia), and infection (in neutropenia or agranulocytosis). Hematopoietic hyperplasia in the bone marrow and reactive leukocytosis in the blood occur in response to various inflammatory stimuli or to certain cellular and metabolic deficiencies and may progress to simulating neoplasia (**leukemoid reaction**). Hematopoietic hyperplasia is accompanied by release from the bone marrow of less mature cells (**shift to the left**) with increased numbers of immature neutrophils, metamyelocytes, or even myelocytes. Different from neoplasia, reactive hyperplasia is usually transient and subsides when the causative stimulus is terminated (Table 10-2).

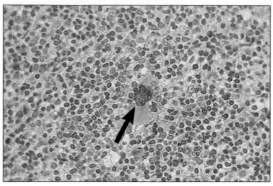

Myelodysplastic syndrome. Bone marrow biopsy specimen showing diffuse marrow hyperplasia with predominance of erythroblasts and dysplastic megakaryocytes (arrow)

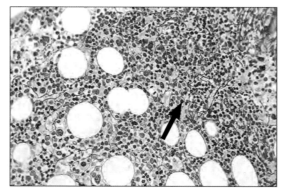

Myelodysplastic syndrome. Showing only slight increase in reticulin fibers (arrow)

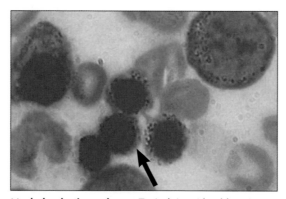

Myelodysplastic syndrome. Typical ring sideroblasts in blood smear (arrow)

FIGURE 10-7   MYELODYSPLASTIC SYNDROME

Myelodysplastic syndrome (MDS) is a form of hematopoietic hyperplasia and dysplasia with peripheral cytopenia. MDS originates from hematopoietic stem cell defects with multiple genetic abnormalities and clonal proliferation of hematopoietic cells, T lymphocytes, and clonal or polyclonal B lymphocytes. Several stages are identified: (1) refractory anemia (RA), with less than 5% blasts in the bone marrow; (2) refractory anemia with ringed sideroblasts (RARS), with less than 5% blasts; (3) refractory anemia with excess blasts (RAEB), with 5% to 20% bone marrow blasts; and (4) refractory anemia with excess blasts in transformation (RAEB-T), with 20% to 30% bone marrow blasts and more than 5% blasts in the blood. Anemia and fatigue are early symptoms, followed by neutropenia, infections, thrombocytopenia, and bleeding. Bone marrow aspirates show a megaloblastic erythropoiesis with ring sideroblasts, increased myeloblasts, and hypolobulated megakaryocytes. Transition to acute myelogenous leukemia (AML) occurs in 40% to 50% of advanced cases.

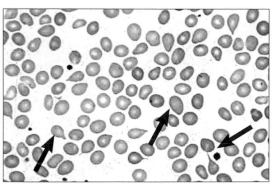

Osteomyelofibrosis. Immature thrombocytes and poikilocytosis (arrows)

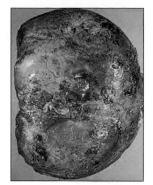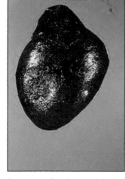

Osteomyelofibrosis. Splenomegaly (normal spleen, right)

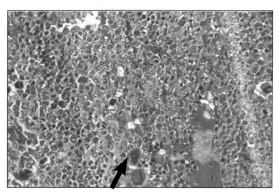

Osteomyelofibrosis. Hyperplastic phase with atypical megakaryocytes (arrow) and mild fibrosis

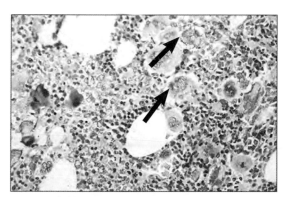

Osteomyelofibrosis. Later phase with many atypical megakaryocytes (arrows)

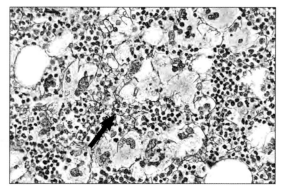

Osteomyelofibrosis. Later phase with prominent reticular fibrosis (arrow) produced by megakaryocytes

FIGURE 10-8   OSTEOMYELOFIBROSIS

Chronic myeloproliferative diseases, clonal neoplastic disorders with variable myelofibrosis and a terminal blastic phase, include **PCV, osteomyelofibrosis, CML, and PTH (primary thrombocythemia).** Osteomyelofibrosis, also referred to as agnogenic myeloid metaplasia, myelosclerosis, and idiopathic myeloid metaplasia, occurs primarily in older populations exposed to viral infections or toxic chemicals. Patients report fatigue, fever and night sweats, weight loss, upper abdominal fullness (splenomegaly, hepatomegaly), and bleeding. Peripheral blood shows "**teardrop**" poikilocytosis (**dacryocytes**), normoblasts, immature myeloid cells and megathrombocytes with the bone marrow in early hematopoietic hyperplasia, and predominance of megakaryocytes and granulocytes. Megakaryocytes include many pleomorphic giant forms with nuclear atypia, naked nuclei, and cytoplasmic fragments. Life expectancy varies according to risk factors (low Hb level and low WBC count) from 93 months to 13 months.

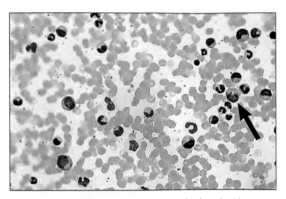

Blood smear of chronic myelogenous leukemia. Showing increased number of metamyelocytes and myelocytes (arrow)

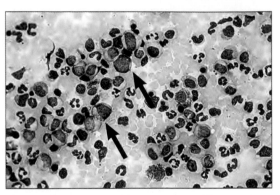

Blood marrow smear. Mild increase in myelocytes and myeloblasts and decreased erythropoiesis (arrows)

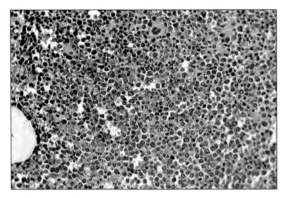

Bone marrow biopsy. Diffuse myelopoietic hyperplasia with delayed maturation (chloroacetate esterase reaction): red cells = myelopoietic cells

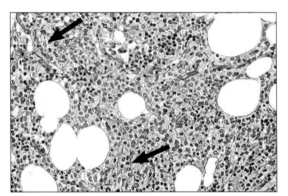

Bone marrow biopsy. Reticulin stain shows increase in fibers (arrows)

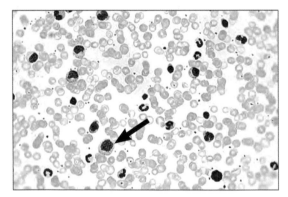

Myelomonocytic variant of chronic myelogenous leukemia (CMoML). Immature monocytoid cells (arrow)

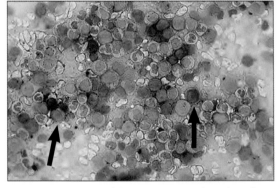

Bone marrow smear of CMoML. Increased number of monocytoid cells (neutral α-naphthyl esterase reaction for monocytes): brown cells (arrow)

FIGURE 10-9   CHRONIC MYELOGENOUS LEUKEMIA

Chronic myelogenous leukemia (CML), another chronic myelo-proliferative disease, is defined by myeloid hyperplasia, leukocytosis, basophilia, and splenomegaly. CML is associated with a characteristic chromosomal t(9,22)(q34;q11) translocation, the **Philadelphia chromosome**, which provides the mutated cells with a proliferative advantage. Clinical features are fatigue, weight loss, sweats, bone pain, anemia, hepatosplenomegaly, and petechial hemorrhages. An initial chronic phase of CML (<10%

blasts in bone marrow) is followed by an accelerated phase with final inevitable and fatal blast crisis (>30% blasts in the bone marrow with promyelocytes). Variants of CML include chronic myelomonocytic leukemia (CMML), which must be distinguished from MDSs. The life expectancy of patients with CML depends on disease progression and type of treatment; 45% to 65% of patients survive 5 years.

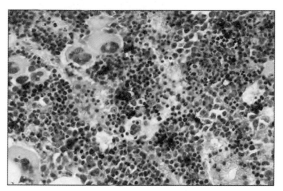

Bone marrow biopsy of primary thrombocythemia (PTH). With diffuse marrow hyperplasia and increased partly immature megakaryocytes (red cells = myelpoiesis)

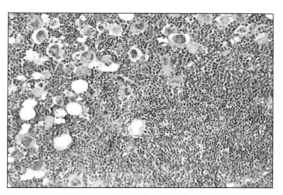

Bone marrow biopsy of PTH. Showing hyperplastic hematopoiesis with increased numbers of megakaryocytes, yet no increased fibroplasia (reticulin stain)

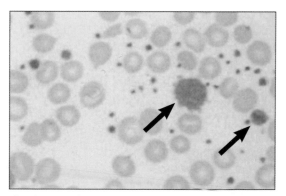

Blood smear of PTH. Showing increased number of immature and giant platelets (arrows)

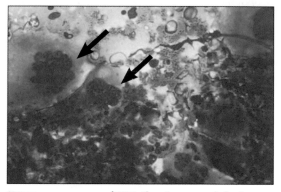

Bone marrow smear of PTH. Showing unusual clotting and increased number of immature giant megakaryocytes (arrows)

FIGURE 10-10   PRIMARY THROMBOCYTHEMIA _____

Primary thrombocythemia (PTH) is a chronic myeloproliferative disease with progressive megakaryocytic hyperplasia, peripheral thrombocytosis (>600,000/mL), splenomegaly, and hemorrhagic and thrombotic complications. The bone marrow contains partially clustered giant megakaryocytes and promegakaryocytes with mitoses, cytoplasmic fragments, and prominent **emperipolesis** (engulfment of a cell by a cell other than phagocytes). Clinical features may include hemorrhagic or thrombotic episodes or both, headache, dizziness, paresthesias, and other neurologic symptoms. Microvascular occlusions cause microinfarcts in several organs and occasional digital gangrene. Large vessel thrombosis occurs most frequently in femoral, renal, coronary, gastrointestinal (GI), and other arteries. In approximately 3% to 10% of patients, blastic transformation with features of myelogenous, myelomonocytic, megakaryocytic, or even lymphoblastic leukemia is reported. The 10-year survival rate for patients with PTH is 65% to 80%.

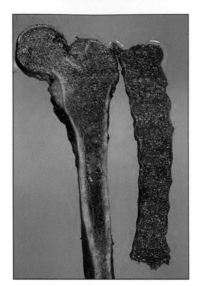

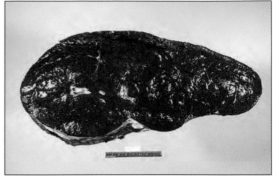

Acute myelogenous leukemia. Leukemic infiltration in bone marrow and spleen

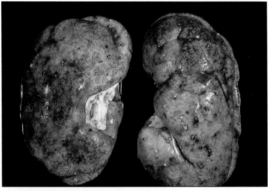

Acute myelogenous leukemia. Leukemic infiltration of kidneys

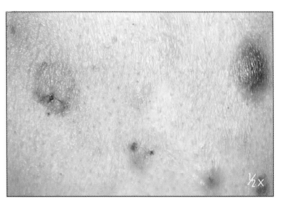

Acute myelomonocytic leukemia. Skin infiltration

TABLE 10-3 CLASSIFICATION IN SUBTYPES OF ACUTE MYELOPROLIFERATIVE DISEASES*

FAB Class	Subtype Name	Abbreviation	Proportion of Acute Myeloproliferative Diseases (%)
M0	Acute myeloblastic leukemia, stem cell (i.e., minimal differentiation)	AML	3-5
M1	Acute myeloblastic leukemia without maturation	AML	15-20
M2	Acute myeloblastic leukemia with maturation	AML	25-30
M3	Acute promyelocytic leukemia	APL	5-20
M4	Acute myelomonocytic leukemia	AMML	20-30
M5	Acute monoblastic leukemia	AMOL	2-9
M6	Acute erythroleukemia	AEL	3-5
M7	Acute megakaryoblastic leukemia		3-12

*Acute myeloproliferative diseases are clonal neoplastic disorders of hematopoietic stem cells, the classification of which is determined by their preferential cytologic differentiation.
FAB indicates French-American-British classification.
Adapted from Hoffman R et al. *Hematology.* Philadelphia: Churchill-Livingstone; 2000.

FIGURE 10-11 ACUTE MYELOGENOUS LEUKEMIA

Acute myelogenous leukemia (AML) is an acute myeloproliferative disease (Table 10-3) representing approximately 90% of all acute leukemias. Approximately 22% of cases develop in patients with MDSs. Patients usually present with malaise and fatigue, frequently after a flulike illness, and may have resistant skin infections, unusual pallor, and bleeding from the gums and the nose. Blood smears show leukopenia of 1000 WBCs/mL or excessive leukocytosis up to 200,000 WBCs/mL with increase in immature cells. The liver and the spleen are enlarged and infiltrated by atypical blasts. Additional symptoms result from metabolic and electrolyte derangements (hypokalemia, hypercalcemia), agranulocytosis (necrotizing enterocolitis), or rapid lysis of leukemic blasts (**tumor lysis syndrome**: urate nephropathy, hyperphosphatemia, muscle cramps, arrhythmias). Survival rates for all AML subtypes combined are 40% at 15 months and approximately 20% at 50 months.

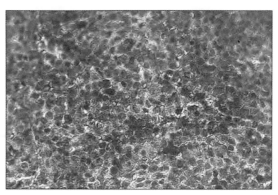

Bone marrow biopsy specimen acute myelogenous leukemia (AML-M1). Diffuse immature myeloid hyperplasia with early maturation (chlorocetate esterase stain; red cells = myeloid differentiation; AML-M0 would show similar picture without red cells)

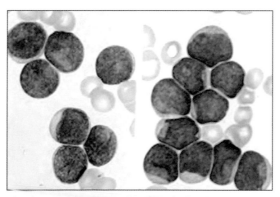

Blood smear of acute myelogenous leukemia (AML-M1). Immature myeloblasts, partly with lymphoid appearance

FIGURE 10-12 ACUTE MYELOGENOUS LEUKEMIA SUBTYPES M0, M1, AND M2

Acute myelogenous leukemia (AML)–M0 and AML-M1 constitute the most immature types of AML and can be difficult to distinguish from acute lymphoblastic leukemia or monoblastic or megakaryoblastic leukemia. They present with more than 30% blasts with hardly any positive myeloperoxidase reaction. AML-M0 cells are usually positive for terminal deoxynucleotidyl transferase (TdT) and CD34 (hematopoietic stem cell marker). AML-M1 types show approximately 10% promyelocytes, suggesting some myelopoietic differentiation. The prognosis is poor. AML-M2 shows signs of maturation beyond promyelocytes. There are more than 30% blasts, and promyelocytes account for 3% to 20% of leukemic cells with occasional maturation of eosinophils and basophils. Maturing cells contain intracytoplasmic red rodlike structures (**Auer rods**) and stain strongly for chloroacetate esterase and peroxidase enzyme activities. The 50% of patients who have t(8;21) chromosomal translocations have a slightly better prognosis than those without translocations.

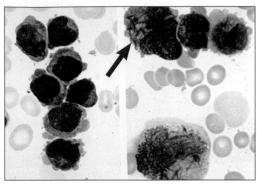

Blood smear of acute promyelocytic leukemia
(**AML-M3**). Showing myeloblasts and promyelocytes
with Auer rods and bundles (arrow)

FIGURE 10-13   ACUTE PROMYELOCYTIC LEUKEMIA SUBTYPE M3

Acute promyelocytic leukemia (AML-M3) is characterized by atypical promyelocytes in the bone marrow and hypergranular cells with multiple Auer rods (**Auer bundles**). Patients with M3 leukemia are generally younger (median age, 31 years) and have lower WBC counts than patients with more common leukemias. They frequently have coagulation disorders with hemorrhage and disseminated intravascular coagulation (DIC). There are diagnos-

tic chromosomal t(15q+;17q-) translocations, which cause a fusion of the retinoic acid receptor-α region on chromosome 17 to a region in chromosome 15 (PML-RARα) and seem to account for a differentiation blockage of the myeloid lineage. Differentiation can be induced by administration of all-*trans* retinoic acid, with complete remission of disease in 70% to 85% of patients.

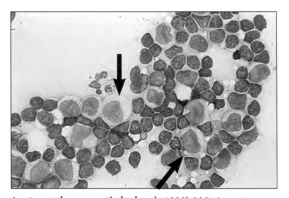

Acute myelomonocytic leukemia (**AML-M4**). Immature monocytoid cells in bone marrow smear

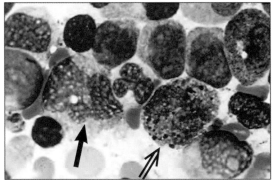

Acute myelomonocytic leukemia (**AML-M4**). Blood smear with monocytes, monoblasts (arrow), and basophils (double arrow)

FIGURE 10-14   ACUTE MYELOMONOCYTIC LEUKEMIA SUBTYPES M4 AND M5

Acute myelomonocytic leukemia (AML-M4) is characterized by cells differentiating toward granulocytes and monocytes. Atypical blasts in the bone marrow (>30%) include myeloblasts, monoblasts, and promonocytes, the latter staining positive for (fluoride inhibitable) nonspecific esterase enzyme activity. There may be abnormal eosinophils with the appearance of monoblasts and eosinophil crystals in the cytoplasm, which may carry CD2+ T-cell markers (M4EO subtype). Clinical features include extramedullary disease with multiple organ involvement includ-

ing the skin and the central nervous system (CNS). Pronounced hepatosplenomegaly and blood cell counts of 30,000 to 100,000 cells/mL are common. Karyotypic changes on chromosome 16 (inversions and translocations) may be found. The response rate to chemotherapy is 65% or greater. **Acute monoblastic leukemia** (AML-M5) is characterized by more than 80% cells of the monocytic series with positive cytoplasmic α-naphthyl acetate esterase reaction. It may occur in young age groups and is associated with a poor prognosis.

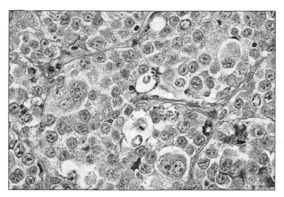

Acute megakaryoblastic leukemia (AML-M7). Bone marrow with diffuse megakaryoblastic proliferation

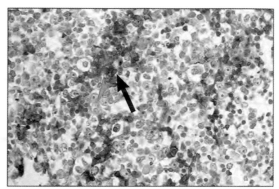

Acute megakaryoblastic leukemia (AML-M7). Bone marrow biopsy with immunostain (red) for glycophorin C (arrow)

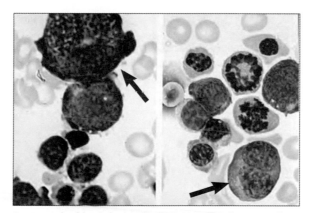

Acute erythroblastic leukemia (AML-M6). Blood smear with immature erythroblastic cells (arrows)

FIGURE 10-15   ACUTE MYELOGENOUS LEUKEMIA SUBTYPES M7 AND M6

Acute megakaryoblastic leukemia (AML-M7) (**acute myelofibrosis** or **malignant myelosclerosis**), follows OMF or CML in up to half of patients. Megakaryoblasts (>30% of cells) are undifferentiated round cells reacting positively with antibodies against platelet glycoproteins or factor VIII–related antigens. WBC counts are usually 5,000 cells/mL or less. Secondary AML-M7 shows prominent hepatosplenomegaly. Advanced marrow fibrosis causes marrow aspirates to be inadequate for diagnosis ("dry tap"). Response to chemotherapy is usually poor. **Acute erythro-**leukemia (**AML-M6**) is characterized by more than 50% abnormal erythroblasts with mixed proportions (30%) of myeloid and monocytic precursors. Peripheral blood smears show abnormal erythrocytes with prominent basophilic granules but rarely atypical blasts. Patients with acute erythroleukemia are usually older than 50 years and have anemia, hepatosplenomegaly, and occasionally rheumatic symptoms, polyclonal gammopathy, and Coombs-positive hemolytic anemia.

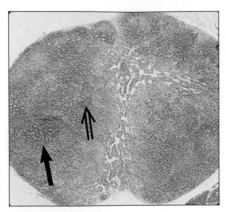

Lymph node. With follicular (arrow) and paracortical (double arrow) hyperplasia representing B- and T-cell activation, respectively

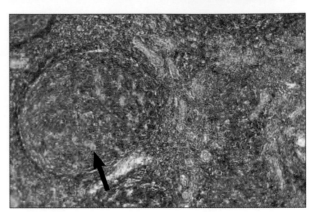

Follicular B lymphocytes, immunostain (arrow)

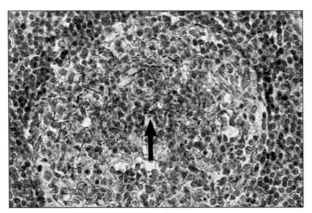

Follicular dendritic cells, immunostain (arrow)

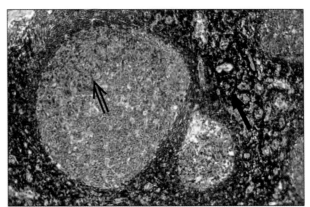

Paracortical T lymphocytes. With some colonization of follicle (double arrow) indicating T- and B-cell cooperation, immunostain

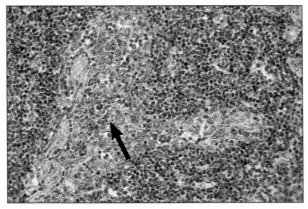

Sinusoidal macrophages, immunostain (arrow)

FIGURE 10-16   LYMPHATIC HYPERPLASIA

After preferred homing of cells in secondary lymphatic tissues and the subdivision of these tissues into functional T- and B-cell units, hyperplasia or aplasia in these units reflects T- or B-cell activities. Functional stimulation of the B-cell system leads to **follicular hyperplasia**, with prominent plasmacytosis in later stages. Stimulation of the T-cell system leads to **paracortical hyperplasia** and activation of phagocytosis to **sinus histiocytosis** or **diffuse reticulohistiocytosis**. Under physiologic conditions of stimulation by compound antigens, these units react together. Loss of reactivity (e.g., hypoplasia or atrophy) of one of these units indicates deficiency. Hyperplastic changes indicating functional activation of lymphatic tissues are found in various viral infections and are most pronounced in infections by **lymphotropic viruses** (e.g., **Epstein-Barr virus**, human herpesvirus types 6 and 7, cytomegalovirus). They cause clinical disorders such as **infectious mononucleosis**.

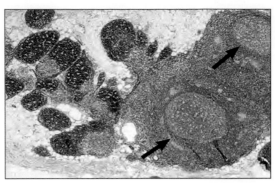

Pathologic follicular B-cell hyperplasia (**arrow**). In the thymus of a patient with systemic lupus erythematosus

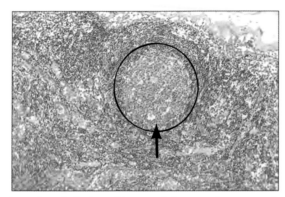

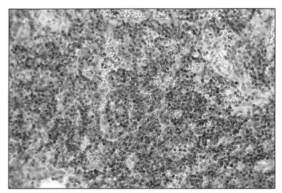

Lymph node. Patient with systemic lupus erythematosus showing paracortical T-cell depletion (arrow) and follicular B-cell hyperplasia (**left**). The paracortical zone also contains increased numbers of B lymphocytes (**right**; immunostain; red cells).

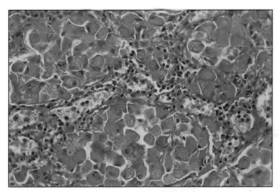

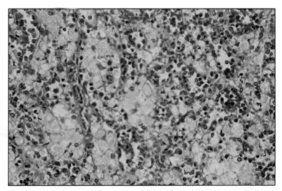

Phagocytic hyperplasia in storage diseases. Gaucher disease (**left**) and Niemann-Pick disease (**right**)

FIGURE 10-17   AUTOIMMUNE DISEASES

Pathologic aberrations from "physiologic" lymphatic hyperplasia are found in **autoimmune diseases** (e.g., **systemic lupus erythematosus** and **rheumatoid arthritis**) and are characterized by B-cell hyperactivity combined with selective T-cell deficiency. Typical lymph node changes consist of prominent follicular hyperplasia and plasmacytosis with paracortical lymphoid depletion. Regressive changes appear and may include degenerating and fibrotic germinal centers (**burnt-out follicles**), atrophy and fibrosis, or postcapillary venules and paracortical zones. Plasmacytosis increases. In some systemic autoimmune diseases, such as lupus erythematosus, the thymus shows an unusual B-cell hyperplastic reaction with follicular hyperplasia, germinal center formation, and plasmacytosis. Excessive and pathologic reactions in lymphatic tissues affect the phagocytic system, as occurs in **storage diseases** (**thesauropathies**, **thesaurismoses**), such as **Niemann-Pick disease** and **Gaucher disease**.

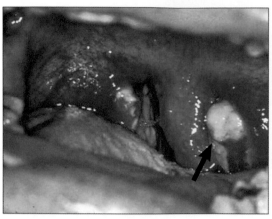 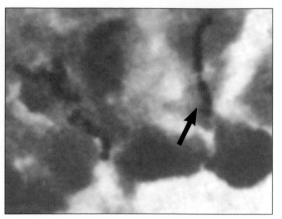

Suppurative tonsilitis. With yellow membranes (**left**, arrow). Touch preparations show streptococcal organisms on Gram stain (**right**, arrow)

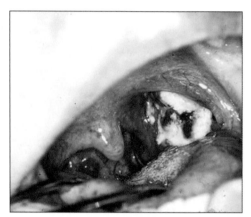 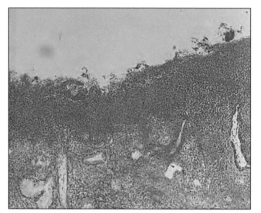

Pseudomembranous and necrotizing tonsillitis. In diphtheria (**left**, arrow) showing typical necroses in microscopy (**right**, arrow)

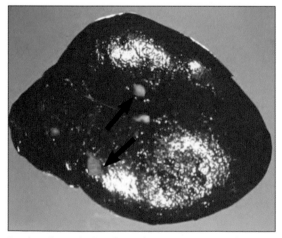

Septicemia. Multiple splenic abscesses (arrows); white color and dryness suggest fungal abscesses

FIGURE 10-18   SUPPURATIVE INFLAMMATION

Bacterial infections (excluding organisms with intracellular replication) commonly cause **suppurative inflammation**; depending on their toxin production, they may cause necrosis, abscess formation, or hemorrhage. These are usually secondary infections after puriform infections in their lymphatic drainage area or septicemia. Lymphadenitis or splenitis with abscess formation is also common in acute fungal infections such as those caused by *Candida* species. If superficial (mucosal) lymphoid organs are involved, localized erosions, ulcerations, and pseudomembranous inflammation may result, as is typically observed in streptococcal and diphtheric tonsillitis or in Peyer patches with salmonella infections (**typhoid fever**).

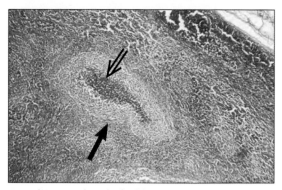

Granulomatous lymphadenitis (arrow). With central abscess (double arrow) in *Yersinia* infection

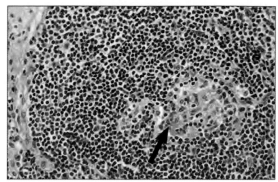

Granulomatous lymphadenitis. In toxoplasmosis (Piringer-Kuchinka lymphadenitis; arrow at granuloma)

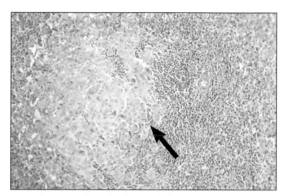

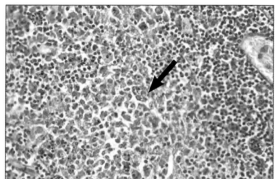

Granulomatous lymphadenitis (**left**) and **splenitis** (**right**). in *Salmonella* infection (i.e., typhoid fever)

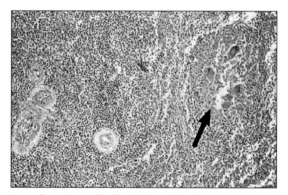

Granulomatous splenitis. With multiple Langhans giant cells in miliary tuberculosis (arrow)

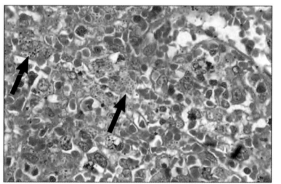

Histiocytic splenitis. In histoplasma infection. Note multiple coccoid organisms in macrophages (arrows)

FIGURE 10-19   GRANULOMATOUS INFLAMMATION

Infections with intracellular organisms persist for a long period, stimulating the T-cell immune system and phagocytosis. Consequently, **granulomatous inflammation** arises in lymphatic tissues just as it would in other organs. Depending on the toxicity of the etiologic agent, necrosis and abscess formation may occur together. **Granulomatous lymphadenitis** caused by *Mycobacterium tuberculosis, Salmonella* species, or fungi of the *Histoplasma*

genus is an example of such a reaction. Combinations of follicular granulomas and centrally located abscesses are found in such diverse infections as ***Yersinia* lymphadenitis, lymphogranuloma venereum, tularemia**, and **catscratch disease**. Some toxic fungal infections, such as histoplasmosis and **mucormycosis**, may cause similarly combined necrotic and granulomatous reactions.

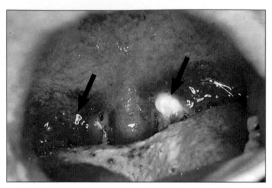

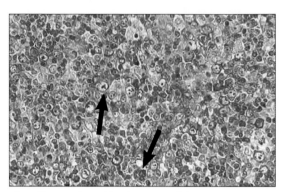

Tonsillitis. In acute infectious mononucleosis with inflamed and swollen tonsils and focal erosions (**left**, arrows). Microscopy shows diffuse paracortical hyperplasia with immunoblasts and plasmacytoid cells (**right**, arrow).

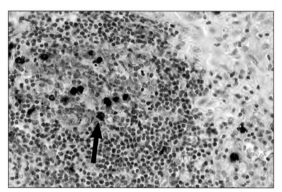

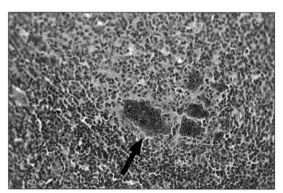

Follicular hyperplasia. In acute adenovirus infection with multiple virus-infected cells (immunostain: red cells with viral antigen; arrow)

Lymph node follicular hyperplasia. In acute measles virus infection. Follicles contain typical Warthin-Finkeldey giant cells (arrow).

FIGURE 10-20   VIRAL INFECTIONS

Viral infections may cause hyperplastic reactions in lymphatic tissues. Specific viral infections can be identified only by characteristic cytopathic effects (e.g., **Warthin-Finkeldey cells** in measles virus infection or **cytomegalic inclusion disease** in cytomegalovirus infection) or by immunologic and molecular techniques for viral antigens and nucleic acids. Except for the lymphotropic viruses, such as Epstein-Barr virus, where such techniques may occasionally be helpful, viral infections are proven by observing their characteristic diseases in nonlymphatic organs and by serologic testing or viral isolation. Lymphotropic viruses cause a prominent paracortical T-zone hyperplasia with release of stimulated T and B cells into the bloodstream (**mononucleosis cells**, **plasmablastoid B cells**). Human immunodeficiency virus (HIV) infection causes rapid loss of cells from the paracortical T-cell zone, structural disruption of cortical follicles, and reactive polyclonal B-cell proliferation.

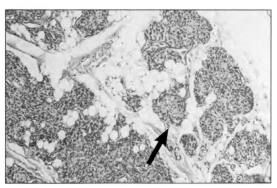

Thymic hypoplasia. In severe combined immune deficiency disorders (SCID) showing immature stromal anlage devoid of lymphocytes (arrow)

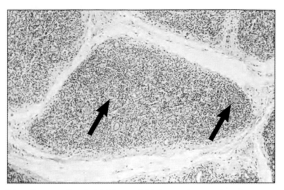

Thymic atrophy. In Wiskott-Aldrich syndrome showing severe depletion of lymphocytes and few small Hassal corpuscles (arrows)

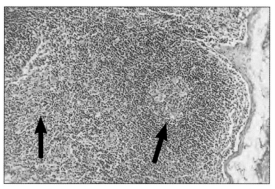

Severe aplasia. Of paracortical T-zone (arrow) of lymph node in DiGiorge syndrome while cortex may contain occasional follicle (arrow)

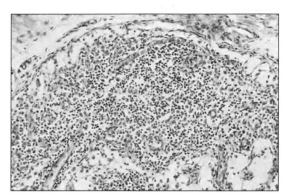

Diffuse hypoplasia. Of lymph node in SCID showing immature lymphoreticular stroma

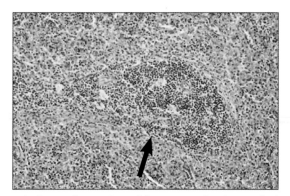

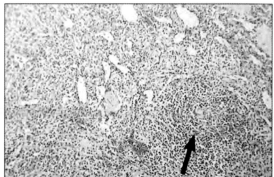

Splenic atrophy. In SCID; (**right**) compared with normal spleen at same age (**left**). Arrows show splenic follicle

FIGURE 10-21   IMMUNE DEFICIENCY DISORDERS

Immune deficiency disorders (IDDs) may be inherited or acquired. Either may affect the B- or T-cell systems or both, with thymic atrophy, paracortical and cortical atrophy of lymph nodes, or follicular atrophy of the spleen and other lymphoid tissues. **Reticular dysgenesis (DeVaal-Seynhaeve syndrome)**, the most extensive form of inherited IDD, affects the T- and B-cell systems and hematopoiesis. Other classic examples, all incompatible with life, are **DiGeorge syndrome** of the T-cell system and of the parathyroid glands, **Bruton disease** of the B-cell system, and **severe combined immune deficiency** (SCID) of T and B cells.

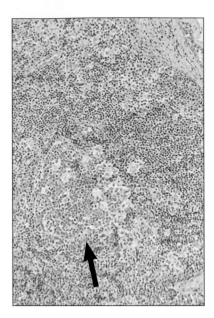

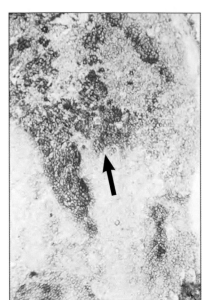

Acquired immune deficiency syndrome (early AIDS) in lymph node. Follicular disruption (arrows) and mixed paracortical hyperplasia (**right**, red cells: B lymphocytes)

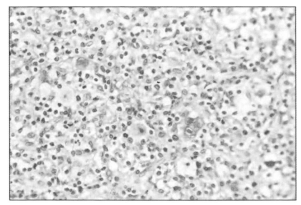

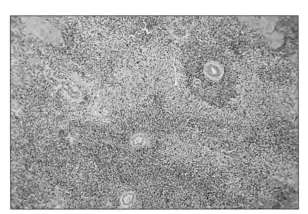

Late AIDS. Diffuse atypical lymphoproliferation in lymph node (**left**) with opportunistic CMV infection (note giant cells with nuclear inclusions) and severe splenic atrophy (**right**)

FIGURE 10-22   ACQUIRED IMMUNE DEFICIENCY DISORDERS

Acquired immune deficiency disorders are caused by toxic drugs (chemotherapeutics, steroids, analgesics, and others), ionizing radiation, endocrine and metabolic disturbances, chronic alcoholism, and viral infections such as congenital rubella and HIV, which is characterized by a combination of T-cell deficiency and polyclonal B-cell proliferation. The diagnosis and classification of IDDs follows detailed immunologic testing.

Pathologic studies with immunologic T- and B-cell quantification show hypoplasia or atrophy of the T-cell system (i.e., thymus and paracortical area of lymph nodes, periarteriolar sheath of spleen), hypoplasia or atrophy of the B-cell system (i.e., lymph node and splenic follicles, plasma cell maturation), or combinations of these features. Clinical consequences of IDDs include **opportunistic infections** and neoplasia (e.g., MLs).

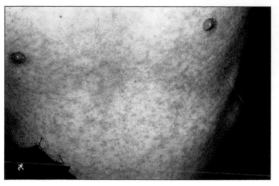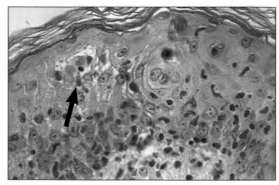

Acute graft-versus-host reaction (GVHR) of skin. Showing a measleslike exanthema (**left**) with T lymphocytes invading and attacking epidermal cells (**right**, arrow)

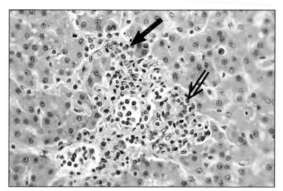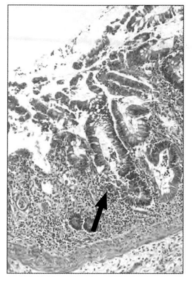

Acute graft-versus-host of liver. Showing lymphoid cells in portal triad invading and attacking parenchymal cells (arrows) and bile duct epithelial cells (double arrow) and vascular endothelial (not shown)

Acute graft-versus-host in duodenum. Showing lymphocytes infiltrating mucosal glands and attacking epithelial cells (arrow)

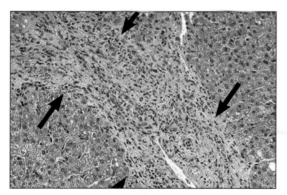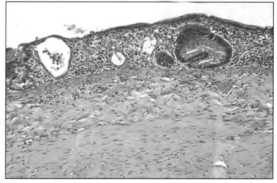

Chronic graft-versus-host in liver. Showing portal lymphocytic infiltration, fibrosis, and loss of bile ducts

Chronic graft-versus-host in colon. Showing scattered lymphocytic infiltration, glandular degeneration, severe mucosal atrophy with loss of glands

FIGURE 10-23   GRAFT-VERSUS-HOST REACTION

Graft-versus-host reaction (GVHR) is the "rejection" of the recipient (host) by a transplant (graft). It may occur whenever genetically foreign immunocompetent cells are transplanted into an immunodeficient recipient, especially in bone marrow allotransplantation. It also may occur in patients with leukemia or other IDDs who receive multiple blood transfusions. Transfused immunocompetent T lymphocytes recognize and destroy such allogeneic host cells as epidermal cells, hepatocytes, bile duct epithelia, intestinal epithelial cells, and cells of hemolymphatic tissues. Microscopically, a typical acute GVHR shows a T-cell immune reaction in the skin, the liver, and the upper intestines combined with growth inhibition and atrophy of hemolymphatic tissues. Severe acute GVHR has a high mortality secondary to severe ulcerating enteritis with superinfection, diarrhea, and fluid loss; severe hepatitis with hepatocellular necroses; or systemic viral disease and bacterial septicemia.

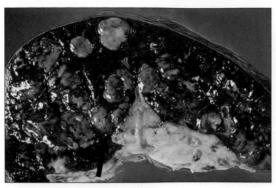

Gross infiltration of spleen in Hodgkin disease

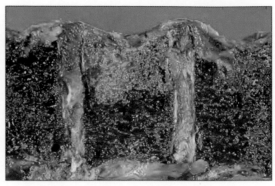

Gross infiltration of spine in Hodgkin disease

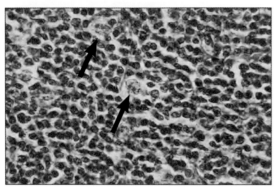

Lymphocyte-predominant type of Hodgkin disease. With only occasional Hodgkin and Reed-Sternberg cells (arrows)

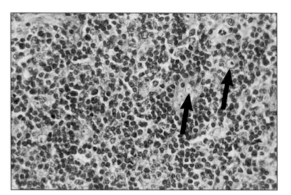

Mixed cellularity type of Hodgkin disease. With mixed population of lymphocytes, histiocytes (which may show epithelioid features), eosinophils, Hodgkin and Reed-Sternberg cells (arrows)

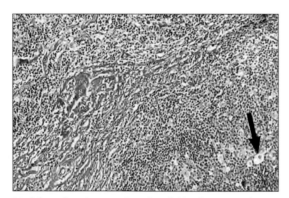

Nodular sclerosis type (C1) of Hodgkin disease. With paracortical atrophy, fibrosis, and typical lacunar-type Hodgkin and Reed-Sternberg cells (arrow)

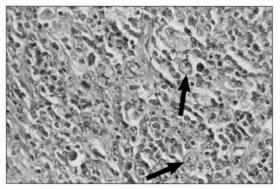

Lymphocyte-depleted type (C2) of Hodgkin disease. Showing predominance of atypical histioid blasts with many Hodgkin and Reed-Sternberg cells (arrows)

FIGURE 10-24   HODGKIN DISEASE

Hodgkin disease is characterized histologically by mixed proliferations of lymphoid cells with various numbers of histiocytes, eosinophils, and the diagnostic **Hodgkin cells** or **Reed-Sternberg cells**. Lymph nodes may show focal or diffuse involvement with effacement of the architecture and invasion beyond their capsule. HD cells are mononuclear histiocytoid blasts with vesicular nuclei and large prominent nucleoli. Reed-Sternberg cells are essentially similar but binucleated blasts.

HD are classified into 4 major groups according to their overall cell composition: lymphocyte-predominant type, mixed-cellularity type, nodular-sclerosing type, and lymphocyte-depleted type. The most frequently affected lymph nodes are in the mediastinum (59%), the neck (55-58%), the axillae (13-14%), and the lung hilus (11-12%). Multimodal radiation therapy and chemotherapy can result in stage-dependent disease-free survival of up to 94% at 10 years.

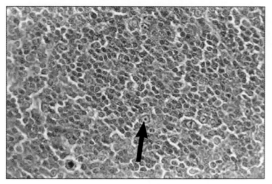

Lymphoplasmacytoid non-Hodgkin lymphoma (NHL). Showing a mixture of lymphocytes, plasmacytoid cells and occasional immunoblast (arrow; Giemsa stain)

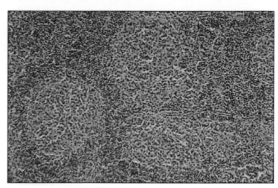

Follicular non-Hodgkin lymphoma (FCC) (follicular center cell lymphoma). Showing nodular, partly follicular, structure with a mixed small and large cell population (Giemsa stain)

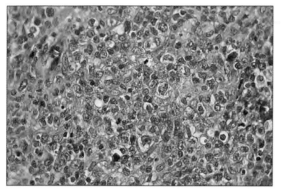

Follicular center cell lymphoma. With predominant large cells. The follicular may be still discernible or completely lost (H & E stain)

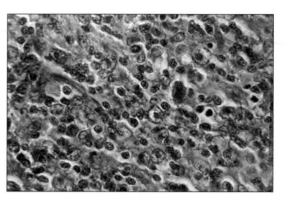

Large cell immunoblastic NHL. Showing predominance of immunoblasts (arrow) with some plasmacytoid features (PAS stain)

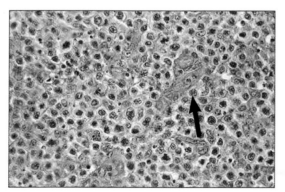

Immunoblastic T-cell–type large cell lymphoma. Showing histiocytoid cells and prominent (partly infiltrated) postcapillary venules (arrow)

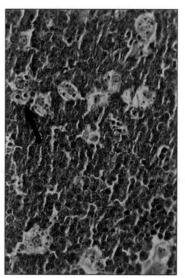

Burkitt-type NHL (here classical Burkitt lymphoma). Showing densely packed lymphoblasts with scattered histiocytes containing nuclear debris (starry sky pattern; arrow)

FIGURE 10-25   NON-HODGKIN LYMPHOMAS, MICROSCOPIC

Non-Hodgkin lymphomas are a diverse group of monoclonal T- or B-cell proliferative diseases recently classified according to the Revised European American Lymphoma (REAL) classification, shown in Table 10-4, which categorizes them based on cytology, histologic growth pattern, immunologic phenotype, and cytogenetic markers and includes consideration of clinical course and prognosis. Immunologically, there are B-cell lymphomas, T-cell lymphomas, T-cell–rich B-cell lymphomas, B-cell–rich T-cell lymphomas, and **natural killer** (NK) **cell** lymphomas. The etiology of most NHLs is unknown. Some are related to viral infection; Epstein-Barr virus is implicated in **Burkitt** and **Burkitt-type lymphoma**, and human T-cell leukemia virus (HTLV-1) is implicated in adult T-cell leukemia (ATL). Many NHLs show genetic mutations with unusual oncogene activation (e.g., *c-myc*, *BCL-2*, *BCL-1*, *BCL-6*, *PAX-5*, *NPM/ALK*) or inactivation of tumor suppressor genes (*p53*, *p16*).

TABLE 10-4 CLASSIFICATION OF LYMPHOMA (NHL) ENTITIES
Revised European American Lymphoma (REAL) Classification

B-Cell Lymphomas	T-Cell and NK-Cell Lymphomas
Precursor B-Cell Neoplasias	*Precursor T-Cell Neoplasia*
1. Precursor B-lymphoblastic lymphoma (B-LBL) 2. Precursor B-lymphoblastic leukemia (B-ALL)	1. Precursor T-lymphoblastic lymphoma (T-LBL) 2. Precursor T-lymphoblastic leukemia (T-ALL)
Peripheral B-Cell Neoplasias	*Pewripheral T-Cell and NK-Cell Lymphomas*

1. B-cell chronic lymphatic leukemia (B-CLL) or prolymphocytic leukemia (B-PLL)
2. Small cell lymphocytic lymphoma
3. Lymphoplasmacytoid lymphoma (LPL) or immunocytoma (IC)
4. Mantle cell lymphoma
5. Follicular center cell lymphoma, follicular pattern (FCCf)
  • Grade I small cell
  • Grade II mixed small and large cell
  • Grade III large cell
6. Follicular center cell lymphoma, small cell, diffuse pattern (FCCd)
7. Marginal zone lymphoma (MZL)
  • Subtype I extranodal MZL of MALT-type with or without monocytoid cells
  • Subtype II nodal MZL with or without monocytoid cells
8. Margonal zone lymphoma of the spleen (SLVL)
9. Hairy cell leukemia (HCL)
10. Plasmacytoma/multiple myeloma
11. Diffuse large cell B-cell lymphoma subtype: primary B-cell lymphoma of mediastinum (of thymic origine)
12. Burkitt lymphoma
13. B-cell lymphoma of high malignancy of Burkitt type
	1. T-cell chronic lymphatic leukemia (T-CLL) or T-cell prolymphocytic leukemia (T-PLL)
	2. Large granular cell lymphocytic leukemia (LGL)
	  • Suptype: T-cell type
	  • Subtype: NK-cell type
	3. *Mycosis fungoides*/Sezary's syndrome (MF/SS)
	4. Peripheral T-cell lymphoma NOS (not otherwise specified)
	  • Subtype: Subcutaneous panniculitic T-cell lymphoma
	  • Subtype: Hepatosplenomegalic gamma/delta T-cell lymphoma
	5. Angioimmunoblastic T-cell lymphoma (AILD)
	6. Angiocentric lymphoma
	7. Intestinal T-cell lymphoma
	8. Adult T-cell lymphoma/leukemia (ATL/L)
	9. Anablastic large cell lymphoma (ALCL), CD30+, T- or 0-Cell Type
	10. Anablastic large cell lymphoma, Hodgkin-like

FIGURE 10-25 NON-HODGKIN LYMPHOMAS, MICROSCOPIC *(CONTINUED)* ━━━━━━━━━

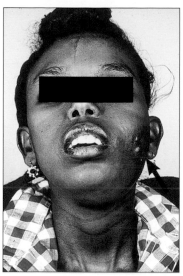

Non-Hodgkin lymphoma. Infiltration of maxilla (Burkitt)

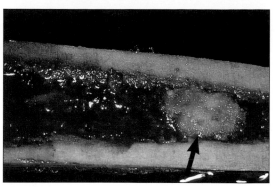

Non-Hodgkin lymphoma. Infiltration of femur marrow (immunoblastic)

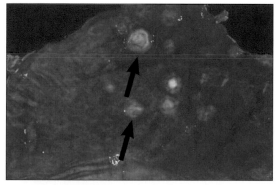

Non-Hodgkin lymphoma. Infiltration of stomach (immunoblastic)

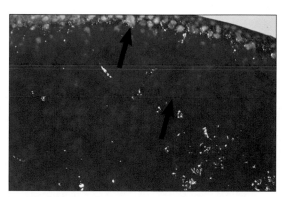

Non-Hodgkin lymphoma. Infiltration of spleen (follicular)

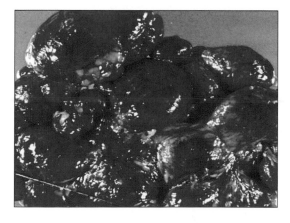

Enlarged, well-demarcated axillary lymph nodes. In small cell lymphocytic lymphoma (same as in chronic lymphocytic leukemia)

FIGURE 10-26   NON-HODGKIN LYMPHOMAS, GROSS VIEW

Patients with NHL present with persistent indolent lymphade-nopathy with or without splenic enlargement and **B-symptoms** (night sweats, fever, weight loss). Internal and extranodal lymphomas cause symptoms only by compression or infiltration of adjacent organs (e.g., abdominal discomfort, uncharacteristic GI problems). Hypersplenism or direct invasion of the bone marrow may be followed by anemia, thrombocytopenia, and pancytopenia. Treatment of NHL is adjusted according to its histologic classification and clinical stage. Follicular lymphomas and small-cell lymphomas are usually less aggressive and have a better prognosis than large-cell and diffuse lymphomas. In certain lymphomas, however, relapses have been described after periods as long as 15 years.

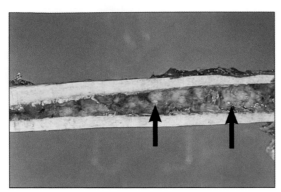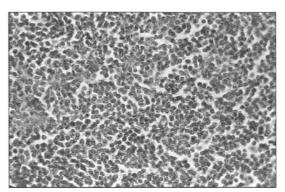

Chronic lymphocytic leukemia (CLL). Showing gross infiltration of bone marrow (**left**) and details of microscopic cell populations (small lymphocytes) in lymph node (**right**; compare also Fig. 10-26)

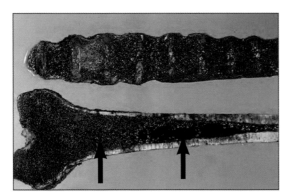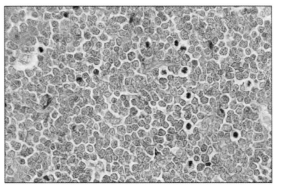

Acute lymphocytic leukemia (ALL). With diffuse infiltration of bone marrow (**left**) lymphoblastic population with much mitoses in lymph node (**right**). Note loss of fat cells from bone marrow and reduction of trabecular bone (arrows)

FIGURE 10-27 LYMPHOCYTIC LEUKEMIAS

Lymphocytic leukemias are characterized by hematogenous circulation of malignant cells and lymphomatous infiltration of bone marrow, lymphatic organs, or extralymphatic sites. CLL, in approximately 90% of cases a B-cell malignancy, is the most common form of leukemia. Immunodeficiency and autoimmune reactions (autoimmune hemolytic anemia) may accompany CLL, rendering the patient susceptible to infections. The disease course is slowly progressive but rapid when chemotherapy becomes necessary. Acute lymphocytic leukemia (ALL; cytologic subtypes L1-L3 according to cell size) is preferentially a childhood leukemia. Approximately 80% of cases of childhood ALL consist of monoclonal B-precursor cells, and approximately 15% consist of cells from the T-cell lineage. Clinical features are anemia (pallor, fatigue), thrombocytopenia (hemorrhage), and mature leukocytopenia (infections). Combination chemotherapy and radiation therapy have resulted in long-term disease-free survival of 70% to 80% of children.

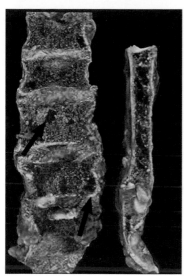

Multiple myeloma infiltration of bone marrow. Causing multiple osteolytic lesions (arrow)

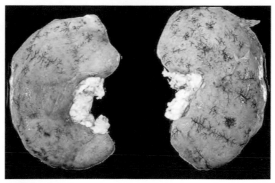

"**Myeloma kidney**." Form of protein nephrosis caused by excessive proteinuria. Note pale color and swelling of kidneys

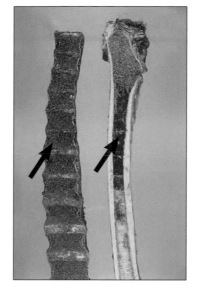

Waldenström disease. Diffuse infiltration of bone marrow. Note pale color of bone marrow and reduction of trabecular bone (arrows)

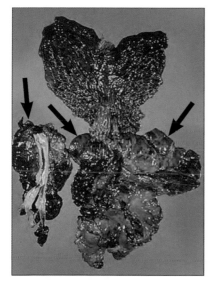

Waldenström disease. Prominent enlargement of paragastric, parapancreatic, and paraaortic lymph nodes caused by atypical lymphoplasmacytoid infiltration in the disease (arrows)

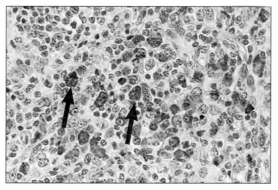

Waldenström disease. Microscopy of atypical mixed lymphoplasmacytoid cell population (immunostain: brown cells containing monoclonal immunoglobulin; arrows)

FIGURE 10-28   MULTIPLE MYELOMA AND WALDENSTRÖM DISEASE

Multiple myeloma is a neoplastic clonal proliferation of plasma cells (**plasmacytoma**) usually at multiple sites in the bone marrow. It frequently is accompanied by the production of unusual immunoglobulin components (**gammopathy**, monoclonal **M protein** in serum, and **Bence Jones protein** in urine). Clinical features include bone pain, anemia, bleeding, hypercalcemia, hyperglobulinemia (**myeloma kidney**), and susceptibility to infection. Systemic **amyloidosis** develops in later stages of the disease. With treatment, the life expectancy is approximately 2.5 to 3 years. **Waldenström disease** (**WD**) is another form of mature B-cell neoplasia with respective lymphoplasmacytic infiltration of the bone marrow and immunoglobulin (Ig) M macroglobulinemia. Other frequently involved sites are lymph nodes, spleen, GI tract, lungs, and skin. Clinical features are **hyperviscosity**, **cryoglobulinemia**, bleeding, renal disease, **peripheral neuropathy**, and **amyloidosis**. The median survival of patients with WD is 5 years.

CHAPTER 11

BONES, JOINTS, AND SOFT TISSUES

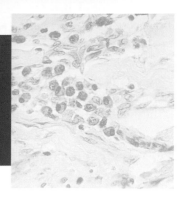

The skeletal system provides structural support and protection to the human body and its internal organs, serves as primary home for blood-forming tissues, and stores several vital minerals, above all, calcium. This chapter focuses on alterations of the bony (structural support) part of the skeletal system. Calcium metabolism is also discussed with the endocrine system (chapter 12), and blood-forming tissues are treated separately in the chapter about hematopoietic and lymphatic tissues (chapter 10).

METABOLIC BONE DISEASES

Metabolic bone diseases include diseases of increased bone resorption, such as osteoporosis, and of calcium metabolism, such as rickets, osteomalacia, hyperparathyroidism, and renal osteodystrophy. Primary osteoporosis is an age-related disorder preferentially affecting women that ultimately may cause a loss of 35% to 50% of cortical or trabecular bone mass. It is related to hormonal influences (e.g., estrogen deficiency), reduced physical activity, and nutritional and genetic factors. Secondary osteoporosis follows a large variety of diseases, including malabsorption or malnutrition, endocrine disorders (e.g., hyperparathyroidism or hypoparathyroidism, hypogonadism, and type 1 diabetes) and neoplastic diseases, such as multiple myeloma and bony metastases. Disorders in calcium homeostasis cause reduced matrix mineralization with osteopenia. Primary and secondary hyperparathyroidism (with the latter related to renal insufficiency) are characterized by increased osteoclastic bone resorption with features of dissecting osteitis and osteitis fibrosa cystica (**von Recklinghausen disease of the bone**).

INFECTIOUS DISEASES

Osteomyelitis (OM), an acute or chronic inflammation of the bone marrow cavity and bone, usually has an infectious cause. OM may originate from hematogenous spread of infectious organisms (i.e., secondary to **pyemia** or **septicemia**) or from their direct invasion through penetrating wounds (including from orthopaedic procedures) or open fractures. Despite readily available antibiotic drugs, infectious OM still constitutes a serious clinical problem for several reasons: First, OM is rarely a primary disease but more often a complication of an undiagnosed or inadequately treated infection. Second, OM responds poorly to antibiotic treatment (causative organisms may be drug resistant) and may run a chronic course with complications such as **amyloidosis**. Third, OM may be the source of additional hematogenous spread causing septic shock, hemorrhage, or abscesses in vital organs (brain, myocardium). Therefore, treatment must be radical, combining antibiotic and surgical intervention.

NONINFECTIOUS ARTHRITIC DISEASES

Osteoarthritis (OA) is an extremely common cause of disability, especially in people aged older than 75 years, 85% of whom show clinical evidence of the disorder. Despite its ubiquity, primary OA is of unknown etiology, although it is thought to result from intrinsic defects of cartilage. Abnormal mechanical forces on the cartilage, decreased water bonding of cartilage, increased stiffness of subcartilaginous bone, and biochemical abnormalities such as decrease in proteoglycans and shortening of glucosaminoglycans have been implicated. The latter decreases cartilaginous water binding in favor of its binding by collagen fibers. Mutations of the collagen type II gene may be involved. Secondary OA occurs in patients with such underlying causes as malformations, trauma, and metabolic diseases with or without crystalline deposits.

PAGET DISEASE

Excessive osteoblastic bone formation with abnormal structure and impaired stability characterize Paget disease (PD; **osteitis deformans**). After the age of 40 years, the disease increases in incidence to affect 4% to 10% of the population, primarily in white populations of Northern Europe, North America, Australia, and New Zealand, more often in men than women. It may occur in a **monostotic** form (in only one bony site) or in **polyostotic** forms (i.e., systemically). Head bones become enlarged; patients report headache, back pain, deafness, and visual disturbances; long bones (especially of the lower extremities) become tender; and deformities and fractures occur. The disease course is complicated by osteosarcoma (OS) in approximately 1% of patients.

TUMORS OF THE SKELETAL SYSTEM

Tumors of the skeletal system comprise a large variety of benign and malignant lesions, including bone cysts. They are classified according to their tissue of origin and are further identified by the age of the patient and the site. Primary tumors of bone are less common than metastatic lesions to the skeletal system, which always should be considered in differential diagnosis (usually, radiographic findings of primary and metastatic lesions are quite characteristic). The extraskeletal malignant neoplasms most likely to metastasize to the skeleton are carcinomas of the prostate, the breast, the lungs, the gastrointestinal tract, the kidneys, and the thyroid. Such metastases may be osteoblastic (e.g., prostate) or osteolytic.

Other primary tumors with secondary involvement of the bony skeleton are those of the hematopoietic bone marrow or lymphatic tissues (e.g., plasmacytoma, Hodgkin disease). They are discussed in chapter 10.

SOFT TISSUE DISORDERS

Soft tissue refers to the widely distributed interstitial tissue of mesodermal origin filling spaces between ectodermal, endodermal, and skeletal structures. It includes differentiated tissues such as fibrous tissue, fat, and skeletal muscle. Although all pathologic reaction patterns are represented in diseases of soft tissue, including necrosis and degeneration, infection and inflammation, and hyperplasia and neoplasia, only a few examples can be discussed here. We focus on such important disorders as **compartment syndrome**, **collagen-vascular diseases** (CVDs), and benign and malignant tumors.

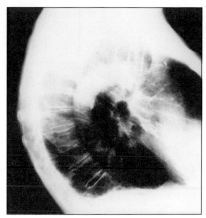
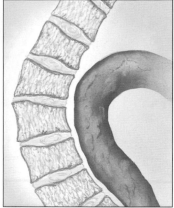

Marked kyphosis is evident. Anterior wedge and biconcave (codfish) deformities are present.

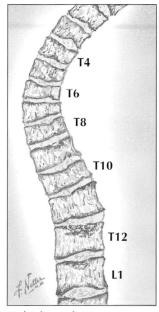
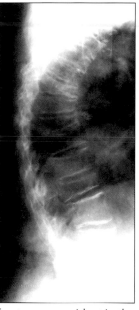

T4
T6
T8
T10
T12
L1

Multiple grade 3 compression fractures are evident in the thoracic vertebral bodies, resulting in marked kyphosis.

TABLE 11-1 PATHOGENETIC FORMS OF OSTEOPOROSIS

Category	Mechanism	Examples
Primary, type 1	Increased osteoclast activity	Postmenopausal (estrogen withdrawal)
Primary, type 2	Decreased osteoblast activity	"Old age" osteoporosis
Secondary	Endocrine disorders	Hyperparathyroidism, hyperthyroidism or hypothyroidism, hypogonadism, Cushing syndrome, Addison disease, acromegaly
	Hematologic diseases	Multiple myeloma, systemic mastocytosis, some leukemias and lymphomas
	Malabsorptive	Malabsorption syndromes, malnutrition, gastrectomy, hepatic diseases, vitamin D and C deficiencies
	Others	Inactivity osteoporosis, chemotherapy and other drugs, chronic alcoholism, certain metabolic diseases

FIGURE 11-1 OSTEOPOROSIS

Osteoporosis refers to a condition of reduced mass of mineralized bone secondary to an imbalance between catabolic ($\uparrow$) and anabolic ($\downarrow$) bone metabolism. The loss of skeletal mass can reach a state where the mechanical stability of affected parts is no longer maintained and fractures occur. There are primary and secondary forms of osteoporosis, and localized or systemic changes are identified. The most well-known and frequent type of primary osteoporosis is old age osteoporosis (**senile osteoporosis**). **Inactivity osteoporosis** (**immobilization osteoporosis**) is a localized form of secondary osteoporosis Other pathogenetic categories of osteoporosis are summarized in Table 11-1.

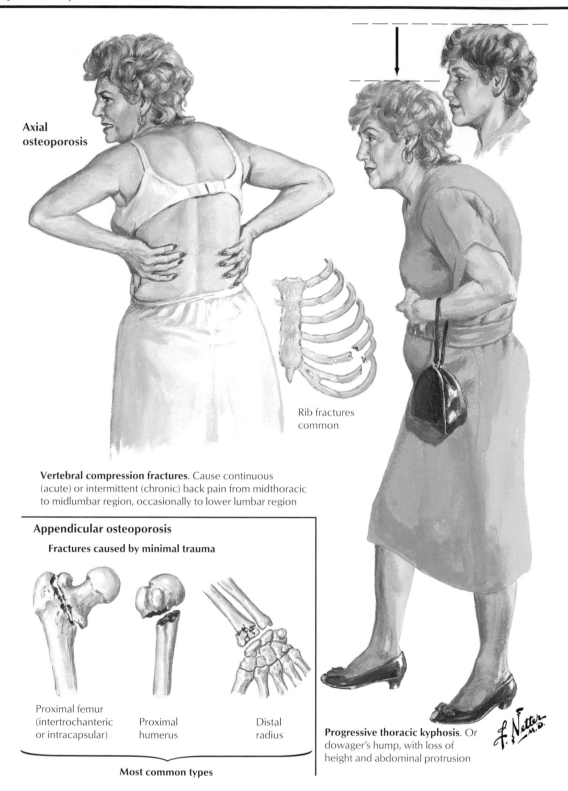

Axial osteoporosis

Vertebral compression fractures. Cause continuous (acute) or intermittent (chronic) back pain from midthoracic to midlumbar region, occasionally to lower lumbar region

Rib fractures common

Appendicular osteoporosis

Fractures caused by minimal trauma

Proximal femur (intertrochanteric or intracapsular)

Proximal humerus

Distal radius

Most common types

Progressive thoracic kyphosis. Or dowager's hump, with loss of height and abdominal protrusion

FIGURE 11-2   OSTEOPOROSIS: CLINICAL MANIFESTATIONS

The anatomical and clinical manifestations of **osteoporosis** are dependent on the maximal bone mass (peak bone mass), which is genetically determined. It is higher in men than in women and lower in white populations than in others. Therefore, a white female is at highest risk. Bone mass is commonly determined by radiographic measurement of bone density, which is highest at the ages of 25 to 35 years and decreases gradually thereafter by approximately 0.7% per year. Gross and microscopic features of osteoporosis show a diffuse rarefaction of trabecular bone and a symmetric thinning of trabecular and cortical bone. The ratio of mineralized bone to osteoid remains normal. In postmenopausal osteoporosis, disruption of trabecular bone adds significantly to the instability of the skeleton. The most common fractures resulting from primary osteoporosis are hip fractures, compression fractures of vertebral bodies (8 times more frequent in females), and fractures of the distal radius.

Childhood Rickets

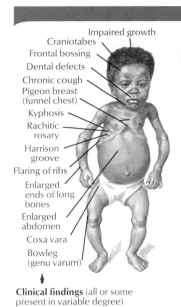

Impaired growth
Craniotabes
Frontal bossing
Dental defects
Chronic cough
Pigeon breast (funnel chest)
Kyphosis
Rachitic rosary
Harrison groove
Flaring of ribs
Enlarged ends of long bones
Enlarged abdomen
Coxa vara
Bowleg (genu varum)

Clinical findings (all or some present in variable degree)

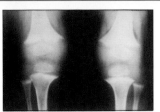
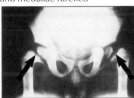

Flaring of metaphyseal ends of tibia and femur. Growth plates thickened, irregular, cupped, and axially widened. Zones of provisional calcification fuzzy and indistinct. Bone cortices thinned and medullae rarefied

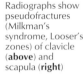

Coxa vara and slipped capital femoral epiphysis. Mottled areas of lucency and density in pelvic bones

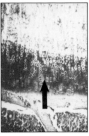

Cartilage of epiphyseal plate in immature normal rat. Cells of middle (maturation) zone in orderly columns, with calcified cartilage between columns

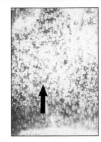

After 6 weeks of vitamin D– and phosphate–deficient diet. Large increase in axial height of maturation zone, with cells closely packed and irregularly arranged

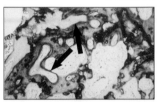

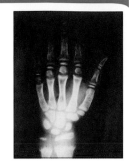

Radiograph of rachitic hand. Shows decreased bone density, irregular trabeculation, and thin cortices of metacarpals and proximal phalanges. Note increased axial width of epiphyseal line, especially in radius and ulna (arrow).

Section of rachitic bone shows sparse, thin trabeculae surrounded by much uncalcified osteoid (osteoid seams) and cavities caused by increased resorption (arrow).

Adult Osteomalacia
Radiographic findings

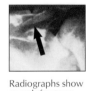
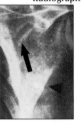
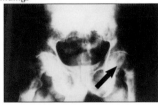

Subtle symptomatology (all or some present)

Generalized muscle weakness and hypotonia

Some weight loss

Variable bone pain

Mild bowing of limbs

Radiographs show pseudofractures (Milkman's syndrome, Looser's zones) of clavicle (**above**) and scapula (**right**)

Variegated rarefaction of pelvic bones. Coxa vara, deepened acetabula, and subtrochanteric pseudofracture of right femur

F. Netter M.D.

TABLE 11-2   PATHOGENETIC MECHANISMS OF RICKETS AND OSTEOMALACIA*

Category	Mechanism	Causes
Vitamin D deficiencies	Decreased synthesis in skin	Insufficient sun exposure from 7-dehydrocholesterol
	Decreased intestinal absorption	Dietary lack, malabsorption syndromes (intestines, pancreas, bile)
	Decreased synthesis of 25(OH)-D	Liver diseases
	Enhanced degradation of 25(OH)-D	Various drugs inducing cytochrome and P450 enzymes
	Decreased synthesis of 1,25(OH)$_2$-D	Advanced renal disease
Phosphate deficiency	Increased excretion	Renal tubular disorders (e.g., *Fanconi* syndromes)
	Decreased absorption	Phosphate-binding drugs (e.g., antacids)
	Disturbed reabsorption	Tumor associated (e.g., prostate cancer, neurofibromatosis)
Mineralization defects	Target organ resistance	Congenital lack of receptors (type II rickets)

*1,25(OH)-D indicates 1,25-dihydroxyvitamin-D, active form after second hydroxylation in renal tubule; 25(OH)-D, 25-hydroxyvitamin-D, major circulating metabolite hydroxylated in the liver.

FIGURE 11-3   RICKETS AND OSTEOMALACIA

In rickets and osteomalacia, mineralization of osteoid is reduced while bone mass remains normal. Rickets affects the growing bones of children, and osteomalacia affects the newly formed bone matrix in adults. Responsible metabolic disturbances are vitamin D deficiency, phosphate deficiency, and mineralization defects (Table 11-2). Growing bone is severely changed in children with rickets because inadequate mineralization of osteoid matrix leads to overgrowth and distortion of epiphyseal cartilage projecting into the medullary space, disruption of osteoid/cartilage replacement, and reactive proliferation of capillaries and fibroblasts. Loss of structural stability causes skeletal bone deformations (thoracic kyphosis, lumbar lordosis, coxa vara, genu varum). Osteocartilaginous thickening of ribs produces characteristic rachitic rosary. Adults with osteomalacia experience only mild bowing of long bones; however, stress resistance of bones is reduced, and gross or microscopic fractures may occur.

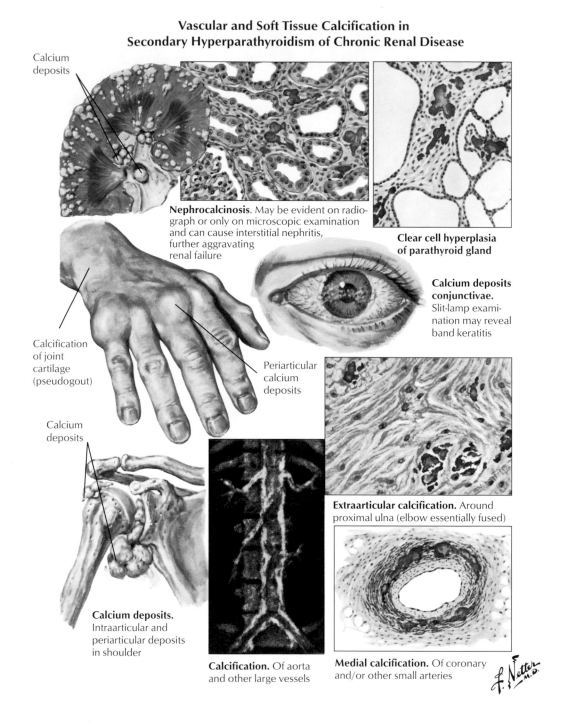

Vascular and Soft Tissue Calcification in Secondary Hyperparathyroidism of Chronic Renal Disease

Calcium deposits

Nephrocalcinosis. May be evident on radiograph or only on microscopic examination and can cause interstitial nephritis, further aggravating renal failure

Clear cell hyperplasia of parathyroid gland

Calcification of joint cartilage (pseudogout)

Calcium deposits conjunctivae. Slit-lamp examination may reveal band keratitis

Calcium deposits

Periarticular calcium deposits

Extraarticular calcification. Around proximal ulna (elbow essentially fused)

Calcium deposits. Intraarticular and periarticular deposits in shoulder

Calcification. Of aorta and other large vessels

Medial calcification. Of coronary and/or other small arteries

FIGURE 11-4   RENAL OSTEODYSTROPHY

Renal osteodystrophy, which is most common in patients undergoing long-term dialysis for chronic renal failure, combines the changes of osteomalacia with focal soft tissue, bone resorption, and vascular calcifications (**metastatic** calcification). Tumorlike calcium deposits are observed in some cases. While osteomalacic changes suggest renal tubular damage, additional focal osteoclastic bone resorption is caused by secondary hyperparathyroidism. Therapeutic planning must focus on treating the chronic renal disease, replacing 1,25(OH)$_2$-D, substituting for hypophosphatemia, and partially resecting hyperplastic parathyroid glands.

Pathology and Clinical Manifestations

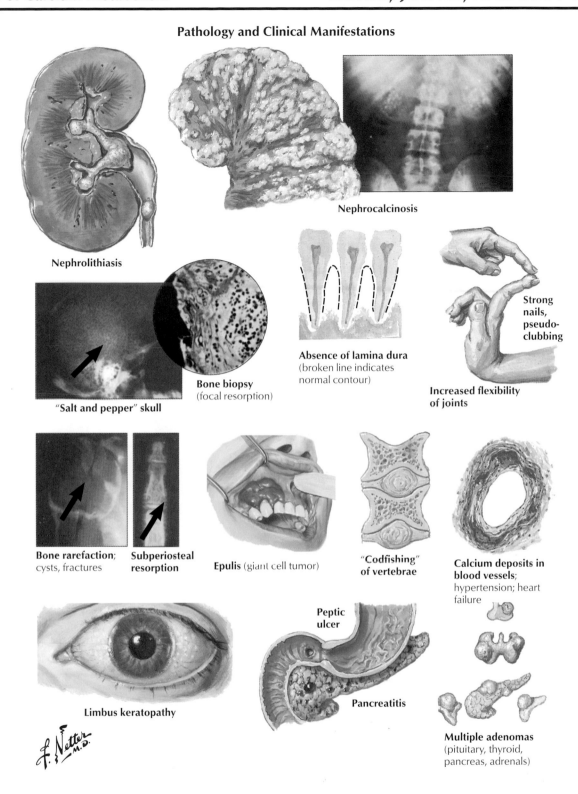

Nephrolithiasis

Nephrocalcinosis

"Salt and pepper" skull

Bone biopsy (focal resorption)

Absence of lamina dura (broken line indicates normal contour)

Strong nails, pseudo-clubbing

Increased flexibility of joints

Bone rarefaction; cysts, fractures

Subperiosteal resorption

Epulis (giant cell tumor)

"Codfishing" of vertebrae

Calcium deposits in blood vessels; hypertension; heart failure

Limbus keratopathy

Peptic ulcer

Pancreatitis

Multiple adenomas (pituitary, thyroid, pancreas, adrenals)

FIGURE 11-5   PRIMARY HYPERPARATHYROIDISM

Primary hyperparathyroidism causes generalized bone resorption by focal osteoclastic activities (as described in **osteitis fibrosa cystica**) combined with an increased incidence of stone formation (e.g., **nephrolithiasis**). Osteoclastic hyperactivity starts at subperiosteal and endosteal surfaces, cutting into the bone and replacing respective splits and holes by connective tissue (**dissecting osteitis**). Areas of hemorrhage and microfracture may occur. Larger cystic spaces occur eventually, hemorrhage

expands, and resorptive giant cell granulomas develop ("**brown tumors**" in osteitis fibrosa cystica). These must be distinguished from **aneurysmal bone cysts** (ABCs), **giant cell tumor** (GCT) **of bone**, and **telangiectatic OS**. Characteristic radiographic changes in hyperparathyroidism are found preferentially in the hands (radial phalanges of the second and third fingers), with signs of focal calcinosis in the spine and the cartilage of major joints.

Clinical Manifestations

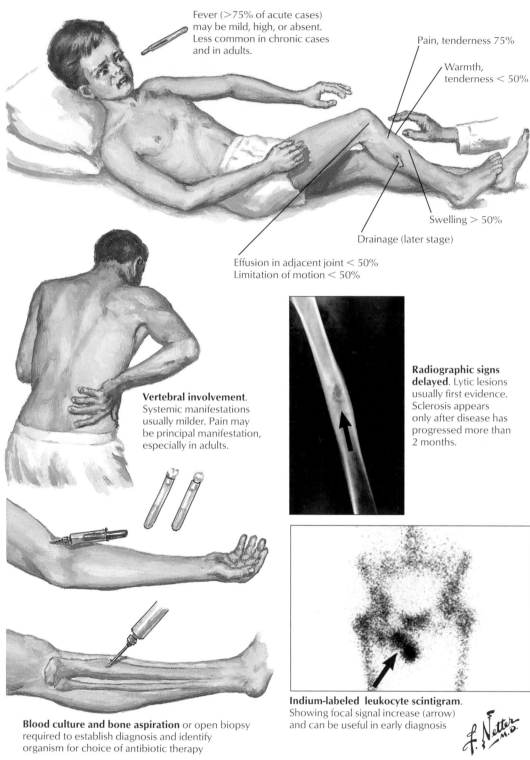

Fever (>75% of acute cases) may be mild, high, or absent. Less common in chronic cases and in adults.

Pain, tenderness 75%

Warmth, tenderness < 50%

Swelling > 50%

Drainage (later stage)

Effusion in adjacent joint < 50%
Limitation of motion < 50%

Vertebral involvement. Systemic manifestations usually milder. Pain may be principal manifestation, especially in adults.

Radiographic signs delayed. Lytic lesions usually first evidence. Sclerosis appears only after disease has progressed more than 2 months.

Blood culture and bone aspiration or open biopsy required to establish diagnosis and identify organism for choice of antibiotic therapy

Indium-labeled leukocyte scintigram. Showing focal signal increase (arrow) and can be useful in early diagnosis

FIGURE 11-6 OSTEOMYELITIS

Although **osteomyelitis (OM)** can easily be suspected from persistent purulent secretion from deep open wounds or fistulas extending to the bone, the clinical manifestations of hematogenous OM are more difficult to identify. Obscure back pain, low-grade fever, malaise, and moderate blood leukocytosis are among uncharacteristic general symptoms. If localized signs appear, such as circumscribed bone pain, reddening and swelling of the covering skin or mucous membranes, or even

fistula formation with purulent discharge, radiographic procedures and tissue biopsies may reveal the real nature of the disease. The most common organisms causing OM are *Staphylococcus aureus* (e.g., after long-standing infected intravenous catheters, endocarditis, or complicated wound healing), various gram-negative rods, pneumococci (in neonates), salmonellae, and *Mycobacterium tuberculosis*.

Pathogenesis

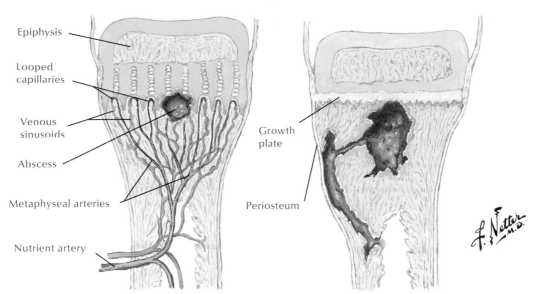

Terminal branches of metaphyseal arteries form loops at growth plate and enter irregular afferent venous sinusoids. Blood flow slowed and turbulent, predisposing to bacterial seeding. In addition, lining cells have little or no phagocytic activity. Area is catch basin for bacteria, and abscess may form.

Abscess, limited by growth plate, spreads transversely along Volkmann canals and elevates periosteum; extends subperiosteally and may invade shaft. In infants under 1 year of age, some metaphyseal arterial branches pass through growth plate, and infection may invade epiphysis and joint.

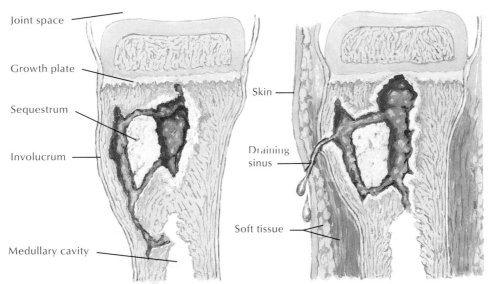

As abscess spreads, segment of devitalized bone (sequestrum) remains within it. Elevated periosteum may also lay down bone to form encasing shell (involucrum). Occasionally, abscess walled off by fibrosis and bone sclerosis to form Brodie abscess.

Infectious process may erode periosteum and form sinus through soft tissues and skin to drain externally. Process influenced by virulence of organism, resistance of host, administration of antibiotics, and fibrotic and sclerotic responses.

FIGURE 11-7 CHRONIC OSTEOMYELITIS

At the site of bacterial nesting in the bone, usually at well-vascularized metaphyseal sites, acute endotheliitis/vasculitis with subsequent neutrophilic exudation and necrosis of adjacent bone develops. Necrosis may follow local vascular occlusion by thrombosis, compression and hypoxemia, or both. Infection spreads through the marrow cavity and cortical bone, extending subperiosteally, transperiosteally, and through soft tissues, creating draining sinuses (fistulas). Progression to **chronic OM** adds focal osteoclastic bone resorption and fibrous repair mechanisms. Bony cavities may contain fragments of necrotic bone (bony **sequester**) surrounded by hyperostotic bone (**involucrum**). Persistent abscesses are surrounded by condensed sclerotic bone (**Brodie abscess**). Periosteal and osteal hyperostosis on radiograph may signal underlying chronic OM. Microscopic features include decreased neutrophils, persistent edematous swelling, scattered plasmacytic infiltrates, and progressive fibrosis.

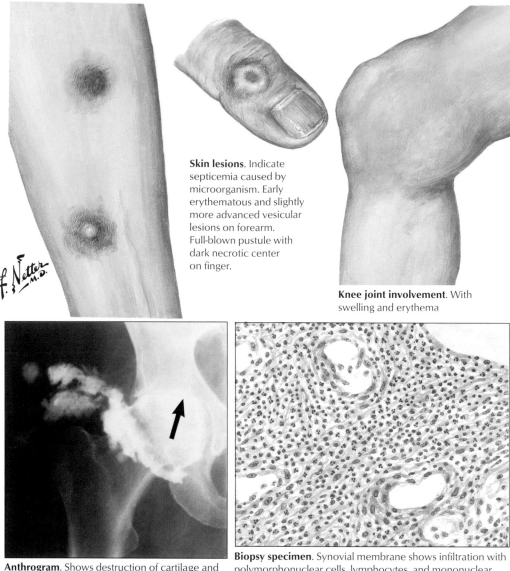

Skin lesions. Indicate septicemia caused by microorganism. Early erythematous and slightly more advanced vesicular lesions on forearm. Full-blown pustule with dark necrotic center on finger.

Knee joint involvement. With swelling and erythema

Anthrogram. Shows destruction of cartilage and bone (aspiration yielded purulent fluid)

Biopsy specimen. Synovial membrane shows infiltration with polymorphonuclear cells, lymphocytes, and mononuclear cells, and tissue proliferation with neovascularization

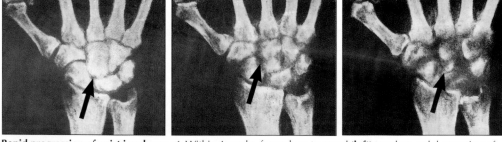

Rapid progression of wrist involvement. Within 4 weeks, from almost normal (**left**) to advanced destruction of articular cartilages and severe osteoporosis (**right**)

FIGURE 11-8 INFECTIOUS ARTHRITIS

Infectious arthritis is an acute or chronic inflammation of a joint or joints, usually caused directly or indirectly by specific infectious organisms. Infectious arthritis is caused directly by seeding of such pyogenic organisms as gonococci, staphylococci, meningococci, and pneumococci. Infection results in a characteristic edematous and neutrophilic infiltration of the synovialis with hemorrhage or necrosis (according to endotoxin or exotoxin activities) and with subsequent lymphoplasmacytic infiltration, capillary proliferation, and fibrosis, depending on the duration of the process. Destruction of cartilage and fibrous adhesions may cause final joint dysfunction and **ankylosis**.

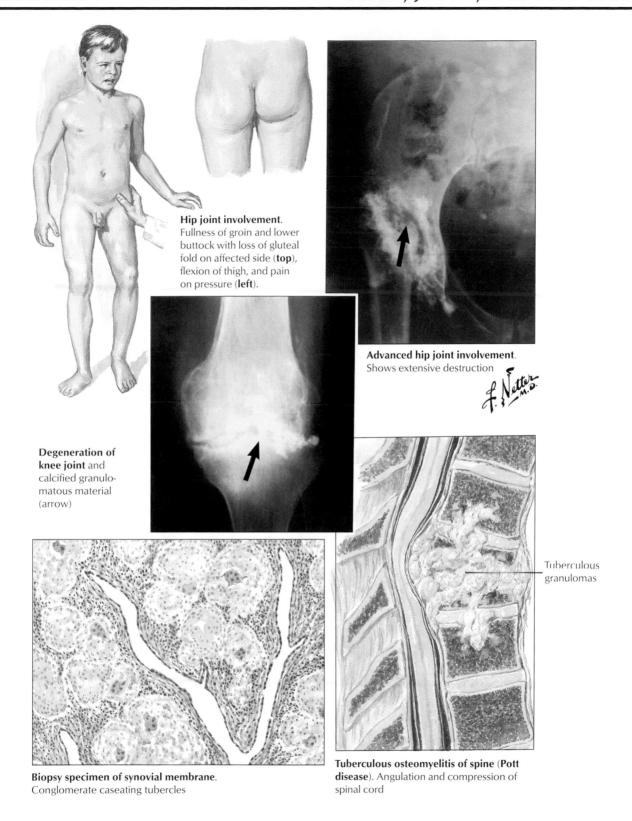

Hip joint involvement. Fullness of groin and lower buttock with loss of gluteal fold on affected side (**top**), flexion of thigh, and pain on pressure (**left**).

Advanced hip joint involvement. Shows extensive destruction

Degeneration of knee joint and calcified granulomatous material (arrow)

Tuberculous granulomas

Biopsy specimen of synovial membrane. Conglomerate caseating tubercles

Tuberculous osteomyelitis of spine (Pott disease). Angulation and compression of spinal cord

FIGURE 11-9 TUBERCULOUS ARTHRITIS

Tuberculous arthritis is characterized by granulomatous reaction and runs a primary chronic course. It is the consequence of hematogenous spread of organisms, usually during early or later phases of stage II tuberculosis (early or late post–primary tuberculosis). Infection usually affects only one joint, most frequently the spine, the hip, the knee, the elbow, or the ankle. The onset of symptoms is insidious; frequent local muscle spasms at night may be the first suspicious sign of the disease. Walking may be problematic if the spine is involved (**Pott disease**). Radiographic changes and strong positive tuberculin skin test results are helpful in establishing the diagnosis. Diagnostic proof is given by tissue biopsy and the demonstration of acid-fast bacilli in the granulomatous inflammation as well as by culture or polymerase chain amplification reaction (PCR) techniques.

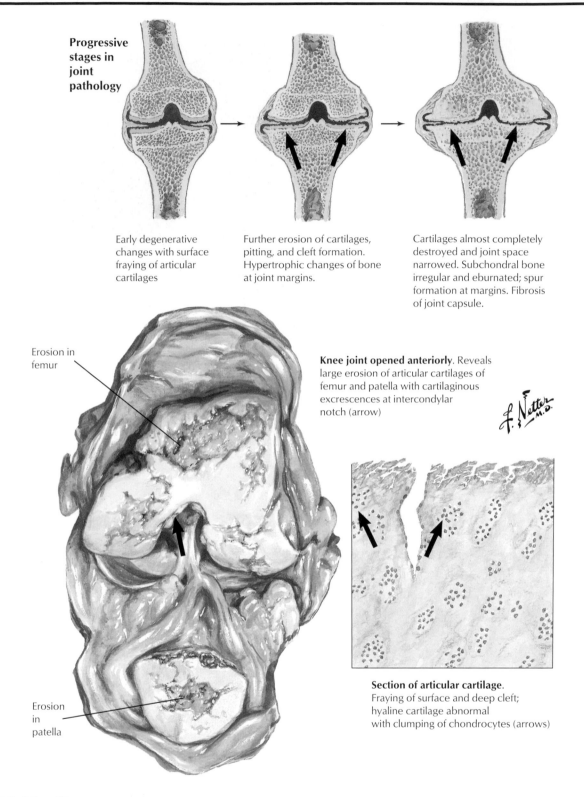

Progressive stages in joint pathology

Early degenerative changes with surface fraying of articular cartilages

Further erosion of cartilages, pitting, and cleft formation. Hypertrophic changes of bone at joint margins.

Cartilages almost completely destroyed and joint space narrowed. Subchondral bone irregular and eburnated; spur formation at margins. Fibrosis of joint capsule.

Erosion in femur

Knee joint opened anteriorly. Reveals large erosion of articular cartilages of femur and patella with cartilaginous excrescences at intercondylar notch (arrow)

Erosion in patella

Section of articular cartilage. Fraying of surface and deep cleft; hyaline cartilage abnormal with clumping of chondrocytes (arrows)

FIGURE 11-10   OSTEOARTHRITIS

Osteoarthritis (OA) is the most common degenerative joint disease causing physical disabilities in persons aged older than 65 years. Initial changes, which become overt by the age of 20 years in 4% of the population, increase steadily to affect more than 85% of persons by the age of 75 years. Primary OA is thought to result from intrinsic defects of cartilage. Secondary OA results from conditions such as malformations, trauma, and metabolic diseases with or without crystalline deposits. Several pathogenetically important factors may contribute to the development of OA: abnormal mechanical forces on the cartilage (increased unit load), decreased water bonding of cartilage (decreased resilience), increased stiffness of subcartilaginous bone, and biochemical abnormalities such as decrease in proteoglycans and shortening of glucosaminoglycans. The latter decreases cartilaginous water binding in favor of binding by collagen fibers. Genetic factors may favor mutations of the collagen type II gene.

Cervical spine involvement

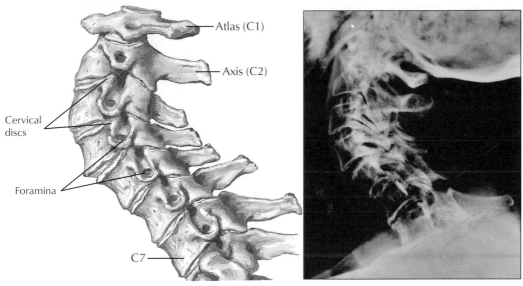

Atlas (C1)

Axis (C2)

Cervical discs

Foramina

C7

Extensive thinning of cervical discs and hyperextension deformity. Narrowing of intervertebral foramina. Lateral radiograph reveals similar changes.

Thoracic spine involvement

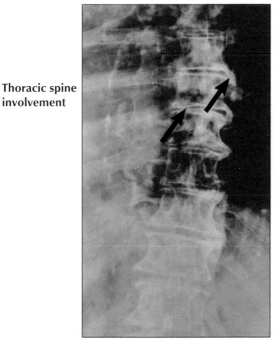

Lumbar spine involvement

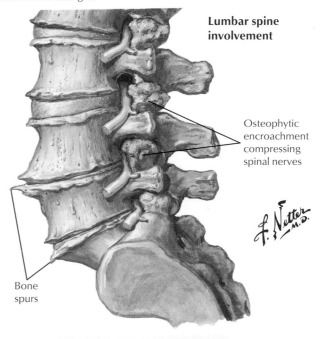

Osteophytic encroachment compressing spinal nerves

Bone spurs

Radiograph of thoracic spine. Narrowing of intervertebral spaces and spur formation (arrow)

Degeneration of lumbar intervertebral discs and hypertrophic changes. At vertebral margins with spur formation. Osteophytic encroachment on intervertebral foramina compresses spinal nerves

FIGURE 11-11   OSTEOARTHRITIS: CLINICAL MANIFESTATIONS

Signs and symptoms of **osteoarthritis** (**OA**)—morning stiffness and pain, rubbing sounds (**crepitus**), and tenderness and swelling of soft tissues covering joints—develop gradually, most often in the knees, the hips, the lumbar and cervical spine, and the finger joints, leading eventually to muscle contracture and compromised joint mobility. Early microscopic findings are loss of cartilaginous metachromatic staining (loss of proteoglycans), loss of chondrocytes, reactive hypertrophy and grouping of residual chondrocytes, and fibrillation and splitting of the cartilage

surface. Fibrillation favors infiltration by synovial fluid with further enzymatic damage, inflammation, and cartilage destruction. Granulation tissue and fibrosis replace cartilage, and erosions result in open bony surfaces. Reactive new bone formation (**osteophytes**) and fibrous adhesions in border zones limit movement. Circumscribed areas of destruction with fragments of cartilage, dead bone, and synovial fluid may expand into the adjacent bone, forming debris-laden subchondral cysts.

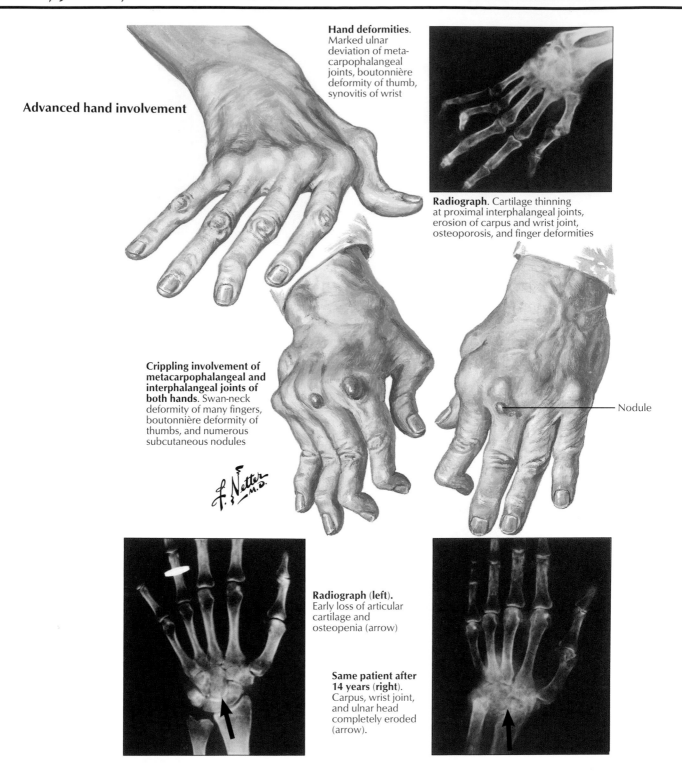

Advanced hand involvement

Hand deformities. Marked ulnar deviation of metacarpophalangeal joints, boutonnière deformity of thumb, synovitis of wrist

Radiograph. Cartilage thinning at proximal interphalangeal joints, erosion of carpus and wrist joint, osteoporosis, and finger deformities

Crippling involvement of metacarpophalangeal and interphalangeal joints of both hands. Swan-neck deformity of many fingers, boutonnière deformity of thumbs, and numerous subcutaneous nodules

— Nodule

Radiograph (left). Early loss of articular cartilage and osteopenia (arrow)

Same patient after 14 years (right). Carpus, wrist joint, and ulnar head completely eroded (arrow).

FIGURE 11-12   RHEUMATOID ARTHRITIS

Rheumatoid arthritis (RA) is a systemic chronic progressive inflammatory disease with symmetric involvement of small joints. Variants are **Still disease** in children (juvenile arthritis) and **ankylosing spondylitis (Bechterew disease)** preferentially involving the vertebral column and the sacroiliacal joints. RA is representative of a group of autoimmune disorders referred to as **collagen–vascular diseases**, which include lupus erythematosus,

primary systemic sclerosis, polymyositis, and dermatomyositis. The etiology of RA is unknown; however, its pathogenesis includes genetic factors (prevalence of HLA-DR4 and HLA-DR1 genes and others), autoimmune reactions (possibly postinfectious), and local factors such as mechanical stress and specifics of tissue reactivity.

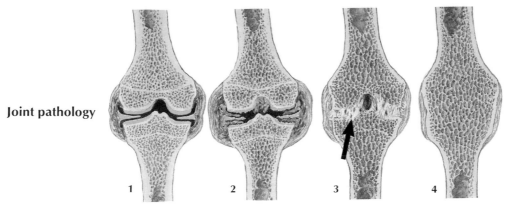

Joint pathology

Progressive stages in joint pathology. 1. Acute inflammation of synovial membrane (synovitis) and beginning proliferative changes. 2. Progression of inflammation with pannus formation; beginning destruction of cartilage and mild osteoporosis. 3. Subsidence of inflammation; fibrous ankylosis (arrow). 4. Bony ankylosis; advanced osteoporosis.

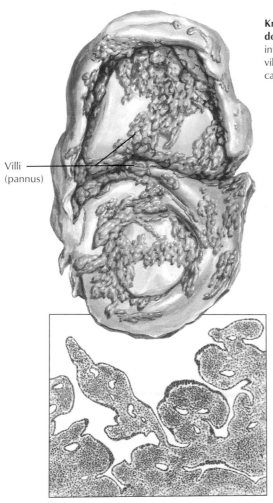

Villi
(pannus)

Knee joint opened anteriorly, patella reflected downward. Thickened synovial membrane inflamed; polypoid outgrowths and numerous villi (pannus) extend over rough articular cartilages of femur and patella

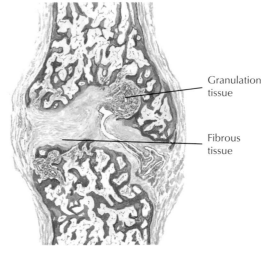

Granulation
tissue

Fibrous
tissue

Section of proximal interphalangeal joint. Marked destruction of both articular cartilages and subchondral bone; replacement by fibrous and granulation tissue, which has obliterated most of joint space and invaded bone

Section of synovial membrane. Villous proliferation with extensive lymphocytic and plasma cells

FIGURE 11-13   RHEUMATOID ARTHRITIS: CLINICAL MANIFESTATIONS

Microscopic features of **rheumatoid arthritis** (**RA**) are progressive villous hypertrophy of the synovialis secondary to fibrinous swelling, proliferation of synovial lining cells, and lymphoplasmacytic infiltration. With increasing chronicity, acute inflammatory reactions are replaced by granulation tissue and fibrosis covering and eroding the cartilaginous surface of the joints (**pannus** formation). Joint mobility is severely inhibited with grossly impressive deviations (subluxation) of joints. End-stage disease is characterized by complete fibrous obliteration of the joints. Adjacent soft tissues may contain focal granulomas with binucleated giant cells (**Aschoff cells**) surrounding soft tissue fibrinoid necrosis (**rheumatic nodule**). Although 25% of patients with RA may recover completely, 50% experience terminal severe incapacitation. Death usually occurs from complications such as infections, gastrointestinal hemorrhage, or cardiovascular or pulmonary involvement.

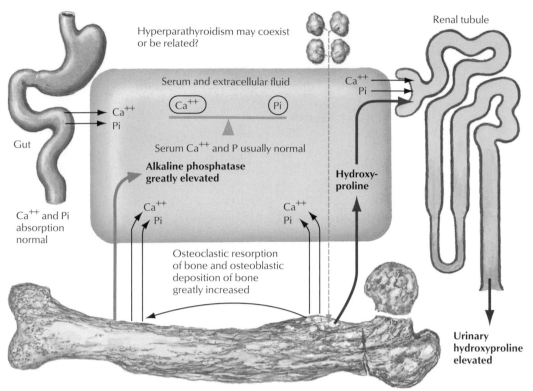

Hyperparathyroidism may coexist or be related?

Renal tubule

Serum and extracellular fluid

Ca⁺⁺

Ca^{++}

Pi

Ca^{++} Pi

Gut

Ca^{++} Pi

Serum Ca^{++} and P usually normal

Alkaline phosphatase greatly elevated

Ca^{++} and Pi absorption normal

Ca^{++} Pi Ca^{++} Pi

Hydroxy-proline

Osteoclastic resorption of bone and osteoblastic deposition of bone greatly increased

Urinary hydroxyproline elevated

Abnormal bone structure, coarse trabeculation, thickening, bowing, pseudofractures, fractures, hypervascularity

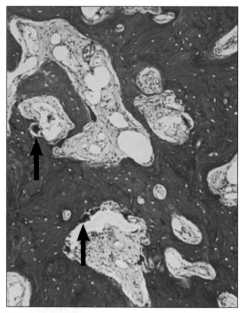

Section of bone. Intense osteoclastic and (arrows) osteoblastic activity and mosaic of lamellar bone

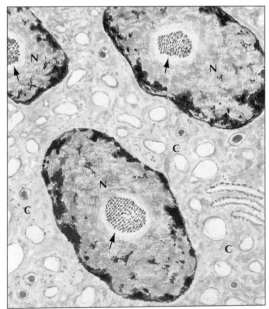

Electron microscopic view. Multinucleated osteoclast with nuclear inclusions that may be viruses (arrows). N = nuclei; C = cytoplasm

FIGURE 11-14   PAGET DISEASE

Paget disease (osteitis deformans) is characterized by excessive osteoblastic bone formation with abnormal structure and impaired stability. It occurs with increasing incidence after the age of 40 years (4-10% of the population), primarily in white populations, more often in men than in women. PD may occur in a **monostotic** form (one bony site) or in a systemic **polyostotic** form. In the initial stage, osteoclast hyperactivity with increased lacunar bone resorption is seen; the presence of respective inclusion bodies and viral transcripts (resembling paramyxovirus) suggests it is stimulated by infection with a **slow virus**. In the second stage, marked osteoblastic hyperactivity compensates and then overcompensates for the osteoclast function, and excessive disorderly new bone with irregular cement lines (**mosaic bone**) is produced. The final stage ("cold" or burnt-out phase) is characterized by marked thickening of densely mineralized bone (**osteosclerotic** phase) with minimal cellular activity.

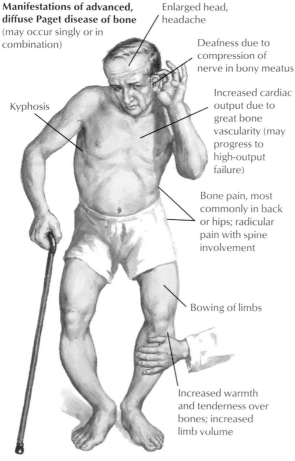

Manifestations of advanced, diffuse Paget disease of bone (may occur singly or in combination)

Enlarged head, headache

Deafness due to compression of nerve in bony meatus

Increased cardiac output due to great bone vascularity (may progress to high-output failure)

Kyphosis

Bone pain, most commonly in back or hips; radicular pain with spine involvement

Bowing of limbs

Increased warmth and tenderness over bones; increased limb volume

Mild cases often asymptomatic (may be discovered incidentally on radiographs taken for other reasons)

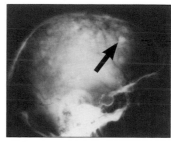

Lateral radiograph. Patchy density of skull (arrow), with areas of osteopenia (osteoporosis circumscripta cranii)

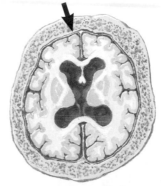

Coronal section of skull and brain. Extremely thickened skull bones, which may encroach on nerve foramina or brainstem and cause hydrocephalus (shown) by compressing cerebral aqueduct

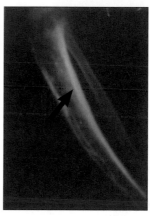

Characteristic radiographic findings in tibia. Thickening, bowing, and coarse trabeculation, with advancing radiolucent wedge

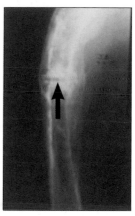

Healing chalk-stick fracture

F. Netter M.D.

FIGURE 11-15   PAGET DISEASE: CLINICAL MANIFESTATIONS

Early phases of **Paget disease** (PD) are asymptomatic, although incidentally increased serum alkaline phosphatase levels may suggest a skeletal disorder. In more advanced cases, incidental radiographic findings may suggest the disease. Typical features are enlargement of head bones, headache, deafness and visual disturbances, deformation and tenderness of long bones (especially of the lower extremities), back pain, and fractures (vertebra, **chalk-stick**–type cross-fractures of long bones). OS develops in approximately 1% of patients.

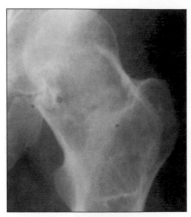

Pathologic fracture of femoral neck.
Typical ground-glass appearance
of bone

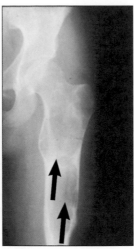
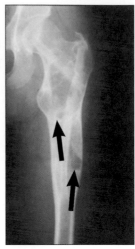

Radiographs of severe monostotic fibrous dysplasia of femur.
Treated for fracture prophylaxis with cortical autograft from
fibula. Preoperative (**left**) and postoperative (**right**)

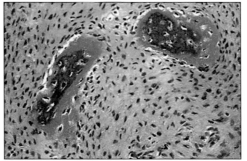

Bone section. Dense fibrous tissue with islands of
trabecular bone without osteoblastic rim (H and E stain)

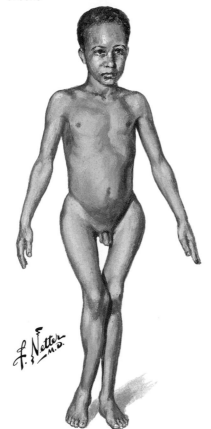

**"Shepard's crook" deformity
of both femoral necks.** Note
also deformity of right tibia.

FIGURE 11-16   FIBROUS DYSPLASIA

Fibrous dysplasia (FD) is a tumor-imitating developmental abnormality of bone that consists of circumscribed mixed fibrous and osseus lesions. FD may be associated with endocrine abnormalities and skin pigmentation such as precocious puberty and **café au lait spots (McCune-Albright syndrome)**, **acromegaly**, and **Cushing syndrome**. Monostotic and polyostotic forms frequently occur in the proximal femur, the tibia, the ribs, and the mandible. Polyostotic forms (25%) also may involve the pelvis,

the hands, or the feet. Growing lesions cause pain, deformation of bones, and pathologic fractures. Characteristic radiographic findings show a ground-glass, slightly "multivesicular" ("soap bubble") appearance with distinct borders. Microscopy shows a dense whorled fibrous tissue containing spicules of woven bone. The prognosis of FD is good, and management should prevent complications such as fractures. Rarely, malignant sarcomas may complicate the course of FD. See Table 11-3.

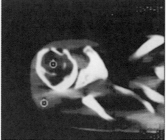

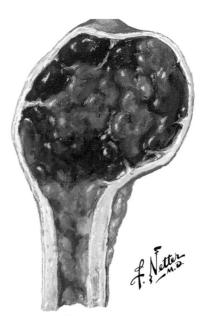

CT scan. Defines margins and density of lesion

Aneurysmal bone cyst in proximal tibia. Anterior (**left**) and lateral (**right**) views

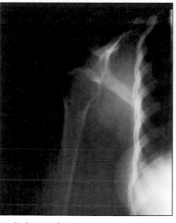

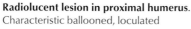

Radiolucent lesion in proximal humerus. Characteristic ballooned, loculated appearance

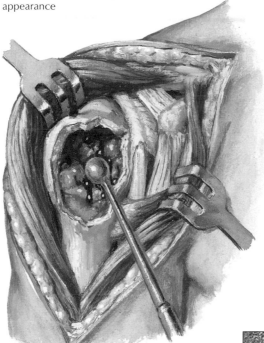

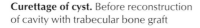

Curettage of cyst. Before reconstruction of cavity with trabecular bone graft

Bone specimen. Ballooned shape, margin of reactive bone, and characteristic multi-loculation. Pockets filled with clotted (cranberry sauce–like) blood.

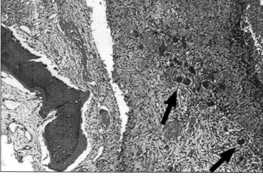

Bone section. Stroma of benign spindle cells, scattered giant cells (arrows), blood, and bone fragments (H and E stain)

FIGURE 11-17 ANEURYSMAL BONE CYSTS

Aneurysmal bone cysts are not a true neoplasm but a reactive tumorlike lesion arising suggestively from previous trauma or degeneration of another underlying disease (e.g., osteoblastoma, FD, GCT, and others). Grossly, ABCs appear as circumscribed masses of spongy, bloody tissue with fibrous septae, thinning the cortical bone, and bulging through the periosteum. Part of the bone may be replaced by granulation tissue with microscopic multinucleated giant cells and osteoid bone formation. Although lesions usually enlarge rapidly, there are slow-growing types of ABC that must be distinguished from the malignant telangiectatic osteosarcoma and giant cell tumor of bones. Bone scans and computed density measurements may be helpful in the differential diagnosis, but biopsy and pathologic investigation are necessary to confirm ABCs. Local curettage with grafting of trabecular bone is the treatment of choice. See Table 11-3.

TABLE 11-3 BENIGN PRIMARY TUMOROUS LESIONS OF THE SKELETAL SYSTEM AND JOINTS

Type of Lesion	Ages	Usual Location	Gross Features
Nonossifying fibroma (fibrous cortical defect)	Children	Metaphysis, long bones (tibia, fibula)	Eccentric cortical lesion with well-demarcated sclerotic margins
Solitary bone cyst	Children, adolescents	Humerus, femur (adjacent to growth plate)	Well-demarcated epi-diaphyseal lesion
Aneurysmal bone cyst	Children, young adults	Long bones, vertebra (essentially everywhere)	Rapidly expanding cyst (previous trauma?)
Fibrous dysplasia (monostotic or polyostotic)	Adolescents, young adults	Long bones	Diaphyseal "soap bubble" translucencies
Osteoma (eburneum) (probably not a real neoplasm)	Adults	Skull, tibia	Exophytic solid mass
Osteoid osteoma	Children, young adults	Tubular bones, lower extremity	Diaphyseal cortex "nidus"
Osteoblastoma	Children, young adults	Vertebra, spinal, transverse process	Similar to osteoid osteoma ("nidus")
Osteochondroma (exostosis)	Young adults	Long bones	Bony exostoses with cartilaginous cap
Chondroma (enchondroma)	Adults	Tubular bones metacarpi, phalanges	Intraosseous, solitary well-circumscribed lesion
Chondroblastoma	Children, young adults	Long bones femur, tibia, humerus	Epiphysis, paraarticular well-circumscribed lesion
Chondromyxoid fibroma	Children, young adults	Femur, tibia	Excentric lucent defect, delicate sclerotic border
Synovial chondromatosis (self-limited)	Young adults (men)	Large joints	Hyaline cartilage nodules and floating free bodies
Villonodular synovitis Pigmented	Young adults	Knee, hip, ankles, feet, fingers	Synovial lining cell proliferation with hemosiderin deposits

TABLE 11-4 MALIGNANT PRIMARY TUMOROUS LESIONS OF THE SKELETAL SYSTEM AND JOINTS

Type of Lesion	Ages	Usual Location	Gross Features
Osteogenic sarcoma (osteosarcoma)	Adolescents, children	Femur, tibia, fibula, and others	Irregular bone destruction, reactive periosteal new bone (see text for variants)
Chondrosarcoma	Adults (fourth to sixth decades of life)	Pelvis, shoulder, proximal femur, ribs	Often bulky destructive lesion with calcification or bone formation (see text for variants)
Giant cell tumor (locally aggressive, potentially malignant)	Adults	Long bones, epimetaphyseal junction	Slowly growing lytic lesion with periosteal reaction, circumscribed, painful
Ewing sarcoma	Children, adolescents	Long bones, mid shaft metaphyseal humerus, femur, tibia	Lytic lesion in medulla and inner cortex, periosteal reaction
Synovial sarcoma	Adolescents, young adults	In vicinity of joints, 10% intraarticular	Soft tissue tumor associated with tendons, bursae, joint capsule

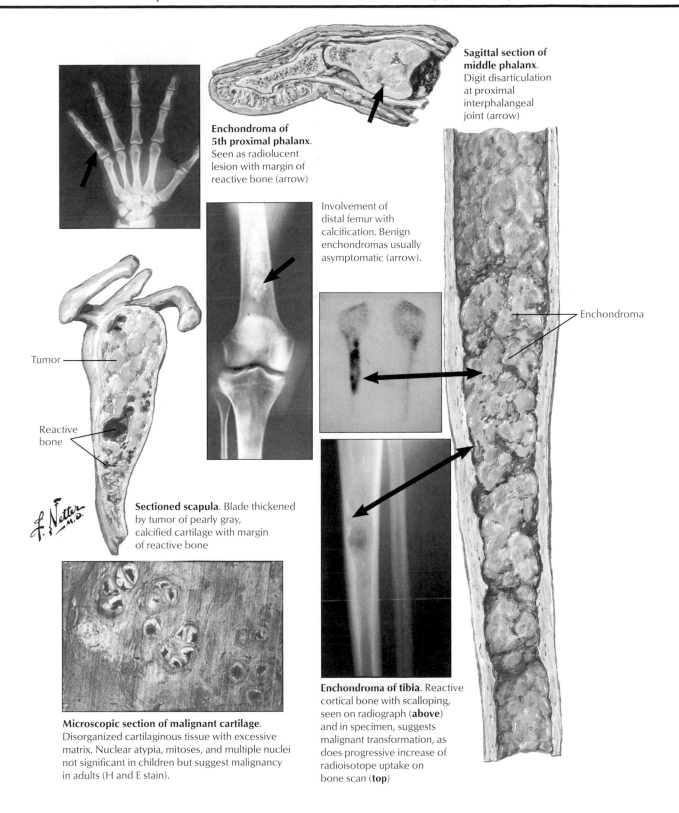

Sagittal section of middle phalanx. Digit disarticulation at proximal interphalangeal joint (arrow)

Enchondroma of 5th proximal phalanx. Seen as radiolucent lesion with margin of reactive bone (arrow)

Involvement of distal femur with calcification. Benign enchondromas usually asymptomatic (arrow).

Enchondroma

Tumor

Reactive bone

Sectioned scapula. Blade thickened by tumor of pearly gray, calcified cartilage with margin of reactive bone

Microscopic section of malignant cartilage. Disorganized cartilaginous tissue with excessive matrix. Nuclear atypia, mitoses, and multiple nuclei not significant in children but suggest malignancy in adults (H and E stain).

Enchondroma of tibia. Reactive cortical bone with scalloping, seen on radiograph (**above**) and in specimen, suggests malignant transformation, as does progressive increase of radioisotope uptake on bone scan (**top**)

FIGURE 11-18   ENCHONDROMA

Enchondroma (EC) is a benign intraosseous tumor of well-differentiated cartilage occurring primarily in adults and adolescents. It most frequently affects small tubular bones of the hands and feet but can develop anywhere in the skeleton. The monoclonality of chondrocytes in EC suggests a benign neoplasm. EC may occur in multiplicity (enchondromatosis, **Ollier disease**). Rarely, EC transforms to secondary chondrosarcoma (CS). EC is usually asymptomatic except for certain "obscure" pain sensations.

Incidental radiographs show well-defined radiolucent lesions with slightly pronounced bony margins and sometimes calcification. Microscopy reveals a somewhat disorganized, well-differentiated cartilage with stippled calcification. Larger lesions may undergo pseudocystic degeneration. The prognosis for small benign ECs is good, and lesions may be followed without intervention. Surgical intervention is suggested for mechanical reasons or when suspicion of malignancy arises. See Table 11-3.

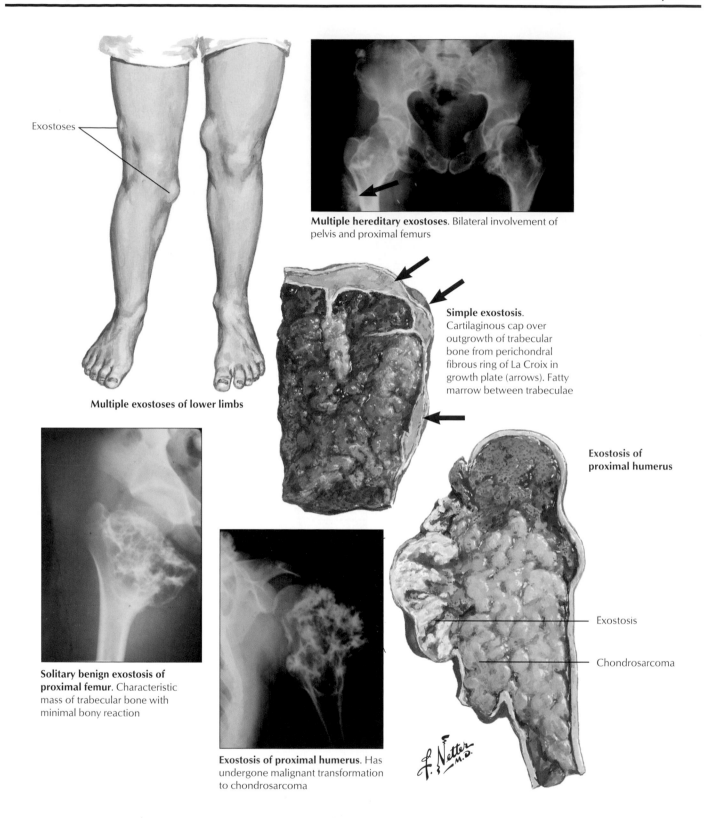

Exostoses

Multiple hereditary exostoses. Bilateral involvement of pelvis and proximal femurs

Simple exostosis. Cartilaginous cap over outgrowth of trabecular bone from perichondral fibrous ring of La Croix in growth plate (arrows). Fatty marrow between trabeculae

Exostosis of proximal humerus

Multiple exostoses of lower limbs

Solitary benign exostosis of proximal femur. Characteristic mass of trabecular bone with minimal bony reaction

Exostosis

Chondrosarcoma

Exostosis of proximal humerus. Has undergone malignant transformation to chondrosarcoma

FIGURE 11-19   OSTEOCHONDROMA

Osteochondroma (osteocartilaginous exostoses), which constitute approximately one third of benign bone tumors, are not tumors as such but rather developmental dysplasias of the growth plate. Osteochondroma presents as a solitary lobulated metaphyseal outgrowth, polyostotic, or rarely as a familial disorder (**multiple hereditary exostosis**) and consists of mature trabecular bone with a cartilaginous cap. Common locations are the proximal and distal femur, the proximal humerus and tibia, and the pelvis and scapula. Radiographic and gross changes are characteristic. Rapidly growing lesions in adults may indicate a (rare) risk of malignant transformation to secondary chondrosarcoma. These lesions must be distinguished from parosteal osteosarcoma. The prognosis of solitary exostosis is excellent, with approximately 5% recurrence after surgical removal. See Table 11-3.

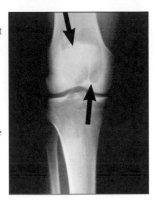

Anteroposterior radiograph. Giant cell tumor of epiphysis and metaphysis of distal femur extending into, but not penetrating, subchondral plate

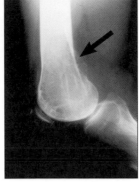

Lateral view radiograph. Radiolucent lesion bulging posteriorly into popliteal fossa

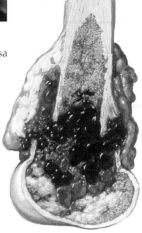

CT scan, right femur. Marked endosteal erosion by intraosseous lesion

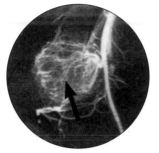

Angiogram. Intense vascularity of tumor area (arrow)

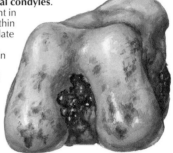

Pathologic fracture. Through giant cell tumor of distal femur

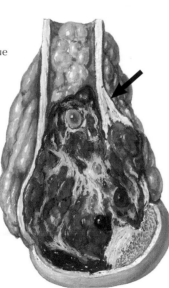

Sectioned distal femur. Meaty, hemorrhagic tissue with lighter, dense, fibrous areas, small cysts and blood clots, and thin margin of reactive bone with Codman triangle (arrow). Tumor has infiltrated soft tissue.

View of femoral condyles. Tumor apparent in spots through thin subchondral plate and articular cartilage; also in intercondylar notch covered by synovial membrane

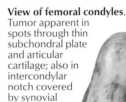

Bone section. Stroma of spindlelike cells with pale-staining cytoplasm and nuclei, many multinucleated giant cells, vascular channels, and free blood (H and E stain)

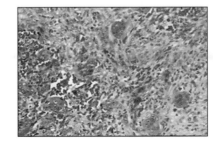

FIGURE 11-20　GIANT CELL TUMOR

Giant cell tumor of bone (osteoclastoma) occurs preferentially between the ages of 20 and 40 years. Typically, the lesion is located at the epimetaphyseal junction of long bones such as the femur, the tibia, the humerus, the radius, and the fibula, presenting as a slowly growing lytic lesion causing persistent intraosseous pain, reactive effusions, and eventual fractures. Radiographs reveal large radiolucent lesions with surrounding reactive bone formation, cortical thinning, trabecularization, and bony separation. Grossly, they appear as soft, friable, reddish-brown tissue resembling a bloody sponge. There may be areas of aneurysmal cavitation. Microscopically, they show a mixed-cell proliferation of stromal mononuclear cells and multinucleated (osteoclastic) giant cells in a markedly vascularized stroma and focal hemorrhages. Up to 10% (usually the incompletely removed tumors) metastasize; the neoplastic component is the mononuclear stromal cells. Treatment by curettage alone results in 50% recurrence. See Table 11-3.

Parosteal osteosarcoma

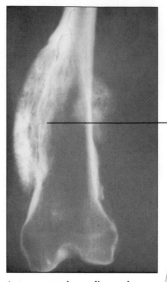

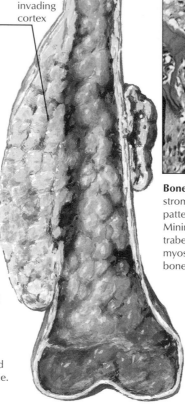

Tumor invading cortex

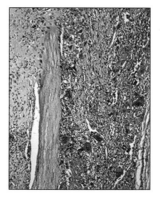

Anteroposterior radiograph. Densely ossified prominence on anterolateral aspect of distal femur; satellite lesion on opposite side characterizes mass as parosteal osteosarcoma rather than osteoma or osteocartilaginous exostosis.

Sectioned femur. Longitudinal tumor has invaded cortex but not medullary canal. Satellite lesion still separated from cortex by cleft; in early stage, primary tumor is also separated from cortex by uninvolved zone.

Bone section. Relatively bland stroma with mature trabecular pattern but without mitoses. Minimal osteoblastic rim on trabeculae helps rule out myositis ossificans or reactive bone (H and E stain).

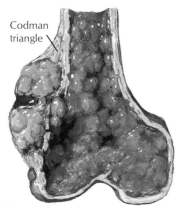

Codman triangle

Periosteal osteosarcoma

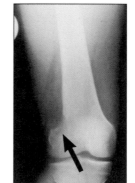

Distal femur. Erosive cartilaginous lesion in periosteum of distal femoral metaphysis. Codman triangles of reactive bone at margins.

Radiograph. Craterlike lesion with margin of reactive bone and faint calcification

Bone section. Highly malignant stroma with cartilaginous and osteoid components (H and E stain)

FIGURE 11-21 OSTEOSARCOMA

Osteosarcoma (**osteogenic sarcoma**) is the most common malignant bone tumor, occurring in endosteal, cortical or parosteal juxtacortical forms, usually during the second decade of life. Most frequent sites (75%) are metaphyseal areas adjacent to knee or shoulder (e.g., tibia, fibula, humerus), hands, feet, skull and jaws. Radiographs show localized lytic or osteoblastic lesions with fuzzy borders and prominent subperiosteal reactive bone formation (**Codman triangle**). The cut surface depends on the histologic variant of the tumor: it is whitish soft or bony hard, pseudocystic with focal necroses or hemorrhages and freely invades into adjacent soft tissues. Parosteal OS may resemble exostoses with well-differentiated bone or fibrous tissue components. Histologic variants include degrees of differentiation of chondroblastic areas or of giant cell components tand overtly telangiectatic or fibroblastic forms. OS readily metastasizes into the lungs and pleura, less frequently to other organs. See Table 11-4.

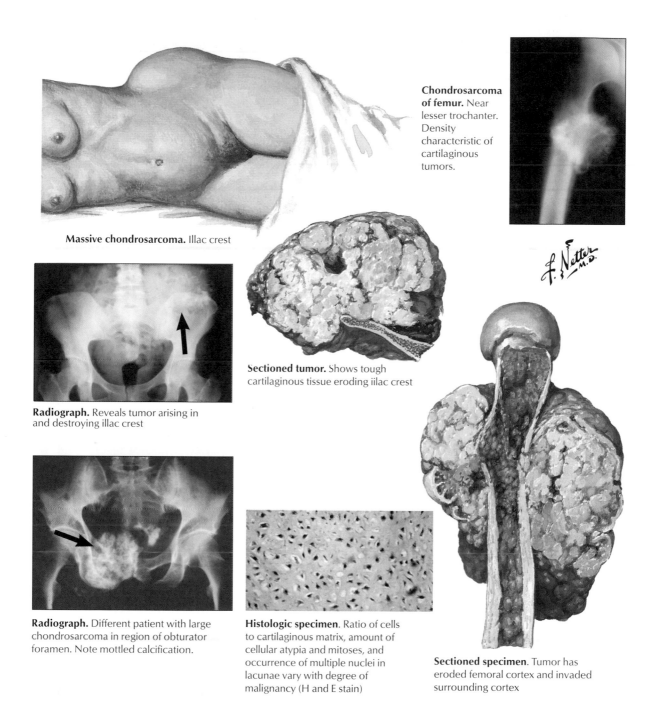

Massive chondrosarcoma. Iliac crest

Chondrosarcoma of femur. Near lesser trochanter. Density characteristic of cartilaginous tumors.

Radiograph. Reveals tumor arising in and destroying illiac crest

Sectioned tumor. Shows tough cartilaginous tissue eroding iiIac crest

Radiograph. Different patient with large chondrosarcoma in region of obturator foramen. Note mottled calcification.

Histologic specimen. Ratio of cells to cartilaginous matrix, amount of cellular atypia and mitoses, and occurrence of multiple nuclei in lacunae vary with degree of malignancy (H and E stain)

Sectioned specimen. Tumor has eroded femoral cortex and invaded surrounding cortex

FIGURE 11-22　CHONDROSARCOMA

Chondrosarcoma arises from cartilage rests or preexisting ECs. There are several gross variants: central, juxtacortical and peripheral (the latter arising outside the bone). CSs occur in older persons with a peak in the sixth decade of life, usually in central portions of the skeleton such as shoulder, pelvis, proximal femur and ribs. Radiographic images show a bulky osteodestructive lesion with a characteristic pattern of calcification ("salt and pepper" or "popcorn"). Gross lesions show a smooth whitish glistening cut-surface that is occasionally lobulated and focally calcified. Histologic appearances vary from well differentiated cartilaginous tumors to undifferentiated and mesenchymal forms. Well-differentiated OS can be hard to distinguish from EC. Criteria of malignancy are the grouping and polymorphism of chondrocytes, their nuclear atypia, multinucleate cells and occasional mitoses. CSs metastasize preferentially to the lungs. See Table 11-4.

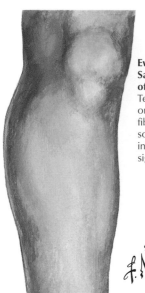

Ewing's Sarcoma of knee. Tender bulge on proximal fibula with some inflammatory signs

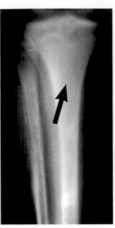

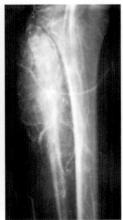

Radiograph. Mottled, destructive, radiolucent lesion (arrow)

Angiogram. Vascular blush extending into soft tissue

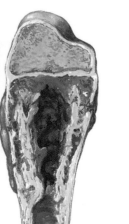

Bone scan. Heavy radioisotope uptake in tumor area; other hot spots related to normal bone growth

Sectioned fibula. Infiltrative, destructive tumor extending into soft tissue seen in sectioned proximal fibula

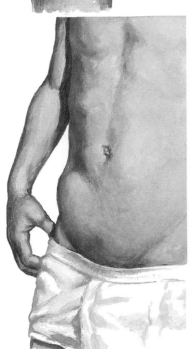

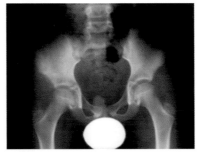

Lesion of mottled density involves anterior superior iliac spine

Sectioned femur. Highly vascular intraosseous and soft tissue tumor components with much reactive bone

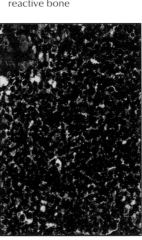

Ewing sarcoma of pelvis. Scarcely visible but palpable mass in right lower quadrant

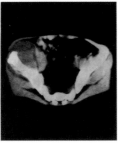

CT scan. Defines mass filling right iliac fossa (arrow)

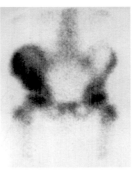

Bone scan. Heavy radioisotope uptake in right iliac wing (arrow)

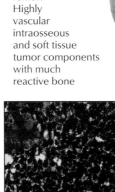

Bone section. Masses of small, round cells with uniform-sized hyperchromatic nuclei (H and E stain)

FIGURE 11-23 EWING SARCOMA

Ewing sarcoma (ES), after OS the second most common bone tumor in children, accounts for approximately 5% of all bone tumors and has a peak incidence in the second decade of life. Although its histogenesis remains unclear, frequent genetic mutations (t[11;22]p13;q12) suggest a relationship of malignant cells in ES to primitive neuroectodermal cells. Unlike other bone tumors, ES frequently presents with fever and pain simulating an inflammatory disease. The diagnosis is confirmed by biopsy and microscopic investigation. The characteristic dense small cell tumors must be distinguished from cell tumors such as neuroblastoma and malignant lymphoma. Long bones including midshaft humerus, tibia and femur are the sites most frequently affected. Grossly, the tumor impresses as osteolytic soft grayish-white masses with focal hemorrhage which may penetrate the periosteum and invade adjacent soft tissues. ES commonly metastasizes to lungs, brain and other bony sites such as the skull. See Table 11-4.

Etiology of compartment syndrome

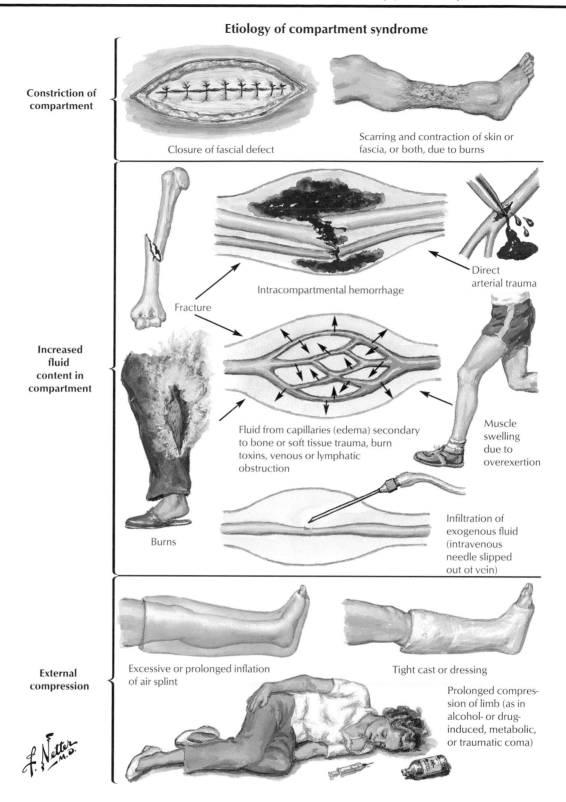

Constriction of compartment

Closure of fascial defect

Scarring and contraction of skin or fascia, or both, due to burns

Increased fluid content in compartment

Fracture

Intracompartmental hemorrhage

Direct arterial trauma

Fluid from capillaries (edema) secondary to bone or soft tissue trauma, burn toxins, venous or lymphatic obstruction

Muscle swelling due to overexertion

Burns

Infiltration of exogenous fluid (intravenous needle slipped out of vein)

External compression

Excessive or prolonged inflation of air splint

Tight cast or dressing

Prolonged compression of limb (as in alcohol- or drug-induced, metabolic, or traumatic coma)

FIGURE 11-24   COMPARTMENT SYNDROME

Compartment syndrome (CS) results from increased pressure in one or more (osteo)fascial compartments. Sustained increase of tissue pressure from local edema reduces capillary perfusion below the level necessary for sustaining tissue viability; irreversible muscle and nerve damage results in a few hours. Partial burial, trauma, burns, or exercise may cause CS. Pathogenetic mechanisms are increased fluid accumulation, decreased tissue volume (compartment constriction), and restricted volume expansion secondary to external compression (e.g., casts). In conscious patients, pain is disproportionate to the obvious injury and increases with passive stretching of muscles. Loss of sensation from nerves running through affected compartments may occur. Microscopic changes are intense soft tissue edema with progressive degeneration and necrosis, hemorrhage, and, in delayed cases, slowly developing granulation tissue and fibrosis. There is high risk of superinfection, and secondary septicemia exists.

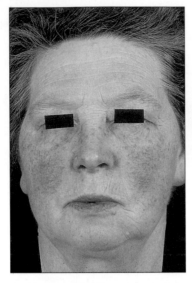

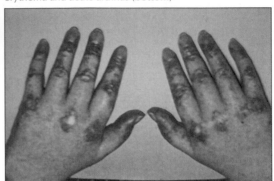

Systemic lupus erythematosus (SLE) (left). Butterfly erythema and acute arthritis (**bottom**)

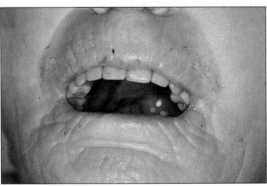

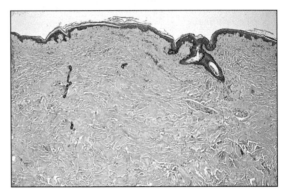

Primary systemic sclerosis (PSS). Atrophy and severe shrinkage of skin. Clinical presentation (**left**) and microscopic presentation (**right**).

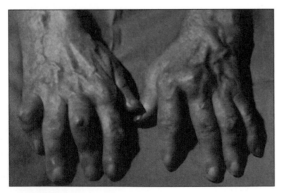

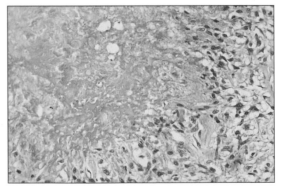

Rheumatoid arthritis (RA). Rheumatoid nodules (**left**), granulomatous inflammation with fibrinoid necrosis (**right**)

FIGURE 11-25 COLLAGEN-VASCULAR DISEASE

Collagen-vascular disease (CVD) refers to a group of systemic autoimmune disorders with overlapping signs and symptoms that affect several organ systems (e.g., skin, kidneys, lungs). CVDs include **systemic lupus erythematosus**, **RA**, **primary systemic** sclerosis, **dermatomyositis**, **polymyositis**, and certain "overlap syndromes" (Table 11-5). Although the etiologies of CVDs are unknown, the pathogenesis is characterized by various autoimmune reactions with demonstration of respective autoantibodies,

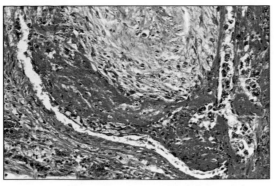
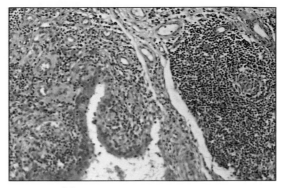

Microscopy of RA. With acute synovialitis (**left**) and chronic tenovaginitis (**right**)

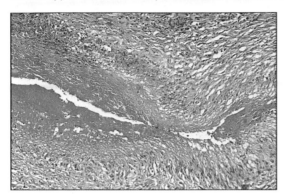
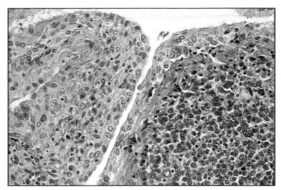

Microscopy of systemic lupus erythematosis. With acute (**left**) and chronic arthritis/synovialitis (**right**)

TABLE 11-5   FEATURES OF EXEMPLARY MEMBERS OF COLLAGEN-VASCULAR DISEASES

Syndrome	Autoimmunity*	Features†
Systemic lupus erythematosus	Autoantibodies against native ds-DNA, denatured ss-DNA, histones, and histone complexes T-, NK-cell, and cytokine abnormalities, circulating immune complexes	Rashes, arthritis/arthralgia, glomerulonephritis, proteinuria, thrombocytopenia, hemolytic anemia, pleural effusions, pulmonary fibrosis, pericarditis, endocarditis, psychosis, seizures Vasculitis and thrombosis
Primary systemic sclerosis	Autoantibodies against small RNA protein (SS-A/Ro), topoisomerase I (Scl-70), 45K RNA protein (SS-B/La)	Hallmark: scleroderma, **Raynaud syndrome,** proliferative arteritis and fibrosis, capillary malformations such as telangiectasia and bleeding; esophagus and lower GI tract: fibrosis and muscular atrophy with motility problems and dysphagia, interstitial pneumonitis, **"shrinking lung disease,"** pulmonary hemorrhage; heart: conductive and ventricular dysfunction, renal vasculitis and hypertension
Polymyositis, dermatomyositis	tRNA synthetases: Jo-1, PL-7; protein complex (PM-Scl)	Muscle weakness: segmental myofiber necrosis with inflammatory infiltrate, fever, myoglobinuria, skin rash, erythema of hands (knuckles), interstitial pneumonitis, approximately 25% associated with malignancies
Rheumatoid arthritis	Denatured ss-DNA Rheumatoid factor, CIC, antikeratin, collagen antibody, T-cell "activation"	Chronic relapsing synovitis, arthritis, small joints of hands, symmetrical, tenosynovitis, soft tissue rheumatic nodules, pleuritis, pericarditis, vasculitis, interstitial pneumonitis, bronchiolitis obliterans, polyneuritis, mononeuritis, **Felty syndrome**

CIC indicates circulating immune complexes; ds, double-stranded; GI, gastrointestinal; ss, single-stranded.

*Selective antibodies only.

†See text for additional microscopy.

FIGURE 11-25   COLLAGEN-VASCULAR DISEASE *(CONTINUED)* ━━━━━━━━━

circulating immune complexes, or both. The essential pathologic features in all CVDs are chronic inflammatory infiltration (lymphoplasmacellular) of connective tissue, edema, fibrinoid necroses, vasculitis, and progressive fibrosis. The extent and composition of these features vary among the different CVDs and with their type of autoimmune reaction (autoantibodies, circulating immune complexes, T-cell immune reaction).

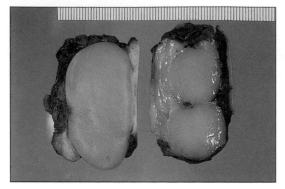

Subcutaneous neurofibroma. Gross appearance

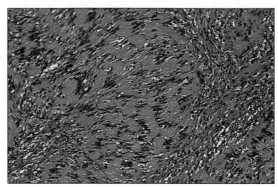

Subcutaneous neurofibroma. Microscopic appearance

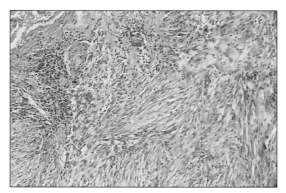

Nodular fasciitis (i.e., "pseudotumor"); microscopic section

FIGURE 11-26   BENIGN SOFT TISSUE TUMORS

Benign tumors of soft tissue may occur at any age and are classified according to the tissue where they arise: **fibromas**, **lipomas**, **rhabdomyomas**, **leiomyomas**, or mixtures of these, and composite tumors with additional tissue components (angiolipomas, fibrous histiocytoma, neurofibroma, myelolipoma). **Subcutaneous lipomas**, the most frequent benign tumors, are slowly enlarging well-circumscribed yellowish masses with a histology indistinguishable from normal fat tissue. Fibrous tumorlike lesions (nodular fasciitis, fibromatosis) are not considered real tumors, although some show locally aggressive behavior. **Fibrous histiocytomas** are dermal tumors of interlacing fibrous strands and collections of lipid- and iron-containing histiocytes. **Benign neurofibromas** occur in dermis and in part in the submucosa of the alimentary tract. They may cause bleeding or mild obstruction. Leiomyomas are common in the uterus but also are found in the gastrointestinal tract or originating from blood vessels.

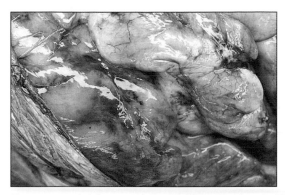

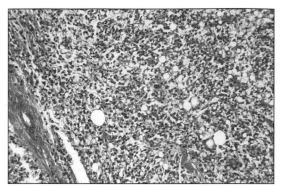

Liposarcoma of abdomen with poorly differentiated atypical lipoblasts, gross (**left**) and microscopic (**right**)

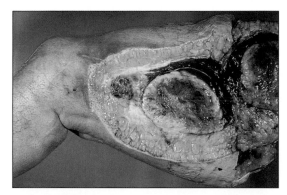

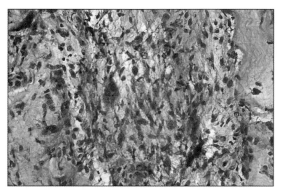

Malignant fibrous histiocytoma (MFH), gross (**left**) and microscopic (**right**)

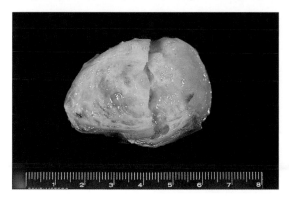

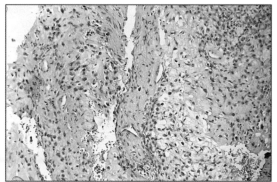

Chondromyxoid neurofibrosarcoma, gross (**left**) and microscopic (**right**)

FIGURE 11-27   MALIGNANT SOFT TISSUE TUMORS

Sarcomas spread by hematogenous metastases rather than through lymphatic channels. They are classified according to the tissue from which they derive, or in a more descriptive way if their histogenesis is unclear. Variants include liposarcomas, fibrosarcomas, **malignant fibrous histiocytoma (MFH)**, neurofibrosarcomas, rhabdomyosarcomas, leiomyosarcomas, and alveolar soft part sarcomas or epithelioid sarcomas. Fibrosarcoma, usually arising from fascia, tendons, periosteum, or scar tissue of the thigh, the knee, or the trunk, is not a common malignancy, but its "pleomorphic cousin," MFH, is the most common soft tissue sarcoma. MFH is a highly malignant tumor of deep fascia, skeletal muscle, and the retroperitoneal space, preferentially occurring in patients aged 50 to 70 years. Postradiation fibrosarcoma is classified as MFH. Prognosis depends on the degree of atypia and the polymorphism of its cells. Approximately 50% of MFHs metastasize early to the lungs. Liposarcomas arise

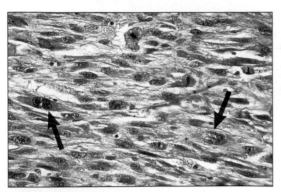

Rhabdomyosarcoma. Microscopy showing atypical spindle cells with occasional cross-striation (arrows) and many mitoses

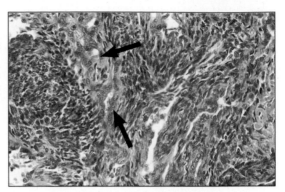

Synovial sarcoma. Microscopy showing atypical biphasic pattern: spindle cells and adenoid structures (arrows)

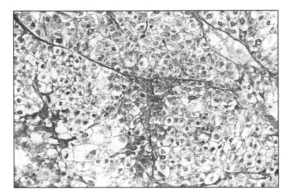

Alveolar soft part sarcoma. Microscopy showing nests of large clear epitheloid cells separated by fine fibrous strands

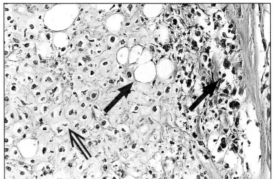

Chondromyxoid liposarcoma. Microscopy showing mixture of atypical lipoblasts (arrow) and chondroid differentiation (double arrow)

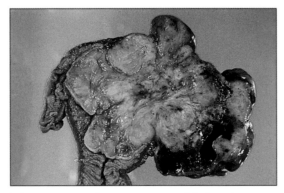

Leiomyosarcoma. Gross appearance of the intestine compressing the lumen, infiltrating and destructing the intestinal wall (intact intestine in lower part of image)

FIGURE 11-27   MALIGNANT SOFT TISSUE TUMORS *(CONTINUED)*

preferentially in the deep subcutaneous tissues of the thighs, the abdomen, and the retroperitoneum of persons aged older than 50 years. There are several morphologic variants (e.g., well-differentiated, myxoid, pleomorphic, and round cell forms), some of which show mutational chromosomal abnormalities of their adipocytes. **Rhabdomyosarcoma** is a tumor of children and young adults. It is thought to derive from primitive mesenchyme or embryonic muscle tissue and has corresponding appearances: embryonal rhabdomyosarcoma, alveolar rhabdomyosarcoma,

and pleomorphic rhabdomyosarcoma. Well-differentiated forms contain plump cells resembling striated muscle. **Leiomyosarcomas** are malignant tumors of smooth muscle, occurring most commonly in the uterus and gastrointestinal tract. **Neurofibrosarcoma** and **neurolemmal sarcoma** (malignant schwannoma) are tumors of peripheral nerves that are more common in adults. **Epithelioid sarcomas** and **alveolar soft part sarcomas** are rare, highly malignant tumors of uncertain histogenesis.

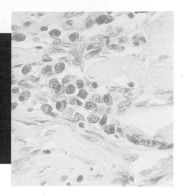

CHAPTER 12

ENDOCRINE SYSTEM

The endocrine system consists of a number of organized glands, groups of cells, and dispersed solitary cells that control the functional balance of internal organs by means of chemical messengers called *hormones*. Organized endocrine glands include the pituitary, the thyroid and parathyroid, the adrenal cortex and medulla, and the endocrine pancreas. In addition, sex organs such as the ovary and testis produce certain hormones (see chapters 7 and 8).

HYPOTHALAMUS-PITUITARY AXIS

Endocrine function responds to feedback control. Because the nervous system "supervises" the endocrine organs, particularly the hypothalamus, it is more appropriate to speak of the **neuroendocrine system**. In fact, almost all neuroendocrine stimuli exert feedback control, so one could speak of, for example, a **neuroendocrine-immunologic axis**. All such actions and reactions follow a circadian rhythm, controlled by light, which is the subject of the science of **chronobiology**.

THYROID GLAND

The thyroid gland, which responds with peripheral feedback control to the hypothalamus and pituitary, is the key endocrine organ controlling energy metabolism (carbohydrate and lipid catabolism, stimulation of protein synthesis). It acts primarily through the effects of 2 hormones, **thyroxin** (**tetraiodothyronine**; T4) and **triiodothyronine** (T3), which bind to receptors on various peripheral cells and stimulate their metabolic activities. These hormones are coupled to thyroglobulin and are stored in follicular colloids. Proteolytic enzymes release T4 and T3 and make it available in the periphery as active hormones. This process is accompanied morphologically by signs of follicular activation such as paraepithelial resorptive vacuoles in the colloid, epithelial swelling (cuboidal size), and proliferation (focal stratification to form **Sanderson cushions** and papillae).

PARATHYROID GLANDS

In most people, 4 separate parathyroid glands lie in close proximity to the posterior part of the thyroid gland. Their hormone, **parathyroid hormone** (PTH), controls the calcium balance of the body as it responds to feedback mechanisms independently of hypothalamic-hypophysial supervision. One third of the normal parathyroid gland consists of fat tissue, and the balance contains the pale PTH-producing **chief cells** and pink **oxyphilic cells**. Any increase in weight above the normal 130 mg or replacement of fat tissue by glandular

cells indicates hyperplasia/hyperfunction. Hyperparathyroidism independent of feedback control (i.e., autonomous) usually is caused by adenomas or carcinomas of the gland. Hypoparathyroidism (lack of PTH) is rare, usually follows surgical resection of the glands in thyroidectomies, and causes severe hypocalcemia. Familial autosomal recessive forms of hypoparathyroidism may occasionally occur as part of a multiglandular deficiency or in combination with T-cell immune deficiency (e.g., **DiGeorge syndrome**). The ionized serum calcium level provides the stimulus for PTH secretion. PTH stabilizes the serum calcium level by inhibiting renal tubular phosphate reabsorption and calcium/phosphate absorption in the bone and by enhancing calcium absorption in the intestines.

ADRENAL CORTEX (SUPRARENAL CORTEX)

The adrenal cortex is composed of 3 microscopically identifiable zones, each of which engages in the production of different hormones: the **zona glomerulosa** (outer zone), the **zona fasciculata** (intermediate zone), and the **zona reticularis** (inner zone adjacent to adrenal medulla). The latter 2 zones respond to stimulation by hypophyseal corticotropin, whereas the **zona glomerulosa** functions independently of it. This zone produces the hormone **aldosterone** in response to increases in potassium levels and angiotensin or decreases in atrial natriuretic peptide or somatostatin. The 2 inner zones produce glucocorticoids and androgens in response to corticotropins. Increased functional activity in either zone is associated with microscopic hyperplasia, adenoma, or carcinoma; decreased functional activity is associated with atrophy (e.g., in malnutrition), necrosis (e.g., in septicemia, tuberculosis, or viral infection), or autoimmune adrenalitis.

ADRENAL MEDULLA

The major organs of the sympathetic neuroendocrine system are the adrenal medulla and less compact collections of neuroendocrine cells in paraganglia, including the carotid body and the **organ of Zuckerkandl**. All consist of **chromaffin cells** (which have an affinity to chromium salts and stain dark on oxidation), which produce the catecholamines **epinephrine** and **norepinephrine**. Several tumors of chromaffin catecholamine-producing cells, such as pheochromocytoma and paragangliomas, exaggerate the physiologic functions of the organs. In addition, ganglionic cells in these regions may give rise to neuroblastomas. Approximately 10% of pheochromocytomas are part of a familial syndrome called **multiple endocrine neoplasia** (MEN). Several forms of MEN are autosomal dominant diseases with mutations on chromosomes 10 and 11. Patients with an identified adenoma or carcinoma at one of these organ sites and their families must therefore be screened for other endocrine abnormalities.

ENDOCRINE PANCREAS

The endocrine pancreas consists of the **islets of Langerhans**. These are composite fabrication sites composed of different cells that produce and secrete several hormones.

The greatest proportion (60-70%) are insulin-producing β cells; α cells (15–20%) produce the "insulin antagonist" glucagon. There are several clones of δ cells (e.g., D cells, D1 cells) which secrete somatostatin or vasoactive intestinal polypeptide (VIP) as well as cells that produce substance P, human pancreatic polypeptide, or gastrin (G cells). Consequently, pancreatic endocrine adenomas or carcinomas (e.g., gastrinoma, vasoactive intestinal polypeptide–secreting tumor [VIPoma], somatostatinoma, and others) can affect multiple endocrine activities. This chapter focuses only on the more common types of hyperinsulinism and hypoinsulinism (**diabetes mellitus**).

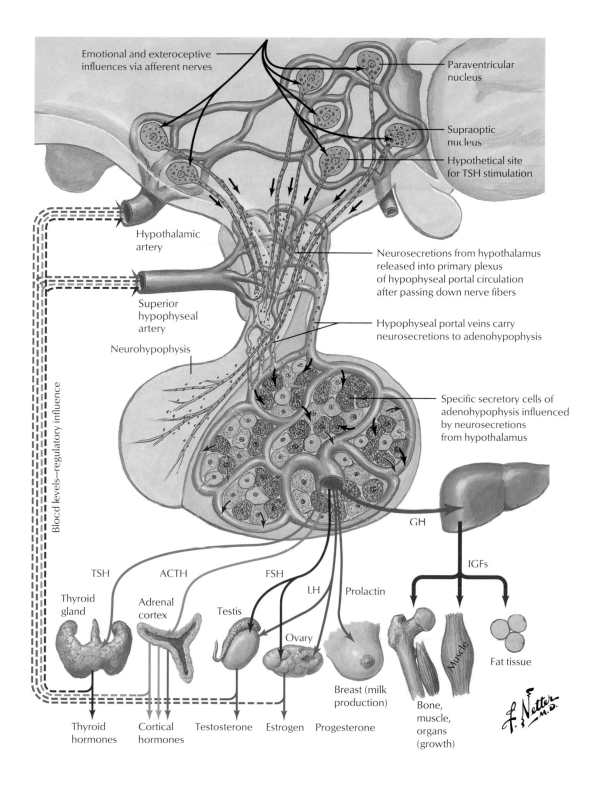

Emotional and exteroceptive influences via afferent nerves

Paraventricular nucleus

Supraoptic nucleus

Hypothetical site for TSH stimulation

Hypothalamic artery

Neurosecretions from hypothalamus released into primary plexus of hypophyseal portal circulation after passing down nerve fibers

Superior hypophyseal artery

Hypophyseal portal veins carry neurosecretions to adenohypophysis

Neurohypophysis

Specific secretory cells of adenohypophysis influenced by neurosecretions from hypothalamus

Blood levels—regulatory influence

GH

IGFs

TSH

ACTH

FSH

LH

Prolactin

Thyroid gland

Adrenal cortex

Testis

Ovary

Breast (milk production)

Bone, muscle, organs (growth)

Muscle

Fat tissue

Thyroid hormones

Cortical hormones

Testosterone

Estrogen

Progesterone

F. Netter M.D.

FIGURE 12-1   ENDOCRINE FUNCTION I

Endocrine function is supervised by the nervous system, especially the hypothalamus. Several nuclei of the hypothalamus secrete hypothalamic hormones that stimulate peripheral endocrine tissues via the pituitary (**hypophysis**). These hormones include **corticotropin-releasing hormone** (CRH), **thyrotropin-releasing hormone** (TRH), **luteinizing hormone-releasing** **hormone** (LHRH), and **growth hormone-releasing hormone** (GHRH). In addition, there are several direct- and indirect-acting hypothalamic hormones, including **arginine vasopressin** (AVP), somatostatin, and dopamine. Hypothalamic function responds to extraneous physical and emotional stimuli as well as to internal feedback control.

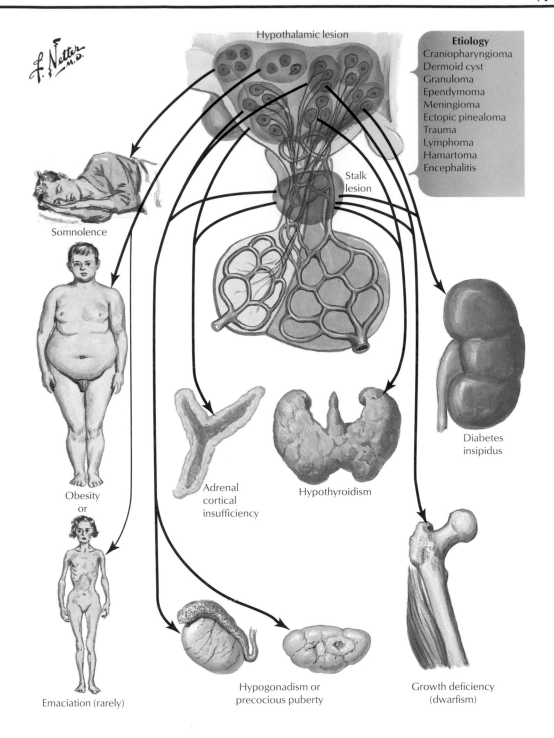

Somnolence

Obesity

or

Emaciation (rarely)

Hypothalamic lesion

Etiology
Craniopharyngioma
Dermoid cyst
Granuloma
Ependymoma
Meningioma
Ectopic pinealoma
Trauma
Lymphoma
Hamartoma
Encephalitis

Stalk lesion

Adrenal cortical insufficiency

Hypothyroidism

Diabetes insipidus

Hypogonadism or precocious puberty

Growth deficiency (dwarfism)

FIGURE 12-2   ENDOCRINE FUNCTION II

The pituitary gland controls the functional activity of peripheral endocrine tissues by secreting a large number of hormones, including **thyroid-stimulating hormone** (TSH), **corticotropin** (adrenocorticotropic hormone [ACTH]), **follicle-stimulating hormone** (FSH), **luteinizing hormone** (LH), **interstitial cell–stimulating hormone** (ICSH), **luteotropic hormone** or **prolactin** (LTH), **somatotropic hormone** (STH), and **melanocyte-stimulating hormone** (MSH). Hypothalamic damage from viral or other infections, granulomatous diseases (e.g., sarcoidosis), degenerative disorders, or tumor metastases has pathologic effects on the function of other peripheral tissues and endocrine organs. Such relations exist in obesity or **anorexia nervosa**, hypogonadism (e.g., **pubertas tarda**, sterility, amenorrhea), and certain rare polysymptomatic syndromes (**Prader-Labhart-Willi syndrome, Laurence-Moon-Bardet-Biedl syndrome**).

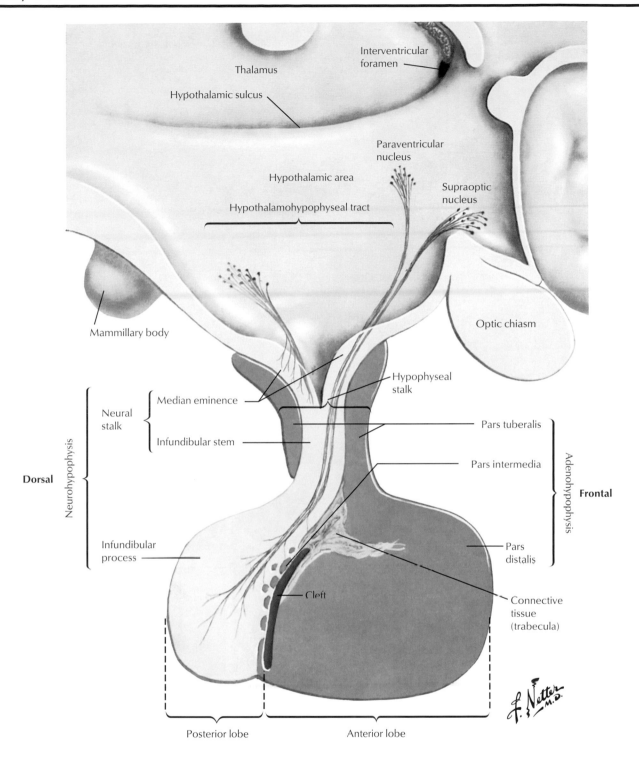

FIGURE 12-3 ANATOMY OF HYPOPHYSIS

The pituitary gland consists of an anterior lobe (**adenohypophysis**) and a posterior lobe (**neurohypophysis**), which has a stalk that connects the organ to the **infundibulum hypothalami**. The anterior lobe develops from an ectodermal outgrowth of the oral cavity, whereas the posterior lobe with the stalk represents a downward extension of the brain. The neurohypophysis (posterior lobe) serves as a reservoir for AVP (**antidiuretic hormone** [ADH])

and oxytocin, both of which are secreted from the hypothalamus by unmyelinated nerve endings. The adenohypophysis, which composes approximately 80% of the organ, is the major hormone-producing part of the pituitary gland. The epithelial cells of the adenohypophysis are classified as acidophilic, basophilic, and chromophobe cells, depending on their hormonal functions.

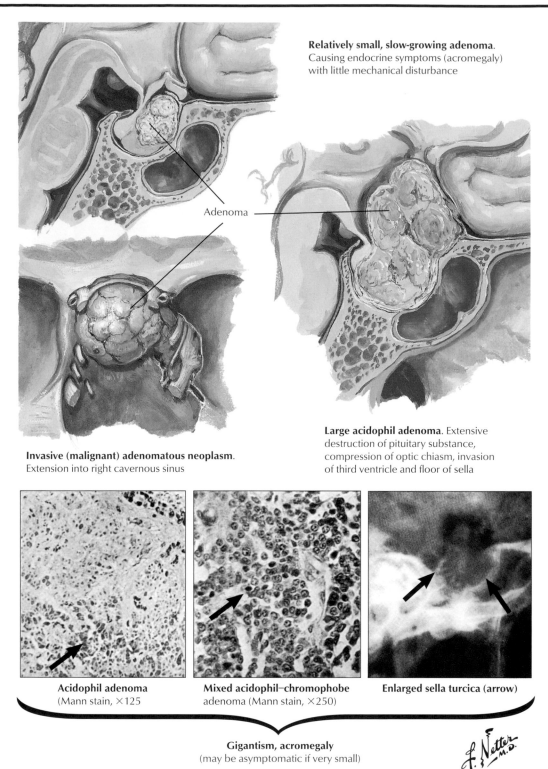

Relatively small, slow-growing adenoma. Causing endocrine symptoms (acromegaly) with little mechanical disturbance

Adenoma

Large acidophil adenoma. Extensive destruction of pituitary substance, compression of optic chiasm, invasion of third ventricle and floor of sella

Invasive (malignant) adenomatous neoplasm. Extension into right cavernous sinus

Acidophil adenoma (Mann stain, ×125

Mixed acidophil–chromophobe adenoma (Mann stain, ×250)

Enlarged sella turcica (arrow)

Gigantism, acromegaly (may be asymptomatic if very small)

FIGURE 12-4   ACIDOPHIL ADENOMA

Acidophilic or **chromophobe adenomas** may secrete excessive somatotropin (growth hormone [GH]), which produces **gigantism** in prepubertal children or **acromegaly** in postpubertal individuals. Exposure to excessive GH before epiphyseal closure leads to symmetric giant growth. After symphyseal fusion, excessive GH causes asymmetrical growth affecting the nose, the chin, the hands, and the toes. Persons with acromegaly show hyperostosis, cardiomegaly and visceromegaly, thickened skin, and other endocrine abnormalities. Clinical features include arthralgia, muscle weakness, neuropathy, and hypertension in approximately one third of patients. Patients are at high risk for cardiovascular and respiratory failure and cerebrovascular death unless the adenoma is removed by surgery or radiation.

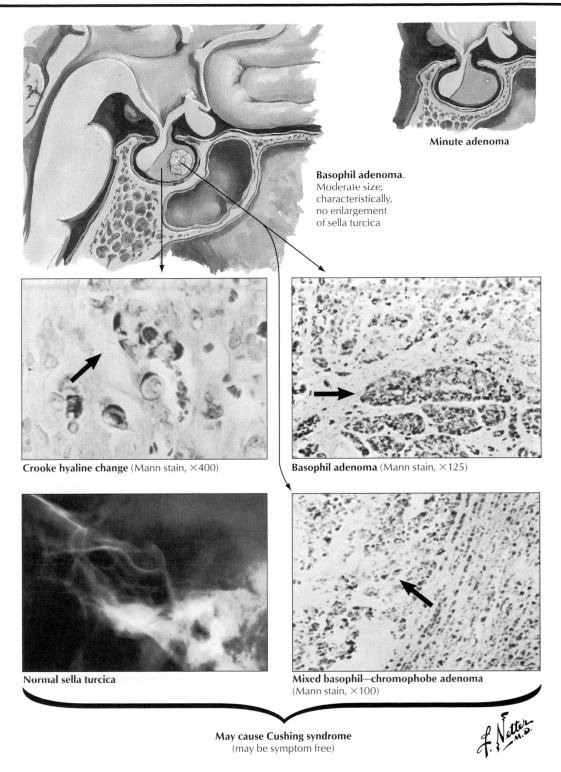

Minute adenoma

Basophil adenoma.
Moderate size;
characteristically,
no enlargement
of sella turcica

Crooke hyaline change (Mann stain, ×400)

Basophil adenoma (Mann stain, ×125)

Normal sella turcica

Mixed basophil—chromophobe adenoma
(Mann stain, ×100)

May cause Cushing syndrome
(may be symptom free)

FIGURE 12-5   BASOPHIL ADENOMA

Basophil adenomas are uncommon, usually small, and located within the normal-sized gland. They may secrete corticotropins (corticotropic adenoma) or related peptides, such as lipotropin and endorphins. **Crooke hyaline**, homogeneous hyaline globules consisting of densely packed, keratin-positive paranuclear intermediate filaments, is characteristic of basophil adenomas. Crooke hyaline is seen when Cushing disease is caused by primary adrenal tumors or in prolonged corticotropin therapy.

Clinical features of functioning corticotropic adenomas are described as **Cushing syndrome**: truncal obesity with **moon facies**, systemic hypertension, muscle weakness (decreased muscle mass), hyperglycemia, and thirst. Osteoporosis, hirsutism (male-type hair distribution in females) and amenorrhea, mood swings, and depression are also characteristic. The diagnosis is further confirmed by elevated free cortisol in the 24-hour urine.

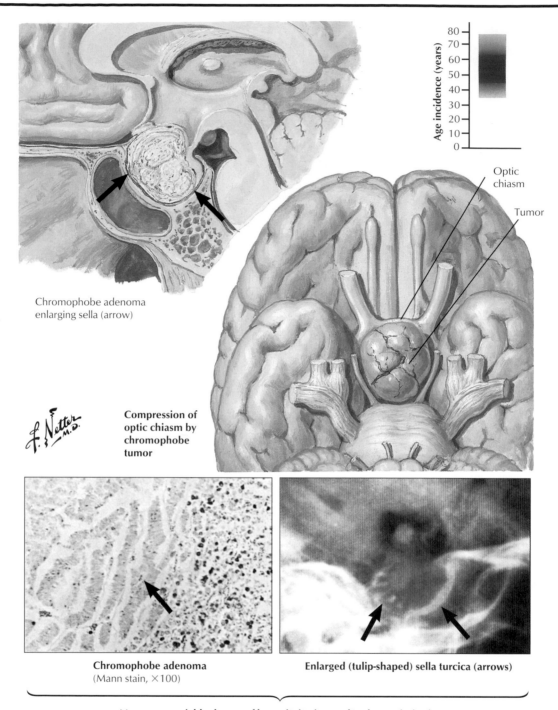

Chromophobe adenoma
enlarging sella (arrow)

Age incidence (years)

Optic
chiasm

Tumor

Compression of
optic chiasm by
chromophobe
tumor

Chromophobe adenoma
(Mann stain, ×100)

Enlarged (tulip-shaped) sella turcica (arrows)

**May cause variable degree of hypopituitarism and/or hyperpituitarism
(Cushing syndrome, acromegaly, adrenal virilism, galactorrhea)**

FIGURE 12-6   CHROMOPHOBE ADENOMA

Chromophobe adenomas, the most common pituitary tumors, constitute approximately 15% of all intracranial tumors. They occur in both sexes, usually in later life (sixth decade). Chromophobe adenomas, which may remain microscopic for long periods, most often compress the optic chiasm, causing subsequent **bitemporal hemianopsia** when they expand. Vision impairment is often the initial clinical sign. Functioning chromo-phobe adenomas produce a variety of hormones, including prolactin (lactotrophic adenomas), somatotropin (somatotropic adenomas), LH and FSH (gonadotropic adenomas), and, rarely, TSH (thyrotropic adenomas). Clinical features differ according to adenoma type with signs of hypogonadism and virilization, acromegaly, hypothyroidism, and others. Some adenomas produce more than 1 hormone including corticotropins.

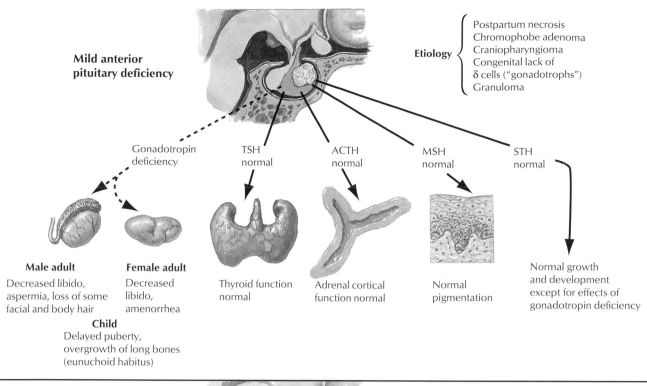

Mild anterior pituitary deficiency

Etiology
- Postpartum necrosis
- Chromophobe adenoma
- Craniopharyngioma
- Congenital lack of δ cells ("gonadotrophs")
- Granuloma

Gonadotropin deficiency

TSH normal

ACTH normal

MSH normal

STH normal

Male adult
Decreased libido, aspermia, loss of some facial and body hair

Female adult
Decreased libido, amenorrhea

Child
Delayed puberty, overgrowth of long bones (eunuchoid habitus)

Thyroid function normal

Adrenal cortical function normal

Normal pigmentation

Normal growth and development except for effects of gonadotropin deficiency

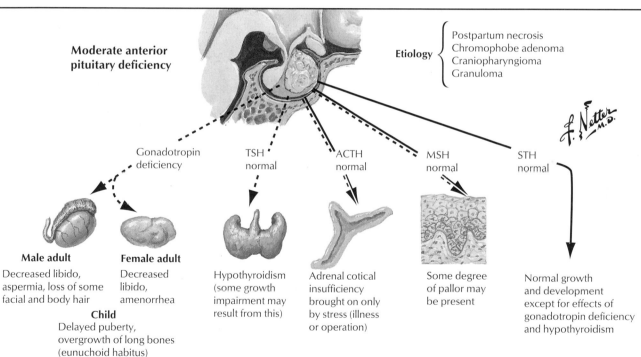

Moderate anterior pituitary deficiency

Etiology
- Postpartum necrosis
- Chromophobe adenoma
- Craniopharyngioma
- Granuloma

Gonadotropin deficiency

TSH normal

ACTH normal

MSH normal

STH normal

Male adult
Decreased libido, aspermia, loss of some facial and body hair

Female adult
Decreased libido, amenorrhea

Child
Delayed puberty, overgrowth of long bones (eunuchoid habitus)

Hypothyroidism (some growth impairment may result from this)

Adrenal cotical insufficiency brought on only by stress (illness or operation)

Some degree of pallor may be present

Normal growth and development except for effects of gonadotropin deficiency and hypothyroidism

FIGURE 12-7   HYPOPITUITARISM

Hypopituitarism refers to deficiencies in hormone production by the adenohypophysis (anterior lobe of pituitary) The lack of hormone affects the function of peripheral endocrine tissues. Hypopituitarism is caused by destruction of the gland by tumor metastases, local tumors extending into the **sella turcica**, infiltrative processes such as infections (e.g., tuberculosis), metabolic disorders (e.g., **hemochromatosis, Hand-Schüller-** **Christian disease**), ischemic postpartum necrosis (**Sheehan syndrome**), hemorrhagic infarction (pituitary **apoplexy**), or, rarely, hypophyseal atrophy secondary to subarachnoid space herniation (**empty sella syndrome**). Symptoms develop slowly and occur when approximately 75% of the adenohypophysis is lost. Hormone replacement is the therapy of choice. The underlying disease causing the hypopituitarism determines the prognosis.

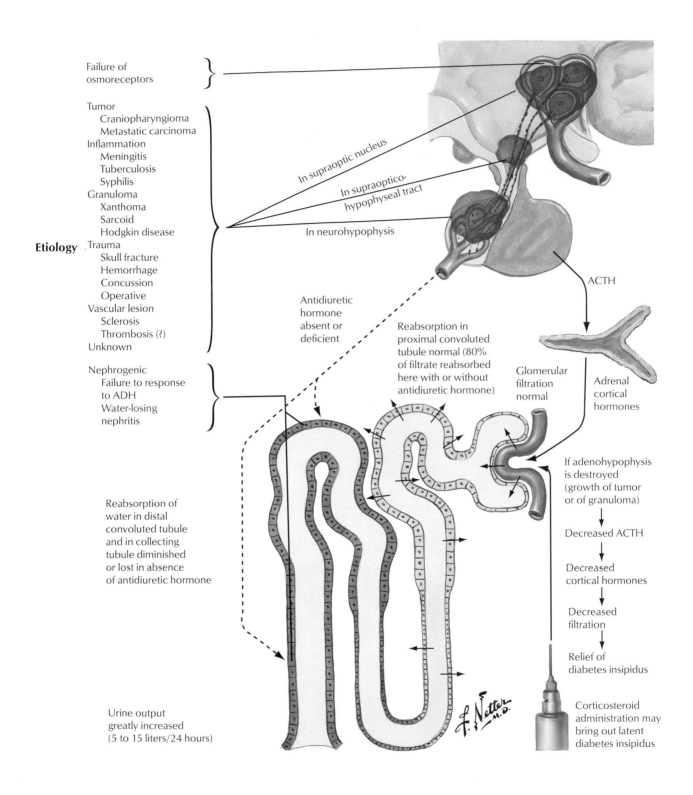

Etiology

Failure of osmoreceptors

Tumor
  Craniopharyngioma
  Metastatic carcinoma
Inflammation
  Meningitis
  Tuberculosis
  Syphilis
Granuloma
  Xanthoma
  Sarcoid
  Hodgkin disease
Trauma
  Skull fracture
  Hemorrhage
  Concussion
  Operative
Vascular lesion
  Sclerosis
  Thrombosis (?)
Unknown

Nephrogenic
  Failure to response
  to ADH
  Water-losing
  nephritis

In supraoptic nucleus

In supraoptico-hypophyseal tract

In neurohypophysis

ACTH

Antidiuretic hormone absent or deficient

Reabsorption in proximal convoluted tubule normal (80% of filtrate reabsorbed here with or without antidiuretic hormone)

Glomerular filtration normal

Adrenal cortical hormones

If adenohypophysis is destroyed (growth of tumor or of granuloma)

Decreased ACTH

Decreased cortical hormones

Decreased filtration

Relief of diabetes insipidus

Reabsorption of water in distal convoluted tubule and in collecting tubule diminished or lost in absence of antidiuretic hormone

Urine output greatly increased (5 to 15 liters/24 hours)

Corticosteroid administration may bring out latent diabetes insipidus

FIGURE 12-8   DIABETES INSIPIDUS

Deficient hormone release by the neurohypophysis (posterior lobe of pituitary) results in inadequate ADH availability. Diabetes insipidus, characterized by uncontrolled water diuresis, **polyuria**, and **polydipsia** (excessive thirst), ensues. Although patients consume large amounts of water daily, they may experience life-threatening dehydration. Diabetes insipidus is caused by a variety of processes (head trauma, infection, neoplasm), but many cases develop without recognizable underlying disease. **Craniopharyngioma**, a **dysontogenetic tumor** derived from displaced epithelium of the **Rathke pouch**, is one of the more common tumors that compresses and destroys the neurohypophysis.

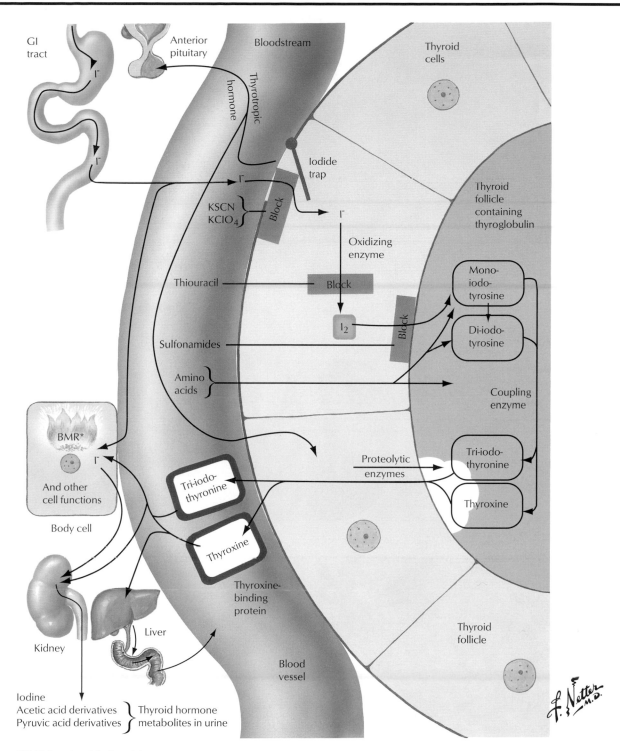

GI tract

Anterior pituitary

Bloodstream

Thyroid cells

Thyrotropic hormone

Iodide trap

Thyroid follicle containing thyroglobulin

KSCN
KClO₄ — Block

Oxidizing enzyme

Thiouracil — Block

Mono-iodo-tyrosine

Di-iodo-tyrosine

Sulfonamides

Amino acids

Coupling enzyme

BMR*

And other cell functions

Body cell

Proteolytic enzymes

Tri-iodo-thyronine

Thyroxine

Tri-iodo-thyronine

Thyroxine

Thyroxine-binding protein

Kidney

Liver

Blood vessel

Thyroid follicle

Iodine
Acetic acid derivatives
Pyruvic acid derivatives
} Thyroid hormone metabolites in urine

*BMR (basal metabolic rate)

FIGURE 12-9   PHYSIOLOGY OF THYROID HORMONES

In the thyroid follicular epithelial cells, iodide, which is absorbed in the gastrointestinal (GI) tract, is oxidized to I_2, which serves for the stepwise iodination of tyrosine. The combination of 2 molecules of diiodotyrosine produces T4 (L-thyroxin). The coupling of 1 molecule of monoiodotyrosine to 1 molecule of diiodotyrosine results in T3. T4 and T3 are the main thyroid hormones. They are coupled to thyroglobulin and are stored in follicular colloids. Proteolytic enzymes release T4 and T3 into the circulation as active hormones when stimulated. **Proteolysis**, the follicular epithelial resorption and release of the hormone by these cells, is accompanied morphologically by such signs of follicular activation as paraepithelial resorptive vacuoles in the colloid and epithelial swelling (cuboidal size) and proliferation (focal stratification to form **Sanderson cushions** and papillae). Various steps in iodine/hormone metabolism can be blocked by chemicals, which thus can be used to treat thyroid functional aberrations.

Thyroid Pathology in Hyperthyroidism With Diffuse Goiter
(Graves Disease)

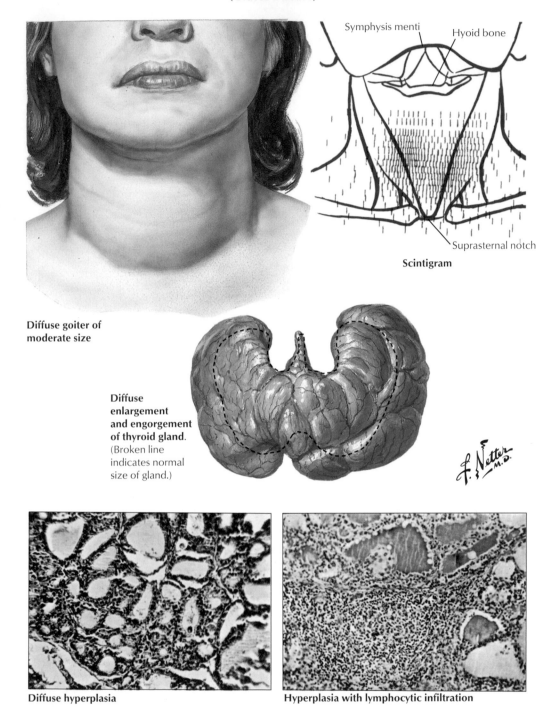

Symphysis menti

Hyoid bone

Suprasternal notch

Scintigram

Diffuse goiter of moderate size

Diffuse enlargement and engorgement of thyroid gland. (Broken line indicates normal size of gland.)

Diffuse hyperplasia

Hyperplasia with lymphocytic infiltration

FIGURE 12-10   HYPERTHYROIDISM

Hyperthyroidism is associated pathologically with diffuse or nodular goiter, **Graves disease (morbus Basedow)**, thyroid adenoma and carcinomas, and certain forms of early thyroiditis. The etiology of Graves disease, the most common cause of hyperthyroidism, remains obscure. The diagnosis is confirmed by scintigraphic demonstration of increased T4, T3 uptake in the thyroid gland. Autoantibodies against follicular epithelial membranes, which may bind to the TSH receptor and thus contribute to thyroid stimulation, are frequently observed. The thyroid, which is grossly enlarged, firm, and red (**struma parenchymatosa**), shows histologically diffuse follicular activation and hyperplasia with resorption of colloid and eventual lymphocytic infiltration. The clinical course is variable, with exacerbations, remissions, and final hypothyroidism after secondary chronic nonspecific thyroiditis.

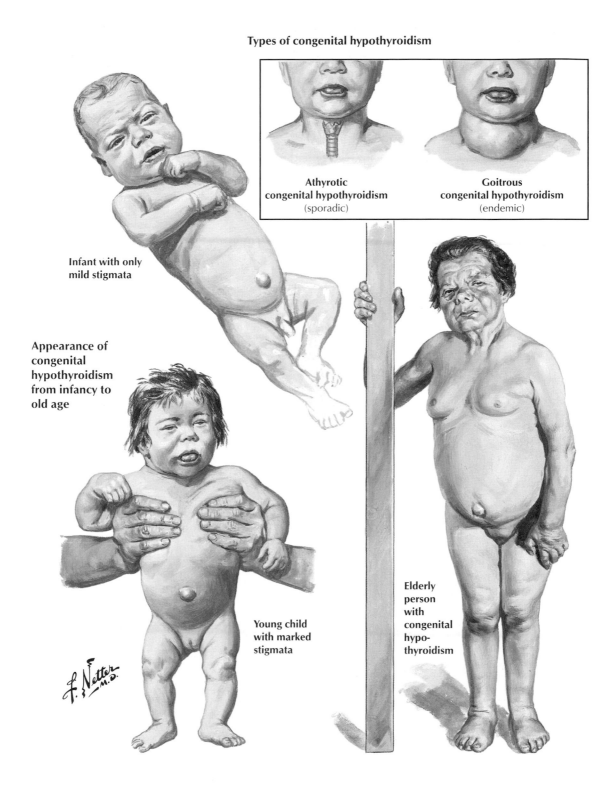

Types of congenital hypothyroidism

**Athyrotic
congenital hypothyroidism**
(sporadic)

**Goitrous
congenital hypothyroidism**
(endemic)

Infant with only
mild stigmata

Appearance of
congenital
hypothyroidism
from infancy to
old age

Young child
with marked
stigmata

Elderly
person
with
congenital
hypo-
thyroidism

FIGURE 12-11　CONGENITAL HYPOTHYROIDISM AND MYXEDEMA

Hypothyroidism is characterized by a reduction of the physiologic thyroid function with respectively reduced thyroid hormone excretion. **Congenital hypothyroidism** is related to developmental defects and may occur endemically. In addition, there exists a sporadic, intrauterine post–inflammatory or post–

toxic hypothyroidism with unresponsiveness of the thyroid gland to TSH stimuli and deficient thyroid hormone synthesis. Patients are of short stature, with thick yellowish skin and a characteristic facial expression. Eyelids are puffy, the nose is flat and thick, and the tongue is enlarged and protruding. The neck is short and

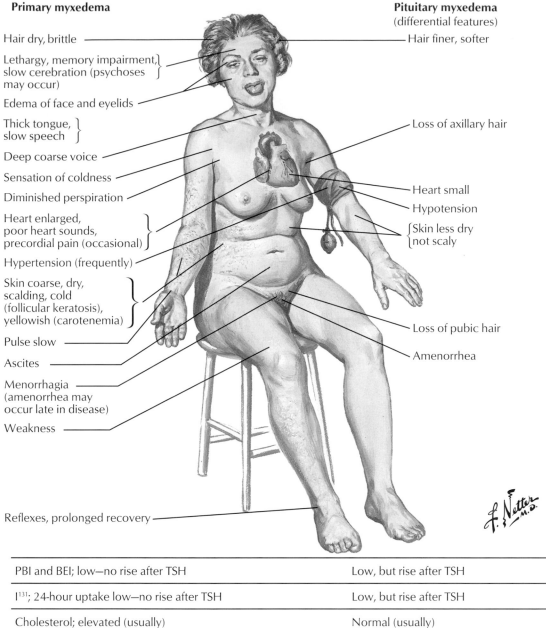

Primary myxedema

Hair dry, brittle

Lethargy, memory impairment, slow cerebration (psychoses may occur)

Edema of face and eyelids

Thick tongue, slow speech

Deep coarse voice

Sensation of coldness

Diminished perspiration

Heart enlarged, poor heart sounds, precordial pain (occasional)

Hypertension (frequently)

Skin coarse, dry, scalding, cold (follicular keratosis), yellowish (carotenemia)

Pulse slow

Ascites

Menorrhagia (amenorrhea may occur late in disease)

Weakness

Reflexes, prolonged recovery

Pituitary myxedema (differential features)

Hair finer, softer

Loss of axillary hair

Heart small

Hypotension

Skin less dry not scaly

Loss of pubic hair

Amenorrhea

PBI and BEI; low—no rise after TSH	Low, but rise after TSH
I¹³¹; 24-hour uptake low—no rise after TSH	Low, but rise after TSH
Cholesterol; elevated (usually)	Normal (usually)
Uric acid; elevated in males and postmenopausal females	Same
Urinary gonadotropins; positive	Absent
17-Ketosteroids; low	Lower
BMR; usually low, but very variable	Same

BMI, basal metabolic rate; BEI, butanol-extractable iodine; PBI, protein-bound iodine; TSH, thyroid-stimulating hormone.

FIGURE 12-11 CONGENITAL HYPOTHYROIDISM AND MYXEDEMA (CONTINUED)

thick. Adult hypothyroidism manifests as myxedema. Patients experience tiredness and lethargy. Their hair is dry and brittle, their skin is thickened (myxedema), and the face resembles to a certain extent that in cretinism. The heart rate is usually de-creased, and some patients have psychotic crises (**myxedema madness**). Laboratory tests show a decrease of T4 levels in the blood, whereas TSH is significantly increased.

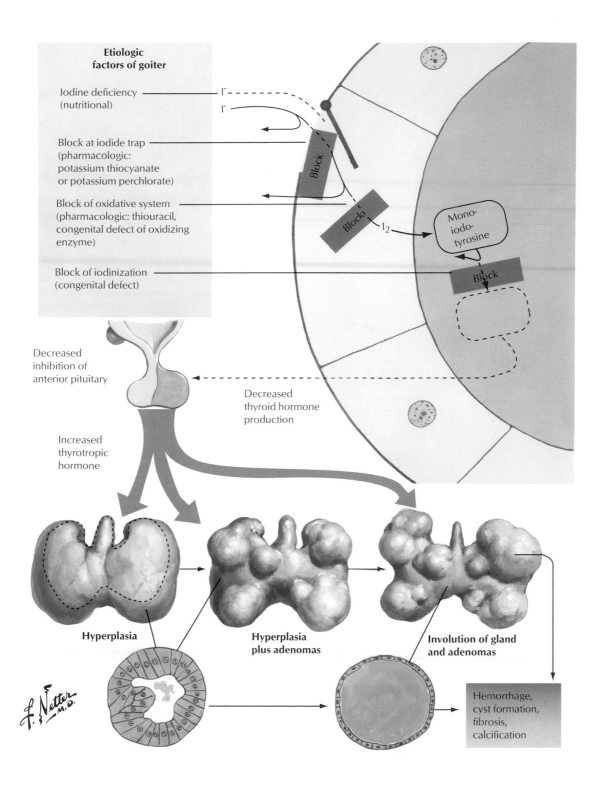

Etiologic factors of goiter

Iodine deficiency (nutritional)

Block at iodide trap (pharmacologic: potassium thiocyanate or potassium perchlorate)

Block of oxidative system (pharmacologic: thiouracil, congenital defect of oxidizing enzyme)

Block of iodinization (congenital defect)

Mono-iodo-tyrosine

I_2

Block

Decreased inhibition of anterior pituitary

Decreased thyroid hormone production

Increased thyrotropic hormone

Hyperplasia

Hyperplasia plus adenomas

Involution of gland and adenomas

Hemorrhage, cyst formation, fibrosis, calcification

FIGURE 12-12　GOITER

Goiter (**struma**) refers to an enlargement (usually nodular) of the thyroid related to either hyperthyroidism or hypothyroidism. **Goiter in combination with hyperthyroidism**, as is seen in Plummer syndrome (toxic goiter), is usually autonomous but not cancerous. Goiter can be caused by low dietary intake of iodine but is usually caused by increased levels of TSH in response to a defect in hormone synthesis in the thyroid gland. Patients with goiter usually remain asymptomatic except for progressive swelling of the neck with potential airway obstruction and dysphagia or compression of the recurrent nerve with hoarseness. Microscopically, there is diffuse or nodular crowding of enlarged follicles. In time, regressive changes with chronic reactive inflammation and fibrosis develop. Focal intrafollicular hemorrhage and siderosis and follicle rupture with signs of colloid resorption and foreign body granulomatous reaction may occur.

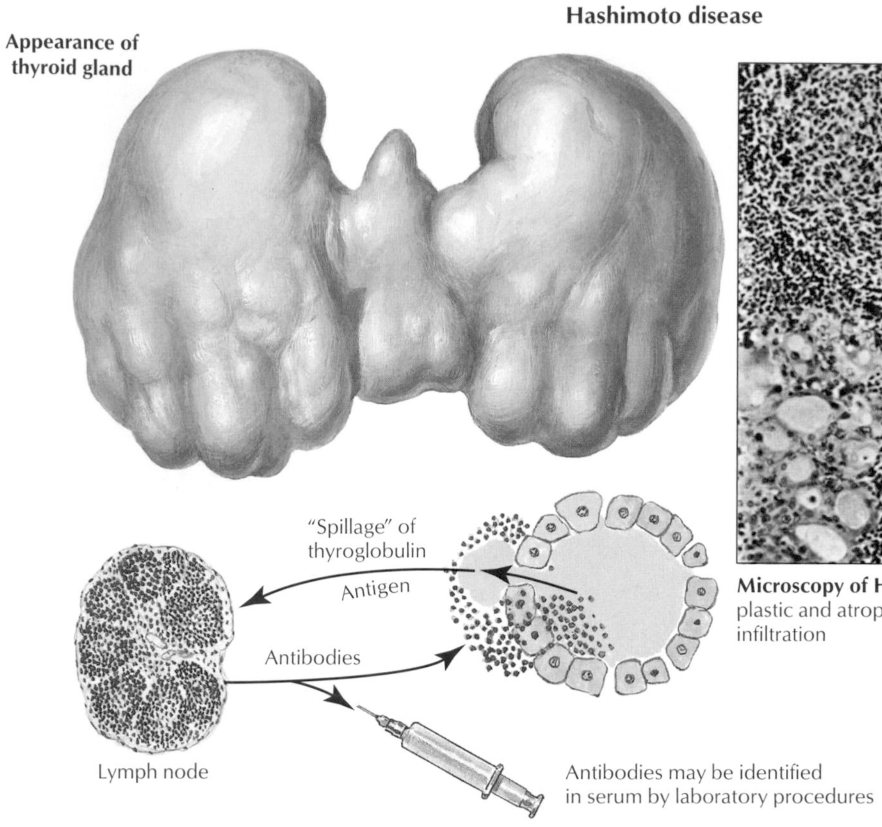

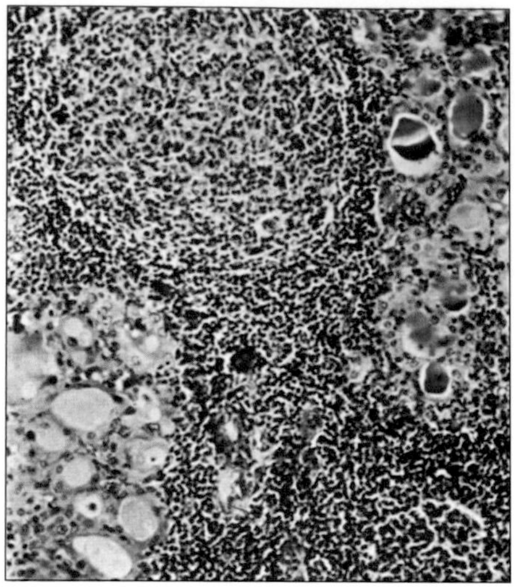

Hashimoto disease

Appearance of thyroid gland

Microscopy of Hashimoto. Mixture of hyperplastic and atrophic follicles with lymphotollicular infiltration

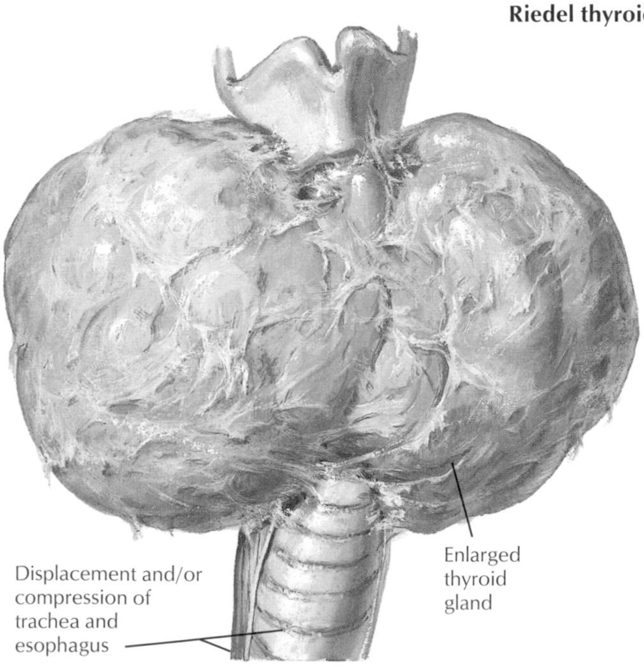

"Spillage" of thyroglobulin

Antigen

Antibodies

Lymph node

Antibodies may be identified in serum by laboratory procedures

Riedel thyroiditis

Displacement and/or compression of trachea and esophagus

Enlarged thyroid gland

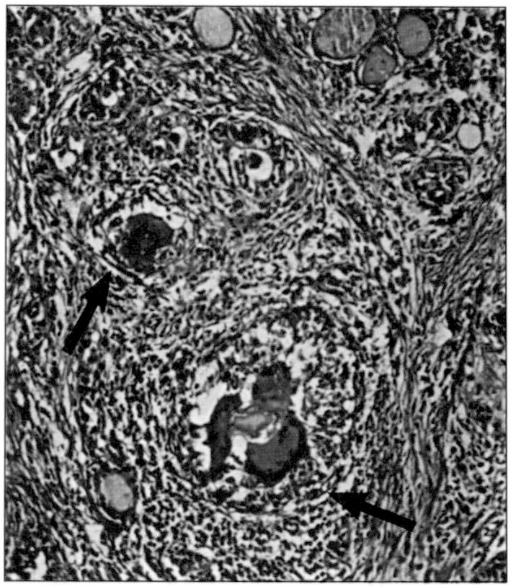

Microscopy of Riedel struma. Lymphocytic and infiltration with atrophy of follicles (arrows) and fibrosis

FIGURE 12-13   THYROIDITIS

There are several forms of primary **thyroiditis** (Table 12-1). The thyroid gland is usually enlarged (except in **Riedel thyroiditis**, in which the gland is small to undetectable) and tender with radiating pain. Regional lymph nodes are enlarged, suggesting an inflammatory disease. Patients may be euthyroid with eventual hyperthyroidism related to follicle destruction (**hashitoxicosis** in **Hashimoto disease**) but eventually have hypothyroidism. Thyroid autoantibodies and cytotoxic T lymphocytes often can be shown.

TABLE 12-1   PRIMARY INFLAMMATION OF THE THYROID GLAND (THYROIDITIS)

Entity	Pathology	Pathogenesis
Lymphofollicular thyroiditis (Hashimoto thyroiditis), chronic	Lymphocytic/plasmacellular infiltrate with lymph follicles, follicle destruction, oxyphilic metaplasia of follicle cells (Hürthle or Askanazy cells)	T-cell autoimmune reaction (TPO, TMA), genetic predisposition
Granulomatous thyroiditis (de Quervain thyroiditis), subacute	Microfocal neutrophilic infiltrates, follicle destruction with secondary giant cell granulomatous reaction, marked lymphoplasmacellular infiltrates	E.g., virus infection: coxsackie, adenovirus, mumps, and others, secondarily autoimmune
Chronic sclerosing thyroiditis (Riedel thyroiditis)	Lymphocytic thyroiditis with progressive glandular atrophy and fibrosis extending to adjacent tissues	Suggestively autoimmune*
Painless subacute thyroiditis	Lymphocytic infiltrates with eventual follicular destruction, usually self-limited, hyperthyroid	Unknown HLA-DR3 associated

TMA indicates thyroid microsomal antigen; TPO, thyroid peroxidase antigen.
*Associated with primary sclerosing cholangitis

FIGURE 12-13   THYROIDITIS (CONTINUED)

Some cases of autoimmune thyroiditis are part of systemic autoimmune disorders such as collagen-vascular diseases. Consequently, careful examination of the patient with primary thyroiditis is recommended. The nature of the autoimmune process usually determines the prognosis of the thyroiditis.

Papillary carcinoma

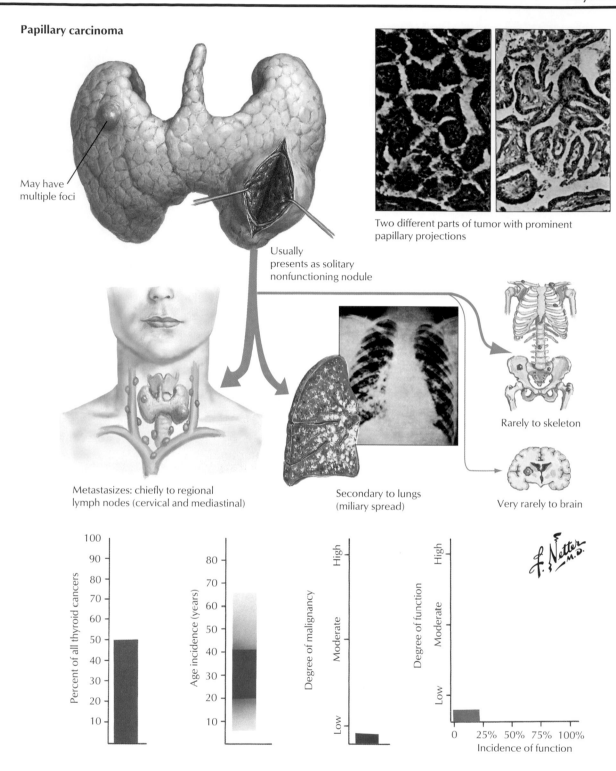

May have multiple foci

Usually presents as solitary nonfunctioning nodule

Two different parts of tumor with prominent papillary projections

Metastasizes: chiefly to regional lymph nodes (cervical and mediastinal)

Secondary to lungs (miliary spread)

Rarely to skeleton

Very rarely to brain

Percent of all thyroid cancers

Age incidence (years)

Degree of malignancy

Degree of function

Incidence of function

FIGURE 12-14 THYROID ADENOMAS AND CARCINOMA

Autonomous proliferative diseases of the thyroid consist of adenomas (benign) and carcinomas (malignant), either of which may be hormone-producing tumors. Adenomas (usually autonomous nodules in a nodular goiter) show signs of hyperthyroidism, tachycardia, shortness of breath, nervousness, weight loss, and emotional instability, although they are usually less pronounced than in Graves disease. Iodine uptake is increased in the ad-

enoma (scintigram), and blood iodine is moderately increased (protein-bound as well as butanol-extractable forms). Certain forms of adenoma are difficult to distinguish from well-differentiated follicular carcinoma (**atypical adenoma** with cellular atypia, mitoses, or even vascular invasion); therefore, adenomas should be removed and studied histologically (see also Table 12-3).

TABLE 12-2   TYPES OF THYROID CARCINOMA

Carcinoma	Frequency*	Pathology and Spread	Prognosis[†]
Papillary carcinoma	Approximately 80%	Solitary or multifocal lesions with papillary structures and **ground glass** "empty" nuclei; preferentially lymphatic spread	10-year survival 90% (in younger persons)
Follicular carcinoma	Approximately 15%	Infiltrative follicular structures without ground glass nuclei; preferentially hematogenous spread	10-year survival 85% (early cancer); 45% in invasive form
Medullary carcinoma originate from C cells	Up to 5%	Solitary or multifocal lesions with pale round or spindle cells and stromal amyloid deposits; hematogenous and lymphatic spread	5-year survival <10%
Anaplastic carcinoma	Rare	Highly anaplastic pleomorphic with giant cells or spindle cells, sarcomatous appearance; rapid hematogenous metastases	5-year survival <10%

*Percentage of all thyroid carcinomas.
[†]Prognosis under optimal conditions of early detection.

FIGURE 12-14   THYROID ADENOMAS AND CARCINOMA (CONTINUED)

The 4 major types of thyroid carcinomas (Table 12-2) differ histologically, in their routes of metastasis, and in their prognosis. **Papillary**, **follicular**, and **anaplastic carcinomas** are derived from follicular epithelial cells. **Medullary carcinoma** is an endocrine tumor from calcitonin-producing interstitial C cells. This tumor may occur in combination with other related endocrine tumors forming familial MEN syndromes, such as MEN-2 with associated pheochromocytoma. The clinical features of such tumors are determined by the combination of different neoplasms. Medullary carcinoma may show symptoms of carcinoids (flushing, watery diarrhea), Cushing syndrome, hyperparathyroidism (HPPT), and episodic hypertension. The life expectancy of patients with MEN is generally shorter than that of patients with solitary medullary carcinoma.

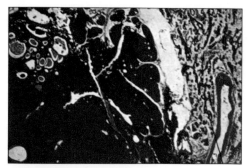

Adenoma. Rim of relatively normal parathyroid tissue about compact adenoma; H and E stain, ×11¹/₂

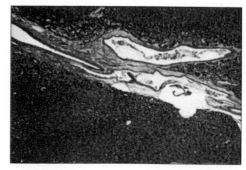

Adenoma. Mixture of oxyphil cells and chief cells in adenoma; H and E stain, ×11¹/₂

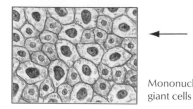

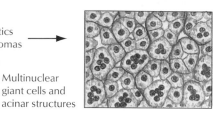

Frequent characteristics
of chief cells in adenomas

Mononuclear
giant cells

Multinuclear
giant cells and
acinar structures

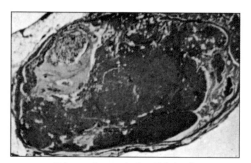

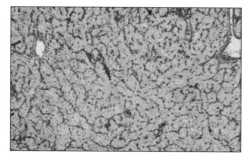

Primary hyperplasia: Chief cell

Primary hyperplasia: Clear cell

Carcinoma

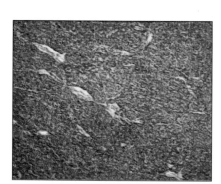

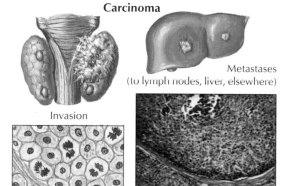

Secondary hyperplasia

Invasion

Mitosis

Metastases
(to lymph nodes, liver, elsewhere)

Fibrous bands
and hyperchromicity

FIGURE 12-15 HYPERPARATHYROIDISM

There are 2 major forms of **hyperparathyroidism** (HPPT), primary and secondary, as well as combinations of the two. Eighty-four percent of **primary HPPT** (autonomous HPPT) is caused by parathyroid adenomas, 12% is caused by hyperplasia, and 4% is caused by parathyroid carcinomas. **Secondary HPPT** follows chronic renal insufficiency (**renal rickets, renal osteodystrophy**) with hyperphosphatemia and decreased ionized serum calcium. Parathyroid glands show diffuse or nodular hyperplasia. Long-standing secondary HPPT may be complicated by development of autonomous adenomas, thus adding a form of primary HPPT. Clinical features of HPPT are variable combinations of serum hypercalcemia with calcium deposits (kidney stones, GI mucosa, blood vessels, soft tissues, etc.) and enhanced bone resorption (**osteitis cystica fibrosa, dissecting fibroosteoclasia**) (see also Table 12-3).

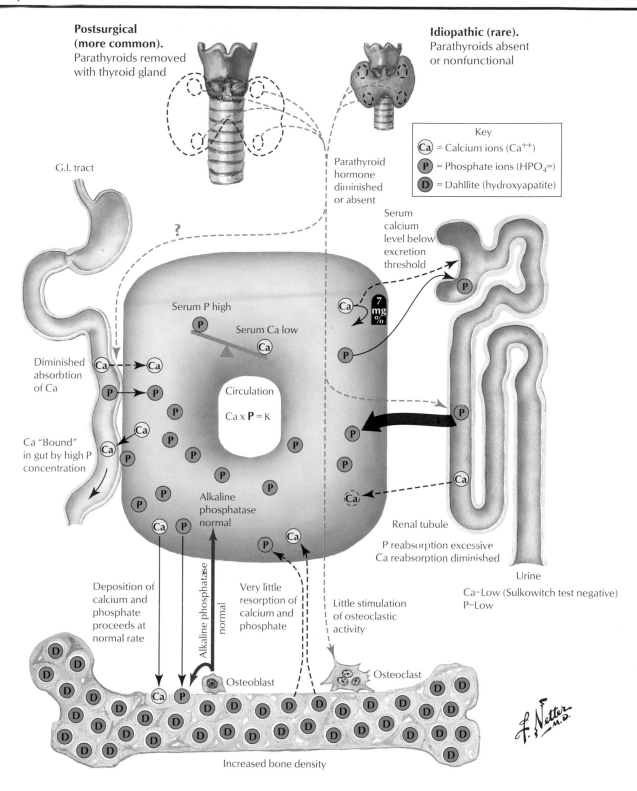

Postsurgical (more common). Parathyroids removed with thyroid gland

Idiopathic (rare). Parathyroids absent or nonfunctional

Parathyroid hormone diminished or absent

Key

Ca = Calcium ions (Ca^{++})

P = Phosphate ions ($HPO_4=$)

D = Dahllite (hydroxyapatite)

G.I. tract

Serum calcium level below excretion threshold

Serum P high

Serum Ca low

7 mg %

Diminished absorbtion of Ca

Circulation

$Ca \times P = K$

Ca "Bound" in gut by high P concentration

Alkaline phosphatase normal

Renal tubule

P reabsorption excessive
Ca reabsorption diminished

Deposition of calcium and phosphate proceeds at normal rate

Very little resorption of calcium and phosphate

Little stimulation of osteoclastic activity

Alkaline phosphatase normal

Urine

Ca–Low (Sulkowitch test negative)
P–Low

Osteoblast

Osteoclast

Increased bone density

FIGURE 12-16   HYPOPARATHYROIDISM

Hypoparathyroidism, the lack of PTH, is a rare condition that may follow surgical resection of parathyroid glands in thyroidectomy. It causes severe hypocalcemia with paresthesias, muscle spasms, and seizures. There are occasional familial autosomal recessive forms of hypothyroidism that occur as part of a multiglandular deficiency or in combination with T-cell immune deficiency (**DiGeorge syndrome**). The ionized serum calcium level provides the stimulus for PTH secretion. PTH stabilizes the serum calcium level by inhibiting renal tubular phosphate resorption and calcium/phosphate absorption in the bone. In addition, calcium absorption in the intestines may be enhanced. Calcitonin or thyrocalcitonin of thyroid interstitial C cells counteracts calcium absorption by decreasing the serum calcium level.

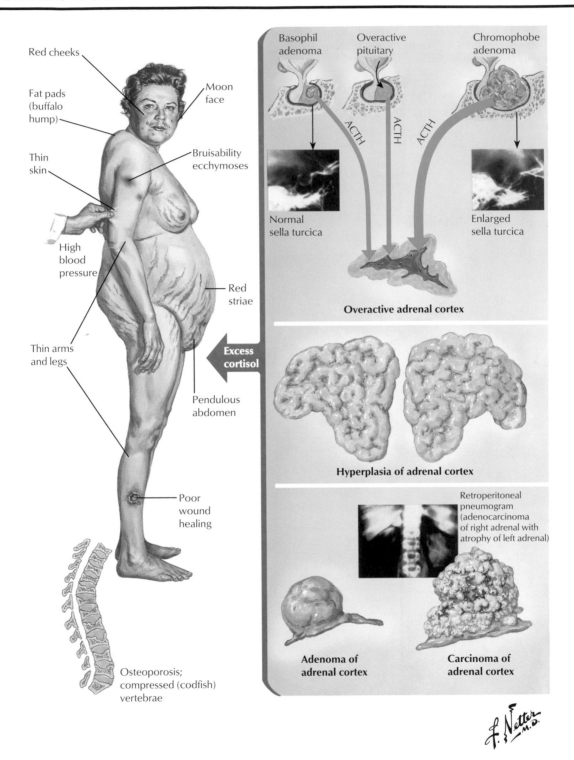

FIGURE 12-17   ADRENAL CORTEX: ANATOMY AND HYPERPLASIA

The **adrenal cortex** is composed of the **zona glomerulosa** (outer zone), the **zona fasciculata** (intermediate zone), and the **zona reticularis** (inner zone adjacent to adrenal medulla). The 2 inner zones respond to stimulation by hypophyseal corticotropin. The outer zone functions independently of corticotropin. This zone produces the hormone **aldosterone** in response to potassium and angiotensin (↑) or atrial natriuretic peptide and somatostatin (↓). The inner zones produce glucocorticoids and androgens in response to corticotropins. Increased functional activity may be caused by hyperplasia, adenoma or carcinoma, and decreased functional activity by atrophy (e.g., in malnutrition), necrosis (e.g., in septicemia, tuberculosis, viral infection), or autoimmune adrenalitis. Hyperplasia of glucocorticoid-producing parts results in **Cushing disease** as caused by excessive corticotropin stimulation. Corticotropin-independent forms of Cushing syndrome occur in autonomous cortical adenomas or carcinomas (see also Table 12-3).

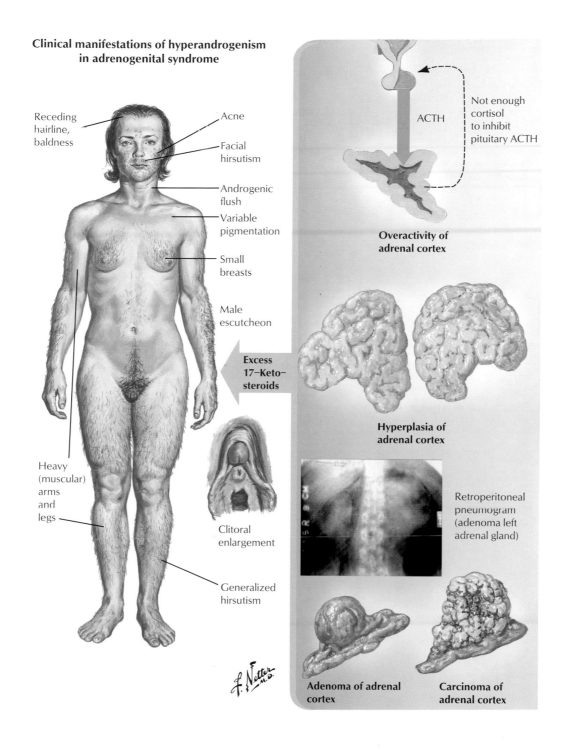

Clinical manifestations of hyperandrogenism in adrenogenital syndrome

Receding hairline, baldness

Acne

Facial hirsutism

Androgenic flush

Variable pigmentation

Small breasts

Male escutcheon

Heavy (muscular) arms and legs

Clitoral enlargement

Generalized hirsutism

Excess 17–Keto– steroids

ACTH

Not enough cortisol to inhibit pituitary ACTH

Overactivity of adrenal cortex

Hyperplasia of adrenal cortex

Retroperitoneal pneumogram (adenoma left adrenal gland)

Adenoma of adrenal cortex

Carcinoma of adrenal cortex

FIGURE 12-18   ADRENOGENITAL SYNDROME

Adrenogenital syndrome (congenital and adult forms) is caused by a form of adrenal cortical hyperplasia or tumors with excessive production of 17-ketosteroids (dehydroepiandrosterone, etiocholanolone, and androsterone). In addition to androgen abnormalities, the syndrome may be complicated by alterations in sodium metabolism, glucocorticoid deficiency, or both. Clinically, there are signs of masculinization in females (**hirsut-**ism, clitoral hypertrophy, oligomenorrhea) and precocious puberty and enlargement of genitalia in males. Some forms of congenital adrenal cortical hyperplasia occur with androgen deficiency and cause pseudohermaphroditism in males. Ninety-five percent of patients with congenital adrenal hyperplasia show defects in 21-hydroxylase, which results from mutations on chromosome 6.

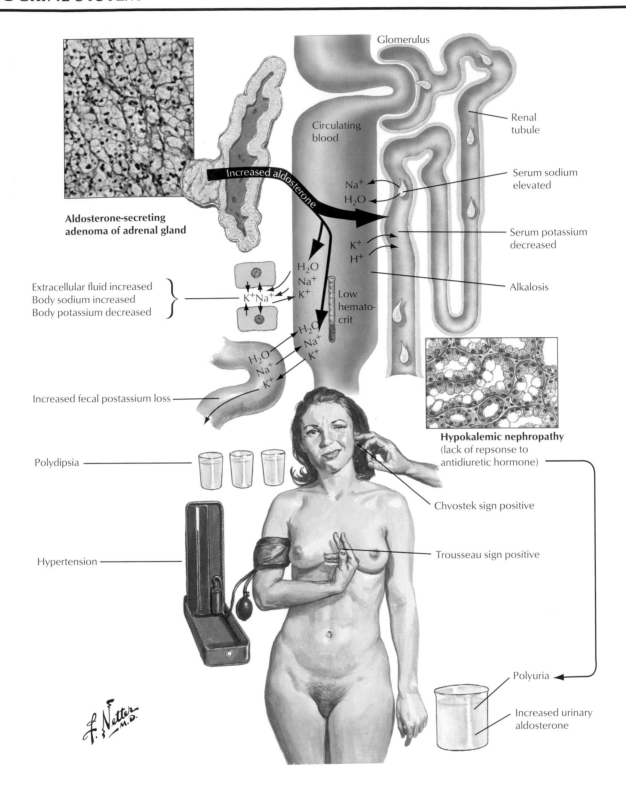

Aldosterone-secreting
adenoma of adrenal gland

Glomerulus

Renal tubule

Circulating blood

Increased aldosterone

Na^+
H_2O

Serum sodium elevated

Extracellular fluid increased
Body sodium increased
Body potassium decreased

K^+Na^+

H_2O
Na^+
K^+

K^+
H^+

Serum potassium decreased

Low hemato-crit

Alkalosis

H_2O
Na^+
K^+

Increased fecal postassium loss

Hypokalemic nephropathy
(lack of repsonse to antidiuretic hormone)

Polydipsia

Chvostek sign positive

Hypertension

Trousseau sign positive

Polyuria

Increased urinary aldosterone

FIGURE 12-19   HYPERALDOSTERONISM

Adrenal cortical adenomas that simulate structures of the zona glomerulosa cause primary **hyperaldosteronism (Conn syndrome)**. Excessive aldosterone secretion causes potassium depletion (increased potassium loss from kidneys and other exocrine glands), sodium retention, decreased plasma renin activity, and hypertension. Secondary hyperaldosteronisms in response to stimulation by the renin-angiotensin mechanisms show increased plasma renin activity. Adenomas in primary hyperaldosteronism usually remain small (less than 6 g) and can be difficult to identify clinically. Patients experience a metabolic alkalosis and muscle weakness.

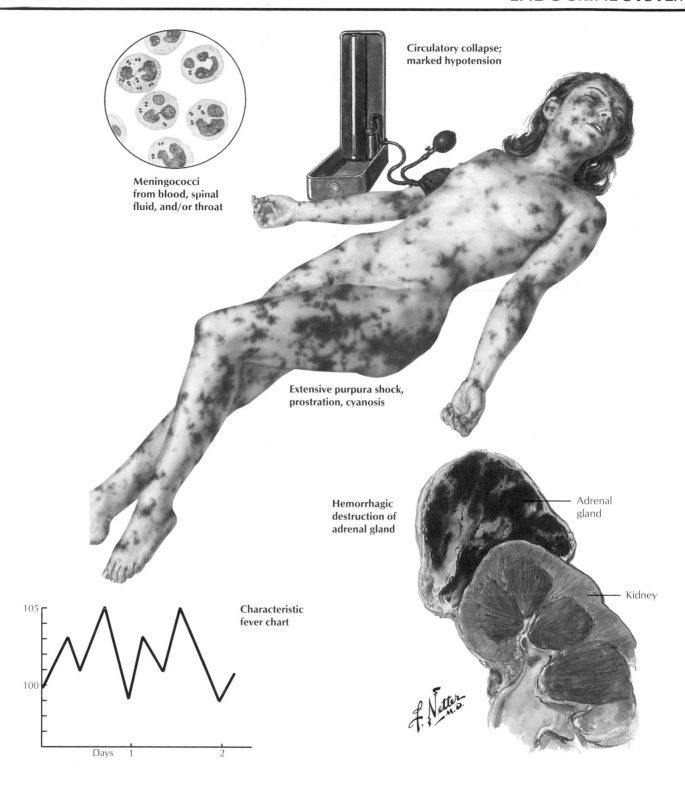

Meningococci from blood, spinal fluid, and/or throat

Circulatory collapse; marked hypotension

Extensive purpura shock, prostration, cyanosis

Hemorrhagic destruction of adrenal gland

Adrenal gland

Kidney

Characteristic fever chart

Days 1 2

FIGURE 12-20 ACUTE ADRENAL CORTICAL INSUFFICIENCY

Acute adrenal cortical insufficiency (adrenal crisis, **Waterhouse-Friderichsen syndrome**) follows the acute necrosis and hemorrhage of the adrenal cortex secondary to bacterial septicemia, usually meningococcal septicemia, and sometimes *Pseudomonas*, pneumococci, and *Haemophilus influenzae*. Bacterial toxins (endotoxins) are thought to cause diffuse vascular damage with intravascular coagulation and hemorrhage, which destroy large parts of the adrenal cortex. Other conditions that may be associated with similar adrenal hemorrhage and necrosis are birth trauma, treatment with anticoagulants, and almost all causes of disseminated intravascular coagulation (DIC). The resulting acute adrenal crisis is attributed primarily to the sudden loss of glucocorticoids.

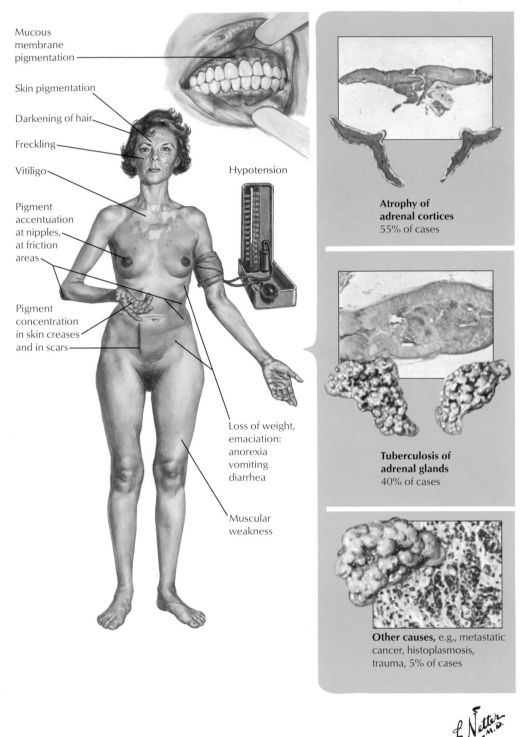

Mucous membrane pigmentation

Skin pigmentation

Darkening of hair

Freckling

Vitiligo

Pigment accentuation at nipples, at friction areas

Pigment concentration in skin creases and in scars

Hypotension

Loss of weight, emaciation: anorexia vomiting diarrhea

Muscular weakness

Atrophy of adrenal cortices
55% of cases

Tuberculosis of adrenal glands
40% of cases

Other causes, e.g., metastatic cancer, histoplasmosis, trauma, 5% of cases

FIGURE 12-21 CHRONIC ADRENAL CORTICAL INSUFFICIENCY

Chronic adrenal cortical insufficiency, **Addison disease**, is a clinical syndrome characterized by progressive weakness and fatigue, hypotension, weight loss, skin and mucosal hyperpigmentation, and abdominal problems. Laboratory test results show hyperkalemia, hyponatremia and volume depletion (decrease in mineralocorticoids such as aldosterone), and, occasionally, hypoglycemia (decrease in glucocorticoids). Patients without adequate replacement therapy die in coma. The underlying disease is a progressive shrinking (collapse) of the adrenal cortex secondary to epithelial atrophy and chronic inflammation (lymphocytic or granulomatous). In approximately two thirds of cases, autoimmune adrenalitis is responsible for these changes. Other cases are associated with infections (tuberculosis, fungal) or tumor metastases. Sarcoidosis, amyloidosis, and hemochromatosis are less frequent causes.

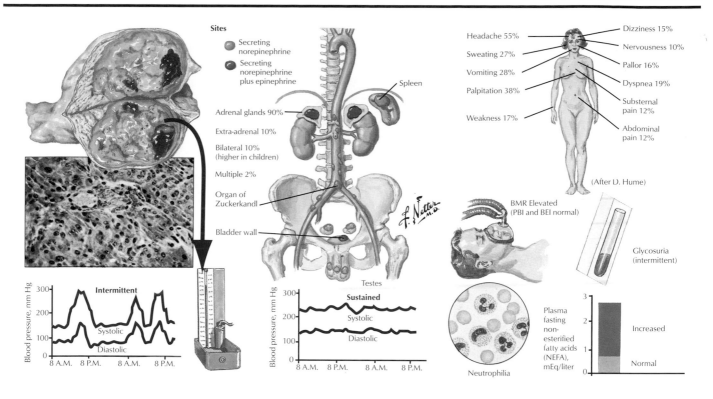

TABLE 12-3   CLASSIFICATION OF MULTIPLE ENDOCRINE NEOPLASIA

Type	Synonym	Pathology*

MEN type I	Wermer syndrome	Adenomas
		  Pituitary
		  Parathyroid
		  Pancreatic islet cells
		    (insulinomas, gastrinomas,
		    Zollinger-Ellison syndrome)
		Hyperplasia
		  Parathyroid
		  Adrenal cortex
		  Thyroid C cells
		Neoplasia
		  Pancreatic islet cell carcinoma

MEN type II (IIa)	Sipple syndrome	Hyperplasia
		  Parathyroid
		Neoplasia
		  Thyroid medullary carcinoma
		  Pheochromocytoma

MEN type III (IIb)	Mucosal neuroma syndrome	Neoplasia
		  Pheochromocytoma
		  Thyroid medullary carcinoma
		  Mucocutaneous ganglioneuroma

MEN indicates multiple endocrine neoplasia.
*With some selectivity in individual patients.

FIGURE 12-22   PHEOCHROMOCYTOMAS

The adrenal medulla consists of typical **chromaffin cells** (affinity to chromium salts with dark staining on oxidation), which produce the catecholamines **epinephrine** (80% in the adrenal medulla) and **norepinephrine**. Tumors of chromaffin, catecholamine-producing cells, include pheochromocytoma and paragangliomas. **Pheochromocytomas**, smooth yellowish-tan nodules or large hemorrhagic masses of several kilograms, may be bilateral. Nests of amphophilic chromaffin cells with a finely granular, silver-stainable cytoplasm are seen microscopically. Approximately 10% of pheochromocytomas are found in extraadrenal locations. Clinical features are headaches, intermittent hypertension, palpitation, and sweating. Approximately 10% of pheochromocytomas are part of a familial syndrome called **multiple endocrine neoplasia**, autosomal dominant diseases with mutations on chromosomes 10 and 11, such as 11q13 (MEN type I) and 10q1.2 (MEN types II and III).

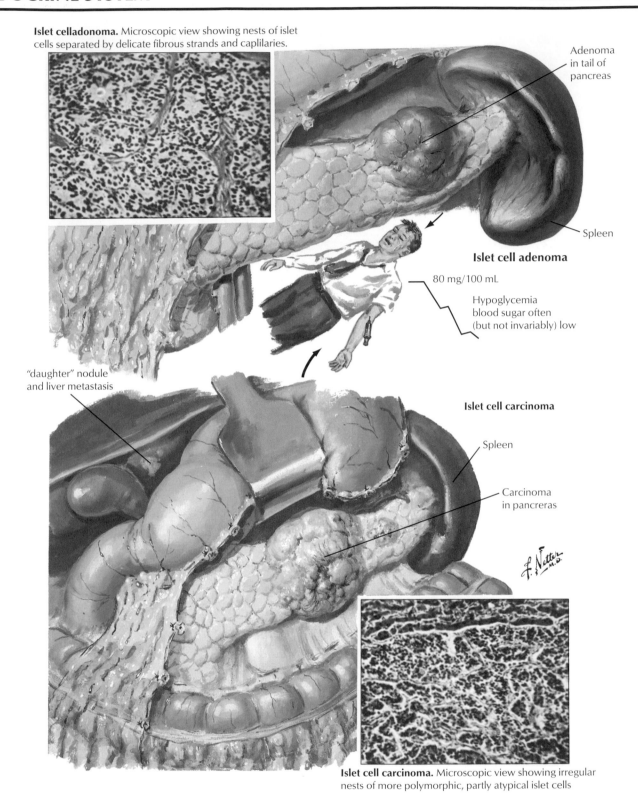

Islet celladonoma. Microscopic view showing nests of islet cells separated by delicate fibrous strands and caplilaries.

Adenoma in tail of pancreas

Spleen

Islet cell adenoma

80 mg/100 mL

Hypoglycemia blood sugar often (but not invariably) low

"daughter" nodule and liver metastasis

Islet cell carcinoma

Spleen

Carcinoma in pancreras

Islet cell carcinoma. Microscopic view showing irregular nests of more polymorphic, partly atypical islet cells

FIGURE 12-23 HYPERINSULINISM

The endocrine pancreas consists of the **islets of Langerhans**, which are composed of insulin-producing β cells (60-70%), α cells (15-20%), which produce the "insulin-antagonist" glucagon, several clones of δ cells (e.g., D cells, D1 cells), which secrete somatostatin or vasoactive intestinal peptide (VIP), and other substances. **Hyperinsulinism** caused by β-cell adenomas or carcinomas constitutes 75% of pancreatic endocrine neoplasms.

Clinical features are spontaneous hypoglycemia with hunger, tremor, perspiration, confusion, anxiety, convulsions, and coma. In **nesidioblastosis**, which occurs in rare cases of reactive hypoglycemia, pancreatic β cells are hypertrophic and increased in number. Islet cell carcinomas (10% of insulin-producing tumors) are less well demarcated, metastasize early, preferentially to the liver, and generally are associated with a poor prognosis.

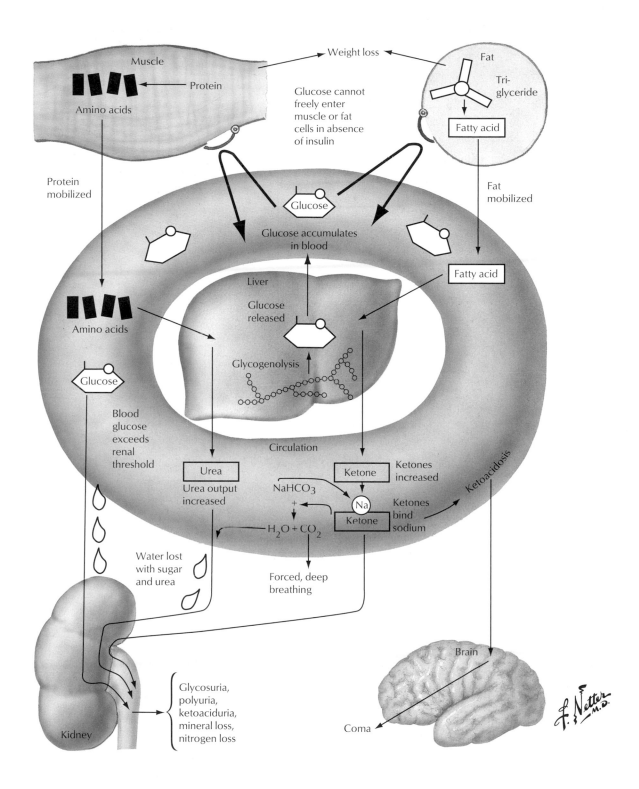

FIGURE 12-24   INSULIN-DEPENDENT DIABETES MELLITUS

Insulin-dependent diabetes mellitus (IDDM, type 1) is a complex disorder of carbohydrate, lipid, and protein metabolism caused by hypoinsulinism and multiorgan disease. In IDDM, the progressive destruction of β cells in pancreatic islets usually begins before the age of 20 years. Microscopically, pancreatic islets show scattered lymphocytic infiltration (predominance of cytotoxic CD8[+] T lymphocytes and anti–islet cell antibodies in up to 80%) with loss of β cells and mild fibrosis. Besides genetic predisposition, virus infections such as coxsackievirus are considered the initiating events for IDDM. The metabolic disturbance is characterized by hyperglycemia with mobilization of fat and protein, negative nitrogen balance, and acidosis. Polyuria leads to loss of electrolytes and dehydration, mobilization of fat and proteins, weight loss, and hunger.

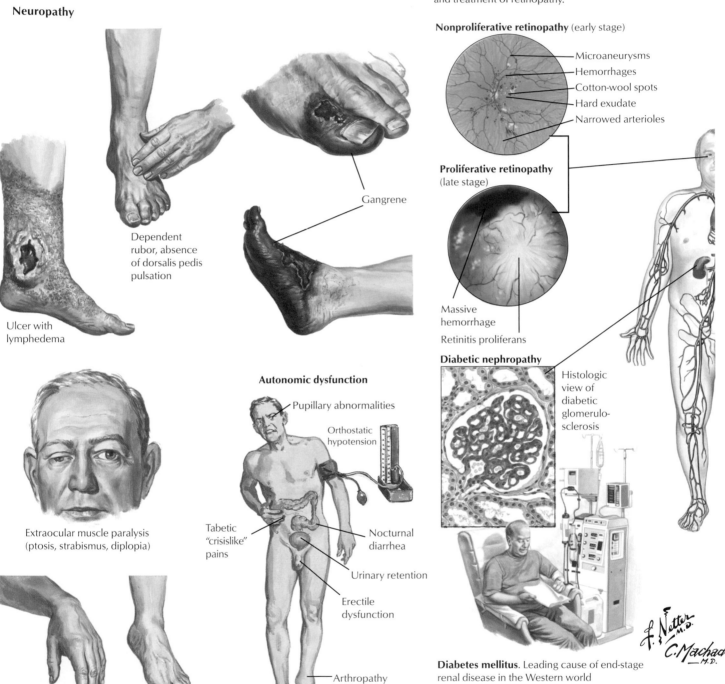

Diabetic retinopathy
Diabetic retinopathy can be easily detected during a dialated eye examination and is the leading cause of blindness among adults in the United States. Visual loss can be prevented with early recognition and treatment of retinopathy.

Nonproliferative retinopathy (early stage)
- Microaneurysms
- Hemorrhages
- Cotton-wool spots
- Hard exudate
- Narrowed arterioles

Proliferative retinopathy (late stage)
Massive hemorrhage
Retinitis proliferans

Neuropathy

Ulcer with lymphedema

Dependent rubor, absence of dorsalis pedis pulsation

Gangrene

Diabetic nephropathy
Histologic view of diabetic glomerulo-sclerosis

Extraocular muscle paralysis (ptosis, strabismus, diplopia)

Autonomic dysfunction
- Pupillary abnormalities
- Orthostatic hypotension
- Tabetic "crisislike" pains
- Nocturnal diarrhea
- Urinary retention
- Erectile dysfunction
- Arthropathy (Charcot joints)

Wrist drop   Ankle drop

Diabetes mellitus. Leading cause of end-stage renal disease in the Western world

FIGURE 12-25   NON–INSULIN-DEPENDENT DIABETES MELLITUS

Non–insulin-dependent diabetes mellitus (NIDDM, type 2), the most common form of diabetes, is characterized by an initial decreased sensitivity of peripheral tissues to insulin (insulin resistance) followed by alterations in insulin secretion by β cells. Pancreatic islets show amyloid deposits, cell atrophy, and progressive fibrosis. The incidence of NIDDM increases with obesity and the consumption of glucose (in all nutritional forms).

Metabolic disturbances, especially hyperglycemia, cause a number of complications and secondary diseases, including progressive microangiopathy with diabetic retinopathy, renal glomerular nephrosclerosis (**Kimmelstiel-Wilson disease**), peripheral neuropathy, ulcus cruris, and gangrene. Many patients have severe hypertensive cardiovascular disease, which is the leading cause of mortality in this population.

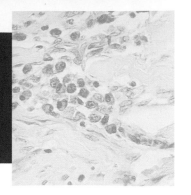

CHAPTER 13

NERVOUS SYSTEM

The **nervous system** is an exceedingly complex entity responsible for the sensory, motor, and cognitive activities of the human body. The nervous system contains groups of neurons organized anatomically and specialized functionally for specific activities. The neurons are supported by the glia—the astrocytes, oligodendroglia, microglia, and ependyma in the central nervous system and the Schwann cells in the peripheral nervous system. This chapter examines a spectrum of diseases of the nervous system and their rule in the differential diagnosis of common neurologic clinical presentations, including headache, vertigo, seizures (epilepsy), hydrocephalus, stroke, and coma.

NEUROLOGIC DISORDERS OF INFANCY AND CHILDHOOD

Many neurologic disorders of infancy and childhood result from birth trauma, prematurity predisposing to hemorrhage within the germinal matrix of the brain, and a wide spectrum of development defects involving abnormalities in the formation of the neural tube (anencephaly, encephalocele), neural proliferation and migration (microcephaly), and neural organization and myelination (porencephaly). The chronic motor dysfunction known as **cerebral palsy** often develops in surviving infants.

CEREBROVASCULAR DISEASE

Cerebrovascular disease presents as a transient ischemic attack or the more severe and persistent neurologic deficit of stroke. It stems from underlying pathology of the extracranial or intracranial cerebral vasculature. The major categories are **ischemic strokes** due to thrombosis, embolism or hypoxia, and hemorrhagic strokes due to rupture of a cerebral vessel. Global cerebral ischemia is caused by hypotension, hypoperfusion, and low flow states and results in multifocal infarcts in the border zones (watershed areas) at the interface between the perfusion zones of 2 major arteries or more diffuse encephalopathy.

Significant obstruction of a component of the carotid or vertebrobasilar arterial trunks leads to focal cerebral ischemia or infarction. *In situ* thrombosis of a cerebral artery is usually secondary to atherosclerosis or, less commonly, arteritis associated with infections or collagen-vascular diseases. Other cases of cerebral infarction are due to emboli to the cerebral vasculature from thrombi formed in a diseased heart, the aorta, or a major extracranial cerebral artery. The effects of arterial occlusion can be mitigated to a variable extent by the collateral circulation, particularly

through the circle of Willis at the base of the brain. Pale, nonhemorrhagic infarcts are produced by in situ thrombosis, whereas hemorrhagic infarcts due to influx of blood from collateral vessels are produced with cerebral emboli. The distinction between infarction due to *in situ* thrombosis versus embolization is important for optimal clinical treatment, which does not call for the use of anticoagulants in cases of hemorrhagic infarcts due to cerebral emboli.

Hypertension is the most common and important cause of primary intracerebral (intraparenchymal) hemorrhage. Other causes include vascular malformations and hematologic disorders. Hypertension produces cerebral arteriolosclerosis and Charcot-Bouchard microaneurysms. Rupture of the microaneurysm leads to hemorrhage into the brain parenchyma, with frequent extension into the ventricles and subarachnoid space. Hypertensive hemorrhages originate in the basal ganglia in approximately 75% of cases and other sites in the remainder. The most common cause of a major primary subarachnoid hemorrhage is the rupture of a saccular (or berry) aneurysm, located at bifurcation sites of the arteries of the circle of Willis.

TRAUMA

Traumatic brain injuries include concussion, contusion, skull fracture, and hemorrhage, which may be epidural, subdural, subarachnoid, or intraparenchymal. **Epidural hematoma** results from rupture of a meningeal artery and follows a hyperacute course, whereas **subdural hematoma** results from rupture of bridging veins and follows an acute or a chronic course, depending on the severity of the injury. Trauma of the spinal cord produces a variety of neurologic deficits not only from direct neurologic trauma, but also from direct and delayed damage to the vasculature, with resultant paraplegia or quadriplegia, depending on the level of injury.

BRAIN TUMORS

Tumors of the central nervous system are either primary or metastatic. The more common metastatic brain tumors may take origin from virtually any primary neoplasm, but the most frequent are lung, breast, melanoma, kidney, and colon. The primary tumors of the central nervous system are classified as gliomas and nonglial neoplasms, including neuronal tumors and meningiomas. The **gliomas** are the most common primary tumors of the brain and include astrocytomas, oligodendrogliomas, and ependymomas. In children, most brain tumors arise in the posterior fossa and include astrocytomas and medulloblastomas of the cerebellum and gliomas of the brainstem, whereas in adults, most brain tumors arise in the cerebral hemispheres. The distinction between benign and malignant lesions is blurred because of the infiltrative growth pattern, frequent involvement of vital structures, and the tendency for lower-grade lesions to transform over time to higher-grade lesions, including the glioblastoma multiforme. **Meningiomas** are typically benign tumors of adults that arise from the meningoepithelial cells of the arachnoid, become attached to the dura, and produce symptoms by compression of adjacent structures. Most tumors of peripheral nerves are derived from Schwann cells. **Acoustic neuroma** is a single lesion that produces a mass effect in the cerebellopontine angle. **Neurofibromatosis**, or **von Recklinghausen disease**, is the prototype of a group of inherited disorders known as phacomatoses, in which defects of the neural crest lead to multifocal lesions of the nervous system and the skin.

DEGENERATIVE DISEASES

Degenerative diseases are characterized by loss of neurons in various regions of the gray matter in selective patterns. These patterns characterize the various clinicopathologic conditions that have obscure etiologies. **Dementia**, or progressive loss of cognitive function, is a major manifestation of the degenerative diseases. **Alzheimer disease** is characterized by cerebral atrophy, most pronounced in the frontal, temporal, and parietal lobes and associated with the microscopic findings of neurofibrillary tangles, senile (neuritic) plaques, and amyloid angiopathy. **Huntington disease** is inherited with an autosomal dominant pattern and is characterized by dementia plus uncoordinated movements (chorea) and by atrophy of the frontal lobes and the caudate nucleus. **Creutzfeldt-Jakob disease** is characterized by spongiform degeneration of the cerebral cortex, with the pathogenesis involving mutated proteins called **prions**. **Parkinsonism**, as seen in idiopathic Parkinson disease and related conditions, is a clinical syndrome with impaired facial and voluntary muscle movements, intention tremor, rigidity, and stuttering gait. The underlying mechanism is impairment of the nigrostriatal dopaminergic system, with prominent neuronal degeneration in the substantia nigra and the locus ceruleus.

INFECTIOUS DISEASES

Infections of the central nervous system may develop as a result of seeding of microorganisms via the hematogenous route, direct implantation from trauma or medical intervention, local spread from a contiguous site such as the paranasal sinuses, or retrograde spread along a peripheral nerve, as is the case with certain viral infections such as herpes simplex and rabies. **Infectious meningitis** of the leptomeninges and the cerebrospinal fluid (CSF) presents with fever, somnolence, and stiff neck. Examination of the CSF is important to differentiate acute pyogenic bacterial meningitis (numerous white blood cells with neutrophil predominance, high protein, low glucose) from aseptic (viral) meningitis (lymphocytic pleocytosis, moderate protein increase,

normal glucose) and chronic forms of meningitis, including tuberculous meningitis (pleocytosis with mononuclear cells or mixed mononuclear cells and neutrophils, markedly increased protein level, and moderately reduced or normal glucose level). Parameningeal infections consist of brain abscess, subdural empyema, and spinal epidural abscess. Neurosyphilis occurs late in the course of approximately 10% of untreated patients and may be manifest as meningeal-meningovascular disease, dementia paralytica (general paresis), or tabes dorsalis. A number of viruses can produce encephalitis or encephalomyelitis, characterized by meningeal and parenchymal, particularly perivascular, inflammation. The viruses include arthropod-borne viruses (e.g., eastern and western equine encephalitis), herpes simplex virus (HSV) types 1 and 2, varicella-zoster virus, cytomegalovirus, poliomyelitis, rabies, human immunodeficiency virus types 1 and 2, and viruses responsible for so-called slow virus infections, including progressive multifocal leukoencephalopathy. Immunosuppressed patients are particularly susceptible to fungal infections such as *Candida albicans*, *Mucor* species, *Aspergillus fumigatus,* and *Cryptococcus neoformans* and protozoal infections such as *Toxoplasma gondii.*

DEMYELINATING DISEASES

Multiple sclerosis is a classic chronic demyelinating disease in which multiple areas of demyelination produce spatially separated plaques in the cerebral white matter that are associated with temporally separated episodes of clinical neurologic deficits. The pathogenesis involves inflammatory damage to the oligodendroglia and white matter, with altered immunity contributing to the process. The disease has a 2 : 1 female-to-male prevalence and is characterized by multiple exacerbations and remissions.

DISORDERS OF THE SPINAL CORD, NERVE ROOT, AND PLEXUS

Spinal cord dysfunction can be produced by primary or metastatic tumors in or about the cord, vascular occlusion, epidural abscess, transverse myelitis (acute demyelinating disorder), cervical or lumbar disc herniation, syringomyelia (a developmental or degenerative defect), and toxic and metabolic disorders, including subacute combined degeneration caused by vitamin B_{12} deficiency. **Amyotrophic lateral sclerosis** combines manifestations of lower motor neuron degeneration leading to muscular weakness with upper motor neuron and corticospinal tract degeneration leading to muscle spasticity.

DISORDERS OF THE MOTOR NEURON, PERIPHERAL NERVE, NEUROMUSCULAR JUNCTION, AND SKELETAL MUSCLES

Peripheral neuropathies manifest as subacute or chronic sensory and motor dysfunction resulting from metabolic, toxic, or nutritional disorders or vasculitis, particularly polyarteritis nodosa (PAN). **Guillain-Barré syndrome** is an acute, rapidly progressive, ascending paralysis due to inflammatory demyelination of peripheral nerves, with potential for reversal. **Myasthenia gravis** is manifest as muscle weakness due to autoimmune attack on acetylcholine receptors at the neuromuscular junction. **Muscular dystrophies** are a heterogeneous group of inherited diseases manifest as progressive muscle weakness and degeneration of skeletal muscle, usually with onset in childhood (e.g., Duchenne muscular dystrophy). **Polymyositis** and **dermatomyositis** are autoimmune, inflammatory disorders producing proximal muscle weakness with or without skin rash.

Inracranial Hemorrhage in Newborn

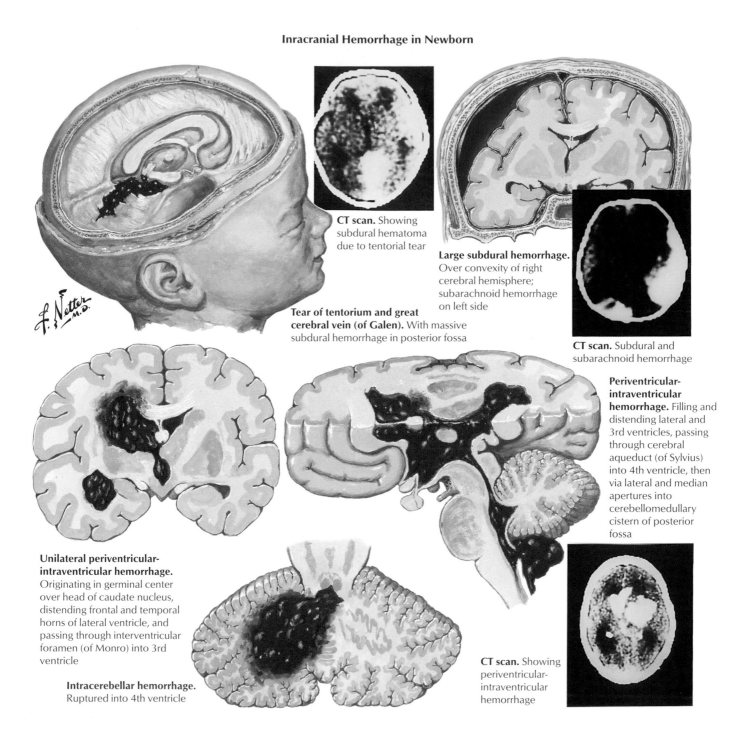

CT scan. Showing subdural hematoma due to tentorial tear

Large subdural hemorrhage. Over convexity of right cerebral hemisphere; subarachnoid hemorrhage on left side

Tear of tentorium and great cerebral vein (of Galen). With massive subdural hemorrhage in posterior fossa

CT scan. Subdural and subarachnoid hemorrhage

Periventricular-intraventricular hemorrhage. Filling and distending lateral and 3rd ventricles, passing through cerebral aqueduct (of Sylvius) into 4th ventricle, then via lateral and median apertures into cerebellomedullary cistern of posterior fossa

Unilateral periventricular-intraventricular hemorrhage. Originating in germinal center over head of caudate nucleus, distending frontal and temporal horns of lateral ventricle, and passing through interventricular foramen (of Monro) into 3rd ventricle

Intracerebellar hemorrhage. Ruptured into 4th ventricle

CT scan. Showing periventricular-intraventricular hemorrhage

FIGURE 13-1 CRANIAL HEMORRHAGE

In the newborn, certain forms of intracranial hemorrhage are usually related to birth trauma, and these include subdural hemorrhage, subarachnoid hemorrhage, and posterior fossa hemorrhage. However, other factors, particularly prematurity and asphyxia, are involved in periventricular and intraventricular hemorrhage. **Periventricular-intraventricular hemorrhage** originates in the germinal matrix and occurs with increasing frequency in relation to the degree of prematurity of the infant. Such bleeding causes a high mortality rate. Surviving infants often develop cerebral palsy.

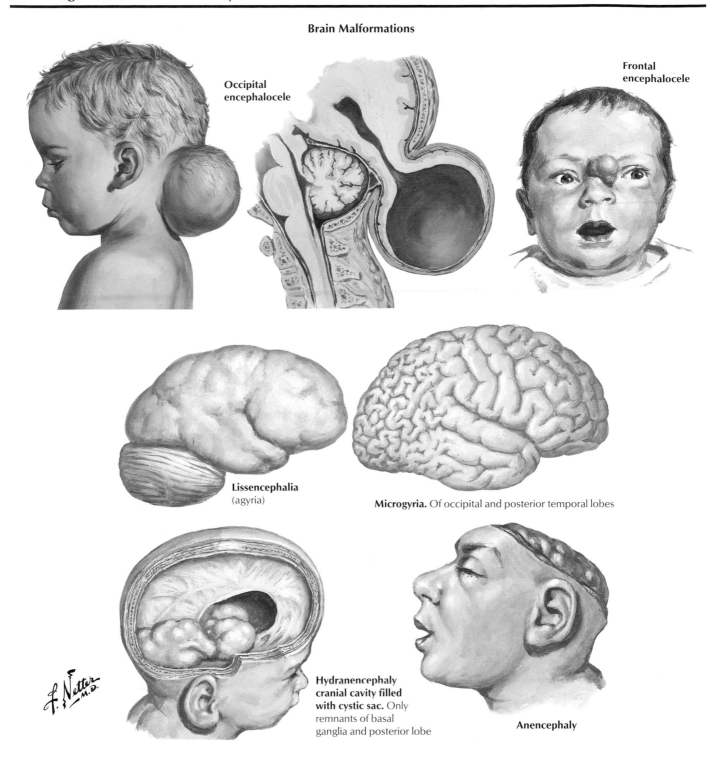

Brain Malformations

Occipital encephalocele

Frontal encephalocele

Lissencephalia (agyria)

Microgyria. Of occipital and posterior temporal lobes

Hydranencephaly cranial cavity filled with cystic sac. Only remnants of basal ganglia and posterior lobe

Anencephaly

FIGURE 13-2   BRAIN MALFORMATIONS

The time of onset of prenatal injury predicts the type of maldevelopment and resultant prenatal encephalopathy characterized by defects in the formation of the neural tube (first trimester), neural proliferation and migration (second trimester), and neural organization and myelination (third trimester). Defects in neural tube formation in the first trimester result in **anencephaly**, **encephalocele**, or **holoprosencephaly** (**arrhinencephalia**), the latter characterized by a single ventricle with defective olfactory and optic systems, and impairment of caudal closure results in meningomyelocele. During the phase of neuronal proliferation, a decrease in number of neurons leads to microcephaly, whereas an increase results in **megalencephaly**. With defective neuronal migration, gyral formation does not occur, resulting in lissencephalia (smooth brain) or other lesions, such as agenesis of the corpus callosum. Abnormalities in intrauterine cerebral blood flow, if severe, can result in the rare disorder of **hydranencephaly** and, if less severe, porencephaly characterized by cystic spaces in the brain parenchyma.

Spina bifida occulta

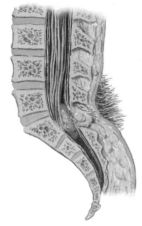

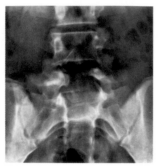

Dermal sinus

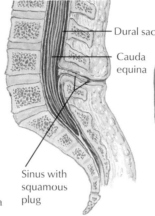

Dural sac

Cauda equina

Sinus with squamous plug

X-ray film. Showing deficit of lamina of sacrum (spina bifida occulta)

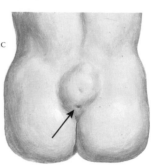

Fat pad overlying spinal bifida occulta. Tuft of hair or only skin dimple may be present, or there may be no external manifestation. Dermal sinus also present in this case (arrow).

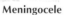

Meningocele   **Meningomyelocele**

Arnold-Chiari malformation

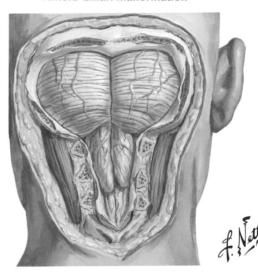

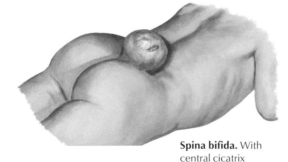

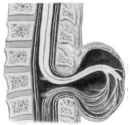

Spina bifida. With central cicatrix

FIGURE 13-3   SPINAL DYSRAPHISM

Spinal dysraphism includes several conditions characterized by congenital failure of fusion of the midline structures of the spinal column. The resultant clinical spectrum ranges from an asymptomatic bony abnormality (spina bifida occulta) to severe and disabling malformation of the spinal column and spinal cord (meningomyelocele). Lesions in the lumbosacral region and higher may produce paraplegia and loss of bowel and bladder control; hydrocephalus develops in approximately 90% of cases. The hydrocephalus is related to a congenital deformity of the hindbrain, known as the **Arnold-Chiari malformation**, in which the posterior fossa structures are downwardly displaced into the spinal canal and interfere with the circulation and absorption of CSF.

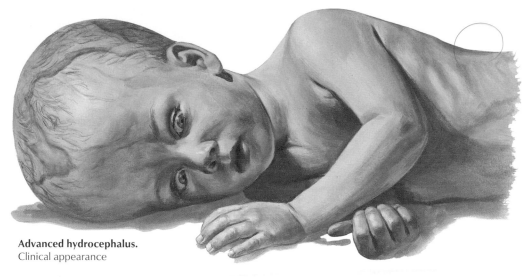

Advanced hydrocephalus.
Clinical appearance

**Potential lesion sites in
obstructive hydrocephalus**

1. Interventricular foramina (of Monro)
2. Cerebral aqueduct (of Sylvius)
3. Lateral apertures (of Luschka)
4. Median aperture (of Magendie)

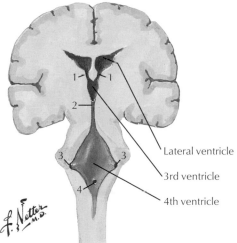

Lateral ventricle

3rd ventricle

4th ventricle

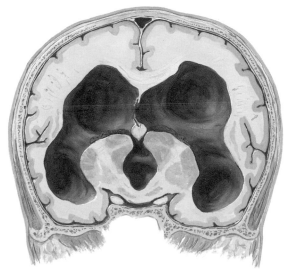

Section through brain. Showing marked
dilation of lateral and 3rd ventricles

FIGURE 13-4   HYDROCEPHALUS

Hydrocephalus, characterized by enlargement of the ventricles of the brain, results from increased formation or decreased absorption of CSF (communicating hydrocephalus) or from blockage of one of the normal outflow paths of the ventricular system (obstructive hydrocephalus). **Obstructive hydrocephalus** often results from a congenital stenosis of the cerebral aqueduct of Sylvius, but a brainstem tumor or a posterior fossa tumor encroaching on the fourth ventricle that obstructs one of the medial or lateral apertures can produce the same effect. In adults,

brain tumors are the usual cause of obstructive hydrocephalus. **Communicating hydrocephalus** may occur in premature infants after intraventricular hemorrhage. In children and adults, communicating hydrocephalus with increased intracranial pressure may follow an intracranial hemorrhage or infection. Adults also may have normal-pressure hydrocephalus, which must be differentiated from ventricular dilatation secondary to brain atrophy (hydrocephalus ex vacuo).

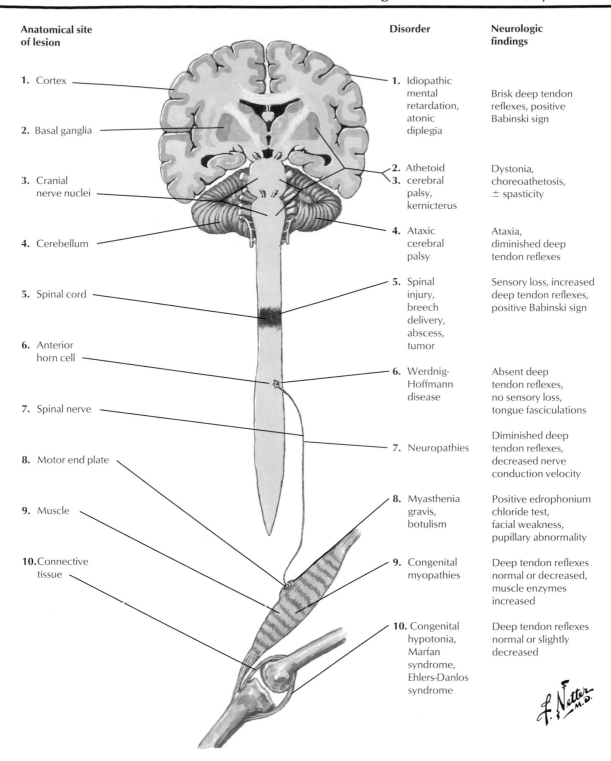

Anatomical site of lesion	Disorder	Neurologic findings
1. Cortex	1. Idiopathic mental retardation, atonic diplegia	Brisk deep tendon reflexes, positive Babinski sign
2. Basal ganglia	2. Athetoid 3. cerebral palsy, kernicterus	Dystonia, choreoathetosis, ± spasticity
3. Cranial nerve nuclei	4. Ataxic cerebral palsy	Ataxia, diminished deep tendon reflexes
4. Cerebellum	5. Spinal injury, breech delivery, abscess, tumor	Sensory loss, increased deep tendon reflexes, positive Babinski sign
5. Spinal cord	6. Werdnig-Hoffmann disease	Absent deep tendon reflexes, no sensory loss, tongue fasciculations
6. Anterior horn cell	7. Neuropathies	Diminished deep tendon reflexes, decreased nerve conduction velocity
7. Spinal nerve	8. Myasthenia gravis, botulism	Positive edrophonium chloride test, facial weakness, pupillary abnormality
8. Motor end plate	9. Congenital myopathies	Deep tendon reflexes normal or decreased, muscle enzymes increased
9. Muscle	10. Congenital hypotonia, Marfan syndrome, Ehlers-Danlos syndrome	Deep tendon reflexes normal or slightly decreased
10. Connective tissue		

FIGURE 13-5   HYPOTONIA

Hypotonia is an important clinical sign of neurologic problems in infants and young children. Classically, the infant hangs like a rag doll when lifted under the abdomen and exhibits weakness and flaccidity of all muscles. Muscle weakness coexisting with hypotonia indicates involvement of the peripheral nervous system, whereas the presence of brisk reflexes and a positive Babinski sign indicate involvement of the central nervous system. **Friedreich ataxia**, which is inherited in an autosomal recessive

fashion, is the most common of the spinocerebellar degenerations in older children. The differential diagnosis includes various congenital myopathies and connective tissue diseases.

Neurologic disease in infants and young children can also result from several inherited single gene defects of lipid metabolism (Niemann-Pick disease, Gaucher disease, and metachromatic leukodystrophy).

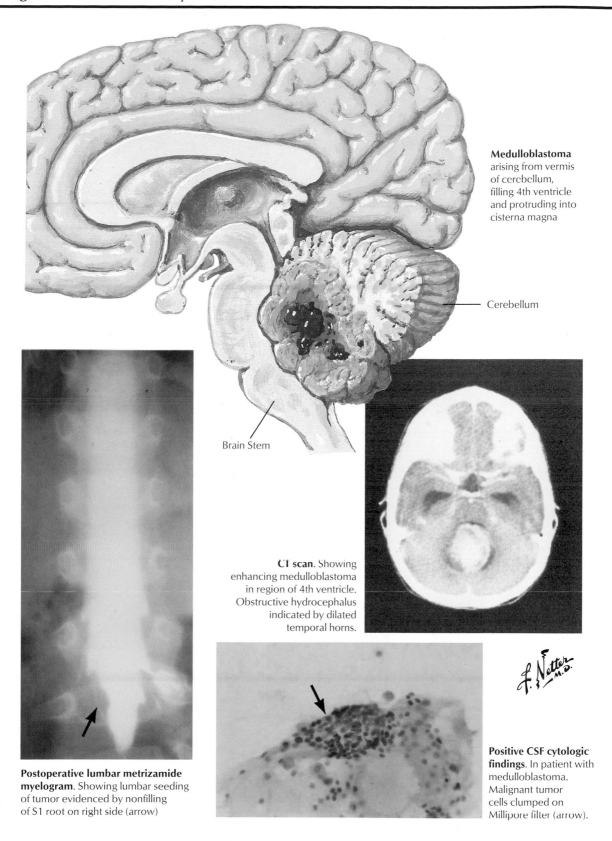

Medulloblastoma arising from vermis of cerebellum, filling 4th ventricle and protruding into cisterna magna

Cerebellum

Brain Stem

CT scan. Showing enhancing medulloblastoma in region of 4th ventricle. Obstructive hydrocephalus indicated by dilated temporal horns.

Postoperative lumbar metrizamide myelogram. Showing lumbar seeding of tumor evidenced by nonfilling of S1 root on right side (arrow)

Positive CSF cytologic findings. In patient with medulloblastoma. Malignant tumor cells clumped on Millipore filter (arrow).

FIGURE 13-6   BRAIN TUMORS IN CHILDREN

Brain tumors in children are found most commonly in the posterior fossa. The more common **astrocytomas** and **medulloblastomas** develop from the parenchyma of the cerebellum. Symptoms include evidence of cerebellar dysfunction (ataxia of the trunk and extremities) and obstruction of CSF flow, leading to headache, nausea, and vomiting. Other tumors include **ependymomas**, which originate from the ependymal cells lining the ventricular system, and **brainstem gliomas**. Treatment of posterior fossa tumors involving a combination of surgery, radiation therapy, and chemotherapy, can yield a favorable prognosis, whereas the prognosis for brainstem gliomas is generally poor.

Tuberous sclerosis

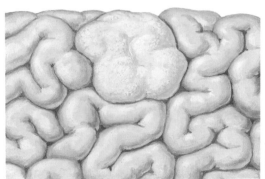

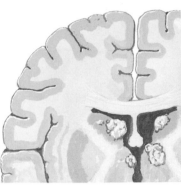

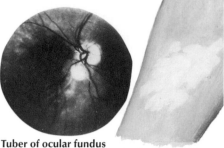

Tuber of ocular fundus

Depigmented skin area

Tuber of cerebral cortex. Consisting of many astrocytes, scanty nerve cells, some abnormal sites

Multiple small tumors. Caudate nucleus and thalamus projecting into ventricles

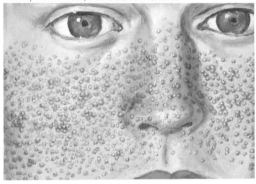

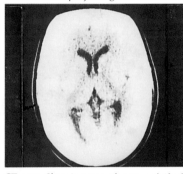

Rhabdomyomas of heart muscle

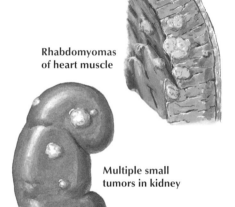

Multiple small tumors in kidney

Adenoma sebaceum. Over both cheeks and bridge of nose

CT scan. Showing one of many calcified lesions in periventricular area

Sturge–Weber disease

Facial nevus

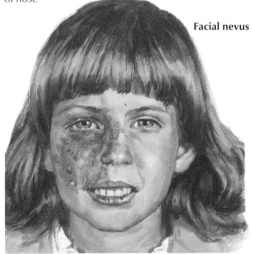

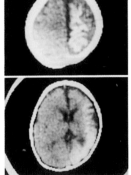

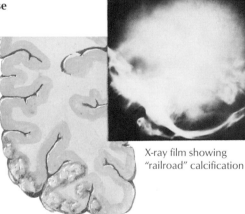

X-ray film showing "railroad" calcification

CT scan. Showing calcifications and atrophy in temporoparietal area

Calcific deposits and hypervascularity. In leptomeninges and gray matter of brain

FIGURE 13-7   NEUROCUTANEOUS SYNDROMES

Tuberous sclerosis is a neurocutaneous syndrome caused by a genetic mutation that occurs spontaneously or is inherited as an autosomal dominant trait. Tubers, foci of abnormal neural tissue growth, form in the nervous system and the retina. The clinical features in childhood are dominated by epilepsy and mental retardation, although some patients may have neither manifestation. Cutaneous manifestations include adenoma sebaceum, depigmented nevi, a shagreen patch in the lumbar

area, and subungual fibromas. Some patients have cardiac tumors, known as *rhabdomyomas,* or angiomyolipomas in the kidneys or both. **Sturge-Weber disease**, which occurs sporadically, presents with a characteristic port-wine nevus that is apparent at birth. Brain lesions consist of hypervascularity and calcification in the leptomeninges and gray matter. The course is progressive, with increasing seizures and hemiparesis.

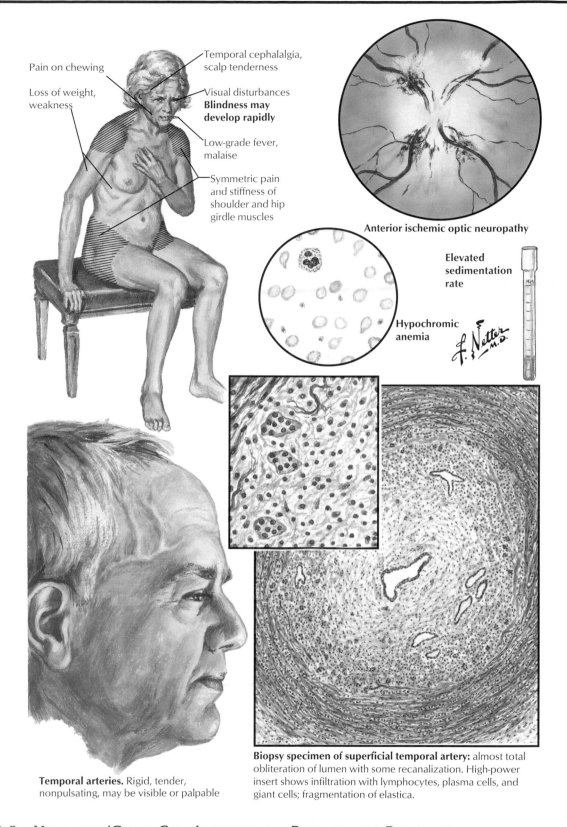

Pain on chewing

Loss of weight, weakness

Temporal cephalalgia, scalp tenderness

Visual disturbances
Blindness may develop rapidly

Low-grade fever, malaise

Symmetric pain and stiffness of shoulder and hip girdle muscles

Anterior ischemic optic neuropathy

Elevated sedimentation rate

Hypochromic anemia

Temporal arteries. Rigid, tender, nonpulsating, may be visible or palpable

Biopsy specimen of superficial temporal artery: almost total obliteration of lumen with some recanalization. High-power insert shows infiltration with lymphocytes, plasma cells, and giant cells; fragmentation of elastica.

FIGURE 13-8 HEADACHE/GIANT CELL ARTERITIS AND POLYMYALGIA RHEUMATICA

The headache syndromes include migraine (vascular headache), cluster headache (a migraine variant), muscle contraction headache (often stress related), and headache due to temporal (giant cell) arteritis. **Temporal (giant cell) arteritis** is an inflammatory disease that occurs in older individuals and affects the temporal branches of the external carotid artery. A steady, aching pain in the temporal and occipital regions, often accompanied by malaise and fever, is symptomatic. The temporal and occipital arteries are firm, tender, and pulseless. Histologically, the arteries are infiltrated by lymphocytes, plasma cells, and giant cells, and the lumen is occluded by organized thrombus. Intracranial vessels are affected occasionally, and blindness can result when ophthalmic arteries are involved. The generalized malaise, muscle pain and stiffness, fever, and other symptoms constitute an associated syndrome of polymyalgia rheumatica.

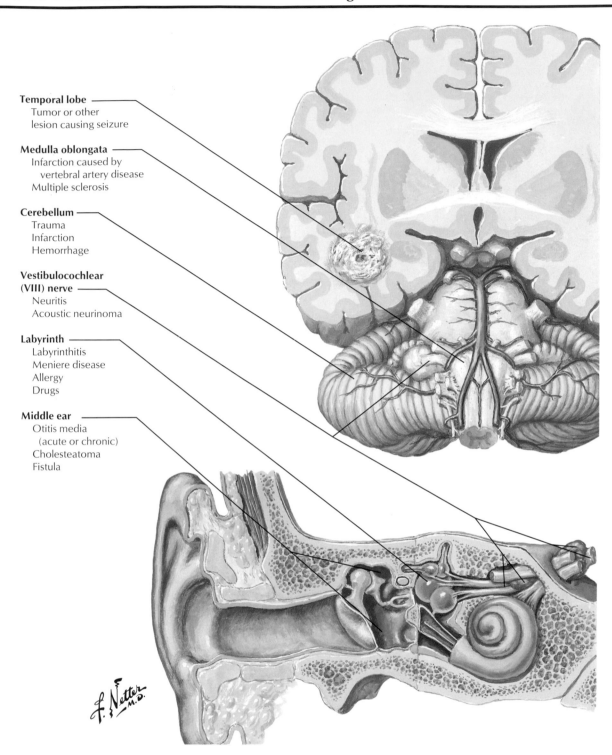

Temporal lobe
Tumor or other
lesion causing seizure

Medulla oblongata
Infarction caused by
vertebral artery disease
Multiple sclerosis

Cerebellum
Trauma
Infarction
Hemorrhage

**Vestibulocochlear
(VIII) nerve**
Neuritis
Acoustic neurinoma

Labyrinth
Labyrinthitis
Meniere disease
Allergy
Drugs

Middle ear
Otitis media
(acute or chronic)
Cholesteatoma
Fistula

FIGURE 13-9   CAUSES OF VERTIGO

Dizziness is a general term used to describe a variety of feelings related to a disturbed sense of relation to space, including unsteadiness and giddiness. **Vertigo** refers more specifically to a sensation of exterior motion, often described as spinning, turning, or rotating of the external environment in relation to the person. Vertigo may be caused by dysfunction of any of the structures that are involved in sound detection or the relay of signals from the vestibular apparatus of the ear to the brain. Useful clues to localization include an analysis of effect of movement or change in position, features of the motion, abnormal symptoms or signs related to dysfunction of adjacent structures, previous attacks, nystagmus, and laboratory tests such as electroencephalography, audiometric tests, computed tomography (CT), and magnetic resonance imaging (MRI).

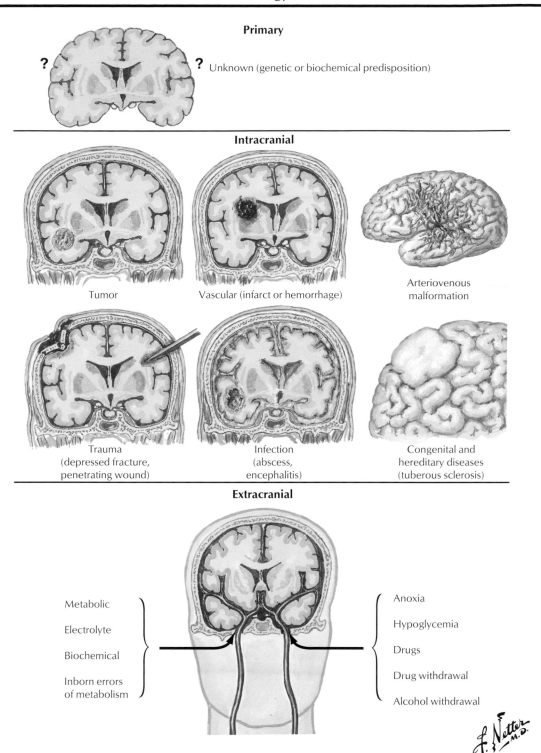

Primary

? ? Unknown (genetic or biochemical predisposition)

Intracranial

Tumor

Vascular (infarct or hemorrhage)

Arteriovenous
malformation

Trauma
(depressed fracture,
penetrating wound)

Infection
(abscess,
encephalitis)

Congenital and
hereditary diseases
(tuberous sclerosis)

Extracranial

Metabolic

Electrolyte

Biochemical

Inborn errors
of metabolism

Anoxia

Hypoglycemia

Drugs

Drug withdrawal

Alcohol withdrawal

FIGURE 13-10 CAUSES OF SEIZURES

Seizures are triggered by the sudden and intense increase in the discharge of neurons and constitute the symptomatic expression of epilepsy. **Primary seizures** are of unknown etiology and are typically generalized without (petit mal) or with tonic-clonic muscle contractions (grand mal). **Secondary seizures**, which may be focal or generalized, result from an identifiable pathologic lesion or disease process, which may be either intracranial or extracranial. The most common intracranial lesions causing seizures are tumors, vascular lesions, head trauma, infectious diseases, congenital defects, and biochemical or degenerative diseases affecting the brain. Extracranial causes of seizures include various metabolic, electrolyte, and biochemical disturbances; fever; inborn errors of metabolism; anoxia; hypoglycemia; toxic processes; and drugs or abrupt withdrawal from drugs or alcohol.

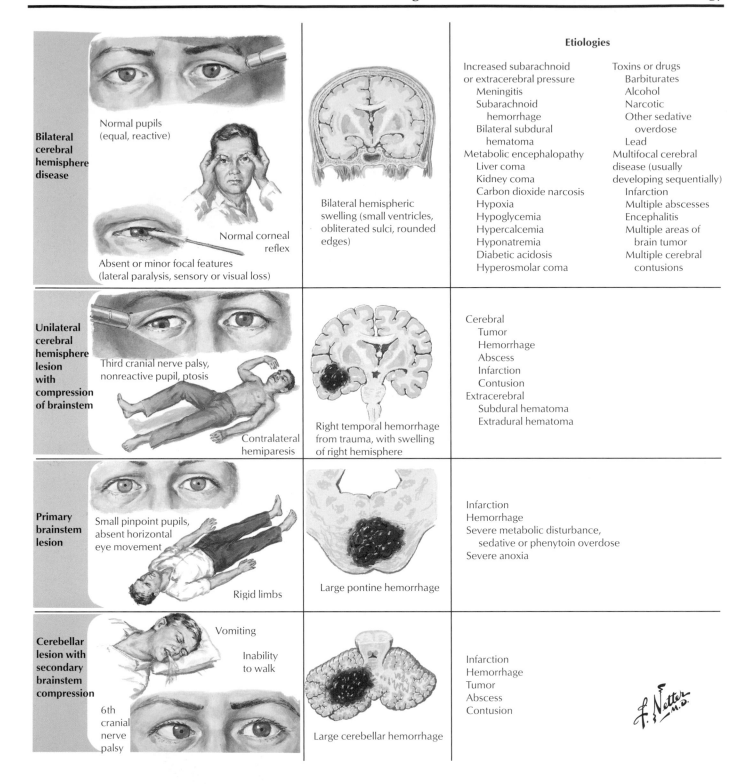

Etiologies

Increased subarachnoid
or extracerebral pressure
Meningitis
Subarachnoid
hemorrhage
Bilateral subdural
hematoma
Metabolic encephalopathy
Liver coma
Kidney coma
Carbon dioxide narcosis
Hypoxia
Hypoglycemia
Hypercalcemia
Hyponatremia
Diabetic acidosis
Hyperosmolar coma

Toxins or drugs
Barbiturates
Alcohol
Narcotic
Other sedative
overdose
Lead
Multifocal cerebral
disease (usually
developing sequentially)
Infarction
Multiple abscesses
Encephalitis
Multiple areas of
brain tumor
Multiple cerebral
contusions

Bilateral cerebral hemisphere disease

Normal pupils (equal, reactive)

Normal corneal reflex

Absent or minor focal features (lateral paralysis, sensory or visual loss)

Bilateral hemispheric swelling (small ventricles, obliterated sulci, rounded edges)

Unilateral cerebral hemisphere lesion with compression of brainstem

Third cranial nerve palsy, nonreactive pupil, ptosis

Contralateral hemiparesis

Right temporal hemorrhage from trauma, with swelling of right hemisphere

Cerebral
Tumor
Hemorrhage
Abscess
Infarction
Contusion
Extracerebral
Subdural hematoma
Extradural hematoma

Primary brainstem lesion

Small pinpoint pupils, absent horizontal eye movement

Rigid limbs

Large pontine hemorrhage

Infarction
Hemorrhage
Severe metabolic disturbance, sedative or phenytoin overdose
Severe anoxia

Cerebellar lesion with secondary brainstem compression

Vomiting

Inability to walk

6th cranial nerve palsy

Large cerebellar hemorrhage

Infarction
Hemorrhage
Tumor
Abscess
Contusion

F. Netter M.D.

Figure 13-11 Differential Diagnosis of Coma

Coma results from loss of consciousness as indicated by the complete absence of awareness of the environment or response to environmental stimuli. Confusion and stupor represent lesser degrees of impairment of consciousness. Consciousness is maintained by coordinated neural activity in both cerebral hemispheres reinforced by the reticular activating system located in the tegmentum of the brainstem. Consciousness is diminished or lost by major impairment of the reticular activating system or

extensive damage to both cerebral hemispheres. The basic pathophysiologic mechanisms for loss of consciousness are (1) bilateral cerebral hemisphere disease, (2) unilateral cerebral hemisphere lesion with compression of the brainstem, (3) primary brainstem lesion, and (4) cerebellar lesion with secondary brainstem compression. These should be differentiated from nonorganic or feigned stupor.

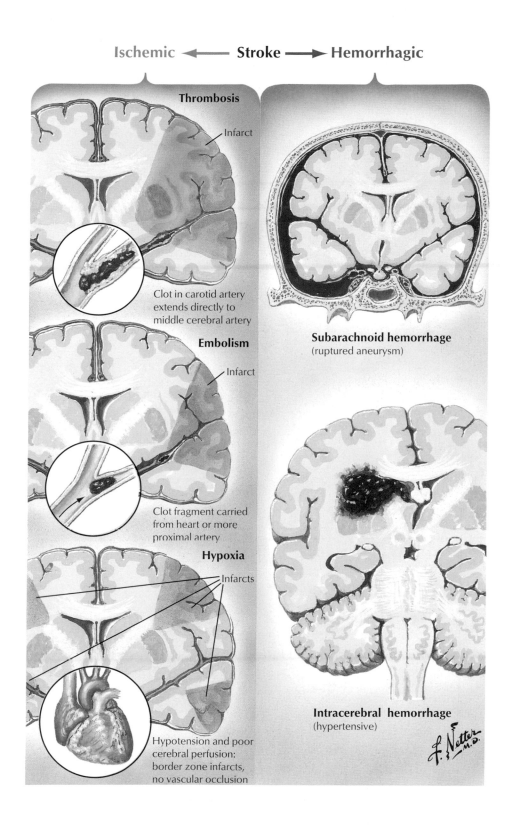

FIGURE 13-12   DIAGNOSIS OF STROKE

Stroke refers to a constellation of disorders in which brain injury is caused by a vascular disorder. The 2 major categories of stroke are ischemic, in which inadequate blood flow due to thrombosis, embolism, or generalized hypoxia causes one or more localized areas of cerebral infarction, and hemorrhagic, in which bleeding in the brain parenchyma or subarachnoid space causes damage and displacement of brain structures. The clinical spectrum of focal cerebral ischemic events includes transient ischemic attacks, residual ischemic neurologic deficit, and completed infarction.

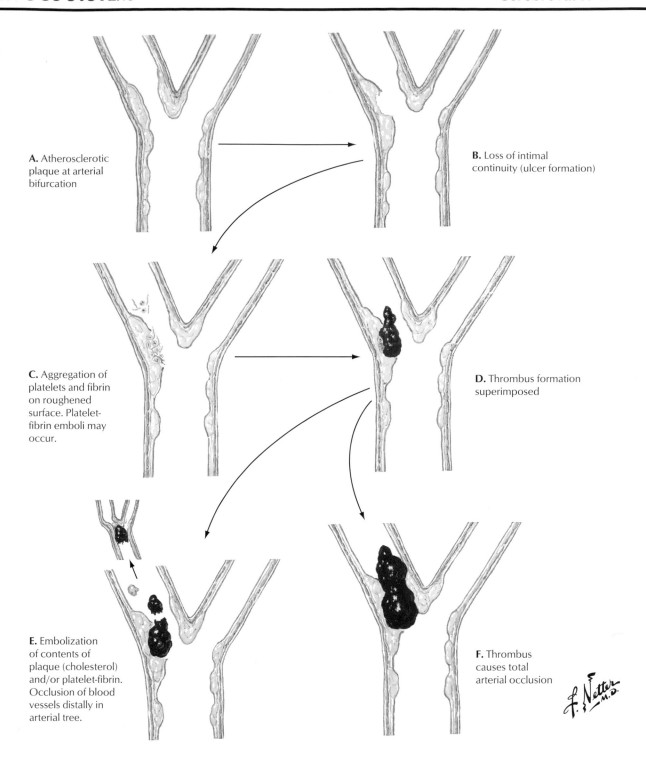

A. Atherosclerotic plaque at arterial bifurcation

B. Loss of intimal continuity (ulcer formation)

C. Aggregation of platelets and fibrin on roughened surface. Platelet-fibrin emboli may occur.

D. Thrombus formation superimposed

E. Embolization of contents of plaque (cholesterol) and/or platelet-fibrin. Occlusion of blood vessels distally in arterial tree.

F. Thrombus causes total arterial occlusion

FIGURE 13-13 ATHEROSCLEROSIS, THROMBOSIS, AND EMBOLISM

Atherosclerosis is characterized by the development of foci of intimal thickening composed of variable combinations of fibrous and fatty material and known as **fibrous** (atheromatous) **plaques**. Such lesions tend to form adjacent to branch points in arteries. The fibrous plaques may remain static, regress, progress, become calcified, or develop into complicated atheromatous lesions called **dangerous** or **vulnerable plaques** because they are responsible for clinical disease. Complications include loss of endothelial integrity, overt surface ulceration, aggregation of platelets and fibrin on the eroded plaque surface, hemorrhage in the plaque, formation of mural thrombi, embolization of plaque contents or thrombotic material or both, and total arterial occlusion by thrombus. The consequences of thrombotic occlusion are variable and unpredictable depending on the extent of disease and the amount of preexisting collateral blood flow. Thrombotic occlusion often results in tissue infarction.

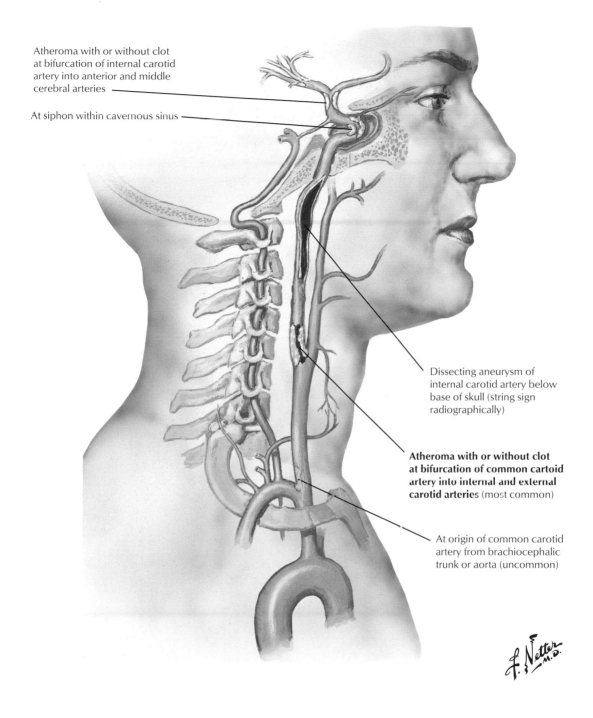

Atheroma with or without clot at bifurcation of internal carotid artery into anterior and middle cerebral arteries

At siphon within cavernous sinus

Dissecting aneurysm of internal carotid artery below base of skull (string sign radiographically)

Atheroma with or without clot at bifurcation of common cartoid artery into internal and external carotid arteries (most common)

At origin of common carotid artery from brachiocephalic trunk or aorta (uncommon)

FIGURE 13-14   STENOSIS OR OCCLUSION OF THE CAROTID ARTERY

Stenosis or occlusion of a carotid artery accounts for a high percentage of strokes. The most common location for atherosclerosis in the carotid system is at the bifurcation of the common carotid artery into the internal and external carotid arteries. Atherosclerotic stenosis at the origin of the common carotid artery is rare, but aortic arch arteritis (Takayasu disease) can occlude the proximal common carotid artery and other aortic branches. The extracranial pharyngeal portion of the internal carotid artery is usually spared of atherosclerosis but is subject to fibromuscular dysplasia and medial dissection. Atherosclerosis can affect the siphon portion of the carotid artery and the site of bifurcation of the internal carotid artery into anterior and middle cerebral arteries after it has begun its intracranial course. Ischemia in the internal carotid territory can lead to visual field defects, language defects, and hemiparesis or hemiplegia.

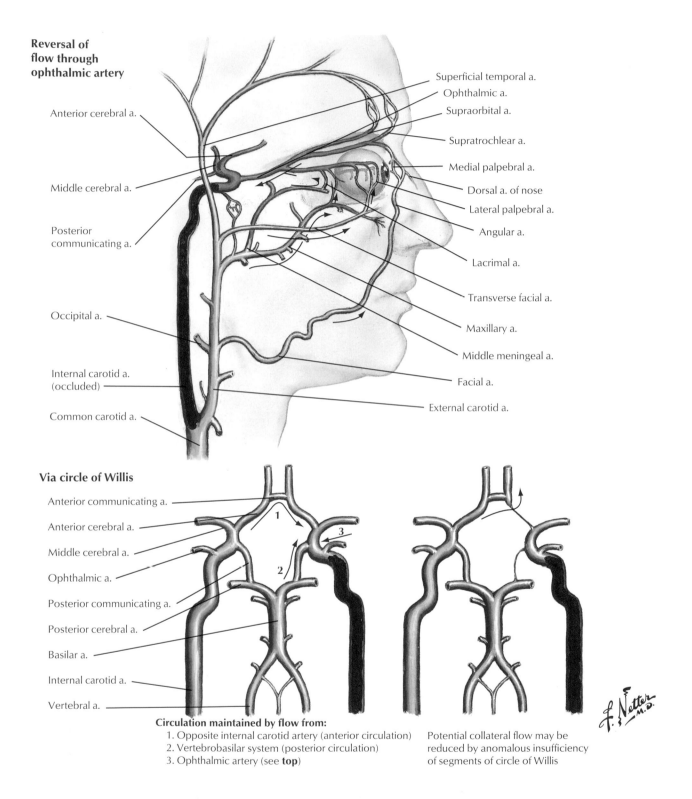

Reversal of flow through ophthalmic artery

Anterior cerebral a.

Middle cerebral a.

Posterior communicating a.

Occipital a.

Internal carotid a. (occluded)

Common carotid a.

Superficial temporal a.

Ophthalmic a.

Supraorbital a.

Supratrochlear a.

Medial palpebral a.

Dorsal a. of nose

Lateral palpebral a.

Angular a.

Lacrimal a.

Transverse facial a.

Maxillary a.

Middle meningeal a.

Facial a.

External carotid a.

Via circle of Willis

Anterior communicating a.

Anterior cerebral a.

Middle cerebral a.

Ophthalmic a.

Posterior communicating a.

Posterior cerebral a.

Basilar a.

Internal carotid a.

Vertebral a.

Circulation maintained by flow from:
1. Opposite internal carotid artery (anterior circulation)
2. Vertebrobasilar system (posterior circulation)
3. Ophthalmic artery (see **top**)

Potential collateral flow may be reduced by anomalous insufficiency of segments of circle of Willis

FIGURE 13-15   COLLATERAL CIRCULATION WITH OCCLUSION OF THE INTERNAL CAROTID ARTERY ___

Collateral circulation occurs by blood flow from the vasculature supplied by one major blood vessel into the vascular branches of another major blood vessel through small vascular channels that connect the two systems. Occlusion of the internal carotid artery can be partially ameliorated through collateral circulation. The major extracranial pathways of collateral circulation are anastomoses between the ophthalmic artery and branches of both external carotid arteries. The major intracranial pathways of collateral circulation are the anastomoses formed by the circle of Willis at the base of the brain. The amount of collateral circulation is determined by the specific anatomy of the vascular connections and the extent and distribution of vascular disease.

Lesion		Artery occluded	Infarct, surface	Infarct, coronal section	Clinical manifestations
Middle cerebral artery	Entire territory	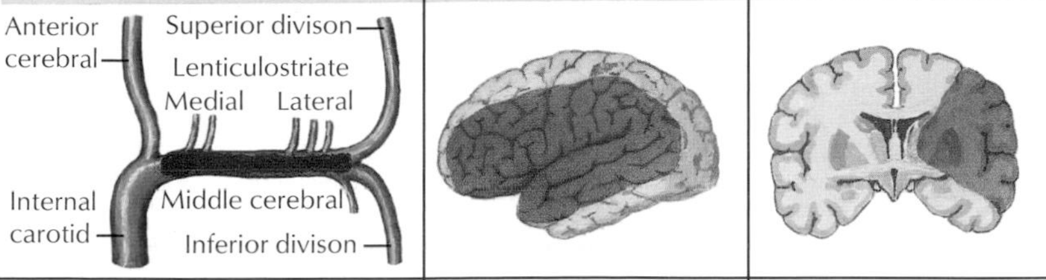 Anterior cerebral — Superior divison — Lenticulostriate — Medial Lateral — Internal carotid — Middle cerebral — Inferior divison			Contralateral gaze palsy, hemiplegia, hemisensory loss, spatial neglect, hemianopsia Global aphasia (if on left side) May lead to coma secondary to edema
	Deep	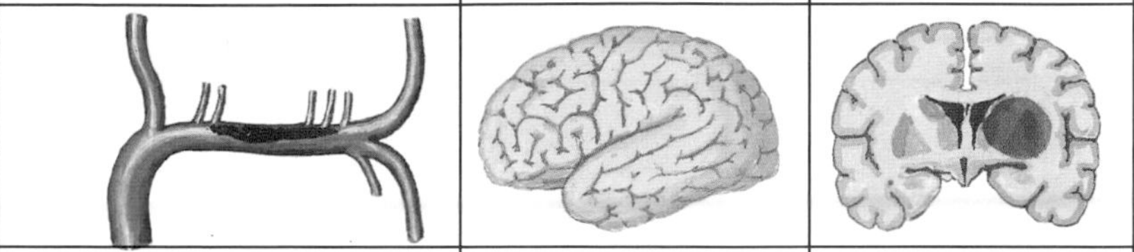			Contralateral hemiplegia, hemisensory loss Transcortical motor and/or sensory aphasia (if on left side)
	Parasylvian	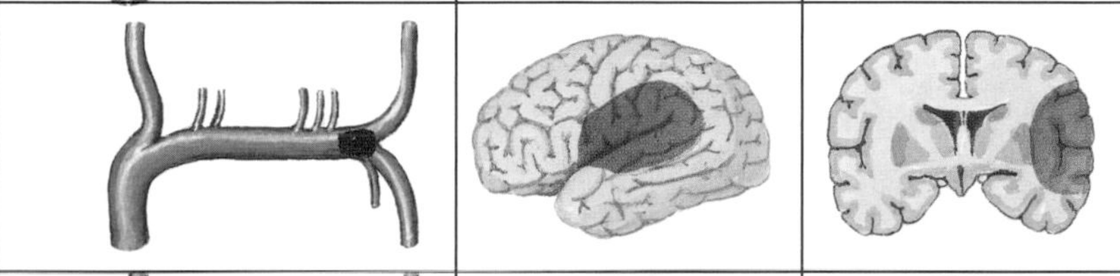			Contralateral weakness and sensory loss of face and hand Conduction aphasia, apraxia, and Gerstmann syndrome (if on left side) Constructional dyspraxia (if on right side)
	Superior division	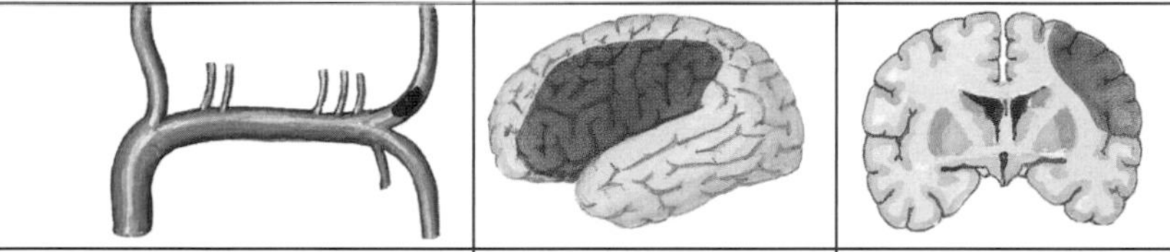			Contralateral hemiplegia, hemisensory loss, gaze palsy, spatial neglect Broca aphasia (if on left side)
	Inferior division	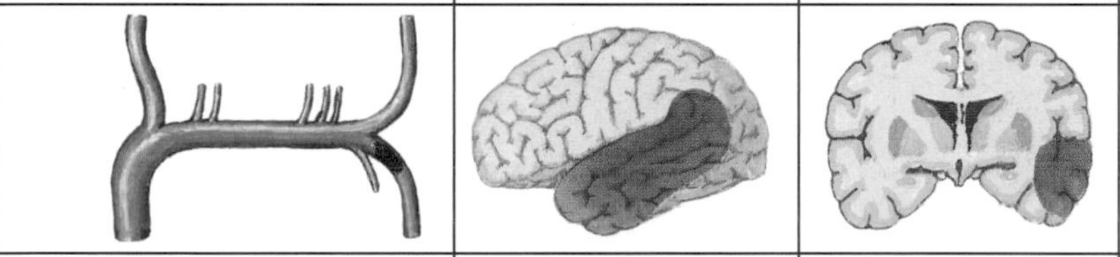			Contralateral hemianopsia or upper quadrant anopsia Wernicke aphasia (if on left side) Constructional dyspraxia (if on right side)
Anterior cerebral artery	Entire territory	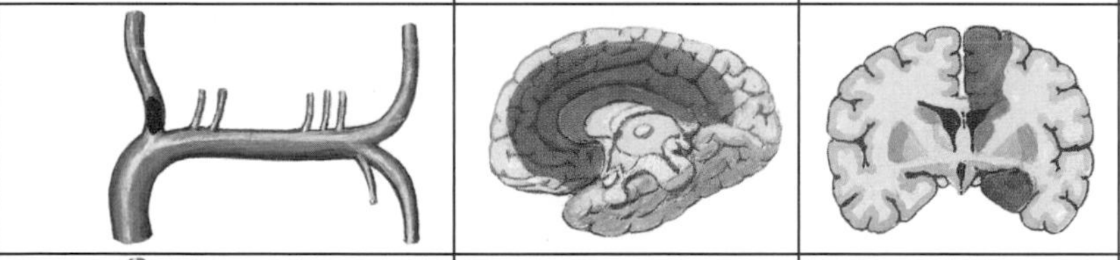			Incontinence Contralateral hemiplegia Abulia Transcortical motor aphasia or motor and sensory aphasia Left limb dyspraxia
	Distal	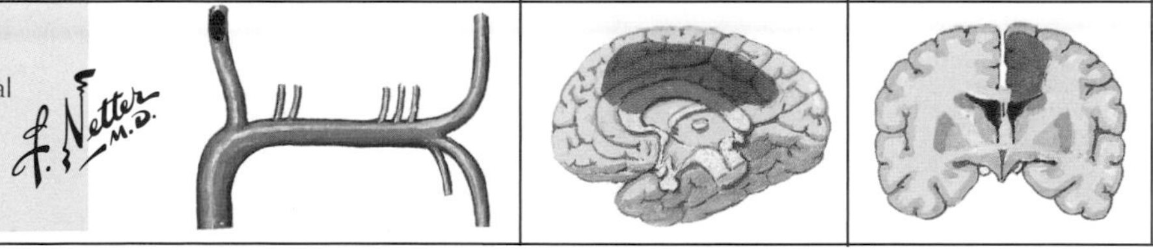			Contralateral weakness of leg, hip, foot, and shoulder Sensory loss in foot Transcortical motor aphasia or motor and sensory aphasia Left limb dyspraxia

FIGURE 13-16   OCCLUSION OF THE MIDDLE AND ANTERIOR CEREBRAL ARTERIES

The internal carotid artery bifurcates within the cranial cavity into the anterior cerebral artery (which supplies the anterior paramedian cerebral hemisphere) and the larger middle cerebral artery (which supplies the lateral cerebral hemisphere and most of the basal ganglia) after giving origin to the ophthalmic, anterior choroidal, and posterior communicating artery branches. The middle cerebral artery contributes penetrating lenticulostriate branches that arise from its horizontal main stem and trifurcates near the lateral cerebral (sylvian) fissure into major superior and inferior trunks and a small anterior temporal artery. Occlusion of the main stem of the middle or anterior cerebral artery or their superficial branches is usually caused by an embolus from the heart or the proximal vessels, particularly the internal carotid artery.

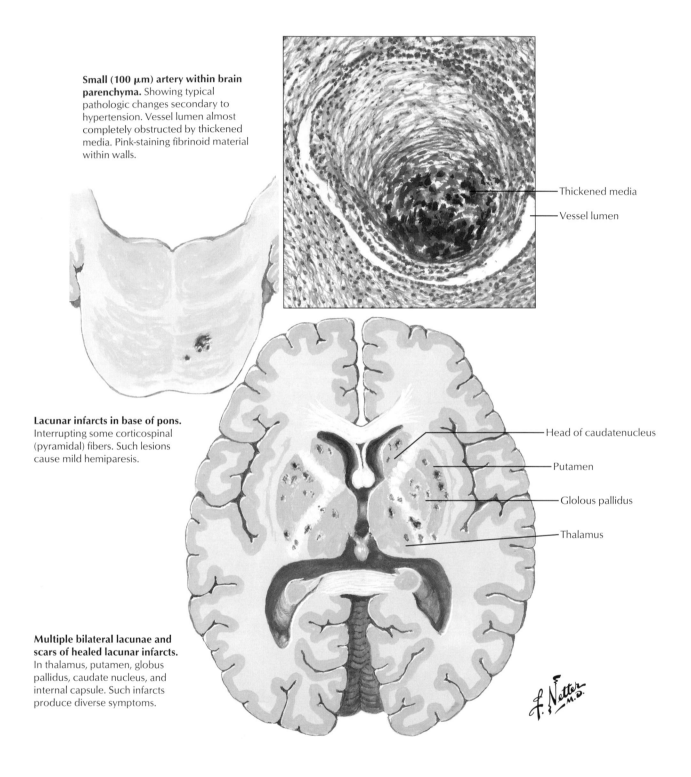

Small (100 μm) artery within brain parenchyma. Showing typical pathologic changes secondary to hypertension. Vessel lumen almost completely obstructed by thickened media. Pink-staining fibrinoid material within walls.

Thickened media

Vessel lumen

Lacunar infarcts in base of pons. Interrupting some corticospinal (pyramidal) fibers. Such lesions cause mild hemiparesis.

Head of caudatenucleus

Putamen

Glolous pallidus

Thalamus

Multiple bilateral lacunae and scars of healed lacunar infarcts. In thalamus, putamen, globus pallidus, caudate nucleus, and internal capsule. Such infarcts produce diverse symptoms.

FIGURE 13-17   LACUNAR INFARCTION

Atherosclerosis involves large- and medium-sized cerebral arteries, whereas hypertension produces disease of small penetrating arteries of the brain. Progressive arteriolosclerosis develops in the small vessels. Hyaline and fibrinoid material thickens the wall and obliterates the lumen. The **lacunae** (holes), the small, round lesions deep in the brain parenchyma, are commonly found in the brain at autopsy. Some lesions are clinically significant. A small infarct in the base of the pons or internal capsule can produce a pure motor hemiplegia with contralateral weakness of the face, the arm, and the leg but no sensory, visual, or intellectual defects. Other lesions can produce pure sensory strokes. Lacunar lesions in the pons can produce several syndromes, including hemiparesis coupled with ataxia.

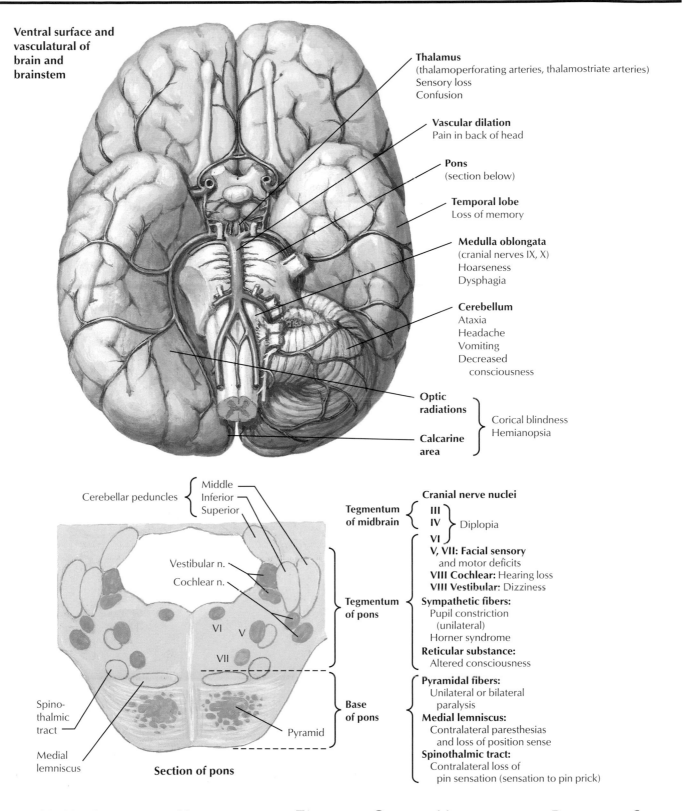

Ventral surface and vasculatural of brain and brainstem

Thalamus
(thalamoperforating arteries, thalamostriate arteries)
Sensory loss
Confusion

Vascular dilation
Pain in back of head

Pons
(section below)

Temporal lobe
Loss of memory

Medulla oblongata
(cranial nerves IX, X)
Hoarseness
Dysphagia

Cerebellum
Ataxia
Headache
Vomiting
Decreased
consciousness

Optic radiations

Calcarine area

Corical blindness
Hemianopsia

Cerebellar peduncles { Middle / Inferior / Superior }

Vestibular n.

Cochlear n.

VI   V

VII

Spino-thalmic tract

Medial lemniscus

Pyramid

Section of pons

Cranial nerve nuclei

Tegmentum of midbrain { III / IV } Diplopia / VI

V, VII: Facial sensory
and motor deficits
VIII Cochlear: Hearing loss
VIII Vestibular: Dizziness

Tegmentum of pons {
Sympathetic fibers:
Pupil constriction
(unilateral)
Horner syndrome
Reticular substance:
Altered consciousness
}

Base of pons {
Pyramidal fibers:
Unilateral or bilateral
paralysis
Medial lemniscus:
Contralateral paresthesias
and loss of position sense
Spinothalmic tract:
Contralateral loss of
pin sensation (sensation to pin prick)
}

FIGURE 13-18   ISCHEMIA IN VERTEBROBASILAR TERRITORY: CLINICAL MANIFESTATIONS RELATED TO SITE

Ischemia in the vertebrobasilar territory accounts for approximately a fifth of all cerebrovascular accidents. Ischemia in the vertebrobasilar system may produce impairment of the brainstem, the cerebellar hemispheres, or the occipital lobes of the cerebral hemispheres. Symptoms and signs include altered consciousness, ataxia, vertigo, motor and sensory deficits of the extremities, visual field defects, and palsy of one or more of the cranial nerves. This illustration shows the relation between areas of the brain affected by various sites of vascular pathology and the associated neurologic symptoms. Atherosclerosis of the basilar artery and posterior cerebral arteries is a common cause of strokes in this region. Also, atherosclerosis and pulseless disease (Takayasu arteritis) may involve the subclavian artery and its right or left vertebral artery branches. Ischemia also can result from trauma of the third segment of the vertebral artery as it enters the posterior fossa.

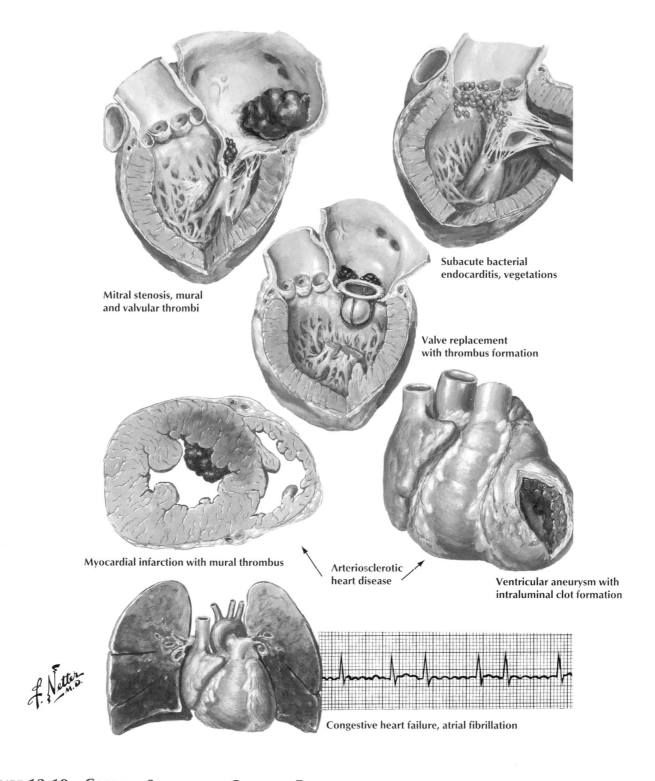

Mitral stenosis, mural and valvular thrombi

Subacute bacterial endocarditis, vegetations

Valve replacement with thrombus formation

Myocardial infarction with mural thrombus

Arteriosclerotic heart disease

Ventricular aneurysm with intraluminal clot formation

Congestive heart failure, atrial fibrillation

FIGURE 13-19 CARDIAC SOURCES OF CEREBRAL EMBOLI

The classic presentation of a stroke of embolic cause is the abrupt loss of neurologic function confined to the distribution of a major cerebral vessel or one of its major branches without previous transient ischemic episodes. In various studies, findings suggestive of an embolic origin have been identified in as many as 50% of patients presenting with stroke. The major sites of origin of cerebral emboli are carotid artery atheromas and a variety of cardiac lesions. Atrial fibrillation is an important

pathophysiologic alteration that can give rise to intracardiac thrombus formation and subsequent cerebral emboli. Atrial fibrillation develops most often in patients with arteriosclerotic heart disease and congestive heart failure of various causes. Emboli also can arise from thrombi forming on prosthetic valves, from vegetations of bacterial endocarditis, and from mural thrombi at sites of acute myocardial infarction or ventricular aneurysms.

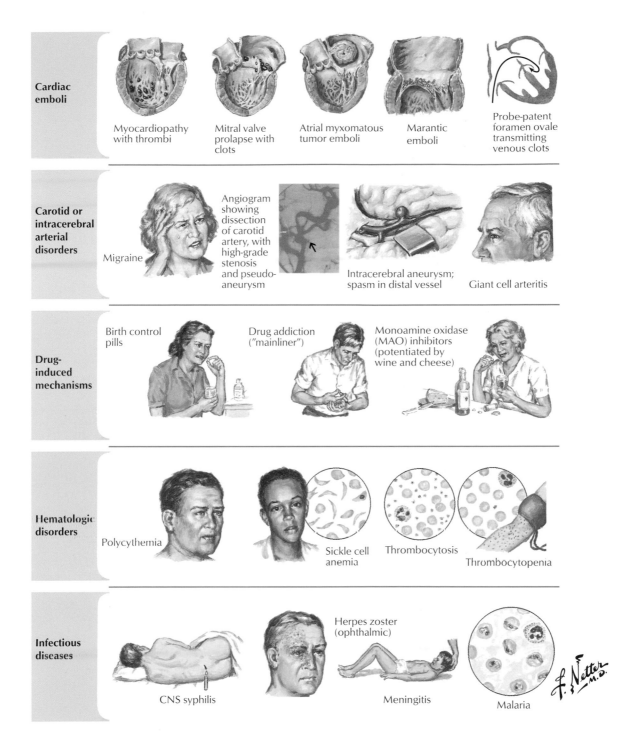

Cardiac emboli

Myocardiopathy with thrombi

Mitral valve prolapse with clots

Atrial myxomatous tumor emboli

Marantic emboli

Probe-patent foramen ovale transmitting venous clots

Carotid or intracerebral arterial disorders

Migraine

Angiogram showing dissection of carotid artery, with high-grade stenosis and pseudo-aneurysm

Intracerebral aneurysm; spasm in distal vessel

Giant cell arteritis

Drug-induced mechanisms

Birth control pills

Drug addiction ("mainliner")

Monoamine oxidase (MAO) inhibitors (potentiated by wine and cheese)

Hematologic disorders

Polycythemia

Sickle cell anemia

Thrombocytosis

Thrombocytopenia

Infectious diseases

CNS syphilis

Herpes zoster (ophthalmic)

Meningitis

Malaria

FIGURE 13-20   UNCOMMON ETIOLOGIC MECHANISMS IN STROKE

Less common but treatable mechanisms should be considered before concluding that stroke is due to cerebral atherosclerosis, including cardiomyopathy, mitral valve prolapse, atrial myxoma, marantic vegetations (nonbacterial thrombotic endocarditis), and paradoxical emboli across a probe-patent foramen ovale. Echocardiography and angiography are important diagnostic procedures to detect cardiac or unusual carotid or intracerebral arterial disorders. Also included in the differential diagnosis are conditions that may be associated with markers of inflammation (erythrocyte sedimentation rate, C-reactive protein), such as intracranial temporal arteritis, other vasculitides, bacterial endocarditis, or atrial myxoma. Abnormal cerebrovascular fluid examination results may lead to a diagnosis of bacterial meningitis or other forms of nervous system infection. Abnormalities affecting platelets or red blood cells may contribute to stroke, and consideration should be given to drug-induced mechanisms of stroke.

Pathogenesis

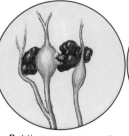

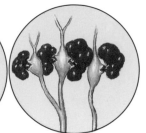

B. Microaneurysm ruptures, causing pressure on adjacent (satellite) vessels

C. Satellite vessels rupture

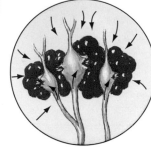

D. Amount of blood extravasated into brain tissue depends on tissue turgor opposed to intravascular blood pressure

A. Microaneurysm formed in parenchymal artery of brain as result of hypertension. Lenticulostriate vessels (shown) most commonly involved, but similar process may occur in other parts of brain, especially lobar white matter, thalamus, pons, and cerebellum.

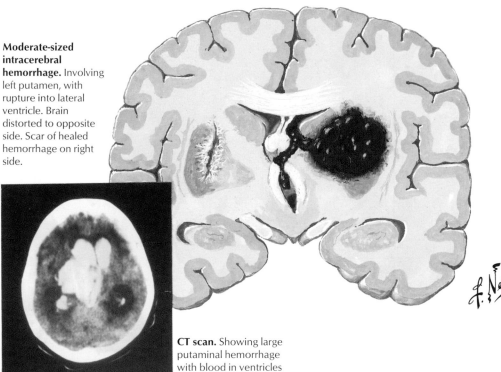

Moderate-sized intracerebral hemorrhage. Involving left putamen, with rupture into lateral ventricle. Brain distorted to opposite side. Scar of healed hemorrhage on right side.

CT scan. Showing large putaminal hemorrhage with blood in ventricles

FIGURE 13-21   INTRACEREBRAL HEMORRHAGE

Hypertension is the most common and important etiologic factor in intracerebral hemorrhage. Over time, degenerative changes of the small arteries lead to the formation of microaneurysms. The penetrating lenticulostriate branches of the middle cerebral artery are most commonly involved, but similar changes can occur in small vessels in other parts of the brain. Hemorrhages tend to dissect through white matter pathways, thereby disrupting the cerebral cortex. The enlarging hematoma may extend onto the cerebral surface, producing subarachnoid hemorrhage or rupture into the ventricles. **Hypertensive hemorrhage** typically occurs in regions where small lacunar lesions develop (see Fig. 13-17) and involve, in descending order of frequency, the putamen, the cerebral white matter, the thalamus, the pons, the cerebellum, and the caudate nucleus. Hemorrhages usually begin while the patient is awake and engaged in daily activity. As the hematoma expands, the focal neurologic deficit gradually increases during a period of minutes or a few hours.

Pathology	CT scan	Pupils	Eye movement	Motor and sensory deficits	Other
Caudate nucleus (blood in ventricle)		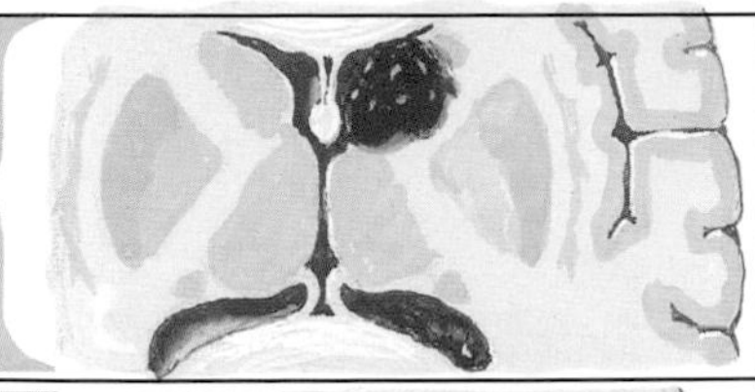 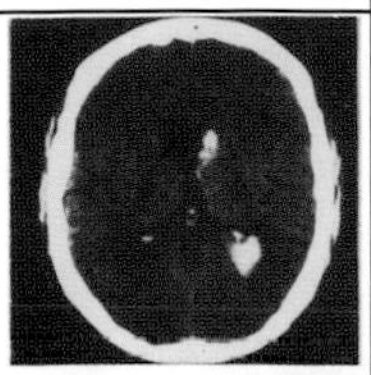 Sometimes ipsilaterally constricted	Conjugate deviation to side of lesion. Slight ptosis.	Contralateral hemiparesis, often transient	Headache, confusion
Putamen (small hemorrhage)		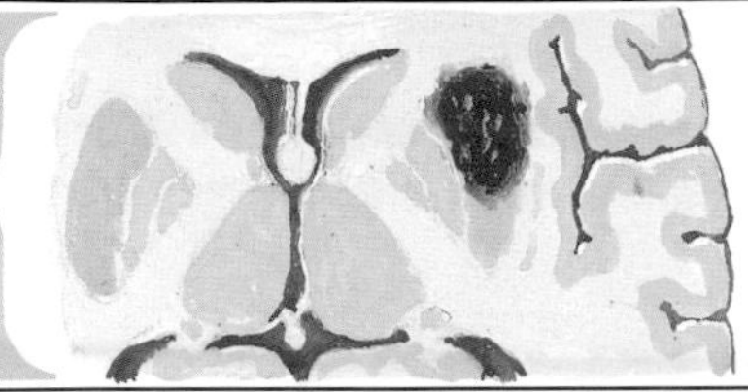 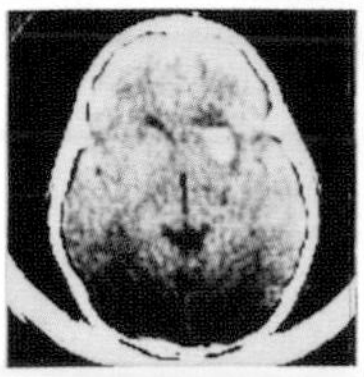 Normal	Conjugate deviation to side of lesion	Contralateral hemiparesis and hemisensory loss	Aphasia (if lesion on left side)
Putamen (large hemorrhage)		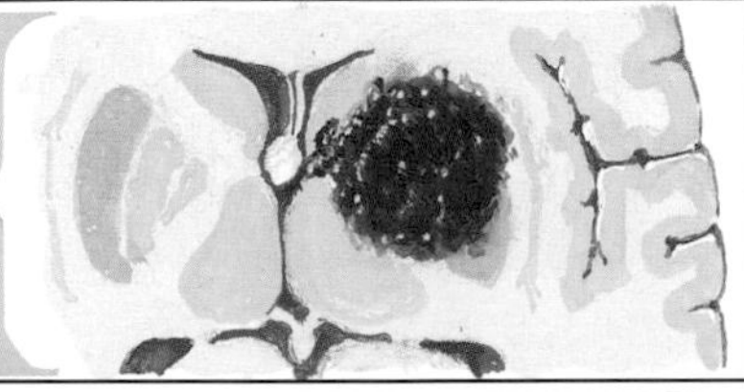 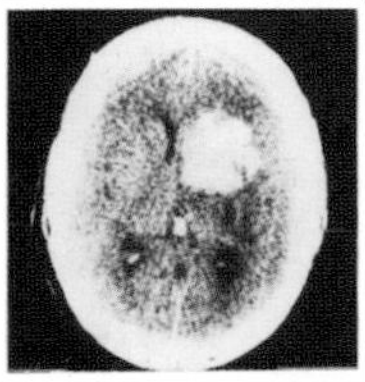 In presence of herniation, pupil dilated on side of lesion	Conjugate deviation to side of lesion	Contralateral hemiparesis and hemisensory loss	Decreased consciousness
Thalamus		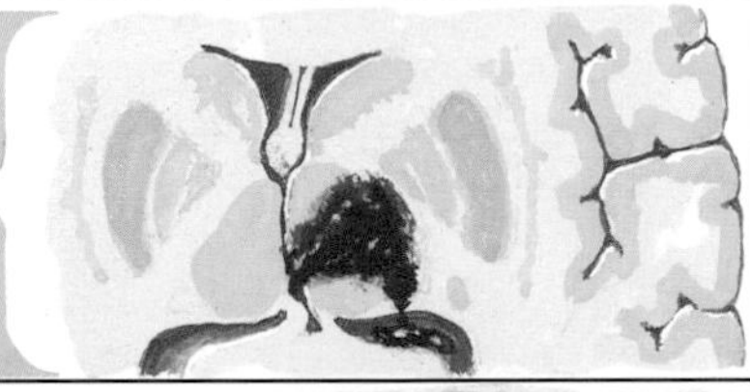 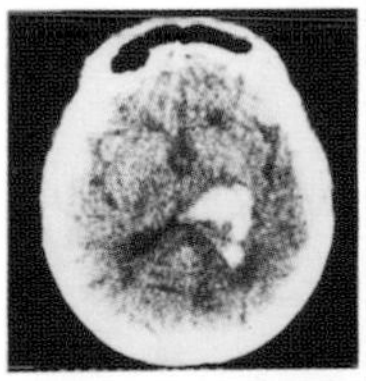 Constricted, poorly reactive to light bilaterally	Both lids retracted. Eyes positioned downward and medially. Cannot look upward.	Slight contralateral hemiparesis, but greater hemisensory loss	Aphasia (if lesion on left side)
Occipital lobar white matter		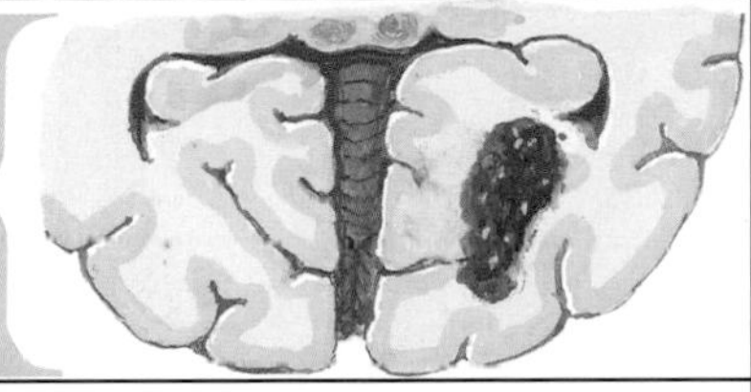 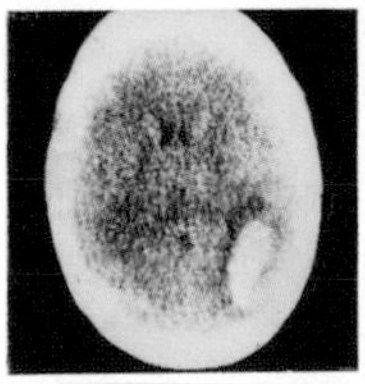 Normal	Normal	Mild, transient hemiparesis	Contralateral hemianopsia
Pons		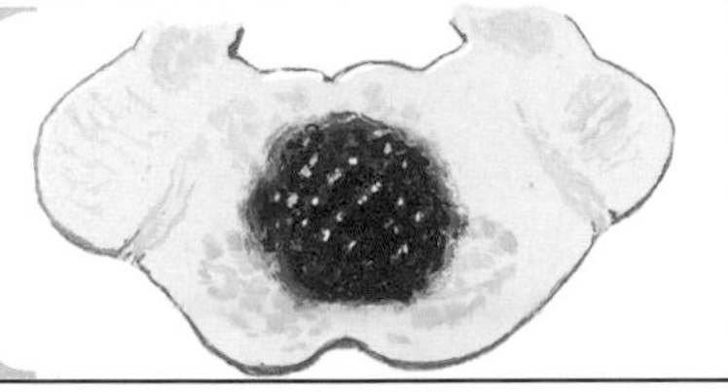 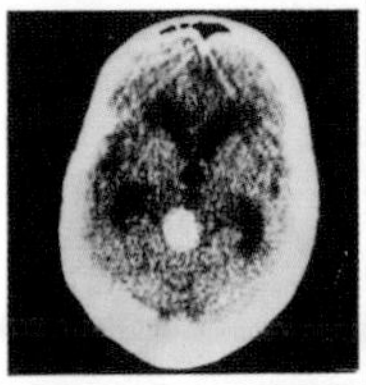 Constricted, reactive to light	No horizontal movements. Vertical movements preserved.	Quadriplegia	Coma
Cerebellum		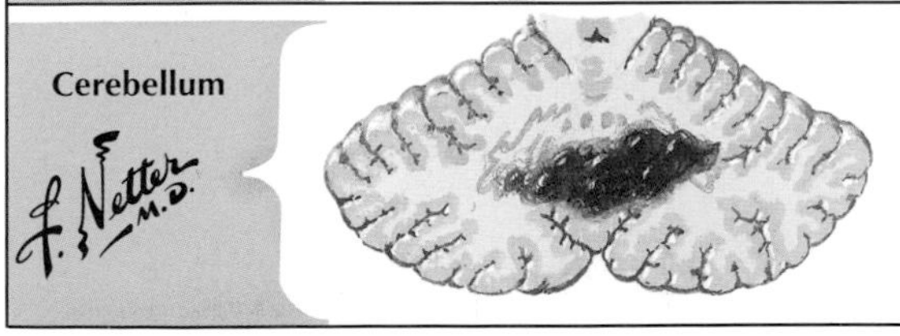 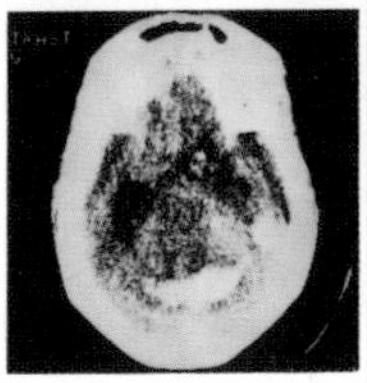 Slight constriction on side of lesion	Slight deviation to opposite side. Movements toward side of lesion impaired, or 6th cranial nerve palsy.	Ipsilateral limb ataxia. No hemiparesis.	Gait ataxia, vomiting

FIGURE 13-22 INTRACEREBRAL HEMORRHAGE: CLINICAL MANIFESTATIONS RELATED TO SITE

Symptoms and specific signs of neurologic deficit relate to the site and size of the intracerebral hemorrhage. Hypertension-induced damage of small arteries is the most common cause of intracerebral hemorrhage. Other causes include arteriovenous malformations (AVMs), bleeding diatheses (natural disease or anticoagulant induced), trauma, drug abuse (amphetamines or cocaine), and amyloid angiopathy (a degenerative vasculopathy seen in elderly patients). CT and MRI confirm the diagnosis of intracerebral hemorrhage. The hemorrhages appear as round, well-circumscribed lesions of uniform high density on CT scans. Large hemorrhages are often fatal. Small hemorrhages can resolve if blood pressure is controlled. Surgical drainage of medium-sized hemorrhages can occasionally be lifesaving.

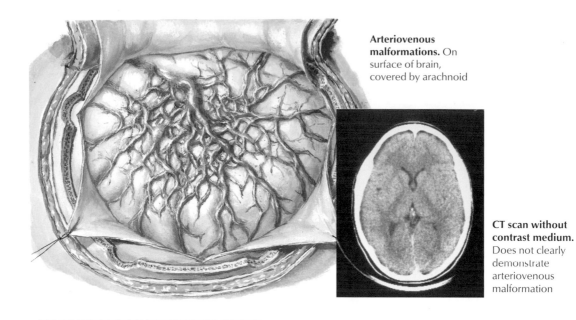

Arteriovenous malformations. On surface of brain, covered by arachnoid

CT scan without contrast medium. Does not clearly demonstrate arteriovenous malformation

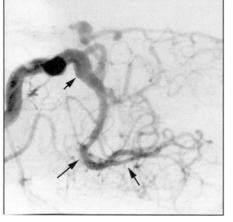

Right internal carotid angiogram. Dense cluster of vessels in sylvian fissure. Main feeding artery (arrowhead), large draining veins (arrows).

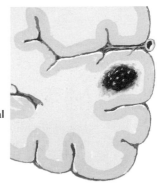

CT scan with contrast medium. Clearly demonstrates arteriovenous malformation

Small angioma. Of superior temporal gyrus

Small intracerebral hemorrhage. Probably resulting from angioma

FIGURE 13-23   VASCULAR MALFORMATIONS

Vascular malformations are congenital anomalies that can cause intracerebral or subarachnoid hemorrhage. There are 4 categories: (1) AVMs characterized by direct connections between arteries and veins, with the veins becoming arterialized by exposure to high pressure; (2) capillary angiomas, or telangiectases, consisting of malformations of arterioles and capillaries; (3) cavernous angiomas, consisting of dilated abnormal vessels of various sizes, with no intervening neural tissue; and (4) venous angiomas, consisting of large aggregates of veins (caput medusae). Complications include headache, epileptic seizures, and bleeding. Treatment may involve surgical ablation or ablation by various interventional neuroradiologic procedures.

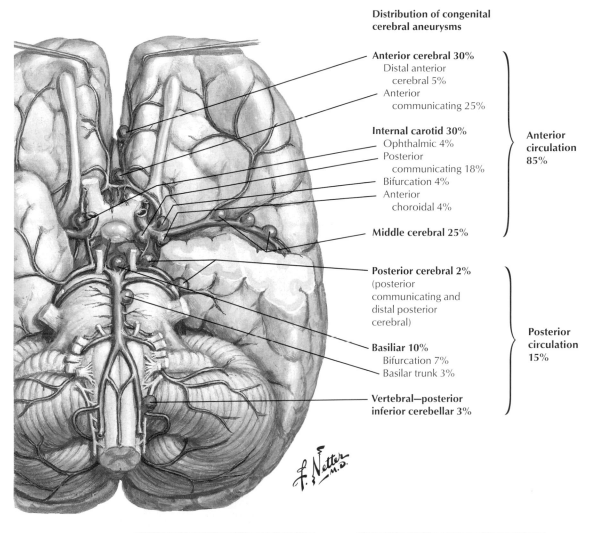

Distribution of congenital cerebral aneurysms

Anterior cerebral 30%
  Distal anterior cerebral 5%
  Anterior communicating 25%

Internal carotid 30%
  Ophthalmic 4%
  Posterior communicating 18%
  Bifurcation 4%
  Anterior choroidal 4%

Middle cerebral 25%

} Anterior circulation 85%

Posterior cerebral 2% (posterior communicating and distal posterior cerebral)

Basiliar 10%
  Bifurcation 7%
  Basilar trunk 3%

Vertebral—posterior inferior cerebellar 3%

} Posterior circulation 15%

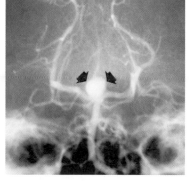

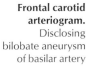

Frontal carotid arteriogram. Disclosing bilobate aneurysm of basilar artery

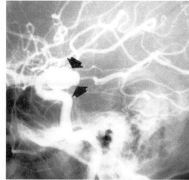

Different patient. Lateral view showing large aneurysm of internal carotid artery at origin of posterior communicating artery

FIGURE 13-24 CONGENITAL INTRACRANIAL ANEURYSMS

Although saccular (berry) aneurysms are generally referred to as **congenital aneurysms**, they are actually caused by a combination of congenital and acquired factors. The congenital defect is a focal absence of the media, particularly at arterial bifurcations. Hemodynamic forces cause the intima to bulge into the adventitia creating the aneurysm, followed by intimal proliferation. Atherosclerosis and hypertension accelerate the process. The relative distribution of aneurysms involving arteries

of the circle of Willis and distributing branches is illustrated. Complications of a rupture include subarachnoid hemorrhage, intracerebral hemorrhage, infarction, and vasospasm. The onset of symptoms after aneurysm rupture is abrupt and rapid, with sudden, severe headache and alteration in consciousness. The mortality rate from rupture is high; rapid diagnosis and surgical intervention are essential to prevent death.

Border zone ischemia (shock, circulatory insufficiency)

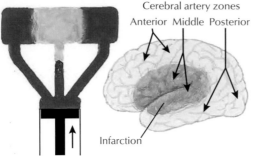

Cerebral artery zones
Anterior Middle Posterior

Infarction

Pump with 3 outflows, 1 outflow blocked; deficit occurs in zone it supplies

If brain artery is blocked, infarction occurs in zone supplied by that vessel

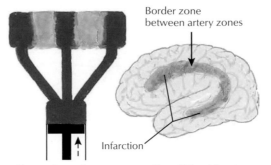

Border zone between artery zones

Infarction

If pump is weak, deficit is between zone supplied by 3 outflows

If total blood flow is inadequate, deficit is mostly at border zone between supply zones

Diffuse cortical necrosis; persistent vegetative state

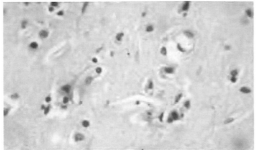

Few anoxic neurons in early anoxia

Extensive laminar necrosis

Brain death

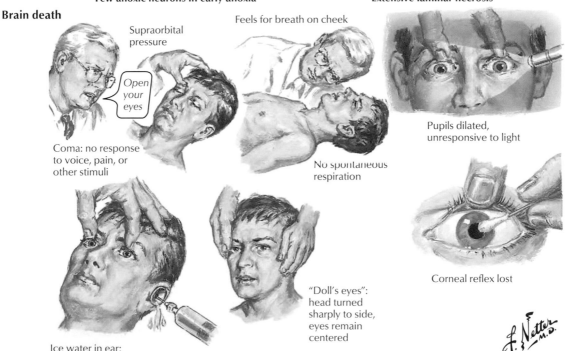

Supraorbital pressure

Open your eyes

Coma: no response to voice, pain, or other stimuli

Feels for breath on cheek

No spontaneous respiration

Pupils dilated, unresponsive to light

Ice water in ear: eyes do not move

"Doll's eyes": head turned sharply to side, eyes remain centered

Corneal reflex lost

FIGURE 13-25   HYPOXIC BRAIN DAMAGE AND BRAIN DEATH

Cardiac arrest or severe cardiac failure leads rapidly to generalized hypoperfusion of the brain and hypoxic brain injury. The extent, severity, and location of hypoxic brain damage are influenced by the degree and duration of circulation collapse (full cardiac arrest or hypotension, with some preserved cardiac pump function) and other factors, such as accompanying respiratory failure. Persistent hypotension usually leads to border zone ischemic lesions, whereas cardiac arrest causes more extensive cortical necrosis, which may include the cerebral gray matter, brainstem nuclei, and the hippocampus. Regions of the brain most susceptible to ischemic damage are the Purkinje cells of the cerebellum, the hippocampus, and border zone (watershed) regions at the boundaries of the territories of major arteries supplying the cerebral cortex. Severe ischemia sets in motion a chain of events leading to irreversible brain death.

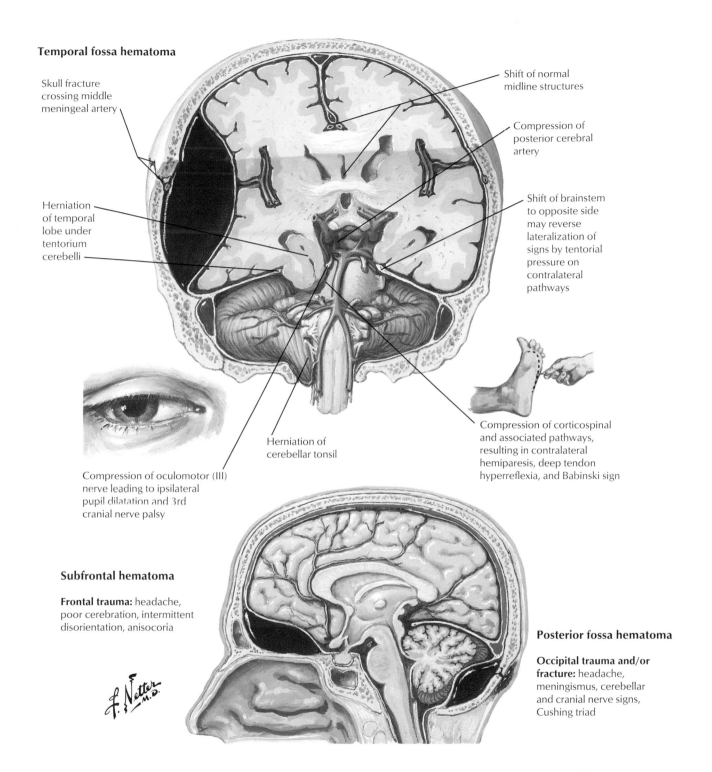

Temporal fossa hematoma

Skull fracture crossing middle meningeal artery

Herniation of temporal lobe under tentorium cerebelli

Shift of normal midline structures

Compression of posterior cerebral artery

Shift of brainstem to opposite side may reverse lateralization of signs by tentorial pressure on contralateral pathways

Compression of corticospinal and associated pathways, resulting in contralateral hemiparesis, deep tendon hyperreflexia, and Babinski sign

Herniation of cerebellar tonsil

Compression of oculomotor (III) nerve leading to ipsilateral pupil dilatation and 3rd cranial nerve palsy

Subfrontal hematoma

Frontal trauma: headache, poor cerebration, intermittent disorientation, anisocoria

Posterior fossa hematoma

Occipital trauma and/or fracture: headache, meningismus, cerebellar and cranial nerve signs, Cushing triad

FIGURE 13-26 EPIDURAL HEMATOMA

Traumatic brain injuries include concussion, contusion, skull fracture, and, in a small percentage of major head injuries, epidural hematomas. Usually, the bleeding is from arterial injury. Common locations of epidural hematomas are the temporal fossa, the subfrontal region, and the occipital-suboccipital area. The **temporal fossa epidural hematoma**, which results from damage to the middle meningeal artery, is the most common epidural hematoma. The classic course is a period of unconsciousness due to a concussion, a period of lucidity as the dura mater initially slows the leakage of blood, and a rapid deterioration of consciousness. An aggressive diagnostic and surgical approach is required to save the patient.

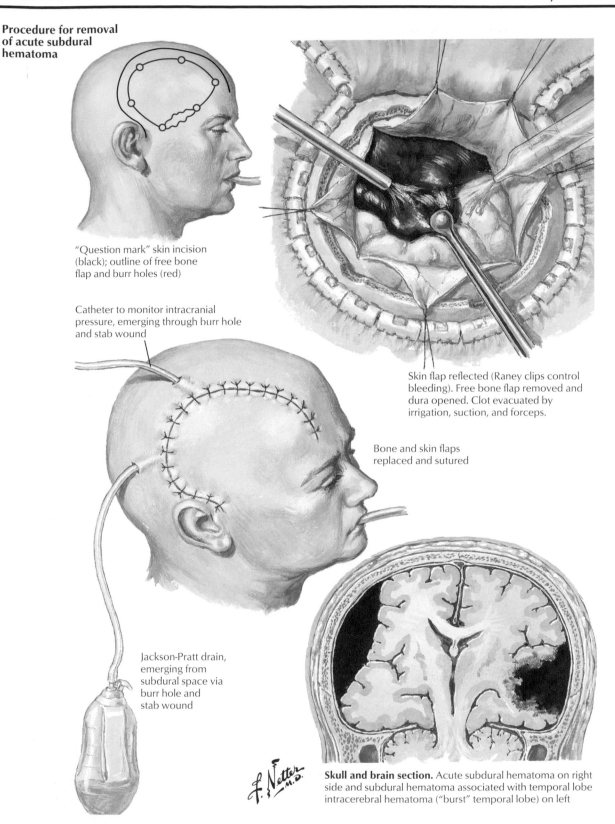

Procedure for removal of acute subdural hematoma

"Question mark" skin incision (black); outline of free bone flap and burr holes (red)

Catheter to monitor intracranial pressure, emerging through burr hole and stab wound

Skin flap reflected (Raney clips control bleeding). Free bone flap removed and dura opened. Clot evacuated by irrigation, suction, and forceps.

Bone and skin flaps replaced and sutured

Jackson-Pratt drain, emerging from subdural space via burr hole and stab wound

Skull and brain section. Acute subdural hematoma on right side and subdural hematoma associated with temporal lobe intracerebral hematoma ("burst" temporal lobe) on left

FIGURE 13-27   ACUTE AND CHRONIC SUBDURAL HEMATOMA

A **subdural hematoma** usually results from an acute venous hemorrhage caused by rupture of cortical bridging veins. Acute subdural hematomas, which are often associated with skull fractures, usually develop within hours after injury. Associated massive cerebral or brainstem contusions or both contribute to a high mortality rate. Common signs are depressed consciousness, ipsilateral pupillary dilatation, and contralateral hemiparesis. Chronic subdural hematomas in infants can occur as a result of birth trauma. In adults, they are more common in the elderly, patients with chronic alcoholism, and patients receiving long-term anticoagulant therapy or who have a blood dyscrasia. The precipitating trauma is often trivial. Brain atrophy with an

Craniostomy for Chronic Subdural Hematoma

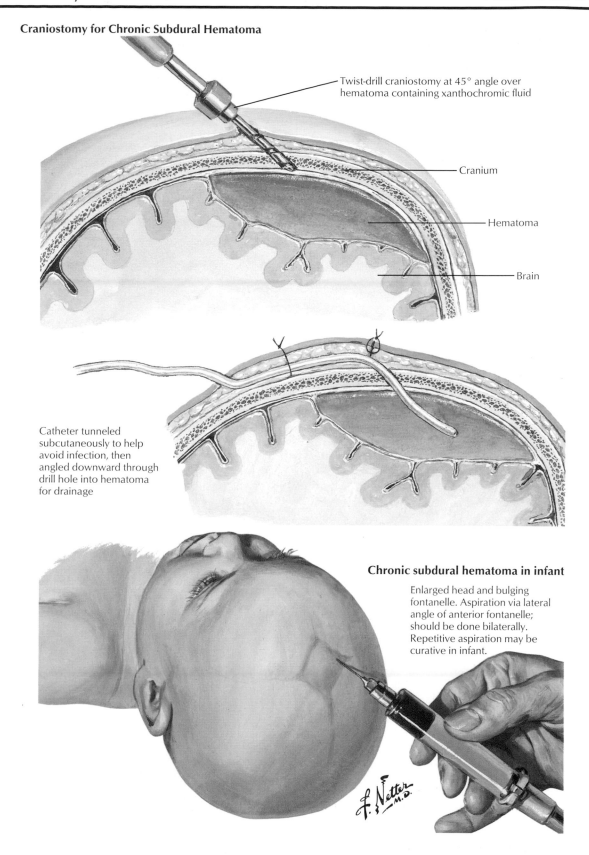

Twist-drill craniostomy at 45° angle over hematoma containing xanthochromic fluid

Cranium

Hematoma

Brain

Catheter tunneled subcutaneously to help avoid infection, then angled downward through drill hole into hematoma for drainage

Chronic subdural hematoma in infant

Enlarged head and bulging fontanelle. Aspiration via lateral angle of anterior fontanelle; should be done bilaterally. Repetitive aspiration may be curative in infant.

FIGURE 13-27   ACUTE AND CHRONIC SUBDURAL HEMATOMA (CONTINUED)

increase in the subdural space is a predisposing factor. A vascular membrane forms around the lesion within 2 weeks after the initial hemorrhage fills the available subdural space. The hematoma enlarges slowly until it produces symptoms. The clinical course can be subtle, with waxing and waning signs and symptoms. The differential diagnosis includes stroke, infection, or psychosis.

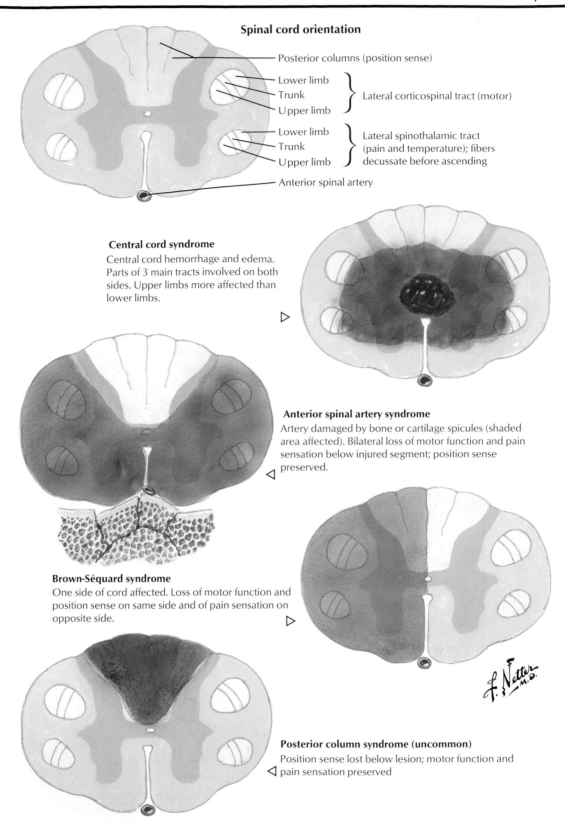

Spinal cord orientation

Posterior columns (position sense)

Lower limb
Trunk
Upper limb
} Lateral corticospinal tract (motor)

Lower limb
Trunk
Upper limb
} Lateral spinothalamic tract (pain and temperature); fibers decussate before ascending

Anterior spinal artery

Central cord syndrome
Central cord hemorrhage and edema. Parts of 3 main tracts involved on both sides. Upper limbs more affected than lower limbs.

Anterior spinal artery syndrome
Artery damaged by bone or cartilage spicules (shaded area affected). Bilateral loss of motor function and pain sensation below injured segment; position sense preserved.

Brown-Séquard syndrome
One side of cord affected. Loss of motor function and position sense on same side and of pain sensation on opposite side.

Posterior column syndrome (uncommon)
Position sense lost below lesion; motor function and pain sensation preserved

FIGURE 13-28   CERVICAL SPINE INJURY: INCOMPLETE SPINAL CORD SYNDROMES

Spinal cord injuries are produced by motor vehicle accidents, other types of accidents, and missile or knife wounds. Spinal cord injury, which involves direct neuronal trauma and direct and delayed injury to the vasculature, can result in a variety of neurologic deficits. The most frequent injuries occur at the levels of the lower cervical vertebrae and the thoracolumbar junction. The resulting neurologic deficits comprise complete functional interruption, partial functional interruption, nerve root deficit, Brown-Séquard syndrome, central cord damage, and other deficits. Initial treatment is aimed at reducing the extent of damage by preventing the delayed component of injury. Currently, there is great expectation that neuronal regeneration can be achieved to treat patients with paraplegia and other deficits from spinal cord injury.

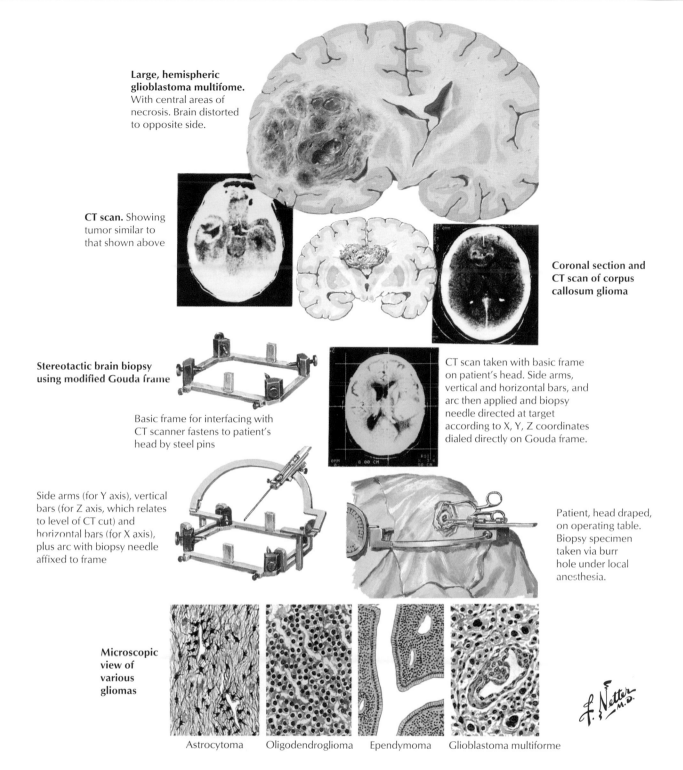

Large, hemispheric glioblastoma multiforme. With central areas of necrosis. Brain distorted to opposite side.

CT scan. Showing tumor similar to that shown above

Coronal section and CT scan of corpus callosum glioma

Stereotactic brain biopsy using modified Gouda frame

Basic frame for interfacing with CT scanner fastens to patient's head by steel pins

CT scan taken with basic frame on patient's head. Side arms, vertical and horizontal bars, and arc then applied and biopsy needle directed at target according to X, Y, Z coordinates dialed directly on Gouda frame.

Side arms (for Y axis), vertical bars (for Z axis, which relates to level of CT cut) and horizontal bars (for X axis), plus arc with biopsy needle affixed to frame

Patient, head draped, on operating table. Biopsy specimen taken via burr hole under local anesthesia.

Microscopic view of various gliomas

Astrocytoma   Oligodendroglioma   Ependymoma   Glioblastoma multiforme

FIGURE 13-29   GLIOMAS

Patients with brain tumors present with symptoms resulting from either increased intracranial pressure or focal brain dysfunction. Gliomas, the most common tumors of the brain, arise from the glial supporting tissue rather than the neurons. The tumors show differentiation toward any of the normal glial components (astrocytoma, oligodendroglioma, ependymoma, and ganglioneuroma). The tumors of each cell type range from moderately well-differentiated, slow-growing neoplasms to pleomorphic,

rapidly growing tumors, the most common of which is the **glioblastoma multiforme**. The glioblastomas are characterized by vascular proliferation and necrosis and cellular pleomorphism. The prognosis, which varies with the location and type of tumor, is difficult to determine because glioblastomas may show a mixed pattern with high-grade areas adjacent to low-grade areas, and low-grade tumors tend to progress over time to high-grade lesions.

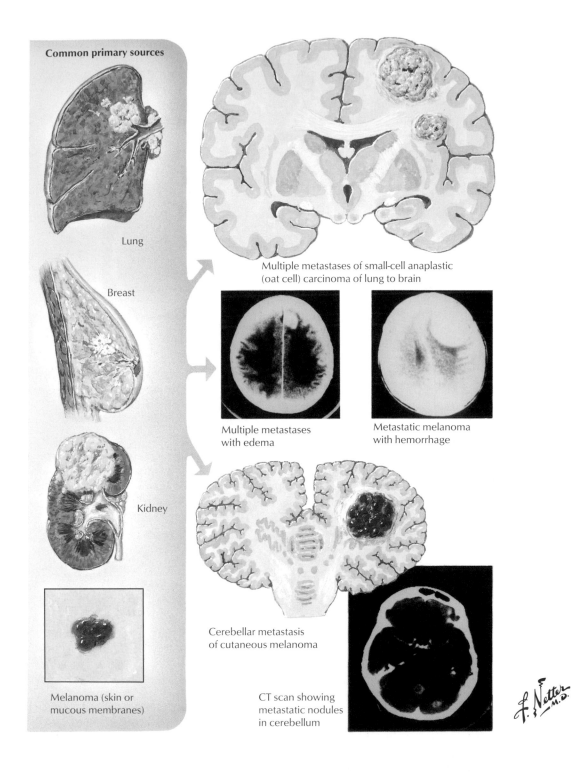

Multiple metastases of small-cell anaplastic (oat cell) carcinoma of lung to brain

Multiple metastases with edema

Metastatic melanoma with hemorrhage

Cerebellar metastasis of cutaneous melanoma

CT scan showing metastatic nodules in cerebellum

Common primary sources

Lung

Breast

Kidney

Melanoma (skin or mucous membranes)

FIGURE 13-30 TUMORS METASTATIC TO THE BRAIN

Certain common neoplasms, particularly carcinomas of the lung and the breast, as well as less common neoplasms, including carcinoma of the kidney and melanoma, have a propensity to metastasize to the brain or spinal cord. Metastatic brain tumors are more common than primary brain tumors. Brain metastases may be the first manifestation of an aggressive tumor such as lung cancer. Most metastatic tumors reach the brain through the bloodstream (hematogenous metastases) and become localized at the border between white and gray matter, although occasionally a tumor may spread directly to the brain by local extension from a head and neck cancer or via Batson venous plexus. Metastatic tumors are usually well demarcated and solid, but they may be cystic. Some tumors may be hemorrhagic at the time of presentation, confusing the real diagnosis. The lesions are frequently multiple. CSF examination may yield evidence of meningeal carcinomatosis.

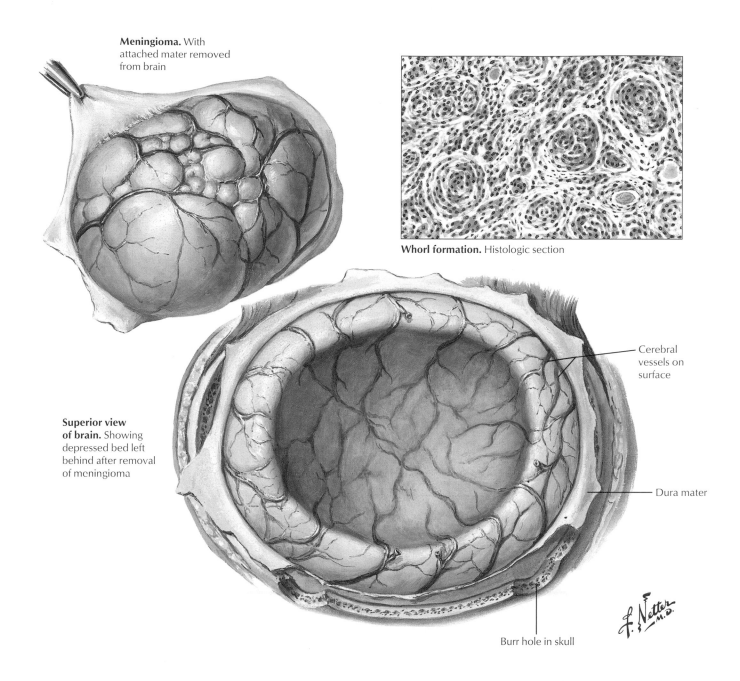

Meningioma. With attached mater removed from brain

Whorl formation. Histologic section

Superior view of brain. Showing depressed bed left behind after removal of meningioma

Cerebral vessels on surface

Dura mater

Burr hole in skull

FIGURE 13-31 MENINGIOMAS

Meningiomas are the most common of the benign brain tumors. Their incidence increases with age, with a moderate female preponderance. Meningiomas, which arise from arachnoid cells in the meninges, are nearly always benign, but rare malignant variants occur. Most meningiomas are composed of groups of cells arranged in a whorled pattern without identifiable cell membranes (syncytial type), sometimes containing large numbers of calcified psammoma bodies (psammomatous type). Fibroblastic and transitional variants also occur. The symptoms depend on location of the tumor, the growth rate, and adherence to adjacent structures rather than on histologic type. Meningiomas may extend into venous structures, such as the superior sagittal sinus, or erode into the bone of the skull.

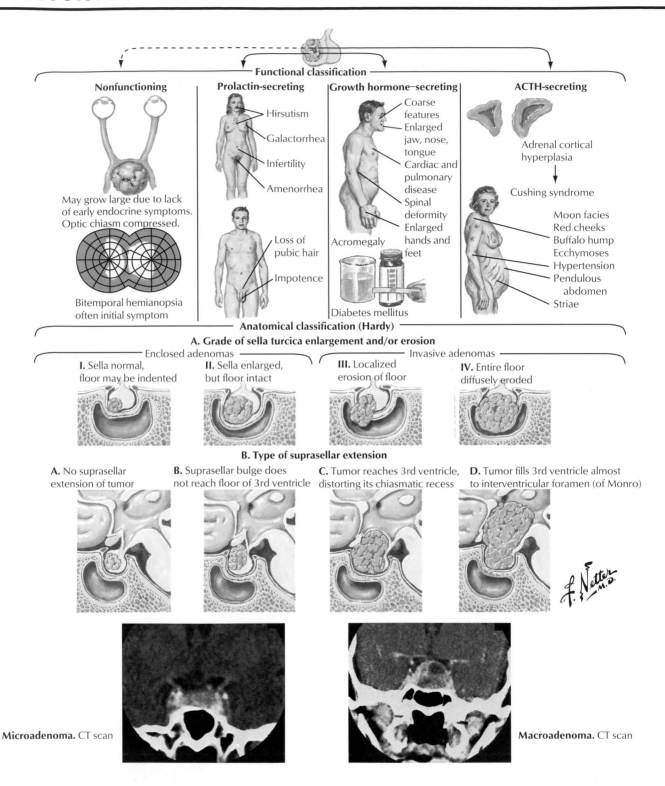

Functional classification

Nonfunctioning

May grow large due to lack of early endocrine symptoms. Optic chiasm compressed.

Bitemporal hemianopsia often initial symptom

Prolactin–secreting

Hirsutism

Galactorrhea

Infertility

Amenorrhea

Loss of pubic hair

Impotence

Growth hormone–secreting

Coarse features
Enlarged jaw, nose, tongue
Cardiac and pulmonary disease
Spinal deformity
Enlarged hands and feet

Acromegaly

Diabetes mellitus

ACTH-secreting

Adrenal cortical hyperplasia

Cushing syndrome

Moon facies
Red cheeks
Buffalo hump
Ecchymoses
Hypertension
Pendulous abdomen
Striae

Anatomical classification (Hardy)

A. Grade of sella turcica enlargement and/or erosion

Enclosed adenomas

I. Sella normal, floor may be indented

II. Sella enlarged, but floor intact

Invasive adenomas

III. Localized erosion of floor

IV. Entire floor diffusely eroded

B. Type of suprasellar extension

A. No suprasellar extension of tumor

B. Suprasellar bulge does not reach floor of 3rd ventricle

C. Tumor reaches 3rd ventricle, distorting its chiasmatic recess

D. Tumor fills 3rd ventricle almost to interventricular foramen (of Monro)

Microadenoma. CT scan

Macroadenoma. CT scan

FIGURE 13-32 PITUITARY TUMORS

Pituitary tumors of the adenohypophysis are classified on both a functional and an anatomical basis. With the use of standard histology, the tumors are classified as eosinophilic adenoma, basophilic adenoma, and chromophobe adenoma. The **eosinophilic adenoma** is associated with acromegaly, and the **basophilic adenoma** is associated with Cushing syndrome. The **chromophobe adenoma**, the most common type of tumor, may be nonfunctioning. A more accurate classification can be obtained by immunocytochemical staining for specific hormones. Clinically important features include the degree of sella turcica enlargement and erosion and the type of suprasellar extension. Precise delineation of tumor extent can be obtained with a combination of CT and MRI scans and angiography.

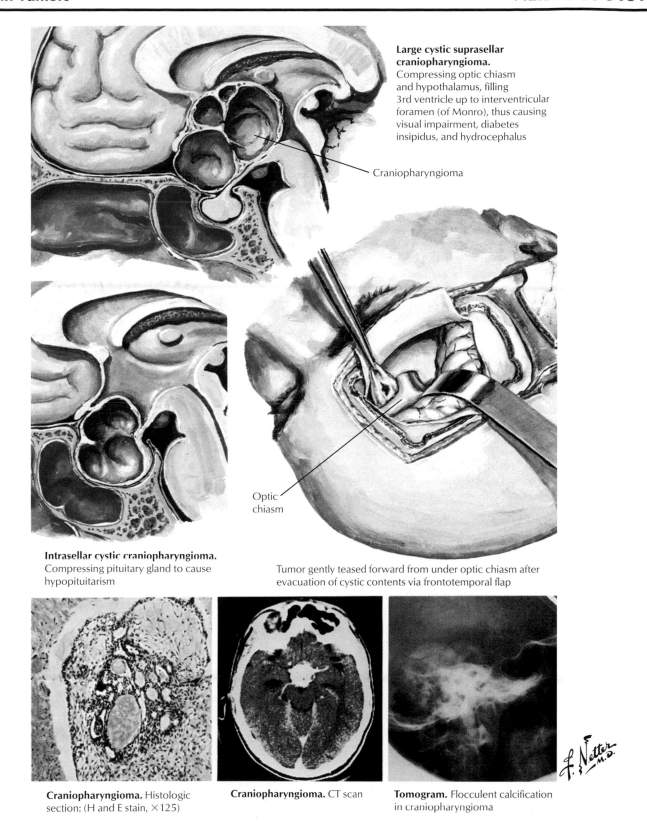

Large cystic suprasellar craniopharyngioma. Compressing optic chiasm and hypothalamus, filling 3rd ventricle up to interventricular foramen (of Monro), thus causing visual impairment, diabetes insipidus, and hydrocephalus

Craniopharyngioma

Optic chiasm

Intrasellar cystic craniopharyngioma. Compressing pituitary gland to cause hypopituitarism

Tumor gently teased forward from under optic chiasm after evacuation of cystic contents via frontotemporal flap

Craniopharyngioma. Histologic section: (H and E stain, ×125)

Craniopharyngioma. CT scan

Tomogram. Flocculent calcification in craniopharyngioma

FIGURE 13-33   CRANIOPHARYNGIOMAS

Craniopharyngiomas are the most common parasellar tumors in children, but they also occur in adults. Craniopharyngiomas arise from remnants of the Rathke pouch derived from the embryonic pharynx. The lesion is composed of clusters of columnar and cuboidal epithelial cells. The tumor may be solid or cystic because of formation of degenerative areas containing oily fluid, calcium, and keratin. The tumor routinely extends to the optic chiasm. A craniopharyngioma produces visual symptoms secondary to compression of the optic tract. Approximately 50% of patients have endocrine dysfunction, with diabetes insipidus, panhypopituitarism, and gonadal deficiency in adults and growth retardation and obesity in children. Hydrocephalus, often with papilledema, also can develop in children with this tumor.

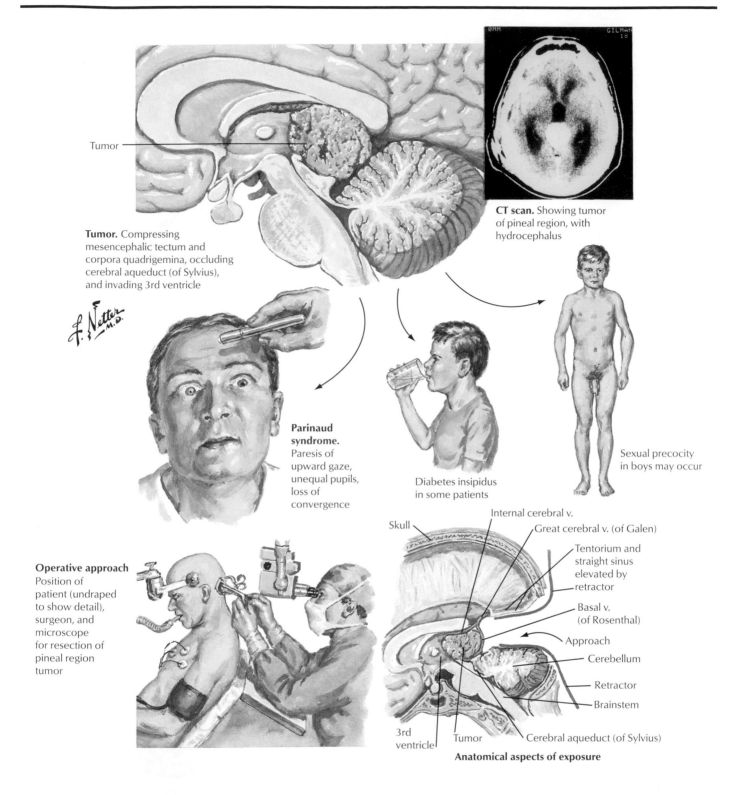

Tumor. Compressing mesencephalic tectum and corpora quadrigemina, occluding cerebral aqueduct (of Sylvius), and invading 3rd ventricle

CT scan. Showing tumor of pineal region, with hydrocephalus

Parinaud syndrome. Paresis of upward gaze, unequal pupils, loss of convergence

Diabetes insipidus in some patients

Sexual precocity in boys may occur

Operative approach Position of patient (undraped to show detail), surgeon, and microscope for resection of pineal region tumor

Skull

Internal cerebral v.

Great cerebral v. (of Galen)

Tentorium and straight sinus elevated by retractor

Basal v. (of Rosenthal)

Approach

Cerebellum

Retractor

Brainstem

3rd ventricle

Tumor

Cerebral aqueduct (of Sylvius)

Anatomical aspects of exposure

FIGURE 13-34   TUMORS OF THE PINEAL REGION

The pineal gland has a strategic central location in the brain surrounded by vital structures, including the posterior third ventricle. Symptoms result from compression or involvement of these vital structures by the pineal tumor. Pineal tumors can be classified into tumors of germ cell origin, tumors of the pineal parenchyma, and a miscellaneous group. **Tumors of germ cell origin** are germinomas and teratomas. **Germinomas**, which comprise approximately half of all pineal tumors, are most common in adolescents and have a marked predilection for

males. **Teratomas** have a similar male predilection. These tumors usually present with endocrine abnormalities. The germinoma usually spreads via the CSF but is radiosensitive, whereas teratomas are not invasive. **Pinealcytoma** is well circumscribed and noninvasive. It occurs at any age and has no sex predilection. The **malignant pineal blastoma** is composed of primitive cells resembling medulloblastoma and spreads within the CSF. Other pineal tumors include benign meningiomas and cysts.

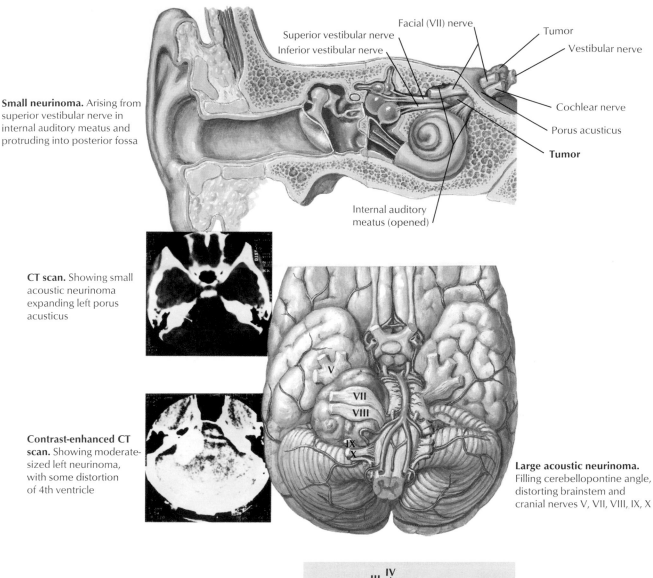

Small neurinoma. Arising from superior vestibular nerve in internal auditory meatus and protruding into posterior fossa

Superior vestibular nerve
Inferior vestibular nerve
Facial (VII) nerve
Tumor
Vestibular nerve
Cochlear nerve
Porus acusticus
Tumor
Internal auditory meatus (opened)

CT scan. Showing small acoustic neurinoma expanding left porus acusticus

Contrast-enhanced CT scan. Showing moderate-sized left neurinoma, with some distortion of 4th ventricle

Large acoustic neurinoma. Filling cerebellopontine angle, distorting brainstem and cranial nerves V, VII, VIII, IX, X

Brainstem auditory evoked response (BAER). In patient with acoustic neurnoma on right side. There is delay in action potentials of cochlear nerve (wave I) and cochlear nuclei (wave II) on affected side.

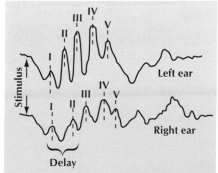

Left ear

Right ear

Delay

FIGURE 13-35 ACOUSTIC NEUROMAS

Acoustic neuromas cause characteristic symptoms resulting from a mass effect in the cerebellopontine angle. The acoustic neuroma typically arises from the Schwann cells of the vestibular nerve, and the tumor slowly impairs the vestibular and cochlear nerves. Undiagnosed, the tumor can continue to expand and produce brainstem compression and **hydrocephalus**. In addition to hearing loss and tinnitus, early symptoms of acoustic neuroma may include tic douloureux, ataxia, facial sensory loss, or, occasionally, even dementia. A hearing loss for high tones, with impaired speech discrimination, frequently occurs. Involvement of the facial (VII) and trigeminal (V) nerves indicates a large tumor.

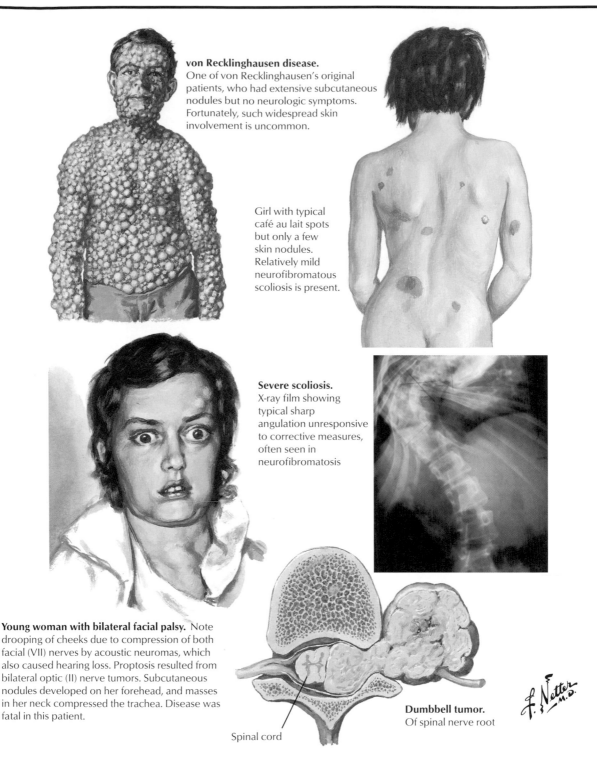

von Recklinghausen disease.
One of von Recklinghausen's original patients, who had extensive subcutaneous nodules but no neurologic symptoms. Fortunately, such widespread skin involvement is uncommon.

Girl with typical café au lait spots but only a few skin nodules. Relatively mild neurofibromatous scoliosis is present.

Severe scoliosis.
X-ray film showing typical sharp angulation unresponsive to corrective measures, often seen in neurofibromatosis

Young woman with bilateral facial palsy. Note drooping of cheeks due to compression of both facial (VII) nerves by acoustic neuromas, which also caused hearing loss. Proptosis resulted from bilateral optic (II) nerve tumors. Subcutaneous nodules developed on her forehead, and masses in her neck compressed the trachea. Disease was fatal in this patient.

Spinal cord

Dumbbell tumor.
Of spinal nerve root

FIGURE 13-36 NEUROFIBROMATOSIS

Neurofibromatosis, or **von Recklinghausen disease**, is the most common of a group of inherited disorders known as *phacomatoses* that involve tissues derived embryologically from the neural crest, including the nervous system and components of the skin. Pathologic lesions of neurofibromatosis consist of café-au-lait spots representing cutaneous patches formed by melanin-containing cells derived from the neural crest and neurofibromas formed from neural crest–derived Schwann cells involving the cranial and peripheral nerves. Gliomas and meningiomas also occur with increased frequency in neurofibromatosis. **Peripheral neurofibromatosis** is characterized by multiple subcutaneous tumors of the peripheral nerves but without apparent central nervous system involvement. The various forms of neurofibromatosis represent a common group of human genetic mutations, with autosomal dominant inheritance. **Bilateral acoustic neuromas** and other intracranial lesions can produce debilitating disease.

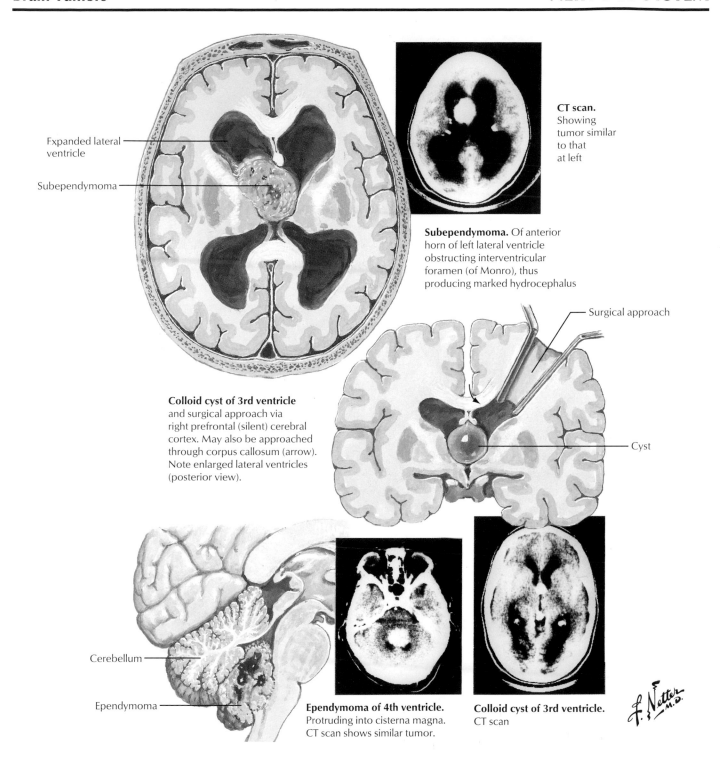

Fxpanded lateral ventricle

Subependymoma

CT scan. Showing tumor similar to that at left

Subependymoma. Of anterior horn of left lateral ventricle obstructing interventricular foramen (of Monro), thus producing marked hydrocephalus

Surgical approach

Colloid cyst of 3rd ventricle and surgical approach via right prefrontal (silent) cerebral cortex. May also be approached through corpus callosum (arrow). Note enlarged lateral ventricles (posterior view).

Cyst

Cerebellum

Ependymoma

Ependymoma of 4th ventricle. Protruding into cisterna magna. CT scan shows similar tumor.

Colloid cyst of 3rd ventricle. CT scan

FIGURE 13-37   INTRAVENTRICULAR TUMORS

Intraventricular tumors are a heterogeneous group that shares a unique position within the brain. These lesions produce symptoms by local pressure and invasion, with the common finding being hydrocephalus. Tumors of the lateral ventricles may arise from the choroid plexus (meningioma and choroid plexus papilloma) or from the brain parenchyma (ependymoma, astrocytoma, subependymoma, and the giant cell tumor of tuberous sclerosis). Anterior third ventricle tumors are colloid cysts, giant craniopharyngioma, and pituitary adenoma. Posterior third ventricle tumors are pineal gland tumors. Tumors of the posterior cranial fossa can be subdivided into 3 groups. The extracerebral tumors are acoustic neuroma, meningioma, and cholesteatoma. Cerebellar hemispheric tumors are cystic astrocytoma and medulloblastoma in children and metastases and astrocytoma in adults. Tumors of the fourth ventricle are ependymoma and subependymoma.

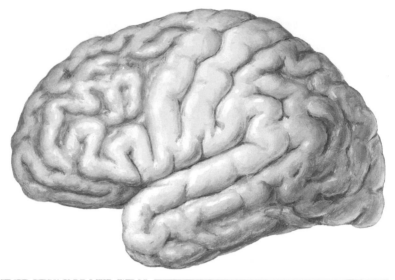

Regional atrophy of brain with narrowed gyri and widened sulci, but precentral and postcentral, inferior frontal, angular, supramarginal, and some occipital gyri fairly well preserved. Association cortex mostly involved.

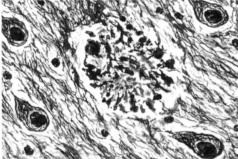

Senile plaque (center) made up of argyrophil fibers around core of pink-staining amyloid (Bodian preparation). Neurons decreased in number, with characteristic tangles in cytoplasm.

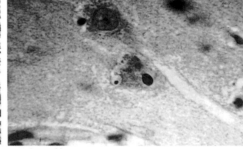

Section of hippocampus showing granulovacuolar inclusions and loss of pyramidal cells

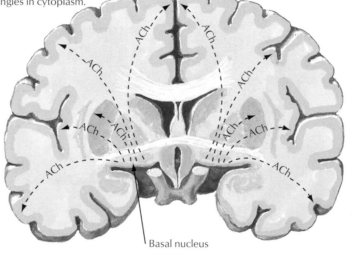

Section of brain schematically demonstrating postulated normal transport of acetylcholine (ACh) from basal nucleus of Meynert (substantia innominata) to cortical gray matter

Basal nucleus

FIGURE 13-38   ALZHEIMER DISEASE: PATHOLOGY

Alzheimer disease, a distinctive form of senile dementia, is a progressive neurologic disorder usually presenting in older adults and characterized by slowly progressive loss of higher intellectual capacity and memory followed by more severe cerebral dysfunction. The distinctive pathologic lesions are the so-called senile plaques, composed of argyrophilic fibers surrounding a central core of amyloid material, and the argyrophilic neurofibrillary tangles in neurons. Granulovacuolar inclusions may also be seen in some neurons. The process results in progressive loss of neurons and cerebral atrophy. The regions of the brain most involved in Alzheimer disease correspond to pathways of neurotransmitter transport, specifically acetylcholine. Certain brain regions, the precentral, postcentral, and some occipital gyri and perisylvian regions, for example, are spared, whereas the prefrontal, superior parietal, and inferior temporal gyri become severely atrophied, eventually involving the frontal lobes.

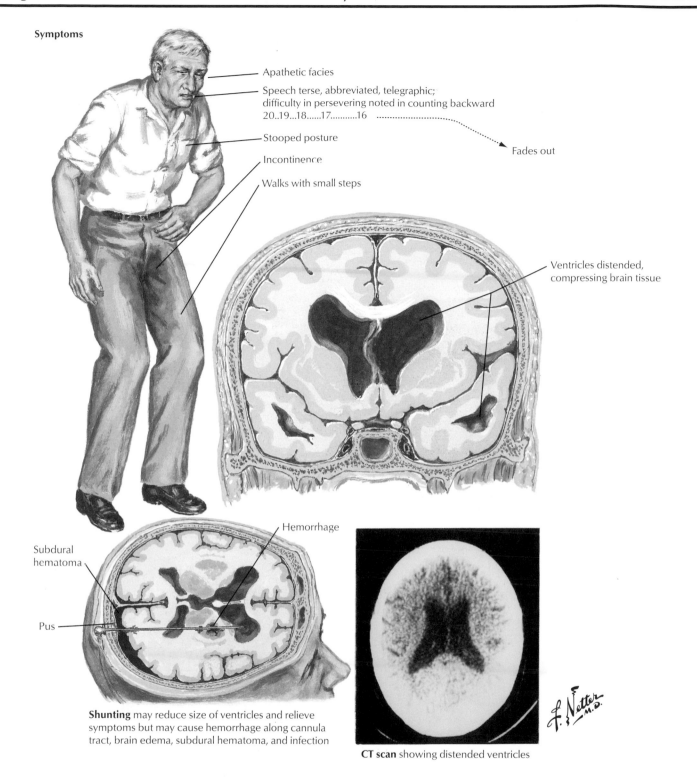

Symptoms

Apathetic facies

Speech terse, abbreviated, telegraphic; difficulty in persevering noted in counting backward 20..19...18......17..........16

Fades out

Stooped posture

Incontinence

Walks with small steps

Ventricles distended, compressing brain tissue

Hemorrhage

Subdural hematoma

Pus

Shunting may reduce size of ventricles and relieve symptoms but may cause hemorrhage along cannula tract, brain edema, subdural hematoma, and infection

CT scan showing distended ventricles

FIGURE 13-39 NORMAL-PRESSURE HYDROCEPHALUS

Normal-pressure hydrocephalus is a disease of the elderly that develops over a period of several months or more insidiously. Most symptoms relate to enlargement of the anterior horns and loss of frontal lobe white matter. The clinical course is dominated by the triad of dementia, abnormalities of gait, and incontinence. If more CSF is produced than is absorbed, the ventricles and subarachnoid space become distended with CSF. Conditions that cause scarring of the piarachnoid membranes, such as meningeal infection, subarachnoid hemorrhage, or bleeding from past traumas, can cause hydrocephalus by decreasing the effectiveness of CSF absorption. However, in most elderly patients, communicating hydrocephalus has no easily identifiable cause.

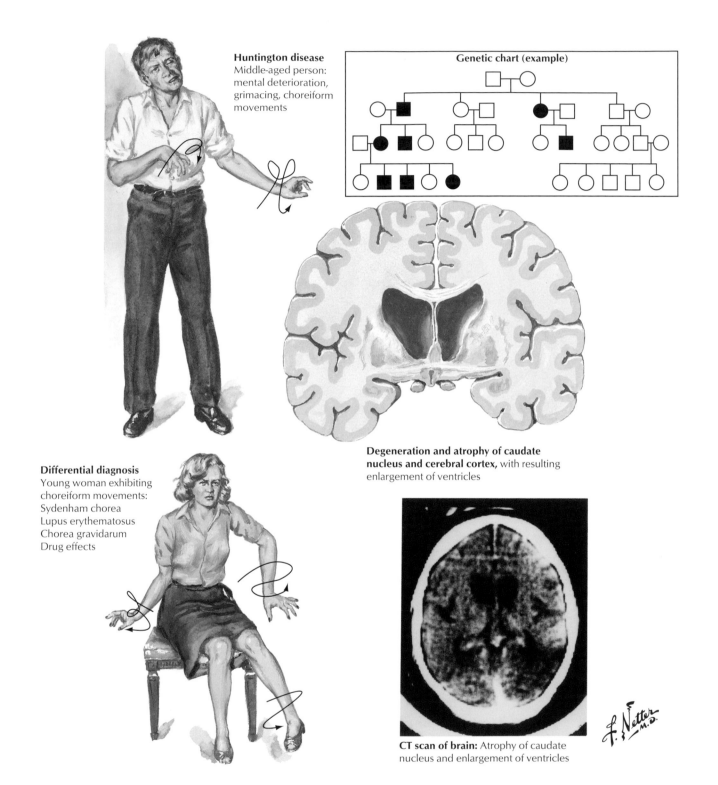

Huntington disease
Middle-aged person: mental deterioration, grimacing, choreiform movements

Genetic chart (example)

Degeneration and atrophy of caudate nucleus and cerebral cortex, with resulting enlargement of ventricles

Differential diagnosis
Young woman exhibiting choreiform movements:
Sydenham chorea
Lupus erythematosus
Chorea gravidarum
Drug effects

CT scan of brain: Atrophy of caudate nucleus and enlargement of ventricles

FIGURE 13-40 CHOREA

Chorea is a term applied to rapid, complex, and varied movements of the body, especially the distal limbs. The differential diagnosis includes Sydenham chorea (acute rheumatic fever), systemic lupus erythematosus, chorea gravidarum (in pregnant women), drug effects, and Huntington chorea. Abnormal facial and limb movements, behavioral disturbances, and progressive dementia characterize Huntington disease, a degenerative disorder with an autosomal dominant inheritance pattern, with onset usually after the age of 40 years. The genetic mutation is carried by approximately 50% of the offspring of an affected individual. Autopsy reveals severe shrinkage of the caudate nucleus and cortical atrophy, especially of the frontal lobes.

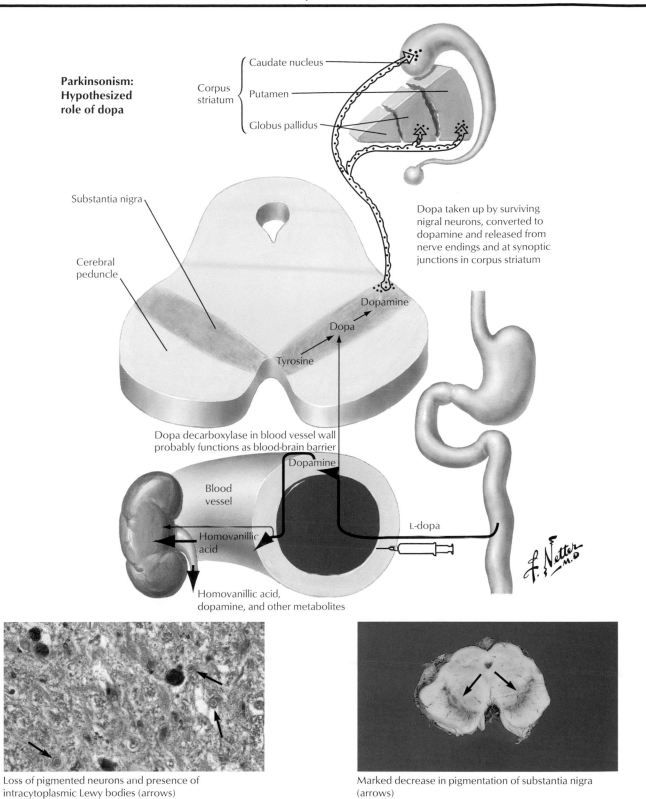

Parkinsonism:
Hypothesized
role of dopa

Caudate nucleus

Corpus striatum

Putamen

Globus pallidus

Dopa taken up by surviving nigral neurons, converted to dopamine and released from nerve endings and at synoptic junctions in corpus striatum

Substantia nigra

Cerebral peduncle

Dopamine

Dopa

Tyrosine

Dopa decarboxylase in blood vessel wall probably functions as blood-brain barrier

Dopamine

Blood vessel

L-dopa

Homovanillic acid

Homovanillic acid, dopamine, and other metabolites

Loss of pigmented neurons and presence of intracytoplasmic Lewy bodies (arrows)

Marked decrease in pigmentation of substantia nigra (arrows)

FIGURE 13-41   PARKINSON DISEASE AND RELATED DISORDERS

Parkinsonism is a clinical syndrome characterized by impaired facial expression, slow voluntary movements, intention tremor, and characteristic gait with increasingly shortened, quickened steps. Impairment of the nigrostriatal dopaminergic system is the underlying mechanism for the variety of conditions that produce the characteristic motor alterations. The pathology of Parkinson disease is characterized by degeneration of the substantia nigra with loss of the normal black pigmentation. Microscopic examination shows loss of neuronal cells and mild reactive gliosis in the substantia nigra, the locus ceruleus, the substantia innominata, and certain reticular nuclei. Many neurons contain distinctive eosinophilic spherical inclusions known as **Lewy bodies**.

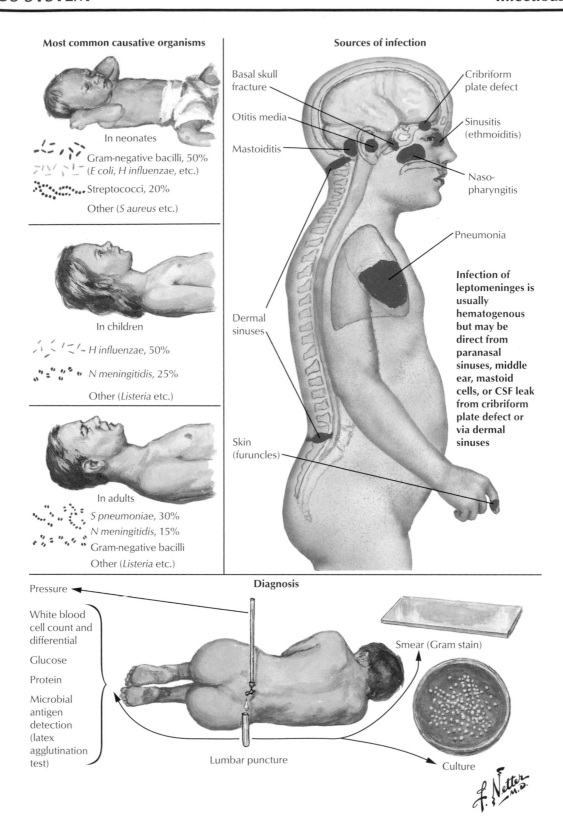

Most common causative organisms

In neonates

Gram-negative bacilli, 50%
(*E coli, H influenzae*, etc.)

Streptococci, 20%

Other (*S aureus* etc.)

In children

H influenzae, 50%

N meningitidis, 25%

Other (*Listeria* etc.)

In adults

S pneumoniae, 30%
N meningitidis, 15%
Gram-negative bacilli

Other (*Listeria* etc.)

Sources of infection

Basal skull fracture

Otitis media

Mastoiditis

Cribriform plate defect

Sinusitis (ethmoiditis)

Naso-pharyngitis

Pneumonia

Infection of leptomeninges is usually hematogenous but may be direct from paranasal sinuses, middle ear, mastoid cells, or CSF leak from cribriform plate defect or via dermal sinuses

Dermal sinuses

Skin (furuncles)

Diagnosis

Pressure

White blood cell count and differential

Glucose

Protein

Microbial antigen detection (latex agglutination test)

Lumbar puncture

Smear (Gram stain)

Culture

FIGURE 13-42 BACTERIAL MENINGITIS

Meningitis, or inflammation of the leptomeningitis and CSF, is usually caused by spread of a microorganism through the bloodstream from another site, such as the ears, the throat, the lungs, or the skin. Less frequent causes include contiguous spread of infection from the paranasal sinuses or the mastoid process or from penetrating trauma. The most likely infectious agents vary according to the age of the patient. Predisposing factors include defects causing leakage of spinal fluid, sickle cell anemia, alcoholism, cirrhosis of the liver, immunodeficient states, and asplenia. The disease usually progresses rapidly with symptoms

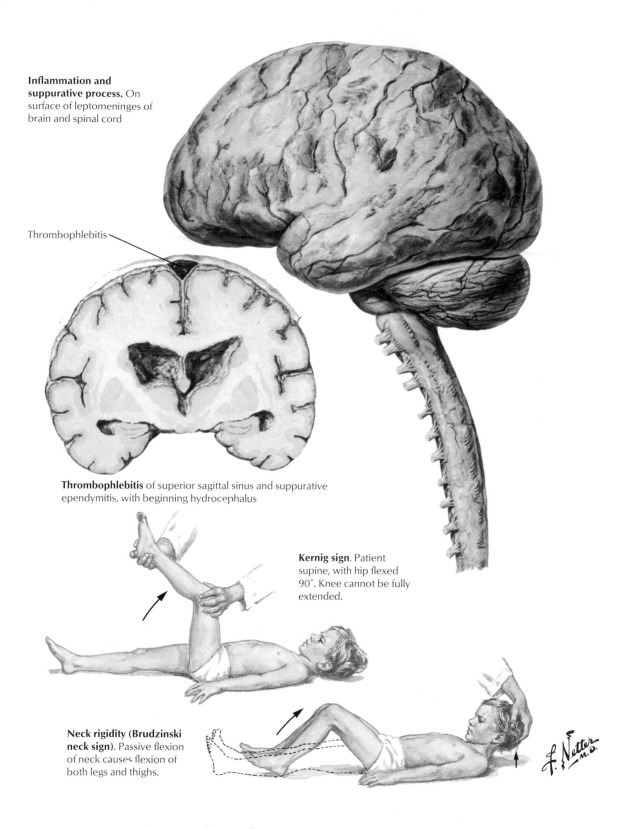

Inflammation and suppurative process. On surface of leptomeninges of brain and spinal cord

Thrombophlebitis

Thrombophlebitis of superior sagittal sinus and suppurative ependymitis, with beginning hydrocephalus

Kernig sign. Patient supine, with hip flexed 90°. Knee cannot be fully extended.

Neck rigidity (Brudzinski neck sign). Passive flexion of neck causes flexion of both legs and thighs.

FIGURE 13-42   BACTERIAL MENINGITIS *(CONTINUED)*

including diffuse headache, fever, vomiting, stiff neck, lethargy, and diminished consciousness. A spinal tap with examination and culture of the CSF can provide definitive information to distinguish suppurative (bacterial) meningitis from other condi- tions. Meningitis can progress to produce severe neurologic damage, particularly if there is obstruction to drainage of CSF, cerebral arteritis, or thrombophlebitis.

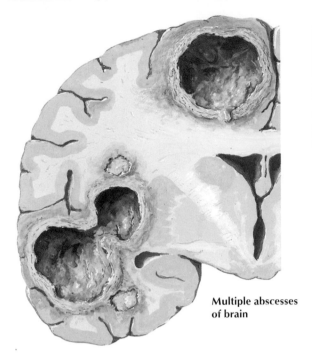

Multiple abscesses of brain

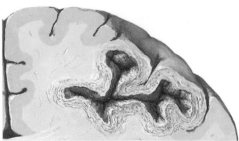

Scar of healed brain abscess, with collapse of brain tissue into cavity

Subdural abscess

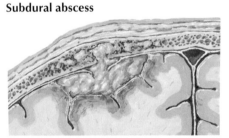

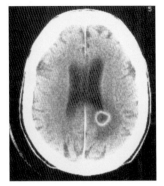

CT scan shows brain abscess with thin enhancing rim and central necrosis

Osteomyelitis of skull, with penetration of dura to form subdural "collar button" abscess

Epidural abscess

Anterior spinal artery

Dura

Arachnoid

Dura

Posterior spinal arteries

Fat in epidural space

Venous plexus

Abscess in epidural space compressing spinal cord and its blood supply

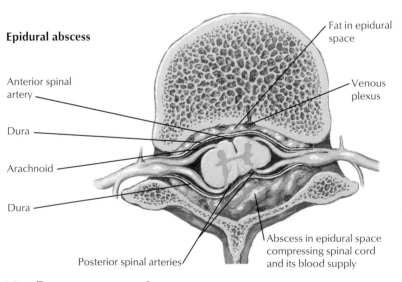

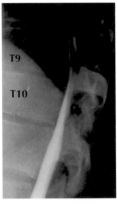

Myelogram: block at T9-10 due to spinal epidural abscess

FIGURE 13-43   PARAMENINGEAL INFECTIONS

Brain abscesses develop from hematogenous spread from a distant site of infection, particularly the heart (infectious endocarditis, congenital heart disease) and the lungs (bronchiectasis, chronic infections), from direct extension from an adjacent focus, such as a middle ear infection, or from penetrating trauma. Direct extension is the usual cause of subdural abscesses as well. Patients with brain abscesses present with severe headache usually accompanied by focal neurologic signs and often with fever. Responsible microbes are usually aerobic bacteria, most

commonly streptococci, staphylococci, or gram-negative bacteria, but some cases involve anaerobic microorganisms or multiple organisms. An epidural abscess is a purulent or granulomatous process within the spinal epidural space that may encroach on the spinal cord, the nerve roots, and the nerves. Predisposing conditions include vertebral osteomyelitis and hematogenous spread of infections from the skin, the mouth, and the respiratory tract.

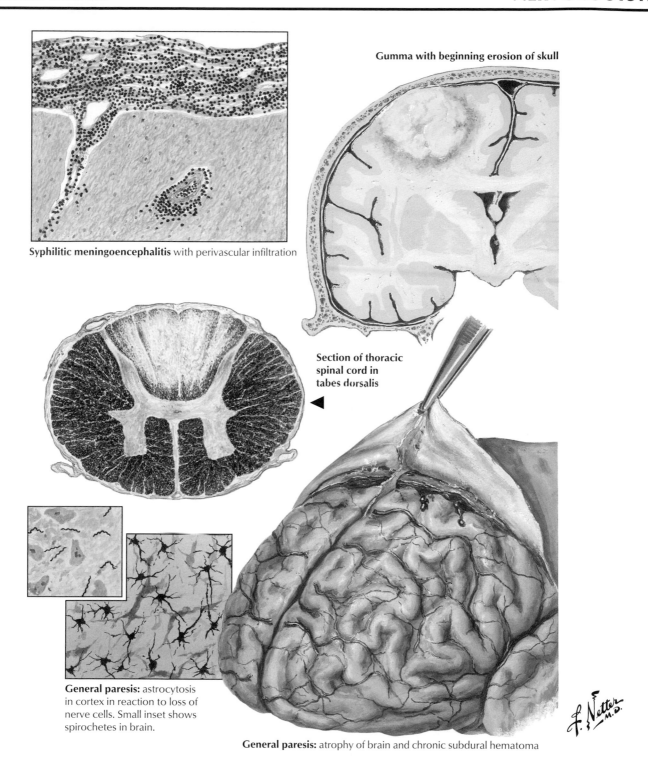

Gumma with beginning erosion of skull

Syphilitic meningoencephalitis with perivascular infiltration

Section of thoracic spinal cord in tabes dorsalis

General paresis: astrocytosis in cortex in reaction to loss of nerve cells. Small inset shows spirochetes in brain.

General paresis: atrophy of brain and chronic subdural hematoma

FIGURE 13-44 NEUROSYPHILIS

Syphilis of the central nervous system occurs late in the course of a primary infection with *Treponema pallidum* in approximately 10% of patients. Invasion of the spirochete elicits a lymphocytic inflammatory process involving the meninges, the brain, and the spinal cord (meningoencephalitis), often accompanied by endarteritis and degenerative and gummatous lesions. Neurosyphilis can occur in several forms: syphilitic meningitis, meningovascular syphilis, tabes dorsalis, dementia paralytica (general paresis), and gumma (rare). CSF analysis shows modest lymphocytosis, a moderately increased protein level, and a normal glucose level. Of key importance, results of serologic tests for syphilis, such as the Venereal Disease Research Laboratory (VDRL) test and the fluorescent treponemal-antibody absorption test, are positive in serum and CSF. Prolonged treatment with penicillin is indicated to arrest the progression of disease.

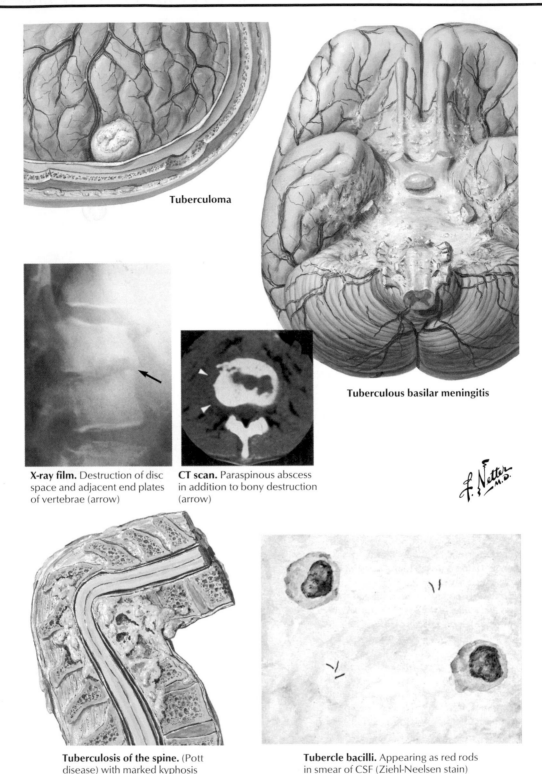

Tuberculoma

Tuberculous basilar meningitis

X-ray film. Destruction of disc space and adjacent end plates of vertebrae (arrow)

CT scan. Paraspinous abscess in addition to bony destruction (arrow)

Tuberculosis of the spine. (Pott disease) with marked kyphosis

Tubercle bacilli. Appearing as red rods in smear of CSF (Ziehl-Neelsen stain)

FIGURE 13-45 TUBERCULOSIS OF THE BRAIN AND SPINE

Tuberculous meninigitis usually begins with a focus of meningeal seeding by hematogenous spread followed by discharge of infection into the subarachnoid space from the caseous focus. The meninginitis sometimes results from contiguous spread from a tuberculoma or parameningeal granuloma with rupture into the subarachnoid space. As the infection spreads, an intensive inflammatory reaction at the base of the brain leads to obliterative endarteritis with thrombosis of small vessels and secondary brain infarction, compression of cranial nerves, and obstruction of the flow of CSF. The clinical course of tuberculous meningitis is usually florid, with rapid progression to neurologic defects and coma. Classically, the CSF glucose level is low, the protein level is high, and the cell count is increased with predominantly lymphocytes. Acid-fast smears may be positive but often are not, so cultures must be performed. Other forms of tuberculous disease are the isolated tuberculoma and vertebral tuberculosis (Pott disease).

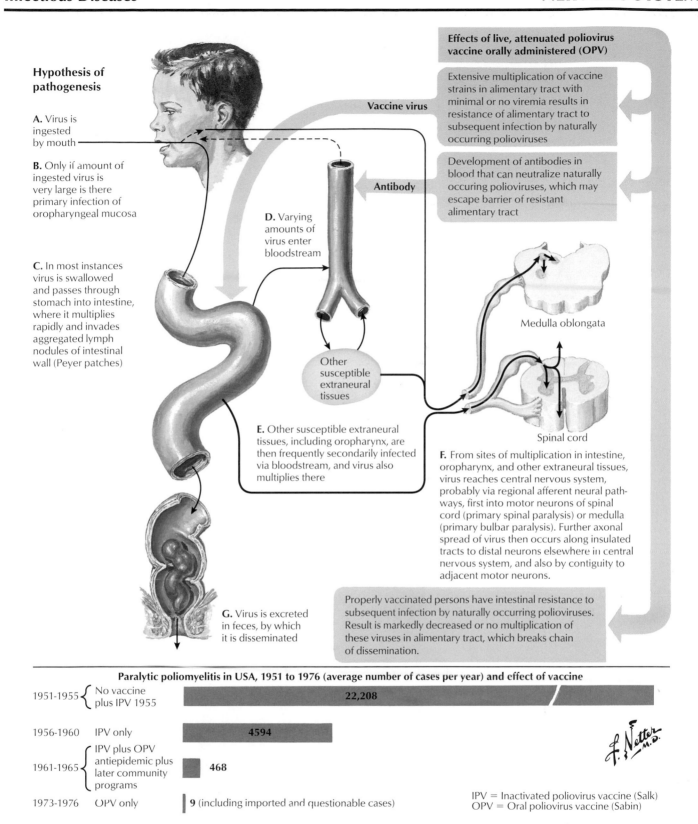

Hypothesis of pathogenesis

A. Virus is ingested by mouth

B. Only if amount of ingested virus is very large is there primary infection of oropharyngeal mucosa

C. In most instances virus is swallowed and passes through stomach into intestine, where it multiplies rapidly and invades aggregated lymph nodules of intestinal wall (Peyer patches)

D. Varying amounts of virus enter bloodstream

E. Other susceptible extraneural tissues, including oropharynx, are then frequently secondarily infected via bloodstream, and virus also multiplies there

Other susceptible extraneural tissues

G. Virus is excreted in feces, by which it is disseminated

Effects of live, attenuated poliovirus vaccine orally administered (OPV)

Vaccine virus

Extensive multiplication of vaccine strains in alimentary tract with minimal or no viremia results in resistance of alimentary tract to subsequent infection by naturally occurring polioviruses

Antibody

Development of antibodies in blood that can neutralize naturally occuring polioviruses, which may escape barrier of resistant alimentary tract

Medulla oblongata

Spinal cord

F. From sites of multiplication in intestine, oropharynx, and other extraneural tissues, virus reaches central nervous system, probably via regional afferent neural pathways, first into motor neurons of spinal cord (primary spinal paralysis) or medulla (primary bulbar paralysis). Further axonal spread of virus then occurs along insulated tracts to distal neurons elsewhere in central nervous system, and also by contiguity to adjacent motor neurons.

Properly vaccinated persons have intestinal resistance to subsequent infection by naturally occurring polioviruses. Result is markedly decreased or no multiplication of these viruses in alimentary tract, which breaks chain of dissemination.

Paralytic poliomyelitis in USA, 1951 to 1976 (average number of cases per year) and effect of vaccine

Period	Vaccine	Cases
1951-1955	No vaccine plus IPV 1955	22,208
1956-1960	IPV only	4594
1961-1965	IPV plus OPV antiepidemic plus later community programs	468
1973-1976	OPV only	9 (including imported and questionable cases)

IPV = Inactivated poliovirus vaccine (Salk)
OPV = Oral poliovirus vaccine (Sabin)

f. Netter M.D.

FIGURE 13-46 POLIOMYELITIS

Poliomyelitis represents a well-characterized neurologic disease caused by poliovirus infection and a disease successfully prevented by vaccination. Poliovirus, an RNA virus of the picorna group of enteroviruses, is propagated by oral-fecal transmission. Poliomyelitis begins as an acute febrile illness. In a small minority of infected individuals, viremia is followed by propagation in the nervous system, leading to a lower motor neuron type of paralysis, which may be accompanied by respiratory and vasomotor disturbances caused by neuronal lesions in the medulla. Outcomes ranging from an abortive minor illness or nonparalytic

Stages in
destruction of
a motor neuron
by poliovirus

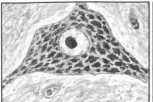
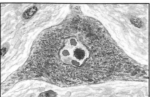
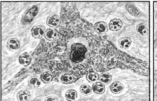
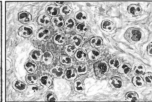

A. Normal motor neuron

B. Diffuse chromatolysis;
three acidophilic nuclear
inclusions around nucleolus

C. Polymorphonuclear cells
invading necrotic neuron

D. Complete neuronophagia

Relative distribution
of neuronal lesions
in spinal and bulbar
poliomyelitis

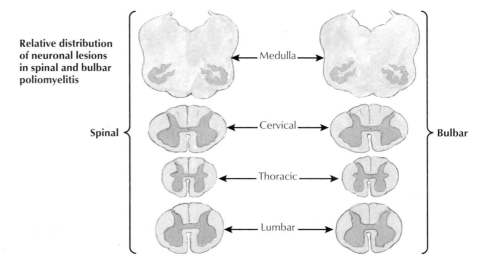

Spinal

Medulla

Cervical

Thoracic

Lumbar

Bulbar

**Paralytic residua of
spinal poliomyelitis**

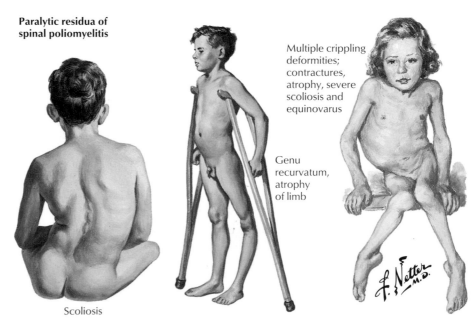

Multiple crippling
deformities;
contractures,
atrophy, severe
scoliosis and
equinovarus

Genu
recurvatum,
atrophy
of limb

Scoliosis

FIGURE 13-46   POLIOMYELITIS (CONTINUED)

illness to paralytic illness depend on individual susceptibility and the neurovirulence of the infecting virus. The incidence of paralytic polio in the United States has progressively and dramatically declined, initially after the introduction of the subcutaneously administered formalin-inactivated poliovirus vaccine (Salk type) and, subsequently, the live, attenuated oral poliovirus vaccine (Sabin type).

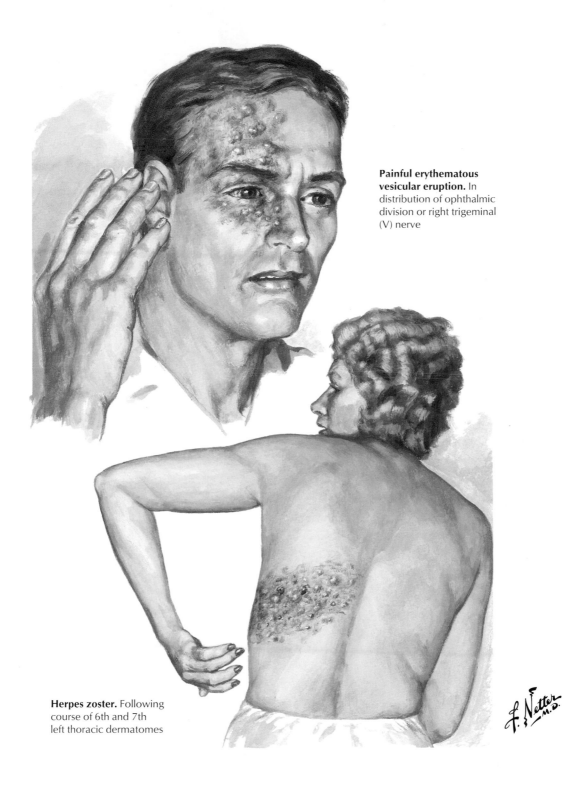

Painful erythematous vesicular eruption. In distribution of ophthalmic division or right trigeminal (V) nerve

Herpes zoster. Following course of 6th and 7th left thoracic dermatomes

FIGURE 13-47   HERPES ZOSTER

Herpes zoster (shingles), a relatively common infection of the peripheral nervous system, occurs most often in immunocompromised individuals. **Herpes zoster** is an acute neuralgia with a characteristic painful vesicular rash confined to the distribution of a specific spinal nerve root or cranial nerve. The primary site of infection is the dorsal root ganglion, and the infectious agent is the DNA-containing varicella-zoster virus, the same virus that causes chickenpox. The virus migrates up the peripheral nerve to the dorsal root ganglion after an attack of chickenpox and then remains dormant until an immunologic imbalance allows it to become active again. On reactivation, an acute inflammatory reaction occurs in the dorsal root ganglion, and the virus then spreads down the nerve root and the peripheral nerve to the skin, producing the characteristic rash. Patients with ophthalmic herpes zoster are at risk for blindness.

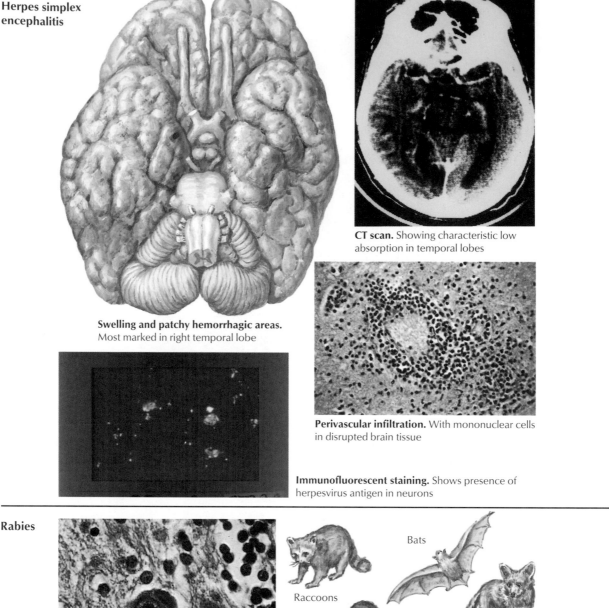

Herpes simplex encephalitis

Swelling and patchy hemorrhagic areas.
Most marked in right temporal lobe

CT scan. Showing characteristic low absorption in temporal lobes

Perivascular infiltration. With mononuclear cells in disrupted brain tissue

Immunofluorescent staining. Shows presence of herpesvirus antigen in neurons

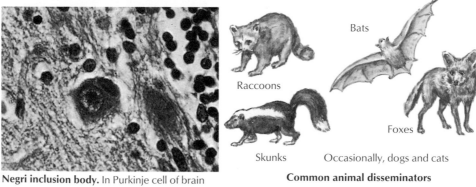

Rabies

Negri inclusion body. In Purkinje cell of brain

Bats

Raccoons

Skunks

Foxes

Occasionally, dogs and cats

Common animal disseminators

FIGURE 13-48   HERPES SIMPLEX ENCEPHALITIS AND RABIES

Herpes simplex encephalitis (HSE) is a relatively common and serious acute viral disease of the brain. The infection is associated with a high mortality, and survivors often have significant neuropsychiatric sequelae. Neonates usually are infected with HSV-2, and children and adults usually are infected with HSV-1. The virus likely reaches the brain via the olfactory tract or the trigeminal (V) nerve and leads to a primary infection or a subsequent reactivation event. Encephalitis most often involves the medial temporal and frontal lobes. The histologic features are hemorrhagic necrosis, inflammatory infiltrates, and neurons containing intranuclear inclusions. *Rabies* is an acute viral disease of the central nervous system caused by an RNA virus of the Rhabdoviridae family transmitted by inoculation of a wound contaminated by saliva of a rabid animal. Paralytic disease begins 1 to 3 months after infection. Although clinical manifestations are severe, neuropathologic findings consist of mild inflammation plus neurons showing the pathognomonic cytoplasmic eosinophilic inclusion, the Negri body.

Slow virus infections

Progressive multifocal leukoencephalopathy (PML)

Coronal section of brain showing many minute demyelinating lesions in white matter, which have coalesced in some areas to form irregular cavitations

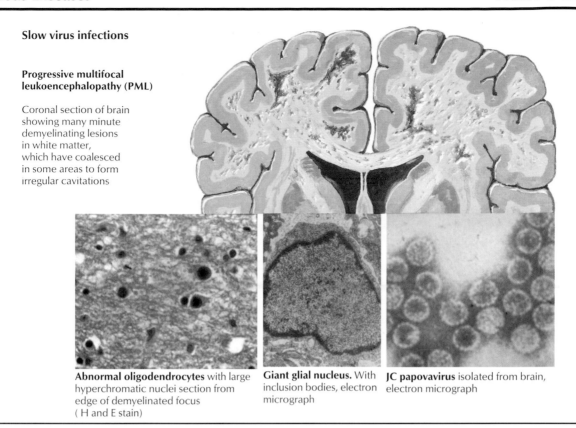

Abnormal oligodendrocytes with large hyperchromatic nuclei section from edge of demyelinated focus (H and E stain)

Giant glial nucleus. With inclusion bodies, electron micrograph

JC papovavirus isolated from brain, electron micrograph

Creutzfeldt-Jakob Disease

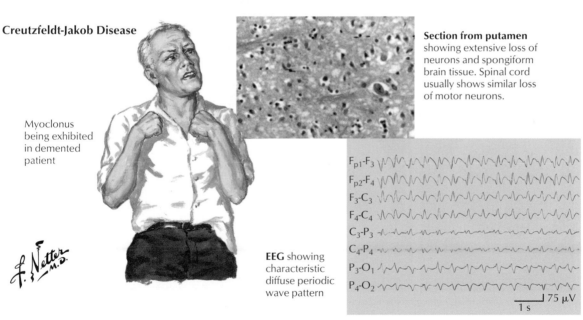

Myoclonus being exhibited in demented patient

Section from putamen showing extensive loss of neurons and spongiform brain tissue. Spinal cord usually shows similar loss of motor neurons.

EEG showing characteristic diffuse periodic wave pattern

F_{p1}-F_3
F_{p2}-F_4
F_3-C_3
F_4-C_4
C_3-P_3
C_4-P_4
P_3-O_1
P_4-O_2

75 μV
1 s

FIGURE 13-49   SLOW VIRUS INFECTIONS AND SPONGIFORM ENCEPHALOPATHIES

Slow virus infections refer to progressive and fatal neurologic syndromes that arise months or years after an initial viral infection. Immunosuppressed patients are particularly susceptible. Examples are progressive multifocal leukoencephalopathy caused by the JC papovavirus and subacute sclerosing panencephalitis caused by reactivation of a measleslike virus. Spongiform encephalopathies are known to be caused not by a virus but by a unique mechanism involving mutated proteins called **prions**. The

human diseases caused by these agents are **Creutzfeldt-Jakob disease**, which has a worldwide distribution, and kuru, linked to cannibalistic practices in the New Guinea highlands. The pathology of both diseases is characterized by neuronal loss, neuronal vacuolization, and astrocytosis without inflammatory infiltrates. The human form of mad cow disease is a variant of Creutzfeldt-Jakob disease. The clinical hallmarks are progressive dementia and myoclonus.

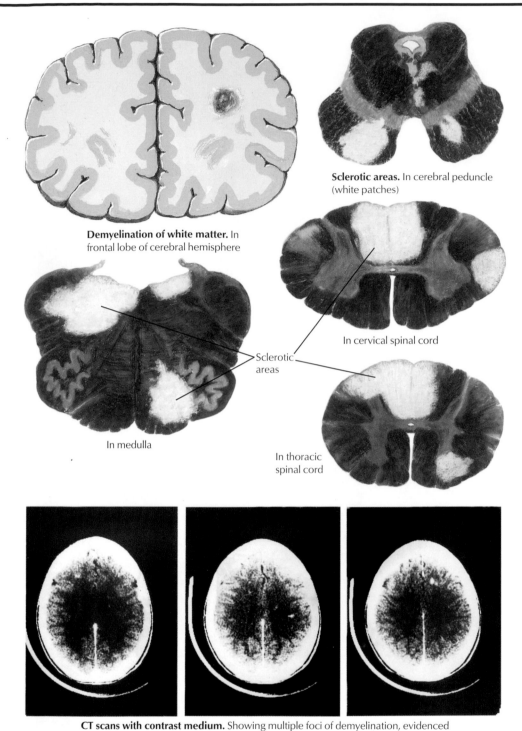

Demyelination of white matter. In frontal lobe of cerebral hemisphere

Sclerotic areas. In cerebral peduncle (white patches)

In cervical spinal cord

Sclerotic areas

In medulla

In thoracic spinal cord

CT scans with contrast medium. Showing multiple foci of demyelination, evidenced by focal enhancing lesions of varying size, located primarily in white matter

FIGURE 13-50   MULTIPLE SCLEROSIS: CENTRAL NERVOUS SYSTEM PATHOLOGY

Multiple sclerosis is a relatively common disease that is characterized by clinical neurologic defects that are separated over time and are linked to the development of demyelinating lesions of the white matter that are separated spatially in the brain. Multiple sclerosis typically occurs in adults aged younger than 50 years and occurs approximately twice as frequently in women as men. The pathogenesis involves inflammation in response to an undefined trigger and possibly involving an autoimmune component. Lymphocytes and macrophages produce focal

destruction of myelin and loss of oligodendroglia while sparing axons, and then microglia and astrocytes phagocytose the myelin. The resulting areas of demyelination with variable amounts of glial scar are known as plaques, and these lesions are the hallmark of the disease. The symptoms and signs of multiple sclerosis depend on the number and the location of the plaques. The course of the disease is characterized by multiple exacerbations and remissions and has highly variable outcomes.

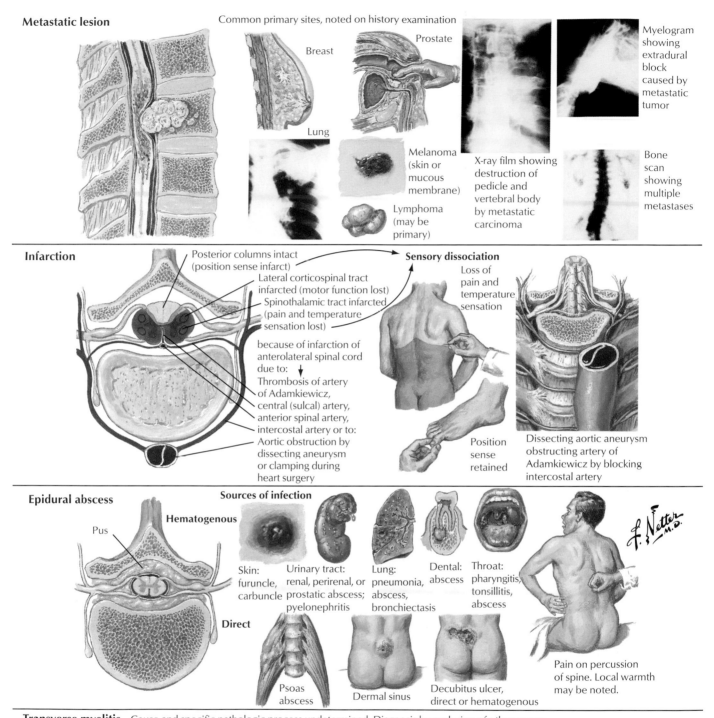

Metastatic lesion

Common primary sites, noted on history examination

Breast

Prostate

Lung

Melanoma (skin or mucous membrane)

Lymphoma (may be primary)

X-ray film showing destruction of pedicle and vertebral body by metastatic carcinoma

Myelogram showing extradural block caused by metastatic tumor

Bone scan showing multiple metastases

Infarction

Posterior columns intact (position sense infarct)
Lateral corticospinal tract infarcted (motor function lost)
Spinothalamic tract infarcted (pain and temperature sensation lost)

because of infarction of anterolateral spinal cord due to:
Thrombosis of artery of Adamkiewicz, central (sulcal) artery, anterior spinal artery, intercostal artery or to:
Aortic obstruction by dissecting aneurysm or clamping during heart surgery

Sensory dissociation

Loss of pain and temperature sensation

Position sense retained

Dissecting aortic aneurysm obstructing artery of Adamkiewicz by blocking intercostal artery

Epidural abscess

Pus

Sources of infection

Hematogenous

Skin: furuncle, carbuncle

Urinary tract: renal, perirenal, or prostatic abscess; pyelonephritis

Lung: pneumonia, abscess, bronchiectasis

Dental: abscess

Throat: pharyngitis, tonsillitis, abscess

Direct

Psoas abscess

Dermal sinus

Decubitus ulcer, direct or hematogenous

Pain on percussion of spine. Local warmth may be noted.

Transverse myelitis   Cause and specific pathologic process undetermined. Diagnosis by exclusion of other causes.

FIGURE 13-51   ACUTE SPINAL CORD SYNDROMES: PATHOLOGY, ETIOLOGY, AND DIAGNOSIS

Acute spinal cord damage is often produced by a mass lesion that reaches a critical size in the confined space of the spinal canal. Differential diagnosis includes metastatic carcinoma, infarction due to a vascular occlusion, epidural abscess, and transverse myelitis. **Transverse myelitis** is a syndrome of acute spinal cord dysfunction due to a demyelinating disorder similar to acute disseminated encephalomyelitis. Prompt diagnosis and treatment of an acute spinal cord lesion may prevent paraplegia.

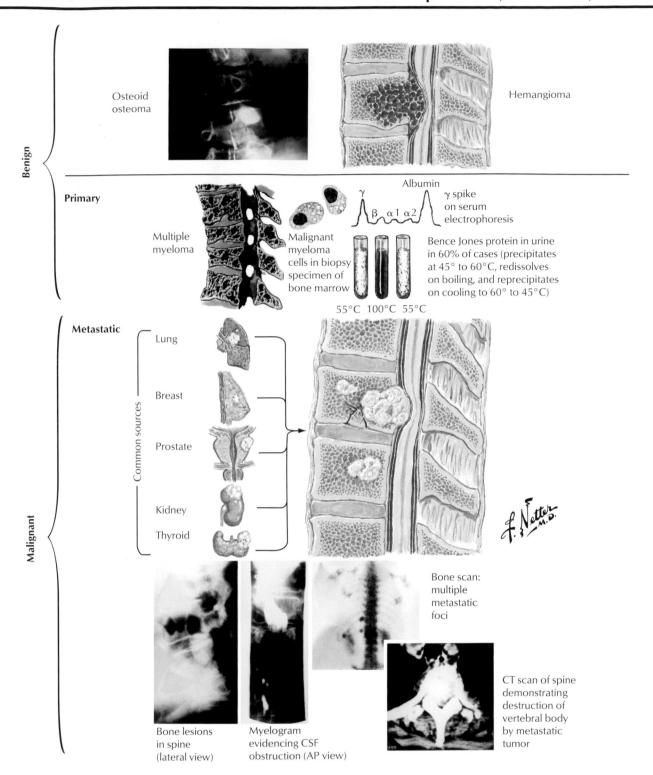

Osteoid osteoma

Hemangioma

Benign

Primary

Multiple myeloma

Malignant myeloma cells in biopsy specimen of bone marrow

Albumin

γ   α1 α2   γ spike on serum electrophoresis

β

Bence Jones protein in urine in 60% of cases (precipitates at 45° to 60°C, redissolves on boiling, and reprecipitates on cooling to 60° to 45°C)

55°C 100°C 55°C

Metastatic

Lung

Breast

Prostate

Kidney

Thyroid

Common sources

Malignant

Bone scan: multiple metastatic foci

CT scan of spine demonstrating destruction of vertebral body by metastatic tumor

Bone lesions in spine (lateral view)

Myelogram evidencing CSF obstruction (AP view)

FIGURE 13-52   TUMORS OF THE SPINAL COLUMN

Tumors involving the spine are found external to the spinal cord (extradural tumors) or they involve the spinal cord (intradural). Extradural tumors are usually metastases to the spine that invade the epidural space. Most occur via hematogenous spread, but direct extension from extravertebral soft tissue also occurs. The most common primary tumors are lung, breast, prostate, kidney, and thyroid. Most produce osteolytic lesions in the vertebrae, but lesions of prostatic cancer are often osteoblastic. There also are primary bone tumors such as osteogenic sarcoma and giant cell tumor and the hemangioma of bone. **Multiple myeloma** is a neoplastic proliferation of plasma cells that typically produces multiple osteolytic lesions in bone. The neoplastic clones typically produce a monoclonal γ-globulin component detectable in serum and in urine as Bence Jones protein.

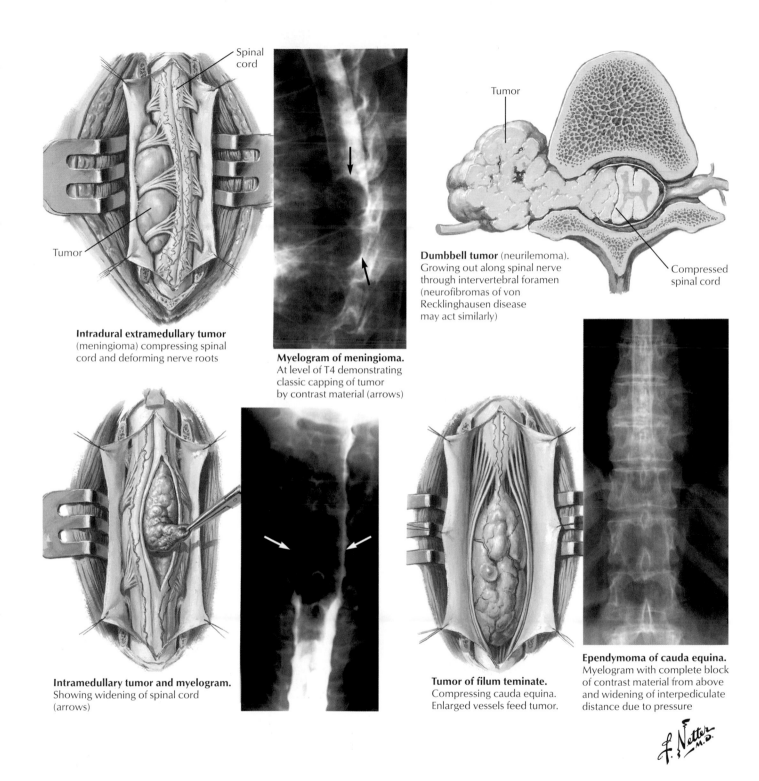

Intradural extramedullary tumor (meningioma) compressing spinal cord and deforming nerve roots

Myelogram of meningioma. At level of T4 demonstrating classic capping of tumor by contrast material (arrows)

Dumbbell tumor (neurilemoma). Growing out along spinal nerve through intervertebral foramen (neurofibromas of von Recklinghausen disease may act similarly)

Intramedullary tumor and myelogram. Showing widening of spinal cord (arrows)

Tumor of filum teminate. Compressing cauda equina. Enlarged vessels feed tumor.

Ependymoma of cauda equina. Myelogram with complete block of contrast material from above and widening of interpediculate distance due to pressure

FIGURE 13-53   TUMORS OF THE SPINAL CORD

Intradural extramedullary tumors arise in the meninges and include the isolated benign meningioma and neurilemmoma and neurofibromas associated with neurofibromatosis. Progressive compression of the spinal cord can lead to local back pain and radicular pain and eventually cause serious spinal cord defects. Intramedullary tumors usually involve a discrete short segment of

499

Myelographic and CT Characteristics of Spinal Tumors

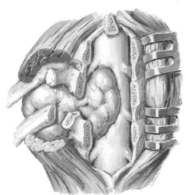

Lymphoma. Invading spinal canal via intervertebral foramen, compressing dura mater and spinal cord

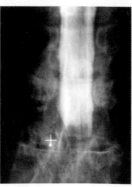
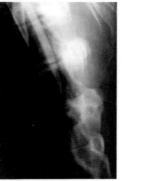

Frontal (left) and lateral (right) metrizamide myelograms. Show complete obstruction just above T6-7. Spinal cord displaced forward and to right, with similar displacement of arachnoid, which suggests that mass is extradural.

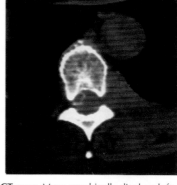

CT scan. More graphically displays left and posteriorly situated soft-tissue mass within spinal canal and its extension through left intervertebral foramen. Absence of bony involvement confirmed.

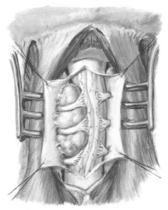

Meningoma. Compressing spinal cord and distorting nerve roots

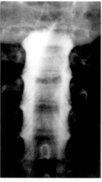
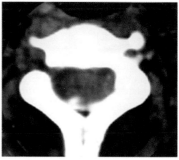

Frontal (left), lateral (center), and oblique (right) metrizamide myelograms. Show right lateral displacement of spinal cord and complete obstruction. Frontal view shows injection from above; lateral and oblique views show interior margin of intradural mass, separate from spinal cord, defined by injection from below.

CT scan. At C2 shows only small amount of contrast medium posteriorly. Tumor is more dense than spinal cord, which is displaced to right and severely deformed and compressed.

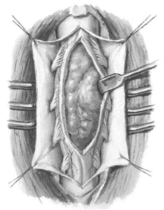

Astrocytoma. Exposed by longitudnal incision in bulging spinal cord

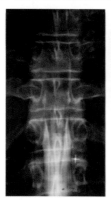
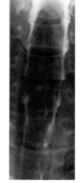

Frontal (left) and lateral (right) metrizamide myelograms. With injection from below show high-grade stenosis caused by nearly symmetric expansion of spinal cord beginning at T12

Myelogram. With injection from above shows extension of tumor to upper cervical level

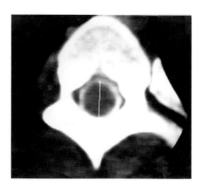

CT scan. Of lower thoracic region showing rounded, expanded spinal cord that is nearly twice normal sagittal diameter

f. Netter, M.D.

FIGURE 13-53   TUMORS OF THE SPINAL CORD *(CONTINUED)*

the spinal cord but may be more extensive, involving much of the length of the spinal cord. The 2 most common intramedullary tumors are the astrocytoma and the ependymoma. Intradural tumors of the lumbar spine can involve the specialized structures of this region, the conus medullaris, the filum terminale, and the cauda equina.

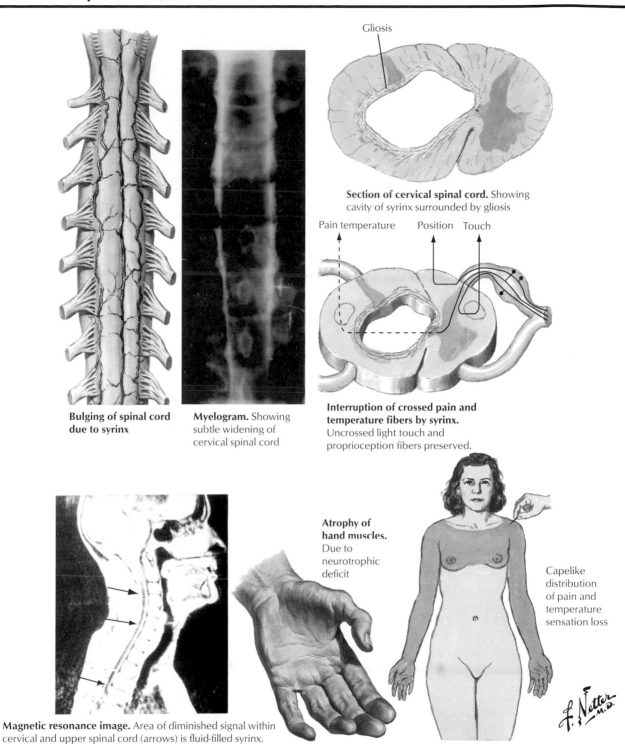

Gliosis

Section of cervical spinal cord. Showing cavity of syrinx surrounded by gliosis

Pain temperature Position Touch

Bulging of spinal cord due to syrinx

Myelogram. Showing subtle widening of cervical spinal cord

Interruption of crossed pain and temperature fibers by syrinx. Uncrossed light touch and proprioception fibers preserved.

Atrophy of hand muscles. Due to neurotrophic deficit

Capelike distribution of pain and temperature sensation loss

Magnetic resonance image. Area of diminished signal within cervical and upper spinal cord (arrows) is fluid-filled syrinx. Cerebellar tonsil extends below foramen magnum.

FIGURE 13-54 SYRINGOMYELIA

Syringomyelia is a rare disorder produced by the development of a cylindrical cavity, or syrinx, in the central area of the spinal cord, most frequently in the cervical and upper thoracic segments. The pathogenesis is poorly understood but seems to be developmental, degenerative, or both in nature. Other defects may be present, including the Arnold-Chiari malformation. Gradual expansion of the syrinx in the central area of the spinal cord produces neuronal and nerve tract damage. Symptoms usually develop in adults aged 20 to 50 years. The classic sign of syringomyelia is a dissociated loss of pain and temperature sensation in the upper extremities with preservation of light touch sensation and proprioception without motor deficits. The disease is characterized by progressive incapacitation due to spinal cord damage.

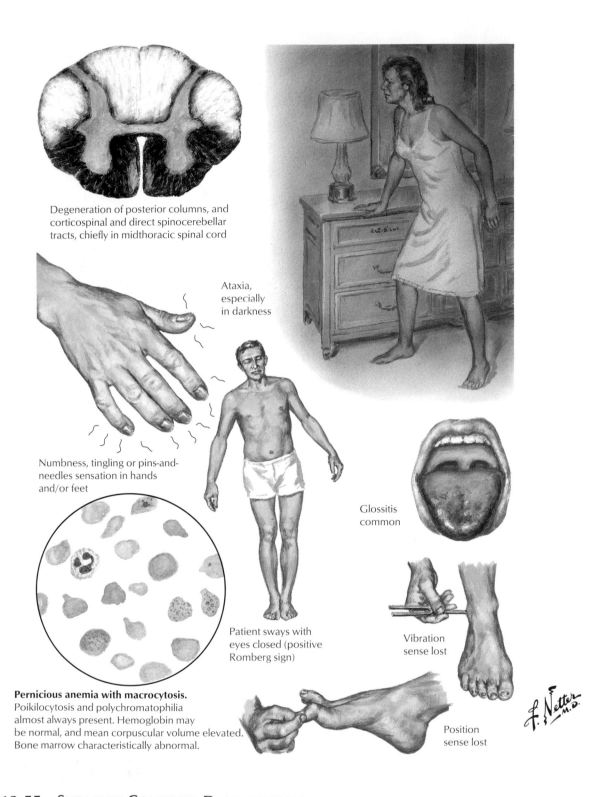

Degeneration of posterior columns, and corticospinal and direct spinocerebellar tracts, chiefly in midthoracic spinal cord

Ataxia, especially in darkness

Numbness, tingling or pins-and-needles sensation in hands and/or feet

Glossitis common

Pernicious anemia with macrocytosis. Poikilocytosis and polychromatophilia almost always present. Hemoglobin may be normal, and mean corpuscular volume elevated. Bone marrow characteristically abnormal.

Patient sways with eyes closed (positive Romberg sign)

Vibration sense lost

Position sense lost

FIGURE 13-55   SUBACUTE COMBINED DEGENERATION

Subacute combined degeneration of the spinal cord is a process of degeneration of the posterior and lateral tracts of the spinal cord resulting from vitamin B_{12} deficiency. Most cases are the result of pernicious anemia due to an autoimmune chronic atrophic gastritis leading to an absence of intrinsic factor needed for vitamin B_{12} absorption or, less often, from other conditions in which vitamin B_{12} absorption is impaired or its dietary intake is insufficient. The most common neurologic symptoms relate to

involvement of the posterior columns with loss of the sense of vibration of particular diagnostic significance. Lateral column dysfunction usually occurs later. The neurologic signs and symptoms may precede the appearance of anemia. Folate ingestion may mask the anemia but may not prevent the progressive neurologic damage. Proper diagnosis and administration of B_{12} is needed to prevent permanent neurologic damage.

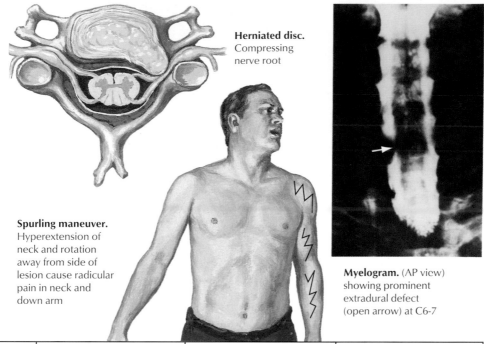

Herniated disc. Compressing nerve root

Spurling maneuver. Hyperextension of neck and rotation away from side of lesion cause radicular pain in neck and down arm

Myelogram. (AP view) showing prominent extradural defect (open arrow) at C6-7

Level	Motor signs (weakness)	Reflex signs	Sensory loss
C5	Deltoid	0	
C6		Biceps brachii — Weak or absent reflex	
C7	Biceps brachii	Triceps brachii — Weak or absent reflex	
C8	Interossei	Horner syndrome	

f. Netter M.D.

FIGURE 13-56 CERVICAL DISC HERNIATION: CLINICAL MANIFESTATIONS

Cervical disc herniation is a common disorder usually caused by degenerative disease (osteoarthritis) rather than trauma. Severe degenerative cervical disc disease (spondylosis) can result in rupture of an intervertebral disc or osteophytes developing on the vertebrae from osteoarthritis. Osteophytes or ruptured discs produce symptoms when they compress the spinal cord or nerve roots against posteriorly located structures of the spinal column, including the posterior nerve root foramen and the ligamentum flavum. Neurologic examination focusing on motor, reflex, and sensory findings in the upper extremities usually reveals a diagnostic grouping of symptoms and signs pointing to the location of the pathologic lesion. Surgical therapy is indicated only if conservative management is unsuccessful.

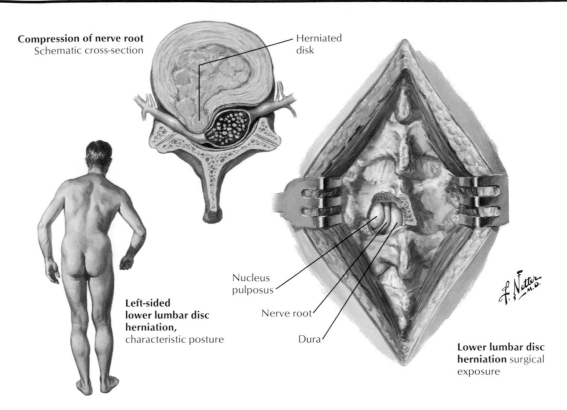

Compression of nerve root
Schematic cross-section

Herniated disk

Left-sided lower lumbar disc herniation, characteristic posture

Nucleus pulposus

Nerve root

Dura

Lower lumbar disc herniation surgical exposure

Clinical features of herniated lumbar nucleus pulposus					
Level of herniation	Pain	Numbness	Weakness	Atrophy	Reflexes
L4–5 disc; 5th lumbar nerve root	Over sacro-iliac joint, hip, lateral thigh, and leg	Lateral leg, first 3 toes	Dorsiflexion of great toe and foot; difficulty walking on heels; foot drop may occur	Minor	Changes uncommon in knee and ankle jerks, but internal hamstring reflex diminished or absent
L5–S1 disc; 1st sacral nerve root	Over sacro-iliac joint, hip, postero-lateral thigh, and leg to heel	Back of calf, lateral heel, foot to toe	Plantar flexion of foot and great toe may be affected; difficulty walking on toes	Gastrocnemi-us and soleus	Ankle jerk diminished or absent

FIGURE 13-57 LUMBAR DISC HERNIATION: CLINICAL MANIFESTATIONS

Lumbar disc disease causing low back pain and nerve root pain is a common problem. The *lumbar spine* is a compact anatomical region composed of the 5 lumbar vertebrae and the sacrum, which are separated by the normally tough and compact intervertebral discs. With aging, the fibrocartilaginous disc degenerates and fragments; in the process, the adherence to the adjacent vertebrae is weakened. Mechanical forces can then cause the fragments to move, usually in a posterolateral direction toward the exit sites of the nerve roots. Pain and neurologic deficits develop from the ensuing pressure on the nerve roots. The various clinical features of a herniated nucleus pulposus of a lumbar intervertebral disc are shown here. Surgical intervention is often needed to relieve the problem.

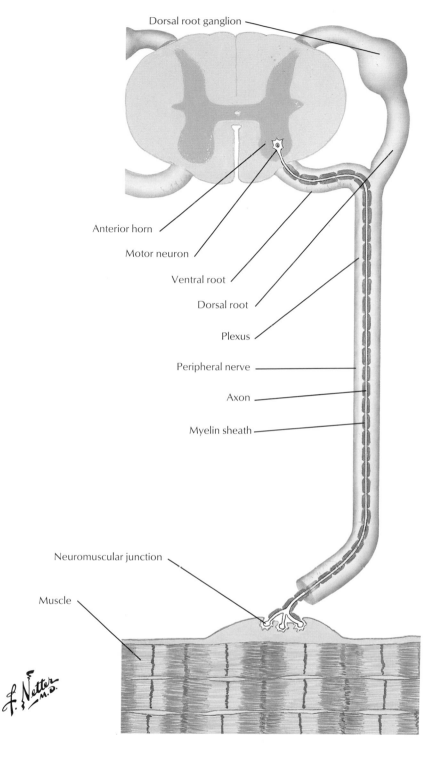

Motor neuron
- Primary motor neuron diseases
  - Progressive muscular atrophy
  - Primary bulbar palsy
  - Amyotrophic lateral sclerosis
  - Werdnig-Hoffman disease
- Poliomyelitis
- Tetanus

Dorsal root ganglion
- Herpes zoster
- Friedreich ataxia
- Hereditary sensory neuropathy

Spinal nerve (dorsal and ventral roots)
- Disc extrusion or herniation
- Tumor

Plexus
- Tumor
- Trauma
- Idiopathic plexopathy
- Diabetic plexopathy

Peripheral nerve
- Metabolic, toxic, nutritional, idiopathic neuropathies
- Arteritis
- Hereditary neuropathies
- Infectious, postinfectious, inflammatory neuropathies (Guillain-Barré syndrome)
- Entrapment and compression syndromes
- Trauma

Neuromuscular junction
- Myasthenia gravis
- Lambert-Eaton syndrome
- Botulism

Muscle
- Duchenne muscular dystrophy
- Myotonic dystrophy
- Limb-girdle muscular dystrophy
- Congenital myopathies
- Polymyositis/dermatomyositis
- Potassium-related myopathies
- Endocrine dysfunction myopathies
- Enzymatic myopathies
- Rhabdomyolysis

Labels on figure: Dorsal root ganglion; Anterior horn; Motor neuron; Ventral root; Dorsal root; Plexus; Peripheral nerve; Axon; Myelin sheath; Neuromuscular junction; Muscle

FIGURE 13-58   DISEASES OF THE MOTOR-SENSORY UNIT: REGIONAL CLASSIFICATION

The motor neurons of the spinal cord and the cranial nerves serve as the final common path for transmission of neural impulses through the axon and neuromuscular junction to the skeletal musculature. Diseases of the motor-sensory unit typically occur without impairment of mental function. In diseases of the neuromuscular junction, particularly in myasthenia gravis, cranial nerve abnormalities, especially those producing diplopia or ptosis or both, occur frequently. Bulbar motor neuron disease may present with dysphagia. Careful evaluation of gait and the pattern of muscle weakness are important in the differential diagnosis. In general, the deep tendon reflexes are either normal or reduced in most disorders of the motor-sensory unit. A sensory examination and pattern of sensory deficit also are important to determine the underlying pathology because sensation is usually intact in motor neuron disease, neuromuscular junction disorders, and primary myopathies, whereas distal sensory loss is typical of peripheral neuropathies.

Motor neuron disease

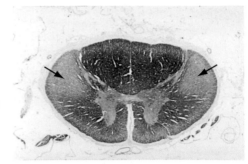

Cross-section of spinal cord. From patient with amyotrophic lateral sclerosis showing bilateral degeneration of corticospinal tracts (arrows)

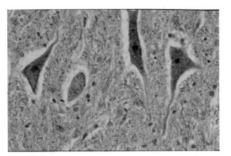

Anterior horn of spinal cord. With normal motor neurons (Luxol fast blue with H and E stain)

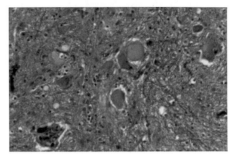

Degeneration of anterior horn cells. In amyotrophic lateral sclerosis (same stain)

Electromyography

At rest   Voluntary contraction

Normal

1 mV

Silent   Motor units closely spaced, 0.5-1.0 mV   0.01 s

Amyotrophic lateral sclerosis

8 mV

Fibrillations and fasciculations   Motor units decreased in number, high amplitude, long duration, polyphasic   0.01 s

FIGURE 13-59   PRIMARY MOTOR NEURON DISEASE

Primary motor neuron diseases have varied clinical manifestations. Patients may present with **progressive muscular atrophy** (primary asymmetric lower motor neuron disease), **primary bulbar palsy** (dysfunction of motor neurons originating in the brainstem), or the syndrome of **amyotrophic lateral sclerosis** (upper motor neuron disease with corticospinal tract involvement superimposed on primary muscular atrophy or primary bulbar palsy). Amyotrophic lateral sclerosis (Lou Gehrig disease) typically presents with manifestations of lower motor neuron disease, particularly dysfunction of muscle movements. These manifestations eventually join with symptoms of degeneration of the corticospinal or corticobulbar tract, including muscle spasticity. Electromyography reveals a characteristic pattern of abnormalities.

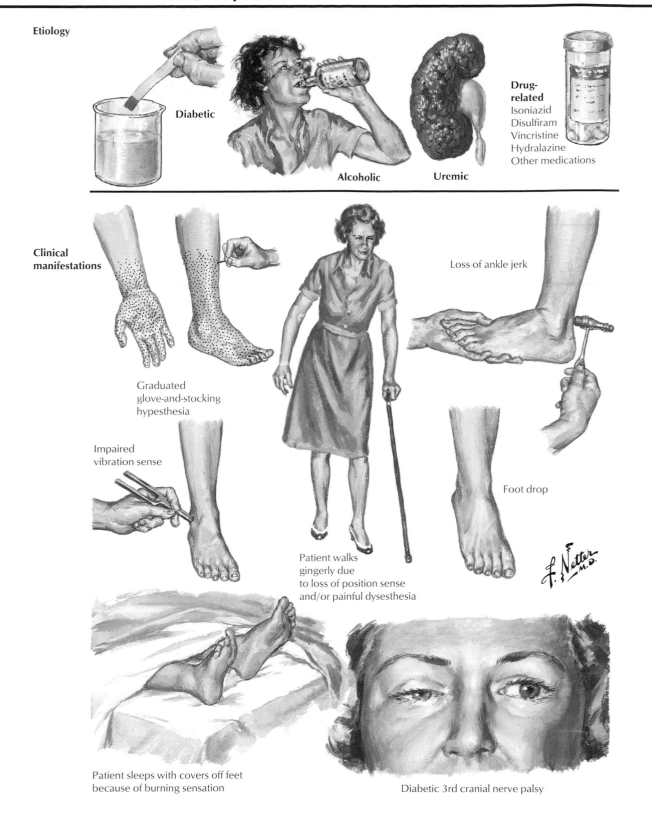

Etiology

Diabetic

Alcoholic

Uremic

Drug-related
Isoniazid
Disulfiram
Vincristine
Hydralazine
Other medications

Clinical manifestations

Graduated glove-and-stocking hypesthesia

Impaired vibration sense

Loss of ankle jerk

Foot drop

Patient walks gingerly due to loss of position sense and/or painful dysesthesia

Patient sleeps with covers off feet because of burning sensation

Diabetic 3rd cranial nerve palsy

FIGURE 13-60   PERIPHERAL NEUROPATHIES: METABOLIC, TOXIC, AND NUTRITIONAL

A variety of metabolic, toxic, or nutritional conditions can produce subacute or chronic peripheral neuropathies that tend to involve multiple nerves in a symmetric pattern. Some cases are idiopathic, and in others, the family history suggests a hereditary basis. Typically, the patient presents with symptoms of symmetric numbness, tingling, burning, or constriction of the extremities and a cautious gait. Physical examination usually shows changes first evident in the legs and feet. There is a symmetric hyporeflexia, with distal weakness. Pathologic changes on nerve biopsy may be nonspecific and consist of patchy foci of demyelination and axonal degeneration or may show more specific findings, such as amyloid deposits and, in patients with diabetes, hyaline arteriolosclerosis.

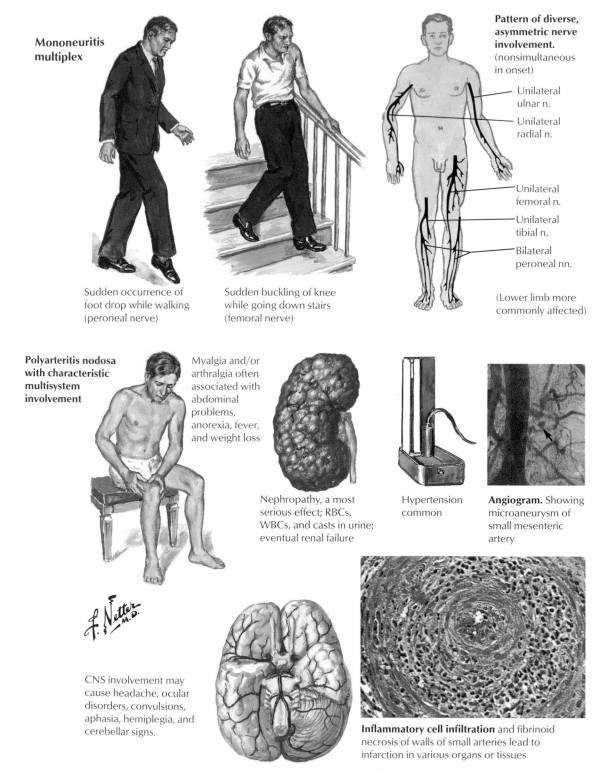

Mononeuritis multiplex

Sudden occurrence of foot drop while walking (peroneal nerve)

Sudden buckling of knee while going down stairs (femoral nerve)

Pattern of diverse, asymmetric nerve involvement. (nonsimultaneous in onset)

Unilateral ulnar n.

Unilateral radial n.

Unilateral femoral n.

Unilateral tibial n.

Bilateral peroneal nn.

(Lower limb more commonly affected)

Polyarteritis nodosa with characteristic multisystem involvement

Myalgia and/or arthralgia often associated with abdominal problems, anorexia, fever, and weight loss

Nephropathy, a most serious effect; RBCs, WBCs, and casts in urine; eventual renal failure

Hypertension common

Angiogram. Showing microaneurysm of small mesenteric artery

CNS involvement may cause headache, ocular disorders, convulsions, aphasia, hemiplegia, and cerebellar signs.

Inflammatory cell infiltration and fibrinoid necrosis of walls of small arteries lead to infarction in various organs or tissues

FIGURE 13-61   MONONEURITIS MULTIPLEX WITH POLYARTERITIS NODOSA (PAN)

There are a number of conditions that compromise the circulation to a specific nerve acutely. The neurologic presentation resembles the acute onset of pressure or traumatic lesions but without evidence of such lesions. The acute onset of foot drop is a common presentation. The illness progresses by recruitment of additional peripheral nerves, usually in an asymmetric fashion. The presentation may even mimic a diffuse, symmetric polyneuropathy but with a much more rapid course. Acute lesions are more commonly caused by disorders affecting small-sized arterioles, and this occurs relatively often in patients with diabetes. Also to be considered are **PAN**, an acute necrotizing vasculitis with multisystem involvement, and the arteritises associated with systemic lupus erythematosus or Churg-Strauss syndrome. Other diagnostic considerations are cardiac embolic lesions from bacterial endocarditis or atrial myxoma; dysproteinemias, a paraneoplastic syndrome associated with some carcinomas; and leprosy.

Etiologic and Pathophysiologic Concepts

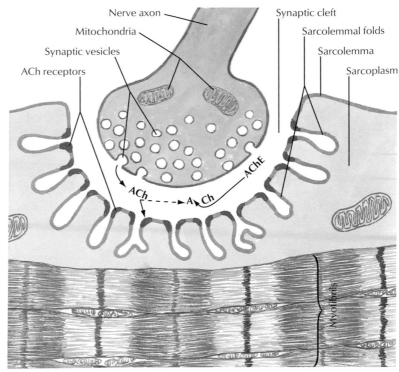

Normal neuromuscular junction

Synaptic vesicles containing acetylcholine (ACh) form in nerve terminal. In response to nerve impulse, vesicles discharge ACh into synaptic cleft. ACh binds to receptor sites on muscle sarcolemma to initiate muscle contraction. Acetylcholinesterase (AChE) hydrolyzes ACh, thus limiting effect and duration of its action.

Myasthenia gravis

Marked reduction in number and length of subneural sarcolemmal folds indicates that underlying defect lies in neuromuscular junction. Anticholinesterase drugs increase effectiveness and duration of ACh action by slowing its destruction by AChE.

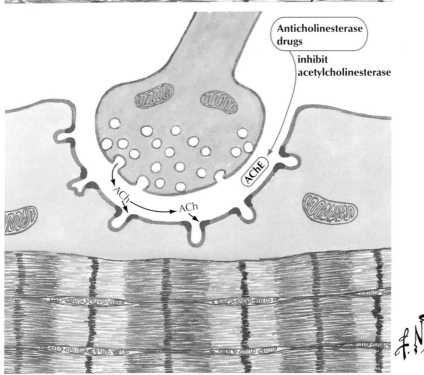

FIGURE 13-62   MYASTHENIA GRAVIS

Myasthenia gravis is an acquired autoimmune disease characterized by production of antibodies to acetylcholine receptors linked to marked reduction of junctional folds and decrease in acetylcholine receptors at the neuromuscular junction, thereby impairing the transmission of nerve impulses. Myasthenia gravis is frequently associated with other autoimmune diseases, such as rheumatoid arthritis, systemic lupus erythematosus, and pernicious anemia. Abnormalities of the thymus are common, which is manifest in most cases as thymic hyperplasia and in approximately 10% as a thymoma. Myasthenia gravis has a worldwide distribution and occurs in all age groups but with a strong female preponderance. Myasthenia gravis may be generalized or limited to ocular myopathy. There also are congenital, neonatal, and drug-induced forms. *Lambert-Eaton syndrome* is a condition resembling myasthenia gravis occurring as a paraneoplastic syndrome in patients with an underlying carcinoma, often oat cell carcinoma of the lung.

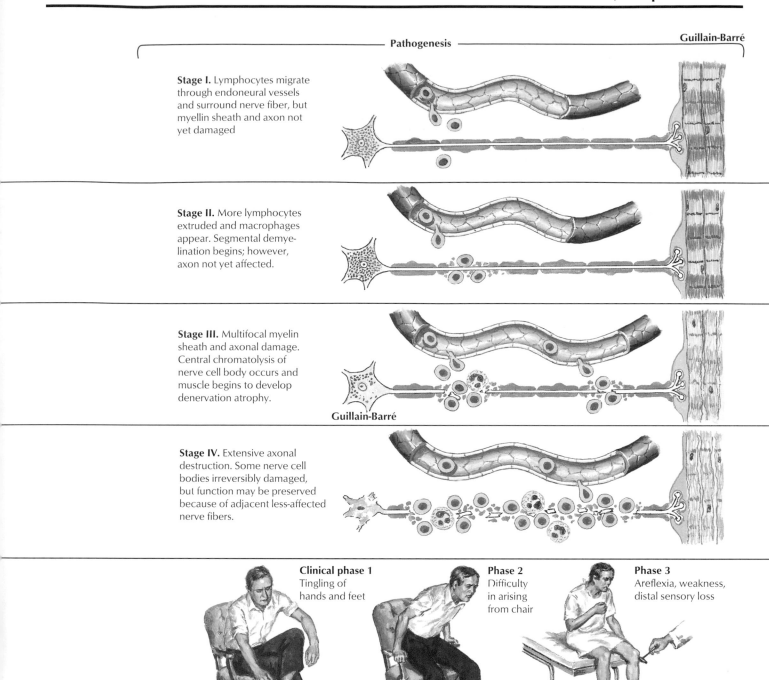

Stage I. Lymphocytes migrate through endoneural vessels and surround nerve fiber, but myellin sheath and axon not yet damaged

Stage II. More lymphocytes extruded and macrophages appear. Segmental demyelination begins; however, axon not yet affected.

Stage III. Multifocal myelin sheath and axonal damage. Central chromatolysis of nerve cell body occurs and muscle begins to develop denervation atrophy.

Stage IV. Extensive axonal destruction. Some nerve cell bodies irreversibly damaged, but function may be preserved because of adjacent less-affected nerve fibers.

Pathogenesis

Guillain-Barré

Guillain-Barré

Clinical phase 1
Tingling of hands and feet

Phase 2
Difficulty in arising from chair

Phase 3
Areflexia, weakness, distal sensory loss

FIGURE 13-63 GUILLAIN-BARRÉ SYNDROME

Guillain-Barré syndrome is an acute, rapidly progressive, ascending paralysis that spreads from the distal limbs to involve more proximal muscle groups, including facial and respiratory muscles. The disease affects motor function primarily, leading to total loss of reflexes and function. Predisposing conditions include a recent viral infection in most patients or impaired immune function. The syndrome results from inflammatory attack of the peripheral nerves, probably triggered by an autoimmune

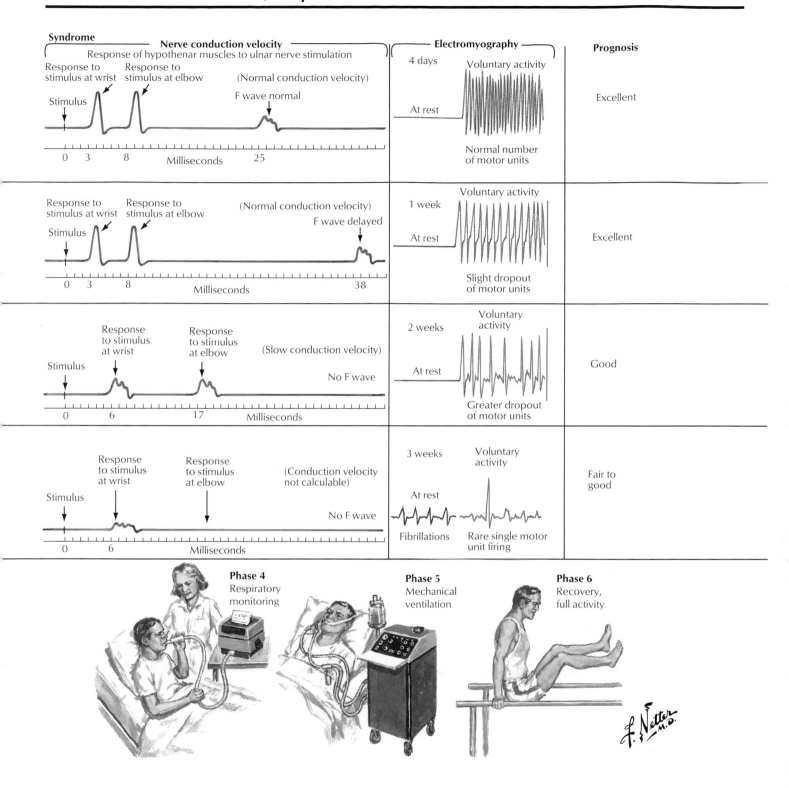

FIGURE 13-63   GUILLAIN-BARRÉ SYNDROME *(CONTINUED)*

reaction. The inflammation leads to demyelination and, in severe cases, secondary axonal damage. Patients may present with progressive symmetric paralysis with cranial nerve dysfunction, particularly Bell palsy, sensory ataxia, or pure autonomic dysfunction. Differential diagnosis includes acute spinal cord lesions; toxic, metabolic, or infectious processes; poliomyelitis; diphtheria; botulism; porphyria; and myasthenia gravis. Guillain-Barré syndrome is self-limiting in most patients.

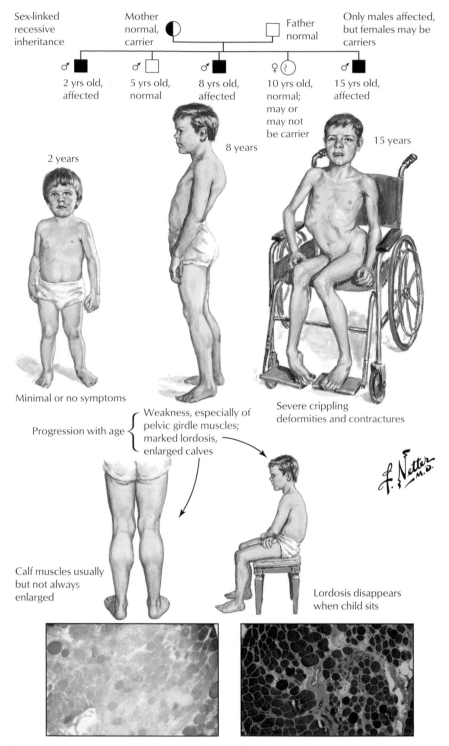

Muscle biopsy specimens showing necrotic muscle fibers being removed by groups of small, round phagocytic cells (left, trichrome stain) and replaced by fibrous and fatty tissue (right, H and E stain)

FIGURE 13-64   DUCHENNE MUSCULAR DYSTROPHY

Muscular dystrophies are a heterogenous group of inherited diseases characterized by progressive muscle weakness due to progressive degeneration of skeletal muscle, often with onset in childhood. There are various inheritance patterns, including the most common X-linked pattern of Duchenne muscular dystrophy and Becker muscular dystrophy, a milder variant. The disease is marked by progressive development of muscle weakness, especially of pelvic girdle muscles, marked lordosis, and

enlargement of the calves, so-called pseudohypertrophy due to muscle swelling. Pathologic changes are those of multifocal muscle fiber degeneration and necrosis, removal of necrotic muscle by phagocytic leukocytes, regenerative changes in surviving muscle fibers, fibrofatty replacement of muscle, and muscle atrophy. The illness progresses relentlessly, and the majority of patients die during the late second or third decade of life.

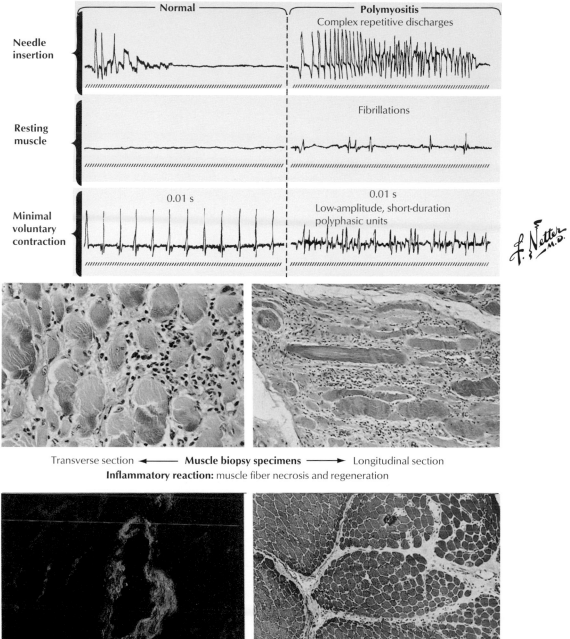

Electromyography

Anti-IgG immunofluorescence of frozen muscle section with positive staining within blood vesssel wall, indicating immunologic basis of dermatomyositis

Perifascicular muscle atrophy in child with dermatomyositis

FIGURE 13-65 POLYMYOSITIS/DERMATOMYOSITIS

Polymyositis is a relatively common condition characterized by weakness of the proximal musculature with usual onset in middle-aged persons. Polymyositis seems to develop on an autoimmune basis, and it can be associated with other connective-tissue diseases, such as systemic lupus erythematosus, rheumatoid arthritis, and systemic vasculitis, or, occasionally, with an underlying malignancy. The onset is often insidious but may be rapid. Many patients have an accompanying rash, and the combination of conditions is known as *dermatomyositis*. In

patients with recent onset of symmetric proximal muscle weakness, with or without a rash, the diagnosis of an inflammatory myopathy can be confirmed by evidence of increased serum markers of muscle damage, especially creatine kinase, typical electromyographic changes, and positive muscle biopsy with inflammatory cellular infiltrates and immunoglobulin deposits by immunofluorescence. The prognosis ranges from complete recovery to frequent recurrence to fatality in approximately 25% patients even with treatment with steroids.

INDEX

Page numbers followed by "f" indicate figures, "t" indicate tables, and "b" indicate boxes.